UNIVERSITY OF IOWA

THE FAMILY PRACTICE HANDBOOK

NOTICE

UNIVERSITY OF IOWA
THE FAMILY PRACTICE HANDBOOK

MARK A. GRABER, M.D.
Assistant Clinical Professor,
Departments of Family Practice and Surgery,
University of Iowa Hospitals and Clinics
Iowa City, Iowa

PETER P. TOTH, M.D., Ph.D.
Former Resident in Family Medicine,
University of Iowa Hospitals and Clinics,
Iowa City, Iowa;
Sullivan Clinic,
Sarah Bush Lincoln Health System,
Sullivan, Illinois

ROBERT L. HERTING, Jr., M.D.
Former Resident in Family Medicine,
Clinical Associate,
Department of Family Medicine,
University of Iowa Hospitals and Clinics,
Iowa City, Iowa

a Mosby handbook

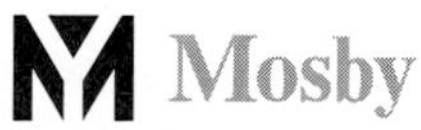

St. Louis Baltimore Boston Carlsbad
Chicago Minneapolis New York Philadelphia Portland
London Milan Sydney Tokyo Toronto

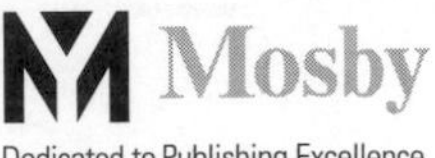

Vice President and Publisher: Anne S. Patterson
Editor: James F. Shanahan
Developmental Editor: Laura C. Berendson
Project Manager: Dana Peick
Production Editor: Carl Masthay
Designer: Renée Duenow
Manufacturing Manager: Betty Mueller

THIRD EDITION

Printed in the United States of America
Composition by Accu-Color, Inc.
Printing/binding by R.R. Donnelly & Sons, Inc.

Mosby–Year Book, Inc.
11830 Westline Industrial Drive
St. Louis, Missouri 63146

Library of Congress Cataloging-in-Publication Data

The family practice handbook / [edited by] Mark A. Graber, Peter P. Toth, Robert L. Herting, Jr. –3rd ed.
p. cm.
At head of title: University of Iowa.
Includes bibliographical references and index.
ISBN 0–8151–2395–7 (alk. paper)
1. Family medicine–Handbooks, manuals, etc. I. Graber, Mark A., MD. II. Toth, Peter P. III. Herting, Robert L. IV. University of Iowa.
[DNLM: 1. Family Practice–handbooks. WB 39 F1985 1997]
RC55.F25 1997
616–dc21
DNLM/DLC 97-2674
for Library of Congress CIP

97 98 99 00 01 / 9 8 7 6 5 4 3 2 1

Contributors

At the time of writing all contributors were residents in the Department of Family Medicine, University of Iowa Hospitals and Clinics, Iowa City, Iowa, unless otherwise specified.

Laura Beaty, M.D.

Nora R. Frohberg, M.D. *(Department of Psychiatry)*

Melissa J. Gamponia, M.D., M.P.H.

Mark A. Graber, M.D. *(Assistant Clinical Professor, Departments of Family Practice and Surgery)*

Robert L. Herting, Jr., M.D.

A. Jothivijayarani, M.D.

Michael Kelly, Pharm.D. *(Assistant Clinical Professor, Division of Pharmacy)*

Viviana Martínez-Bianchi, M.D.

Michelle Rejman-Peterson, M.D.

James Schlichtmann, M.D.

Peter P. Toth, M.D., Ph.D.

Hajime Toyoshima, M.D., Ph.D.

Elizabeth Valdes, M.D.

To my family, Hetty B. Hall, M.D., Rachel Ilana Graber and Abraham David Graber.
To the teachers who made a big difference including Mrs. Ruth Jackson (first grade), Mr. Raymond Hartman (sixth grade), Mary Kelly (eleventh grade), Stan Hoegerman, Ph.D., and Gary Bluemink, M.D.

M.A.G.

To my lovely wife, Karen, my beautiful daughters, Martha Ilona and Mary Elizabeth, my parents, John and Ilona Toth, and Skip and Jane Ireland for their love and support.

P.P.T.

To my wife, Nora, my children, Erika and Robert (born April 9, 1997), and my parents, Bob and Claireen. Their loving support and encouragement have been essential to my success as a physician and to writing this book. Also a sincere thanks to my high school teachers, Fred Wagner and Lynn Dieter, who shaped my career goals and whose teachings continue to influence my day-to-day life.

R.L.H. Jr.

Preface

Everything you need to know about Family Practice in a handbook? To cover all that would require a library! But we hope we have covered most of the common situations you will encounter.

There are several improvements in this third edition. All the therapies have been updated, and the number of illnesses covered in each chapter has been expanded significantly. A new chapter has been added that contains the pediatric and adult dosages of many of the most common drugs that family physicians prescribe. A new Infectious Disease chapter that discusses emerging entities such as ehrlichiosis and babesiosis has been added. The Pediatrics chapter has been expanded, and the General Surgery chapter now includes information about the medical evaluation of the presurgical patient. Overall, about 30% of the information is new, and the rest is updated.

The nature of information retrieval in medicine is changing, and one of the most significant additions is something you cannot hold in your pocket. We have set up a World Wide Web site at "http://www.uiowa.edu/~famprac/index.html" at which we will keep a list of links to other information sites on the web. You also can now write to us by e-mail at "mgraber@blue.weeg.uiowa.edu". See something in the book you like? Let us know. If there is something you believe to be important that we have not covered, let us know this, too. Our goal is to make a book you feel is applicable to your practice and easy to use. Thank you for your continued support.

Mark A. Graber, M.D.

Acknowledgments

The authors would like to thank Pam Hoogerwerf for her help in manuscript preparation. Mark can in good faith let you know that he checked, and indeed her fingers, having been no more than nubbins after typing the *last* edition, have regained their previous length. Thanks also to Boo-Kheat Chong, John Hamiel, Monika Totaraitis, Pharm.D., and Michael Kelly, Pharm.D., for their attention to the details of drug dosing and also to Dedra Diehl for help with procuring journals and articles.

Mark would like to thank Hetty B. Hall, M.D., for her clinical insights and Rachel and Abraham Graber for their support; nobody could ask for better children. Finally, thanks to coffee and tea for keeping me awake through the long process and "They Might Be Giants" for the background music.

Contents

Abbreviations

A/a	alveolar-arterial oxygen gradient
ABCs	airway, breathing, circulation
ABG	arterial blood gas
AC	before meals *(ante cibum)*
AC	acromioclavicular
ACE	angiotensin-converting enzyme
aCL	anticardiolipin (antibody)
ACLS	Advanced Cardiac Life Support
ACOG	American College of Obstetrics and Gynecology
ACTH	adrenocorticotropic hormone
AD	Alzheimer's dementia or disease
A Fib	atrial fibrillation
AFB	acid-fast bacilli
AFP	alpha-fetoprotein
AFV	amniotic fluid volume
AGCUS	atypical glandular cells of undetermined significance
AI	amnioinfusion
AIDS	acquired immunodeficiency syndrome
ALT	alanine aminotransferase
ANA	antinuclear antibody
ANCA	antineutrophil cytoplasmic antibody
AP	anteroposterior
APS	antiphospholipid syndrome
APSAC	anistreplase, anisoylated plasminogen-streptokinase activator complex
APTT	activated partial thromboplastin
ARC	AIDS-related complex
ARDS	adult respiratory distress syndrome
ARF	acute renal failure

ASA	acetylsalicylic acid
ASAP	as soon as possible
ASCUS	atypical squamous cells of undetermined significance
ASO	antistreptolysin O antibody
AST	aspartate aminotransferase
Atg	anti–human thymocyte globulin
ATN	acute tubular necrosis
AV	arteriovenous; atrioventricular
AZT	zidovudine (Azidothymidine)
B_{12}	vitamin B_{12}
BAER	brainstem auditory evoked responses
BBT	basal body temperature
BCG	bacille Calmette-Guérin
BCP	birth control pill
BHCG	beta human chorionic gonadotropin
BID	twice a day (*bis in die*)
BiPAP	bilevel positive airway pressure
BOOP	bronchiolitis obliterans–organizing pneumonia
BP	blood pressure
BPAD	bipolar affective disorder
bpm	beats per minute
BPP	biophysical profile
BPPV	benign paroxysmal positional vertigo
BSA	body surface area
BUN	blood urea nitrogen
BV	bacterial vaginosis
BVM	bag valve mask
C&S	culture and sensitivity
C-peptide	insulin chain C-peptide
C-section	cesarean section
C-spine	cervical spine
CABG	coronary artery bypass graft
$CACl_2$	calcium chloride
CAD	coronary artery disease
cap	capsule
c-ANCA	central antineutrophil cytoplasmic antibody
CBC	complete blood cell count
cc	cubic centimeter (for solids and gases but *ml* for liquids)

CD4+	helper T cell (cluster of differentiation no. 4+)
CDC	Centers for Disease Control and Prevention, Atlanta, Ga.
CEA	carcinoembryonic antigen
CFU	colony-forming unit
CHF	congestive heart failure
Chol	cholesterol
CIN	cervical intraepithelial neoplasia (1 to 3: mild to severe)
CK	creatine kinase
CLL	chronic lymphocytic leukemia
cm	centimeter
CMV	cytomegalovirus
CNS	central nervous system
CO_2	carbon dioxide
COPD	chronic obstructive pulmonary disease
CPAP	continuous positive airway pressure
CPD	cephalopelvic disproportion
CPK	creatine phosphokinase
CPPD	calcium pyrophosphate dihydrate (crystals) (pseudogout)
CPR	cardiopulmonary resuscitation
Cr	creatinine
CRF	chronic renal failure
CRP	C-reactive protein
CSF	cerebrospinal fluid
CST	contraction stress fluid
CT	computerized tomography
CVA	cerebrovascular accident
CVAT	costovertebral-angle tenderness
CVD	cerebrovascular disease
CVN	central venous nutrition
CVP	central venous pressure
CVS	cardiovascular system
c/w	consistent with
CXR	chest x-ray film or radiograph
D&C	dilatation and curettage
DBP	diastolic blood pressure
DDAVP	1-deamino-8-D-arginine vasopressin

DDC, ddC	dideoxycytidine, zalcitabine, Hivid
DDI, ddI	dideoxyinosine, didanosine
D_5W	5% dextrose in water
D4T	stavudine
DHE	dihydroergotamine
DHT	dihydrotestosterone
DIC	disseminated intravascular coagulation
DIP	distal interphalangeal joint
DKA	diabetic ketoacidosis
dl	deciliter
DM	diabetes mellitus
DPL	diagnostic peritoneal lavage
DPT	diphtheria-pertussis-tetanus (vaccine)
DS	double strength
DSM	Diagnostic and Statistical Manual [of Mental Disorders]
dsDNA	double-stranded deoxyribonucleic acid
DTR	deep tendon reflexes
DTs	delirium tremens
DVT	deep venous thrombosis
D/W	dextrose in water
EBV	Epstein-Barr virus
ECF	extracellular fluid
ECG	electrocardiogram
ECMO	extracorporeal membrane oxygenation
ED	emergency department
EDC	estimated date of confinement
EEG	electroencephalogram
EES	erythromycin ethylsuccinate
EGD	esophagogastroduodenoscopy
EIA	enzyme immunoassay
ELISA	enzyme-linked immunosorbent assay
EM	erythema multiforme
EMG	electromyogram
ENG	electronystagmography
ENT	ear, nose, throat
ER	emergency room
ERCP	endoscopic retrograde cholangiopancreatography

ESR	erythrocyte sedimentation rate
ET	endotracheal tube
FB	foreign body
FDA	U.S. Food and Drug Administration
Fe	iron
FE_{Na}	fractional excretion of sodium
FEF	forced expiratory flow
FEV_1	forced expiratory volume at 1 second
FFP	fresh frozen plasma
FH	family history
FHR	fetal heart rate
FSH	follicle-stimulating hormone
FTA	fluorescent treponemal antibody
FTA-ABS	fluorescent treponemal antibody absorption (test)
5-FU	5-fluorouracil
F/U	follow-up (study, exam, test, care)
FUO	fever of unknown origin
G	gauge
G6PD	glucose-6-phosphate dehydrogenase
GBS	group B *Streptococcus* bacteria, or group B streptococcal infection
GC	gonococcus
GCS	Glasgow Coma Scale
GCT	glucose challenge test
GDM	gestational diabetes mellitus
GE	gastroesophageal
GFR	glomerular filtration rate
GI	gastrointestinal
g	gram
GM-CSF	granulocyte-macrophage colony-stimulating factor
GN	glomerulonephritis
GnRH	gonadotropin-releasing hormone
GODM	gestational onset diabetes mellitus
gtt	drops *(guttae)*
GTT	glucose tolerance test
GU	genitourinary
GXT	graded exercise stress test
GYN	gynecologic

h, hr	hour
H&P	history and physical examination
HA	headache
Hb	hemoglobin
HC/AC	head circumference–to–abdominal circumference (ratio)
HCG	human chorionic gonadotropin
HCT	hematocrit
HCTZ	hydrochlorothiazide
HDL	high-density lipoprotein
HELLP	hemolysis, elevated liver enzymes, and low platelet count (syndrome)
HepBsAg	hepatitis B surface antigen
HGE	human granulocytic ehrlichiosis
HIV	human immunodeficiency virus
HME	human monocytic erlichiosis
HMG	human menopausal gonadotropin
h/o	history of
HPF	high-power field
HRT	hormone replacement therapy
HS	at bedtime *(hora somni)*
HSV	herpes simplex virus
ht, Ht	height
HTN	hypertension
HUS	hemolytic uremic syndrome
HZV	herpes zoster virus
I&D	incision and drainage
I&O	intake and output
ICF	intracellular fluid
ICP	intracranial pressure
ICU	intensive care unit
ID	infectious disease
IDDM	insulin-dependent diabetes mellitus
IFA	immunofluorescence assay
IgG	immunoglobulin G
IHSS	idiopathic hypertrophic aortic stenosis
IM	intramuscular
IMV	intermittent mandatory ventilation

IN	intranasally
INH	isoniazid, isonicotinc acid hydrazide
INR	International Normalized Ratio
IO	intraosseous
IPPV	intermittent positive-pressure ventilation
ISA	intrinsic stimulating activity
ITP	idiopathic thrombocytopenia purpura
IU	International Unit
IUD	intrauterine device
IUFD	intrauterine fetal demise
IUGR	intrauterine growth retardation
IUP	intrauterine pregnancy
IV	intravenous
IVDA	intravenous drug abuser
IVP	intravenous pyelogram
JRA	juvenile rheumatoid arthritis
JVD	jugular venous distension
kg	kilogram
K, K^+	potassium
KOH	potassium hydroxide
KS	Kaposi's sarcoma
LA	lupus anticoagulant
LAT	preparation of lidocaine, epinephrine (adrenaline), tetracaine
LBBB	left bundle branch block
LDH	lactate dehydrogenase
LDL	low-density lipoprotein
LE	lupus erythematosus
LES	lower esophageal sphincter
LFT	liver function tests
LGI	lower GI (gastrointestinal)
LH	luteinizing hormone
LLQ	left lower quadrant
LMP	last menstrual period
LMW	low molecular weight
LOC	loss of consciousness
LP	lumbar puncture
LR	lactated Ringer's solution

L/S	lecithin-to-sphingomyelin (ratio)
LSIL	low-grade squamous intraepithelial lesion
LUQ	left upper quadrant
LV	left ventricular
MAI/MAC	*Mycobacterium avium-intracellulare/M. avium* complex
MAO	monoamine oxidase
MAOI	monoamine oxidase inhibitors
MAST	military antishock trousers
MCP	metacarpophalangeal joint
MCV	mean corpuscular volume
MDD	major depressive disorder
MDI	metered dose inhaler
MEE	middle ear effusion
mEq	milliequivalent
mg	milligram
μg	microgram
MI	myocardial infarction
min	minute
mm Hg	milliliters of mercury
mmol	millimole
MMPI	Minnesota Multiphasic Personality Inventory
MMR	measles-mumps-rubella (vaccine)
MMSE	Mini–Mental State examination
mOsm	milliosmole
MR	measles and rubella (vaccine)
MRI	magnetic resonance imaging
MS	multiple sclerosis
MTP	metatarsophalangeal joint
MVP	mitral valve prolaspe
N&V	nausea and vomiting
NCV	nerve conduction velocity
NG	nasogastric
NHL	non-Hodgkin's lymphoma
NIDDM	non–insulin dependent diabetes mellitus
NPH	neutral protamine Hagedorn
NPO	nothing by mouth *(nulla per os)*
NS	normal saline solution
NSAID	nonsteroidal anti-inflammatory drug

NST	nonstress test
NSVD	normal spontaneous vaginal delivery
NTD	neural tube defect
NTG	nitroglycerin
O&P	ova and parasites
OA	osteoarthritis
OCD	obsessive-compulsive disorder
OCP	oral contraceptive pill
17-OHS	17-hydroxysteroid (that is, 17-hydroxycorticosteroid)
OM	otitis media
OPV	oral poliovirus
ORS	WHO oral rehydration solution
osm, Osm	osmole; osmolality
OTC	over the counter
PA	posteroanterior
PAC	premature atrial contraction
PALS	Pediatric Advanced Life Support
Pap	Papanicolaou test or smear
PAS	*para*-aminosalicylic acid
PCA	patient-controlled analgesia
PCN	penicillin
PCOD	polycystic ovarian disease
PCP	*Pneumocystis* pneumonia
PCR	polymerase chain reaction
PCWP	pulmonary capillary wedge pressure
PD	Parkinson's disease
PDA	patent ductus arteriosus
PE	physical examination
PE	pulmonary embolism
PEEP	positive end-expiratory pressure
PEFR	peak expiratory flow rate
PET	positron emission tomography
PFTs	pulmonary function tests
PG	phosphatidylglycerol
pH	hydrogen-ion concentration; pH 7, normal; less is acidic; more is alkaline (or basic)
PID	pelvic inflammatory disease
PIH	pregnancy-induced hypertension

PIP	proximal interphalangeal joint
plt	platelet
PMNs	polymorphonuclear lymphocytes
PMR	polymyalgia rheumatica
PMS	premenstrual syndrome
PO	per mouth (*per os*)
POD	postoperative day
PPD	protein purified derivative
PR	*per rectum*
PRN	as needed *(pro re nata)*
PROM	premature rupture of membranes
PSA	prostate specific antigen
PSVT	paroxysmal supraventricular tachycardia
PT	prothrombin time
PTCA	percutaneous transluminal coronary angioplasty
PTL	premature labor
PTSD	post–traumatic stress disorder
PTT	partial thromboplastin time
PTU	propylthiouracil
PUD	peptic ulcer disease
PVC	premature ventricular contraction
QD	every day *(quaque die)*
QHS	properly 'every hour of sleep,' but usually 'at every bed time' *(quaque hora somni)*
QID	four times per day *(quater in die)*
QOD	every other day *(tertio quoque die)*
RA	rheumatoid arthritis
RBC	red blood cell
RCA	right coronary artery
REM	rapid eye movement
RF	renal failure
RFI	renal failure index
RIA	radioimmunoassay
RIND	reversible ischemic neurologic deficit
RLQ	right lower quadrant
RMSF	Rocky Mountain spotted fever
R/O, r/o	rule out
ROM	rupture of membranes; range-of-motion (exercise)

RPR	rapid plasma reagin
RSI	rapid-sequence intubation
RSV	respiratory syncytial virus
rt-PA	tissue-type plasminogen activator (recombinant) [Alteplase, Recombinant]
RUQ	right upper quadrant
RVMI	right ventricular myocardial infarction
SAARD	slow-acting antirheumatic drug(s)
SAH	subarachnoid hemorrhage
SBP	systolic blood pressure
SCIWORA	spinal cord injury without radiologic abnormality
SGA	small for gestational age
SGOT	See AST
SGPT	See ALT
SIL	squamous intraepithelial lesions
SK	streptokinase
SL	sublingual
SLE	systemic lupus erythematosus
SLR	straight-leg raising (test)
SOB	shortness of breath
sp. gr.	specific gravity
SPECT	single-photon emission computerized tomography
SQ	subcutaneous
SR	slow release
SROM	spontaneous rupture of membrane
SS	single strength
SSKI	saturated solution of potassium iodide
SSRI	selective serotonin reuptake inhibitors
STD	sexually transmitted disease
T_3	triiodothyronine
T_4	thyroxine
TAC	preparation of tetracycline, epinephrine (adrenaline), cocaine
Tb, TB	tuberculosis
TBG	thyroxine-binding globulin
TBSA	total body surface area
TBW	total body water
3TC	lamivudine

TCA	tricyclic antidepressant
TEDS	thromboembolic disease support (stockings, hose)
TEE	transesophageal echocardiography
TENS	transcutaneous electical nerve stimulation
TFT	thyroid function test
TG	triglycerides
3TC	lamivudine
TIA	transient ischemic attack
TIBC	total iron-binding capacity
TM	tympanic membrane
TMJ	temporomandibular joint
TMP/SMX	trimethoprim-sulfamethoxazole (complex)
TORCHS	toxoplasmosis, rubella, cytomegalovirus, herpes simplex, syphilis (infection)
TPA	tissue plasminogen activator
TPN	total parenteral nutrition
TRH	thyrotropin-releasing hormone
TSH	thyroid-stimulating hormone
TTP	thrombotic thrombocytopenic purpura
TURP	transurethral prostatectomy
TWAR	Taiwan acute respiratory disease
U	unit
UA	urinalysis
UC	ulcerative colitis
UGI	upper gastrointestinal (tract)
U/P	urine-to-plasma ratio
URI	upper respiratory infection
U/S	ultrasound, ultrasonogram, ultrasonography
UTI	urinary tract infection
UV	ultraviolet (radiation); B refers to the shorter-wave, more damaging range
V Fib	ventricular fibrillation
V Tach	ventricular tachycardia
VBAC	vaginal birth after cesarean section
VCUG	voiding cystourethrogram
VDRL	Venereal Disease Research Laboratories (test)
V/Q	ventilation-perfusion ratio
VSD	ventricular septal defect

Vt	tidal volume
VT	vestibular training
vWF	von Willebrand's factor
WBC	white blood cell (count)
wt, Wt	weight

1

Emergency Medicine

MARK A. GRABER

ADVANCED CARDIAC LIFE SUPPORT

We strongly suggest taking an ACLS course certified by The American Heart Association. The information below is intended only as a reference in an emergency and will not take the place of ACLS training.

General

The ABCs common to all emergency situations:
A–Airway including relieving obstruction, positioning.
B–Breathing, including 100% O_2 by bag-valve mask or preferably intubation.
C–Circulation, CPR.
D–Drugs

Lidocaine, atropine, naloxone, and epinephrine may be given via endotracheal tube. Give 10 ml of sterile water (best) or saline after drug.

Specific Rhythms and their treatment (Figs. 1-1 to 1-6)

I. VENTRICULAR FIBRILLATION OR PULSELESS VENTRICULAR TACHYCARDIA (Fig. 1-1)

- **A.** Defibrillation is the first priority once diagnosis is established.
- **B.** If greater than 4 minutes to CPR or 8 minutes to ACLS, there is a poor prognosis. If not resuscitated in field or if downtime >30 minutes, almost no long-term survival.
- **C.** Amiodarone is now approved for the treatment of life-threatening ventricular tachycardia and ventricular fibrillation unresponsive to other measures. The initial dose is 150 mg IV over 10 minutes followed by 360 mg over the next 6 hours. The most common side effects are hypotension and bradycardia. Hypotension seems to be related to speed of infusion.

II. BRADYCARDIA

Usually rated <60 beats/min but may have inappropriate bradycardia with pulse >60 but still inappropriately low for current clinical condition (Fig. 1-4).

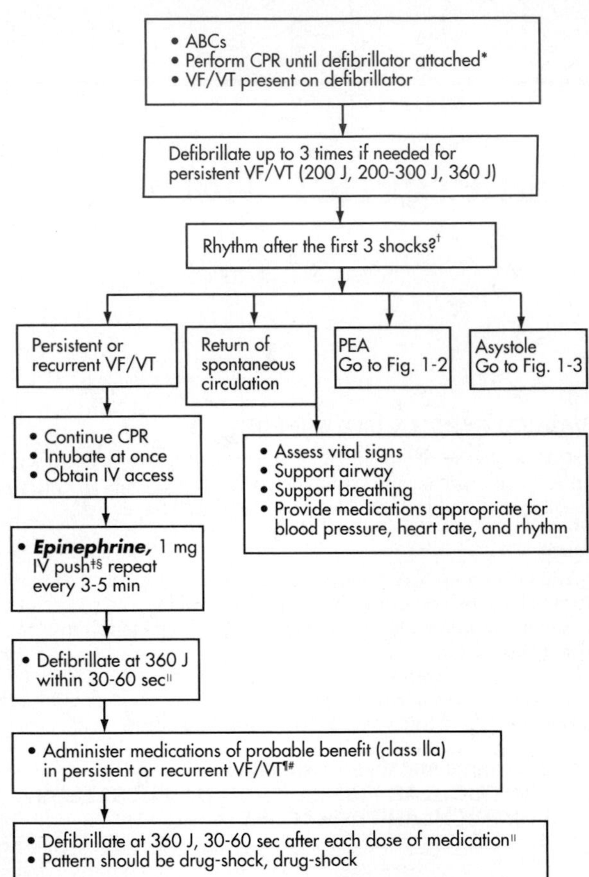

FIG. 1-1 Algorithm for ventricular fibrillation and pulseless ventricular tachycardia (VF/VT). (From Emergency Cardiac Care Committee and Subcommittees, American Heart Association: Guidelines for cardiopulmonary resuscitation and emergency cardiac care, *JAMA* 268:16, 1992.)

Class I: definitely helpful
Class IIa: acceptable, probably helpful
Class IIb: acceptable, possibly helpful
Class III: not indicated, may be harmful

[*] Precordial thump is a class IIb action in witnessed arrest, no pulse, and no defibrillator immediately available.

[†] Hypothermic cardiac arrest is treated differently after this point. See section on hypothermia.

[‡] The recommended dose of ***epinephrine*** is 1mg IV push every 3-5 min. If this approach fails, several class IIb dosing regimens can be considered:
- Intermediate: ***epinephrine,*** 2-5 mg IV push every 3-5 min
- Escalating: ***epinephrine,*** 1 mg, 3 mg, then 5 mg IV push (3 min apart)
- High: ***epinephrine,*** 0.1 mg/kg IV push every 3-5 min

[§] ***Sodium bicarbonate,*** (1 mEq/kg)—class I if patient has known preexisting hyperkalemia.

[||] Multiple sequenced shocks (200 J, 200-300 J, 360 J) are acceptable here (class I), especially when medications are delayed.

[¶]
- ***Lidocaine,*** 1.5 mg/kg IV push. Repeat in 3-5 min to total loading dose of 3 mg/kg; then use
- ***Bretylium,*** 5 mg/kg IV push. Repeat in 5 min at 10 mg/kg
- ***Magnesium sulfate,*** 1-2 g IV in torsades de pointes of suspected hypomagnesemic state or severe refractory VF
- ***Procainamide,*** 30 mg/min in refractory VF (maximum 17 mEq/kg)

[#] ***Sodium bicarbonate,*** (1 mEq/kg IV):
Class IIa
- If known preexisting bicarbonate-responsive acidosis
- If overdose with tricyclic antidepressants
- To alkalinize the urine in drug overdoses

Class IIb
- If intubated and continued long arrest interval
- Upon return of spontaneous circulation after long arrest interval

Class III
- Hypoxic lactic acidosis

FIG. 1-1, cont'd

A. Criteria for treatment. Hypotension, dyspnea, CHF, evidence of poor CNS perfusion.

B. Types of bradycardia.
1. Sinus bradycardia.
2. First-degree AV block with fixed PR interval >0.20 second.
3. Second-degree AV block.
   a. Mobitz type I (Wenckebach). Progressive prolongation of PR interval until there is a nonconducted P wave.
   b. Mobitz type II. Fixed PR interval with dropped beats (may require a pacer).
4. Third-degree AV block: no consistent relationship between P waves and QRS complexes. Will eventually require pacer.

C. Treatment as per algorithm (Fig. 1-4).
1. If secondary to calcium-channel blocker overdose, use calcium chloride 0.5 to 1 g slow IV push.
2. If secondary to beta-blocker overdose, give glucagon 2 to 5 mg IV (can use up to 10 mg), followed by a drip at 1 to 5 mg/hr.

PEA includes
- Electromechanical dissociation (EMD)
- Pseudo-EMD
- Idioventricular rhythms
- Ventricular escape rhythms
- Bradyasystolic rhythms
- Postdefibrillation idioventricular rhythms

- Continue CPR
- Intubate at once
- Obtain IV access
- Assess blood flow by using Doppler ultrasound

↓

Consider possible causes:
(Parentheses = possible therapies and treatments)
- Hypovolemia (volume infusion)
- Hypoxia (ventilation)
- Cardiac tamponade (pericardiocentesis)
- Tension pneumothorax (needle decompression)
- Hypothermia
- Massive pulmonary embolism (surgery, ***thrombolytics***)
- Drug overdoses such as tricyclics, digitalis, β-blockers, calcium-channel blockers
- Hyperkalemia*
- Acidosis†
- Massive acute myocardial infarction

↓

- ***Epinephrine***, 1mg IV push*† Repeat every 3-5 min

↓

- If absolute bradycardia (<60 beats/min) or relative bradycardia, give ***atropine***, 1 mg IV
- Repeat every 3-5 min up to a total of 0.04 mg/kg§

FIG. 1-2 Algorithm for pulseless electrical activity (PEA) (electromechanical dissociation, EMD). (From Emergency Cardiac Care Committee and Subcommittees, American Heart Association: Guidelines for cardiopulmonary resuscitation and emergency cardiac care, *JAMA* 268:16, 1992.)

3. If secondary to digoxin, can use Digibind (see section on digoxin overdose).

III. ELECTROMECHANICAL DISSOCIATION (EMD)/ PULSELESS ELECTRICAL ACTIVITY (PEA) (Fig. 1-2)

A. Defined as absence of a pulse despite organized complexes on a monitor at an adequate rate.

B. Causes include hypovolemia, cardiac tamponade, tension pneumothorax, hypoxia, acidosis, massive infarction with pump failure, pulmonary embolism.

C. Treat underlying cause!

1. *Treat as per protocol* (Fig. 1-2).

Class I: definitely helpful
Class IIa: acceptable, probably helpful
Class IIb: acceptable possibly helpful
Class III: not indicated, may be harmful
* **Sodium bicarbonate**, 1 mEq/kg—class I if patient has known preexisting hyperkalemia
† **Sodium bicarbonate**, 1 mEq/kg:
Class IIa
- If known preexisting bicarbonate-responsive acidosis
- If overdose with tricyclic antidepressants
- To alkalinize the urine in drug overdoses

Class IIb
- If intubated and long arrest interval
- Upon return of spontaneous circulation after long arrest interval

Class III
- Hypoxic lactic acidosis

‡ The recommended dose of **epinephrine** is 1 mg IV push every 3-5 min. If this approach fails, several class IIb dosing regimens can be considered:
- Intermediate: **epinephrine**, 2-5, mg IV push every 3-5 min
- Escalating: **epinephrine**, 1 mg, 3 mg, then 5 mg IV push (3 min apart)
- High: **epinephrine**, 0.1 mg/kg IV push, every 3-5 min

§ Shorter **atropine** dosing intervals are possibly helpful in cardiac arrest (class IIb).

FIG. 1-2, cont'd

2. If *sure* there is massive pulmonary embolism, may try streptokinase if other measures fail (see Chapter 3).

IV. ASYSTOLE (Fig. 1-3)

A. Defined as the absence of any organized electrical activity.
B. Prognosis poor.
C. Make sure to check two leads and their placement (loose or unattached leads may look like asystole on the monitor).
D. 8.8% of "asystole" is really fine ventricular fibrillation; so, if not making progress, can try defibrillation, *but not recommended as routine treatment.*
- Before trying defibrillation, make sure that the monitor is hooked up properly. Defibrillation in some other rhythms may be unnecessary or detrimental.

E. Treatment as per algorithm (Fig. 1-8).
F. Aminophylline, 250 mg IV in a rapid bolus, has been effective in an uncontrolled trial. This is not standard of care and should be used only when conventional therapy has failed.

V. SUSTAINED VENTRICULAR TACHYCARDIA WITH A PULSE (Fig. 1-5)

A. 81% of wide complex tachycardia represents ventricular tachycardia (see PSVT below for diagnostic approach).
B. Notes on algorithm (Fig. 1-5).

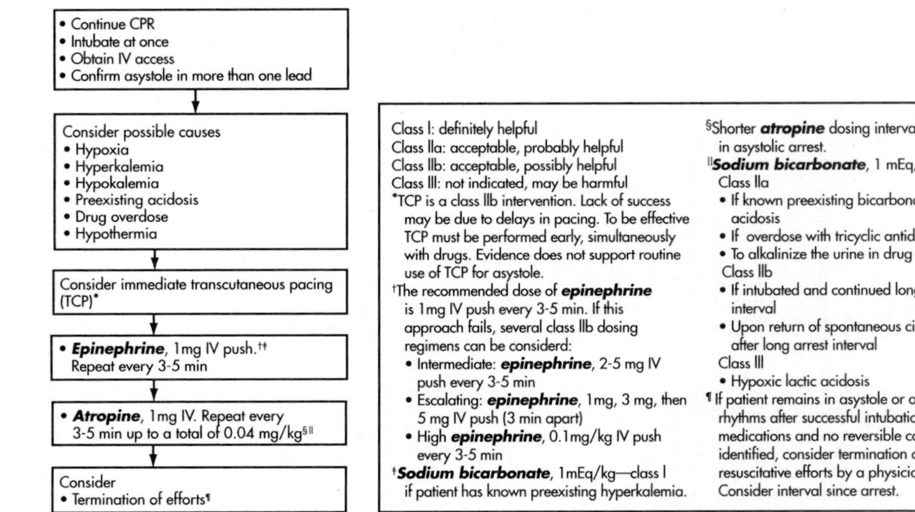

FIG. 1-3 Asystole treatment algorithm. (From Emergency Cardiac Care Committee and Subcommittees, American Heart Association: Guidelines for cardiopulmonary resuscitation and emergency cardiac care, *JAMA* 268:16, 1992.)

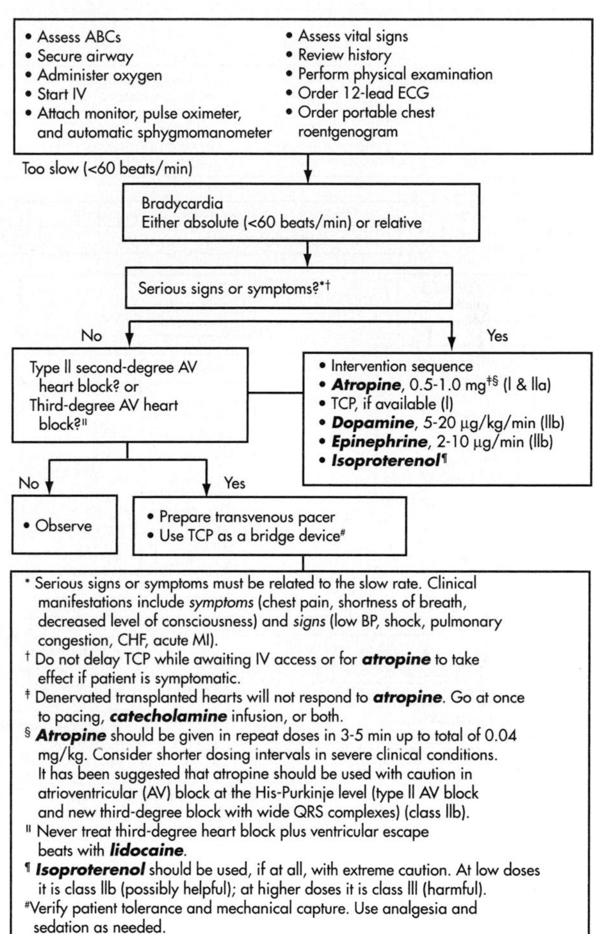

FIG. 1-4 Bradycardia algorithm (with the patient not in cardiac arrest). (From Emergency Cardiac Care Committee and Subcommittees, American Heart Association: Guidelines for cardiopulmonary resuscitation and emergency cardiac care, *JAMA* 268:16, 1992.)

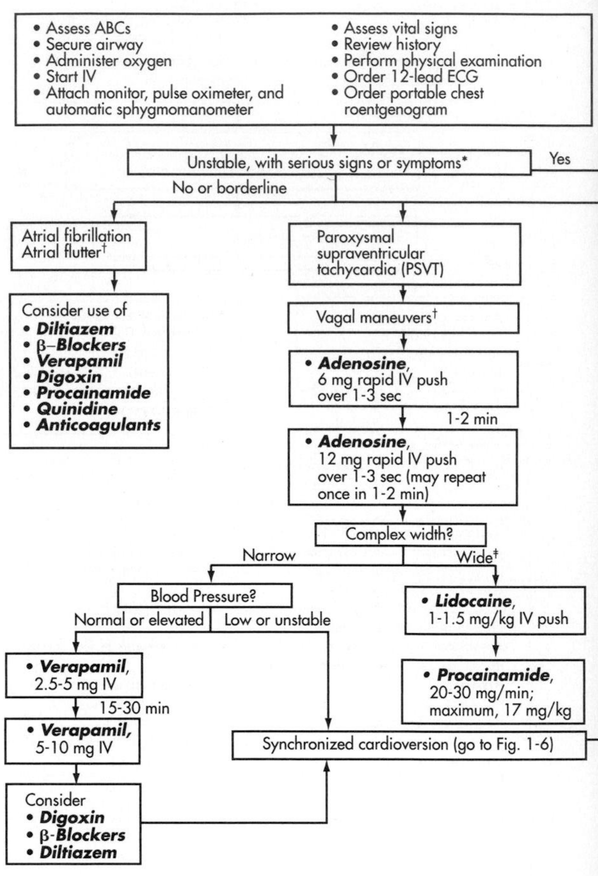

FIG. 1-5 Tachycardia algorithm. (From Emergency Cardiac Care Committee and Subcommittees, American Heart Association: Guidelines for cardiopulmonary resuscitation and emergency cardiac care, *JAMA* 268:16, 1992.)

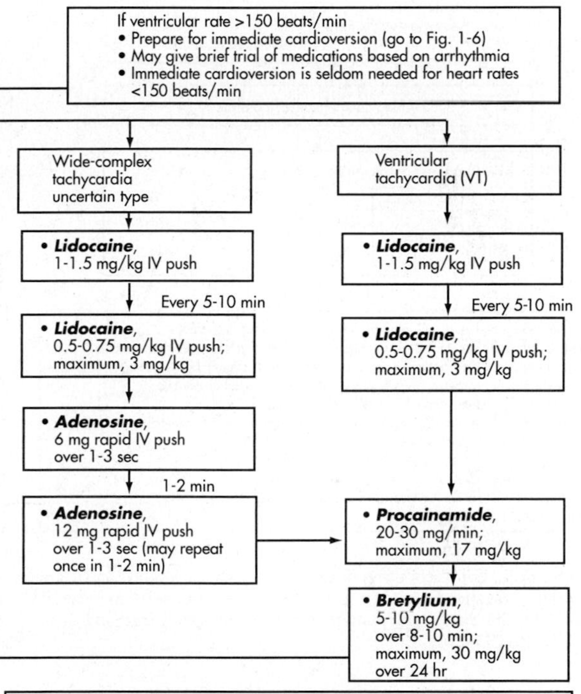

* Unstable condition must be related to the tachycardia. Signs and symptoms may include chest pain, shortness of breath, decreased level of consciousness, low blood pressure (BP), shock, pulmonary congestion, congestive heart failure, acute myocardial infarction.

†Carotid sinus pressure is contraindicated in patients with carotid bruits; avoid ice water immersion in patients with ischemic heart disease.

‡If the wide-complex tachycardia is known with certainty to be PSVT and BP is normal/elevated, sequence can include ***verapamil***.

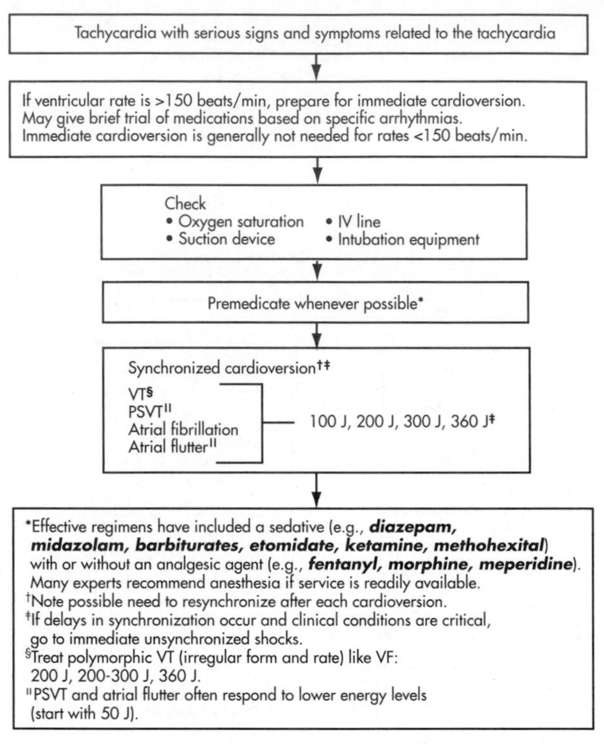

FIG. 1-6 Electrical cardioversion algorithm (with the patient not in cardiac arrest). (From Emergency Cardiac Care Committee and Subcommittees, American Heart Association: Guidelines for cardiopulmonary resuscitation and emergency cardiac care, *JAMA* 268:16, 1992.)

1. An *unstable* patient is one with dyspnea-hypoxia, hypotension, chest pain, or congestive failure. (See Fig. 1-6.)
2. See above under pulseless ventricular tachycardia for information on amiodarone IV.

VI. PAROXYSMAL SUPRAVENTRICULAR TACHYCARDIA (PSVT) (Figs. 1-5 and 1-6)

Notes on protocol:

A. Treat as unstable if CHF, chest pain, hypotension, hypoxia/dyspnea (synchronized cardioversion) (Fig. 1-6).

B. 81% of wide complex tachycardia represents ventricular tachycardia; so make sure that what you are treating is PSVT.

C. Verapamil is contraindicated in ventricular tachycardia and will cause hemodynamic deterioration.

D. Therapeutic options for PSVT.

1. ***Vagal maneuvers.*** Ice bag to face most effective. Can also try Valsalva maneuver, cough, carotid massage.
2. ***Adenosine.***
   a. Give 6 mg rapid IV push (in antecubital or central line) followed by 30 ml saline bolus to flush. Follow by 12 mg rapid IV push if needed.
   b. Half-life is 9 seconds. Will frequently get slowing of rhythm including ventricular tachycardia, allowing a more accurate diagnosis. Will not cause deterioration in ventricular tachycardia.
   c. Frequently get several seconds of asystole.
   d. Many get chest pain because adenosine is a neurotransmitter.
   e. Is less effective in those receiving theophylline.
3. ***Verapamil.***
   a. Can give 1 mg/min IV total dose up to 10 or to 15 mg. This avoids giving more drug than is needed and minimizes side effects. Or 5 mg bolus over 1 to 2 minutes and then 10 mg 10 minutes later.
   b. Can pretreat with calcium chloride (CaCl), 3.3 ml IV of 10% solution over 3 to 5 minutes. This helps to prevent verapamil-induced hypotension but does not affect the antiarrhythmic efficacy.
   c. *Verapamil contraindicated in CHF. Do not use verapamil and beta-blockers together.*
   d. Serum half-life 45 minutes; so should start verapamil orally to prevent recurrence.
   e. For recurrent PSVT, can use verapamil drip at 10 mg/hr.
   f. Verapamil-induced hypotension can be treated with calcium chloride 0.5-1 g IV slowly.
4. ***Diltiazem*** 0.25 mg/kg IV over 2 minutes followed by 0.35 mg/kg IV in 15 minutes.
   a. Safer than verapamil in patients with CHF.
   b. Same precautions regarding ventricular tachycardia apply to diltiazem as those to verapamil.
   c. Can use calcium to reverse hypotensive effects as noted with verapamil.

VII. ATRIAL FIBRILLATION WITH A RAPID VENTRICULAR RESPONSE (Fig. 1-5)

(See tachycardia protocol.)

A. Digoxin. If the rate needs to be sharply slowed, digoxin will not work. Digoxin can be administered if it is to be used to help with long-term rate control but takes at least 1 to 4 hours to have maximal effect.

B. Treat with verapamil as noted under PSVT (Fig. 1-6).

C. If CHF, can try diltiazem 0.25 mg/kg IV followed by 0.35 mg/kg IV in 5 minutes (see under PSVT).

D. Cardiovert only as last resort because of risk of stroke in those who have had the rhythm for >24 hours. See Chapter 2 for details.

1. If CHF caused by rapid rate, verapamil may still be helpful.

VIII. TORSADES DE POINTES (Fig. 1-1)

See ventricular tachycardia, p. 1.

A. Defined as form of ventricular tachycardia often as result of prolonged QT interval.

B. Causes.

1. Digitalis toxicity, erythromycin, (astemizole) Hismanal, (terfenadine) Seldane, lidocaine, tricyclic, antidepressants, quinidine, procainamide, mexiletine, tocainide, amiodarone, nifedipine, cisapride, and others.
2. Toxins including arsenic and organophosphate poisoning.
3. Hypothermia.
4. Hypocalcemia, hypomagnesemia, hypokalemia.
5. Neurologic processes including stroke and subarachnoid bleeding.

C. Treatment.

1. Often hard to terminate; frequently will recur.
2. Avoid drugs that may prolong the QT interval further such as quinidine, lidocaine, and disopyramide.
3. Correct underlying metabolic abnormality if possible.
4. Drug therapy includes:
   a. Cardioversion as per ventricular tachycardia protocols (Fig. 1-6).
   b. Lidocaine usually ineffective.
   c. Isoproterenol 2 to 8 µg/min while making arrangements for overdrive pacing at 90 to 120 beats per minute.
   d. Temporary pacing is the most effective method of treating this arrhythmia.
   e. Magnesium, though not standard treatment, is probably the best pharmacologic approach though may get recurrence.
      (1) Give 2 g bolus of $MgSO_4$ (10 ml of a 20% solution) over 1 to 2 minutes (can push if not perfusing).
      (2) May follow with a second or third bolus if necessary at 5 to 15 minutes. Infusions of 3 to 20 mg/min for 7 to 48 hours or until the QT interval has decreased to less than 0.50 second.
      (3) Magnesium toxicity is heralded by areflexia, bradycardia, coma, respiratory depression, but shouldn't be a problem in doses noted above.
      (4) Magnesium relatively contraindicated in renal failure.
   f. Can try bretylium tosylate 5 to 10 mg/kg IV and drip at 2 to 4 mg/min.

g. Can try phenytoin 250 mg IV in normal saline over 10 minutes followed by 100 mg IV Q5min as needed. Most will respond to 250 mg. Maximum loading dose of phenytoin is 10 to 15 mg/kg in adults. Do not infuse at a rate exceeding 50 mg/min.
h. Amiodarone is now approved for the treatment of life-threatening ventricular tachycardia and ventricular fibrillation unresponsive to other measures.
   (1) Initial dose is 150 mg IV over 10 minutes, but this may be accelerated in critical situations.
   (2) Most common side effects are hypotension, bradycardia. Hypotension seems to be related to speed of infusion.

THE MANAGEMENT OF ACUTE CHEST PAIN IN THE EMERGENCY ROOM SETTING

A. Obtain an ECG as well as a CXR film, CBC count, cardiac enzymes (troponin T or I and myoglobin may be appropriate depending on your institutional standard), and electrolytes. A metabolic cause for angina may be found such as anemia or pneumonia. Do not withhold treatment until laboratory results are available; transfuse as needed.

B. Differential diagnosis of chest pain is complex. Partial list provided in Table 1-1.

C. Administer oxygen to all patients with chest pain.

D. For cardiac pain:

1. Nitrates, either SL nitroglycerin 0.4 mg or IV nitroglycerin 10 to 300 µg/min, should be administered by titration up by 20 µg/min every 5 minutes until pain is relieved or the blood pressure begins to be unacceptably low. Occasionally a patient will get quite hypotensive after the SL administration of NTG, and so prior establishment of an IV dose is prudent though not mandatory. Hypotension will respond to fluids and is self-limited. This is not a contraindication to the judicial use of IV NTG. Prolonged or severe hypotension related to the use of nitrates should be suggestive of a right ventricular infarction, which is often associated with an inferior wall MI and can be diagnosed by the use of right chest leads (see Chapter 2). Hypotension from nitrates in a ventricular infarction will respond to fluid as well. Tolerance to nitrates may develop within 24 hours.
2. Aspirin 325 mg (non–enteric coated) should be administered to any patient with angina that does not have a contraindication such as active bleeding.
3. Morphine given in 2 to 4 mg aliquots IV can be helpful in relieving chest pain and cardiac ischemia. The total dose should not exceed 12 to 14 mg in the usual circumstance.
4. Heparin 5000 units as an IV bolus with a drip at 1000 units/hour is helpful in the patient with unstable angina or

TABLE 1-1
Partial Differential Diagnosis of Acute Chest Pain

Diagnosis	Cardinal symptoms	Diagnosed by	Treated by	Commonly mistaken for	Pitfalls and comments
Angina–myocardial infarction (A-MI)	Substernal pressure with radiation to arms, neck, jaw, dyspnea; occurs with exertion	History and ECG may show evidence of ischemia but may be normal in up to 50% with A-MI	See text	Multiple illnesses including gastric pain, musculoskeletal pain, etc.	Pain may be of any type, and sharp or burning pain does not exclude cardiac ischemia. Diabetics and elderly often have atypical presentation with only dyspnea or epigastric pain.
Anxiety and hyperventilation	May feel chest pain, shortness of breath, feeling as though will die. May have associated circumoral and acral paresthesias	Diagnosis of exclusion Generally have increased stress, history of similar episodes	Reassurance, diazepam IV	Cardiac disease	May have syncope secondary to CNS vasospasm
Esophageal spasm	May mimic MI or angina May respond to nitrates or calcium-channel blockers	Barium swallow or manometry	See Chapter 4	Cardiac disease	Need to rule out cardiac causes, since can mimic well

Gastritis/esophagitis	Burning chest pain	Endoscopy, upper GI, clinically	See text	Cardiac disease and vice versa	May be relieved by "GI cocktail" (i.e., Maalox 30 ml, lidocaine 2% 15 ml but not diagnostic, since some of those with cardiac disease will also respond with pain relief
Musculoskeletal including costochondritis, muscle strain, intercostal strain, rib fracture	Usually tender over specific point that reproduces pain May be history of injury; may be respirophasic (pleuritic in nature)	History, physical			Presence of musculoskeletal disease does not rule out other causes of chest pain
Pericarditis	Pleuritic, radiates to shoulder, worse when lying down, better sitting up May have a rub	ECG shows diffuse ST elevation, but 20% are false negative	See Chapter 2		May be viral, associated with renal failure, TB, or may be carcinomatous from breast or lung cancer

Continued

TABLE 1-1
Partial Differential Diagnosis of Acute Chest Pain—cont'd

Diagnosis	Cardinal symptoms	Diagnosed by	Treated by	Commonly mistaken for	Pitfalls and comments
Pleurisy	Respirophasic (pleuritic) chest pain generally sharp in nature	Diagnosis of exclusion	Anti-inflammatory such as indomethacin		May be viral or associated with pulmonary embolism, pericarditis, pneumonia, etc. Must rule out "serious" cause
Pneumonia	Generally have associated cough, fever	CXR, CBC, clinical picture	Antibiotics (see Chapter 3)		May have associated RLQ abdominal pain
Pulmonary embolism	Sudden onset, respirophasic (pleuritic in nature), dyspnea (see Chapter 3)	Tachycardia, hypoxia, tachypnea. Need V/Q scan or angiogram	See Chapter 3		Keep high clinical suspicion, since any symptom or sign may be absent (see Chapter 3)

Spontaneous pneumomediastinum	Sudden onset, severe pleuritic pain	CXR	Observation		Commonly associated with Valsalva maneuver, especially with smoking crack, marijuana from bong
Spontaneous pneumothorax	Sudden-onset severe pain (pleuritic in nature), dyspnea	CXR (expiratory)	Chest tube (see text)	Pulmonary embolism, substernal catch, pneumonia, PE	May be spontaneous to bleb rupture or secondary to trauma
Thoracic aortic aneurysm	Sudden-onset tearing pain radiating to back, arms, jaw, neck	Angiogram, computerized tomography or transesophageal echocardiography	See text	MI, gastritis, esophageal spasm, etc.	May have unequal pulses and BP in upper extremities, but this is not an absolute finding in all patients with aneurysm

evidence of MI and can be used in addition to aspirin in the patient without contraindications. More recently, weight-based nomograms that are more likely to reach therapeutic levels have been developed. Start with a bolus of 80 U/kg followed by a drip of 18 U/kg/hr. Enoxaparin shows promise in this setting but cannot be recommended at this time.

5. Beta-blockers such as metoprolol 15 mg IV in 5 mg aliquots every 5 minutes can be helpful in patients without failure and a hyperdynamic state. Contraindications include heart block, COPD, bradycardia, and hypotension among others.
6. Calcium-channel blockers.
   (a) Diltiazem. Recent evidence indicates that IV diltiazem 25 mg over 2 minutes followed by a drip at 5 mg/hr may be useful for refractory angina. IV diltiazem should not be used in combination with IV beta-blockers. May cause AV conduction disturbances.
   (b) Nifedipine (Procardia) as a 10 mg capsule chewed and swallowed may result in the relief of angina pain. However, it may exacerbate tachycardia and cause hypotension. Nifedipine is not absorbed through the buccal mucosa and overall does not have any effect on the progression to MI. Other therapies are more effective.
7. Thrombolytics may be indicated in the event of an MI. See section on myocardial infarction in Chapter 2 for management details.
8. Patients should be admitted for unstable angina as well as for R/O or actual MI. The decision should be based on the history, since the ECG may not reflect an abnormality in 50% of those with an acute MI. Enzymes are also *not* helpful in deciding who to admit, since the CPK and troponin-T may not be elevated for up to 6 hours after an infarction.

ACUTE PULMONARY EDEMA AND CARDIOGENIC SHOCK

See Chapter 2.

PEDIATRIC LIFE SUPPORT

We strongly suggest taking a PALS course certified by The American Heart Association. The information below is intended only as a reference in an emergency and will not take the place of PALS training.

I. NEONATAL RESUSCITATION.

See Chapter 10.

II. PEDIATRIC ADVANCED LIFE SUPPORT

A. Breathing. (Remember positioning, suctioning, airway.)

1. Pediatric cardiac arrest almost always secondary to respiratory insult.
   a. Treat any signs of respiratory distress such as tachypnea, retractions, or stridor immediately. (See section on asthma/COPD/dyspnea for differential, p. 27.)
   b. Immediately provide humidified oxygen in highest concentration possible. Treat underlying cause!
   c. For suspected epiglottitis, do not move patient or apply oxygen. Any agitation to the child may precipitate airway obstruction. See Chapter 10 for discussion of epiglottitis.
2. Aspiration of a foreign body especially prevalent in those less than 5 years of age.
   a. Present with sudden-onset dyspnea, stridor, gagging.
   b. Treatment: Observe as long as moving air well and coughing. If there is increased respiratory difficulty, or cough is ineffective, can try Heimlich maneuver or direct visualization of cords, and removal of foreign body if necessary.
3. Bag-valve-mask with 100% O_2 usually adequate even in situations such as epiglottitis.
4. If must intubate, see Table 1-2.

B. Cardiac assessment.

1. Tachycardia usual response to stress.
2. Bradycardia is evidence of impending cardiac arrest.
3. Blood pressure may remain normal until cardiopulmonary arrest imminent. (See blood pressure table in pediatrics chapter and Figs. 10-4 to 10-6.)

TABLE 1-2
Endotracheal tube sizes for children

Age	Endotracheal tube size
Premature	2.5, 3.0 uncuffed
Newborn	3.0, 3.5 uncuffed
6 months	3.5 uncuffed
12 to 18 months	4.0, 4.5 uncuffed
2 years	4.5, 5.0 uncuffed
4 years	5.0, 5.5 uncuffed
6 years	5.5 uncuffed
8 years	6.0 cuffed or uncuffed
10 years	6.5 cuffed
12 years	7.0 cuffed
>12 years	7.0-8.0 cuffed

To calculate: Approximate tube size = (Age/4) + 4

4. Observe level of consciousness, urine output, capillary refill, color, as gauge of end-organ perfusion.
5. For fluid resuscitation: 20 ml/kg IV of NS or LR. May repeat twice or even more if needed.
6. The efficacy of high-dose epinephrine (0.1 mg/kg) has recently been called into question but is still standard of care.
7. Drugs for pediatric resuscitation (Table 1-3).

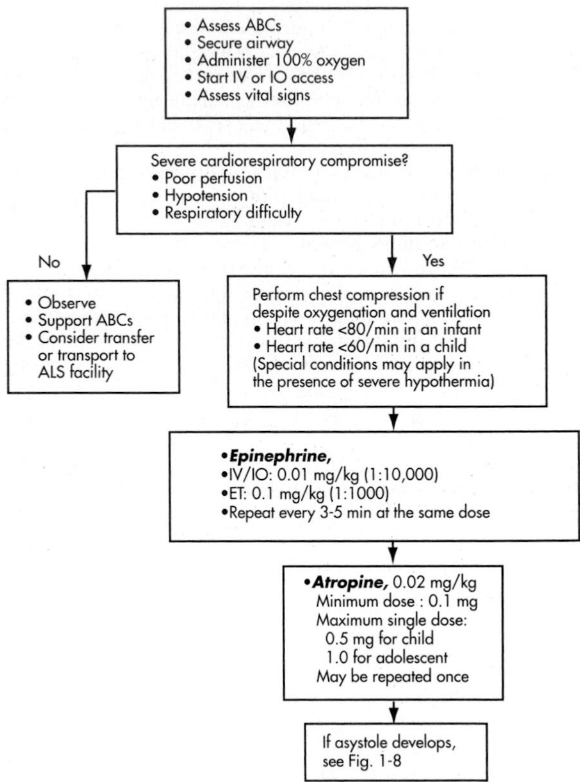

FIG. 1-7 Bradycardia decision tree. (*ABCs,* Airway, breathing, and circulation; *ALS,* advanced life support; *ET,* endotracheal; *IO,* intraosseous; *IV,* intravenous.)

TABLE 1-3
Drug doses for pediatric resuscitation

Drug	Dose	Remarks
Adenosine	0.1 to 0.2 mg/kg Maximum single dose: 12 mg	Rapid IV bolus
Atropine sulfate	0.02 mg/kg per dose	Minimum dose: 0.1 mg Maximum single dose: 0.5 mg in child 1.0 mg in adolescent
Bretylium tosylate	5 mg/kg; may be increased to 10 mg/kg	Rapid IV
Calcium chloride 10%	20 mg/kg per dose	Give slowly
Dopamine hydrochloride*	2 to 20 μg/kg/min	Adrenergic action dominates at ≥15 to 20 μg/kg/min
Dobutamine hydrochloride*	2 to 20 mg/kg/min	Titrate to desired effect
Epinephrine for bradycardia	IV/IO: 0.01 mg/kg (1:10,000) = 0.1 ml/kg of 1:10,000 ET: 0.1 mg/kg (1:1000) = 0.1 ml/kg of 1:1000	Be aware of effect of preservatives administered (if preservatives are present in epinephrine preparation) when high doses are used
Epinephrine for asystolic or pulseless arrest	*First dose:* IV/IO: 0.01 mg/kg (1:10,000) = 0.1 ml/kg of 1:10,000 ET: 0.1 mg/kg (1:1000) = 0.1 ml/kg of 1:1000 Doses as high as 0.2 mg/kg may be effective *Subsequent doses:* IV/IO/ET: 0.1 mg/kg (1:1000) = 0.1 ml/kg of 1:1000 Doses as high as 0.2 mg/kg may be effective	Be aware of effect of preservatives administered (if preservatives present in epinephrine preparation) when high doses are used

Continued

TABLE 1-3
Drug doses for pediatric resuscitation—cont'd

Drug	Dose	Remarks
Epinephrine infusion	Initial at 0.1 μg/kg/min Higher infusion dose used if asystole present	Titrate to desired effect (0.1 to 1.0 μg/kg/min)
Lidocaine	1 mg/kg per dose	
Lidocaine infusion	20 to 50 μg/kg/min	
Sodium bicarbonate	1 mEq/kg per dose, or 0.3 × kg × Base deficit	Infuse slowly and only if ventilation is adequate

*Run these drugs in rapidly at first to clear the line and ensure drug delivery. When there is a clinical response (increase in heart rate, blood pressure), decrease drip rate to desired infusion rate.

ET, Endotracheal; *IO*, intraosseous; *IV*, intravenous.

Defibrillation: Energy dose = 2 J/kg. If this not effective, use 4 J/kg × 2.

Dilutions: For dopamine and dobutamine: 6 × Body weight (kg) = # of mg in 100 ml D_5W and then 1 ml/hr = 1.0 μg/kg/min.

Adapted from American Heart Association: *JAMA* 268:16, 1992.

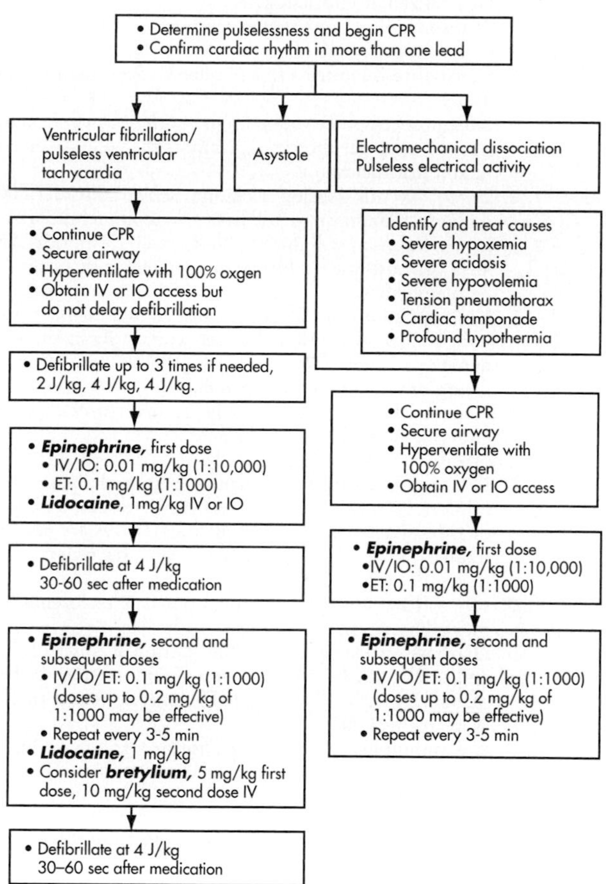

FIG. 1-8 Asystole and pulseless arrest decision tree. *CPR*, Cardiopulmonary resuscitation. (From Emergency Cardiac Care Committee and Subcommittees, American Heart Association: Guidelines for cardiopulmonary resuscitation and emergency cardiac care, *JAMA* 268:16, 1992.)

SEIZURES

I. FEBRILE SEIZURES

A. Salient features.

1. Generalized, nonfocal seizure.
2. Autosomal dominant transmission.
3. 6 months to 5 years of age.
4. Generally self-limited 4 to 5 minutes and less than 15 minutes.
5. Little postictal phase with prompt return of baseline mental status. If postictal, drowsy, or has more than one seizure, see "grand mal" below.
6. 2% to 5% will develop a chronic seizure disorder. 48% under 15 months of age will have a recurrent febrile seizure in the future as will 30% of those over 15 months, and 45% of those with a first-degree relative with history of febrile seizures.
7. Consider admission for focal signs, altered mental status, poor follow-up study, or further workup for meningitis, metabolic abnormality. Consider CT/MRI or EEG if suspicion of underlying structural illness.
8. Finger-stick glucose test should be done unless patient clinically normal.

B. Therapy.

1. No specific therapy for seizure; treat underlying cause of fever. Always evaluate patient clinically for meningitis, or other bacterial infection. It is not necessary to do a lumbar puncture in simple febrile seizures unless otherwise indicated.
2. No evidence that phenobarbital prevents recurrence and may adversely affect learning.
3. Diazepam 0.33 mg/kg PO Q8h starting at onset of fever and continuing for 24 hours after the fever reduced febrile seizures by 82% in those treated (intention to treat analysis = decrease of 44%).
4. Acetaminophen and ibuprofen use are a good idea but up to now there is no convincing evidence that their use reduces febrile seizures.

II. GRAND MAL SEIZURES AND STATUS EPILEPTICUS

A. Salient features.

1. Prolonged >15 minutes (if still seizing by time reach emergency department, by definition that is status if you include transport time).
2. May have focal signs or symptoms.
3. Prolonged postictal state.
4. May have presence of a fever, but this is not a simple febrile seizure.
5. May have prior history of seizures.

B. Etiology.

1. ***Metabolic.*** Check electrolytes, glucose, Ca^{++}, Mg^{++}, CBC.
2. ***Toxins.*** Look for pinpoint pupils, dilated pupils, excess salivation, etc. (See section on overdosage and toxindromes, p. 50). Get drug (prescription and illegal usage) history from family or drug screen.
3. ***Hypoxia.*** Check respiratory status.
4. ***Infection.*** If clinically indicated, perform LP.
   a. Do CT to rule out mass lesion (abscess) before doing LP.
5. ***Space-occupying lesions*** (that is, subdural hematoma, subarachnoid bleed, tumor). Work-up with noncontrast CT/contrast CT for tumor.
6. ***Poor compliance with medications.***

C. Work-up as indicated by history. It is not necessary to repeat all labs on a patient with a known seizure disorder with a simple exacerbation caused by poor compliance. Watch for a change in type or frequency of seizure to guide your work-up.

1. Drug levels are indicated in any patient using antiepileptics or theophylline, other seizure-inducing agent.
2. See above for specific work-ups.

D. Treatment. Because of the short half-life of benzodiazepines, will usually need a drug besides benzodiazepine for management, and so a longer-acting agent (phenytoin or phenobarbital) should be given to most seizure patients. Make sure to get levels in those already taking drugs.

1. Be prepared to manage the airway.
   a. Seizures may cause hypoxia.
   b. Benzodiazepines, phenobarbital may cause apnea.
2. Correct the underlying metabolic problem if possible.
3. ***Treatment of choice.*** *Lorazepam* (Ativan) 0.03 to 0.05 mg/kg (2 to 4 mg in adult) IV or double this rectally if IV access not possible.
   - Advantage over diazepam is longer clinical half-life (hours of seizure suppression versus minutes) with less respiratory depression and need for intubation.
4. Alternative is *diazepam* (Valium) 0.1 to 0.3 mg/kg IV (5 to 10 mg in adult but may need 20 to 30 mg) or double this rectally if no IV access. If above does not work, try the medications below.
5. *Phenobarbital* 15 mg/kg IV at 25 to 50 mg/min. May give IM.
   - Respiratory depression additive to that of benzodiazepines and so need for intubation probable if adding this.
6. *Phenytoin* (Dilantin) 15 mg/kg IV (1 mg/kg/min IV not to exceed 50 mg/min). Do not exceed 1 g in adults; mix with NS (50 ml/500 mg in adults); use in-line filter.

a. Monitor for QT prolongation and stop infusion if increases by >50% (risk of torsades de pointes)
b. An alternative to phenytoin is fosphenytoin (Cerebryx). There is little advantage to fosphenytoin; cardiotoxicity, local irritation, etc. are comparable. However, fosphenytoin is absorbed IM and can be administered rapidly. Fosphenytoin should be infused at ≥100 to 150 mg/min; subtherapeutic levels may occur if infused slowly. Therapeutic blood levels occur in 10 minutes if drug rapidly infused. Dosing is the same as that for phenytoin. The fosphenytoin dose is expressed as the phenytoin equivalent. Use in those with hepatic and renal disease is problematic because of their slower than normal metabolism to active drug and should be avoided.

If above does not work (lidocaine and midazolam are not approved for these indications but are well tested):

7. *Lidocaine.* 1.5 to 2 mg/kg IV over 2 minutes and repeated in 5 minutes if necessary with a drip at 3 to 4 mg/min.
   - Same class of drugs as phenytoin and an excellent membrane stabilizer.
8. *Midazolam* has been found to be useful in those unresponsive to full loading doses of lorazepam, phenobarbital, and phenytoin. Give midazolam bolus of 170 to 220 μg/kg followed by maximal infusion rates of 0.9 to 11 μg/kg/min.
9. *Pyridoxine.* A very rare patient (generally children or those with an isoniazid overdose) will be pyridoxine responsive, and so, if no other measures work, consider pyridoxine (vitamin B_6) 100 mg IV. If suspect isoniazid overdose, give 4 g IV and then 1 g IV Q30 min until equal to amount INH ingested; may give IV push if patient seizing. For children with INH overdose give 40 mg/kg IV. Most vitamin B_6 responsive seizures occur in infants, but they have rarely been reported de novo in older children.

   If above does not work:
10. *Barbiturate coma.* Call anesthesia department.

III. NEONATAL SEIZURES

A. May be atypical in physical presentation because of CNS immaturity.
1. Grand mal may present with sequential clonic-tonic movements of extremities or only focal symptoms.
2. Autonomic seizures noted by changes in respirations, heart rate, pupils.
3. Myoclonic seizures. Single clonic motions throughout day.

B. Is important to pursue a cause, since frequently have specific treatment available.

1. In ED, check electrolytes, calcium, glucose, magnesium, CBC, blood culture, and LP.
2. EEG, CT, skull radiograph, long bone radiograph, as indicated.
3. Bilirubin, ABG, urine amino acids as indicated.

C. **Treatment** for neonatal seizures (in absence of known correctable cause).
1. Pyridoxine (vitamin B_6) 100 mg IV/IM.
2. Glucose 2 ml/kg of $D_{25}W$.
3. Calcium gluconate (10%) 30 to 60 mg/kg (max. 1 g), slow IV, preferably over 1 hour.
4. Magncsium sulfate 20% solution, 0.2 ml/kg IM or IV
5. Phenobarbital. Premature infant 10 to 20 mg/kg IM or IV; term infant 10 to 15 mg/kg IM or IV. Infuse no faster than 30 mg/min.
6. Phenytoin 10 to 15 mg/kg IV. Infuse no faster than 1 mg/kg/min.
7. Lorazepam 0.05 to 0.15 mg/kg IV.
8. Diazepam 0.2 mg/kg repeat twice. Maximum dose 5 mg age <5 years, 10 mg if age >10 years.
   - Diazepam and lorazepam will increase hyperbilirubinemia by uncoupling albumin-bilirubin complex. Therefore be careful in children with jaundice.

ASTHMA/COPD/DYSPNEA

(See also Chapter 3)

A. **Causes of dyspnea.** (See appropriate chapters for in-depth discussions.)
1. ***Upper airway disease/obstruction*** (presents with stridor).
   a. If foreign body above cords, can use direct laryngoscopy and Magill forceps to remove FB if necessary (procedure of choice in the ED).
   b. Think of epiglottitis (in adults as well), croup, retropharyngeal abscess, angioedema. See the section on stridor in Chapter 10.
2. ***Pneumothorax.*** (See chest trauma, p. 42.)
3. ***CHF, "cardiac asthma."*** Look for basilar rales, peripheral edema, JVD, frothy sputum. (See Chapter 2.)
4. ***Pulmonary embolism.*** See Chapter 3 for work-up.
5. ***Pneumonia.*** Fever, chills, purulent sputum, infiltrate on localized rales. (See Chapter 3.)
6. ***COPD.*** Generally have prior history. (See Chapter 3.)
7. ***Central hyperventilation and metabolic acidosis.*** Lungs clear, ABG reflects metabolic acidosis or primary respiratory alkalosis. (See Chapter 5.)
8. ***Anemia.*** (See Chapter 5.)

B. **Acute asthma.**
1. Diagnose by history and physical examination.

a. History.
   (1) Onset, trigger of current exacerbation.
   (2) Severity of symptoms, including limitation of exercise tolerance, interference with sleep.
   (3) Medications.
   (4) Prior hospitalizations, ER visits, especially recent visits.
   (5) Severe exacerbations in past, requiring ICU admissions, intubation.
   (6) Any other chronic medical conditions.
b. Physical examination.
   (1) Severity of respiratory compromise: speech difficult because of breathlessness, use of accessory muscles of respiration, inability to lie supine, pulsus paradoxus >12 mm Hg fall in systolic BP during inspiration, tachycardia, tachypnea (see cardiac tamponade section for procedure to determine pulsus paradoxus, p. 42).
   (2) Complications: pneumonia, pneumothorax, pneumomediastinum.
   (3) Cyanosis, level of alertness, air movement, wheezing. Wheezing can be an unreliable guide to degree of obstruction; severe obstruction may be associated with a "silent chest" because of little or no air movement.
   (4) Beware if patient seems too calm. This may represent CO_2 retention and narcosis.
c. Functional assessment. Monitor PEFR or FEV_1. Check pulse oximetry. Infants become hypoxemic earlier than adults do, and physical assessment of respiratory status in children is less reliable. Check O_2 saturations on all infants and children by pulse oximetry. Room air saturation should be >93%. A room air saturation <91% in infants usually is predictive of the need for hospitalization. Check an arterial or capillary blood gas level on infants with O_2 saturation <90%.
d. Lab tests. Do not delay initial treatment waiting for lab tests and radiographs. After initial stabilization, consider:
   (1) CBC if patient has fever or purulent sputum.
   (2) CXR if suspect complication such as pneumonia or pneumothorax.
   (3) Serum theophylline concentration in all patients taking theophylline.
   (4) ABG in patients with severe distress, poor response to treatment, or abnormal pulse oximetry.
e. High-risk patients. Patients at high risk of asthma-related death or life-threatening deterioration.
   (1) Prior intubation for asthma, or prior ICU admission.

(2) Two or more hospitalizations for asthma in past year.
(3) Three or more ER visits in past year.
(4) Hospitalization or ER visit in past month.
(5) Using or withdrawing from systemic corticosteroids.
(6) History of syncope or seizure related to hypoxia from asthma.
(7) Poor social situation or psychiatric disease.
(8) Infant <1 year old.
(9) $<10\%$ improvement in PEFR or FEV_1 in ER.
(10) PEFR or FEV_1 $<25\%$ predicted.
(11) Pco_2 40 mm Hg or more. A normal Pco_2 is abnormal in the setting of asthma exacerbations where the patient should be hyperventilating, resulting in a low Pco_2. A normal Pco_2 may herald impending respiratory failure.

f. **Treatment for asthma or COPD.**
(1) Oxygen may be needed to support patient and should not be withheld even to do a blood gas analysis.
(2) Hydration is without benefit if the patient is euvolemic, and aggressive IV hydration may precipitate CHF.
(3) If severe asthma, consider cardiac monitoring.
(4) Beta-agonists are the mainstay of treatment.
  (a) *Albuterol.* 2.5 mg in 3 ml of NS by nebulizer (adults). May give up to 4 treatments per hour. Some studies suggest that continuously nebulized albuterol works better.
  (b) In children, can use *albuterol* 0.15 to 0.3 mg/kg by nebulizer every hour (ideally divided every 20 minutes or given continuously over 1 hour). The 0.3 mg/kg dosing is significantly better in moderate to severe asthma.
  (c) Can use nebulized albuterol almost continuously if needed.
    - Tachycardia does not increase further after first several doses.
    - May cause hypokalemia by shifting K^+ intracellularly.
    - Metered-dose inhaler by means of a spacer is just as good as nebulizer if you give about 6 to 8 activations by a spacer to equal one nebulized treatment.

(5) **Steroids.**
  (a) Reduces return visits, admission rates.
  (b) Should be used in most patients: always in those already receiving steroids and in most of

those previously receiving medications who fail to clear after one nebulizer treatment.

(c) *Methylprednisolone.* For adults 125 mg IV and 40 mg IV Q6h. For children 1 to 2 mg/kg IV followed by 2 mg/kg/24 hours divided into Q6h doses.

(d) *Prenisone.* For adults 60 mg PO. For children 0.5 to 2.0 mg/kg Q24h for 3 to 7 days.

- All evidence indicates that steroids given orally are just as effective as IV in acute exacerbations of asthma.
- There is no need for a steroid taper in those not previously receiving steroids *if* only 5- to 7-day course. There is no increase in relapse without taper and no adrenal suppression with a 1-week course.

(6) *Anticholinergics* seem to work better in COPD than asthma but do have some bronchodilating effect.

(a) *Atropine* 0.4 to 2 mg (adult 0.025 mg/kg) *by nebulizer.* May mix with beta-agonists in same nebulizer. May increase heart rate and may cause pupils to dilate from contact with mist.

(b) *Ipratropium* can be used by metered-dose inhaler and is available in a nebulized form. The dose is 0.5 mg by nebulizer. This is preferred over atropine, since there is little systemic effect.

(7) Theophylline-aminophylline. There is little evidence that adding theophylline-aminophylline to maximized beta-adrenergic therapy is helpful in the treatment of acute asthma.

(a) Is arrhythmogenic.

(b) Has a very low therapeutic threshold.

(c) *Always* check a drug level if you feel compelled to use this drug.

(d) Takes 2 to 3 hours to peak effect after IV administration.

(e) Although frequent, optimal doses of beta-blockers are more effective, if you choose to use aminophylline, it is a 6 mg/kg loading dose to maximum of 350 mg over 30 to 45 minutes followed by a drip at 0.6 mg/kg/hr not to exceed 50 to 60 mg/hr. Levels should be checked. Maintenance dose dependent on patient's smoking status, presence of cor pulmonale, and age.

(8) *Magnesium sulfate* is shown in some studies to produce transient improvement in asthma.

- Reasonable if patient has failed conventional therapy; less toxic than theophylline.
- Dose: In adults 2 g IV over 15 to 20 minutes (may mix in 50 ml of normal saline). Very safe but do not use in renal failure. May get flushing, transient hypotension but rare.
- Magnesium sulfate has been successfully used in children. The dose is 25 mg/kg.

(9) Intubation and nasal CPAP (continuous positive-pressure ventilation) are a last resort and may not work well in the asthmatic patient.

(10) Admit if persistent respiratory distress, O_2 saturation <94% after treatment (children), peak expiratory flow of <60% of predicated value in children or failure to increase by 15% above baseline or absolute value of 200 L/min in adults, failure of FEV_1 to increase by 500 cc or produce a total of <1.6 liters (adults), hypercapnia (retaining CO_2 over baseline value), or pneumothorax. Additionally, clinical judgment is important. If the patient does not look well or still feels dyspneic, consider admission to hospital.

AIRWAY MANAGEMENT

A. Adequate anesthesia is critical for intubation in the awake patient.

1. If you have time, lidocaine 4% at 5 ml by hand-held nebulizer facilitates intubation by blocking the gag reflex and providing excellent topical anesthesia.
2. In nasal intubation, cetacaine-lidocaine spray and lidocaine jelly are helpful.

B. Nasal intubation.

1. Simple to do blindly.
2. Contraindicated in bleeding disorders or where you might want to use thrombolytics. Also contraindicated in basilar skull fracture and midface trauma.
3. The patient must be breathing to use this technique.
4. Almost all patients intubated nasally develop a sinusitis and should be given antibiotics if prolonged intubation is required.

RAPID SEQUENCE INTUBATION (RSI)

Before you try this technique, be sure that you are able to control the airway, since the patient will be paralyzed and unable to breathe for himself or herself.

A. Indications. Acute intracranial lesions, some overdoses, status epilepticus, combative trauma patients where behavior threatens life, possible cervical spine fracture where immobilization not possible because of delirium, etc.

B. Drug side effects.

1. Succinylcholine.
   a. Bradycardia
   b. Increased intraocular and intracranial pressure
   c. Contraindicated in penetrating globe trauma
   d. Increased gastric pressure and emesis
   e. Rarely hyperthermia
2. Vecuronium has almost no known side effects.

C. RSI using a depolarizing agent.

Time (minutes)

−3.00 Preoxygenate, IV lines, monitor, oximetry, equipment including that for emergency surgical airway control
−2.00 Lidocaine 1 mg/kg (100 mg*)†
−1.45 Atropine 0.01 mg/kg (0.5 mg*)‡
−1.00 Vecuronium 0.01 mg/kg (1 mg*)§ prevents fasciculation
−1.00 Begin Sellick maneuver (cricothyroid pressure to prevent vomiting and aspiration)
−0.55 Midazolam 0.1 mg/kg (7 mg*)‖
−0.45 Succinylcholine 1.5 mg/kg (100 mg*)¶
0.00 Intubation
+0.30 Assess tube placement
+8.0 Check patient's temperature

D. RSI using nondepolarizing agent.

Time (minutes) to intubation

−3.00 Preoxygenate, IV lines, monitor, oximetry, equipment
−2.00 Lidocaine 1 mg/kg (100 mg*)†
−1.45 Atropine 0.01 mg/kg (0.5 mg*)‡
−1.00 Vecuronium 0.10 mg/kg (10 mg*)
−1.00 Begin Sellick maneuver
−0.55 Midazolam 0.1 mg/kg (7 mg*)‖
0.00 Intubation
+0.30 Assess tube placement

Usual adult dosage. †May be omitted in non–head injury cases. ‡May be omitted in adults if no preexistent bradycardia. §May use pancuronium (same dose). ‖May use thiopental 3 to 5 mg/kg (300 mg). ¶Dose in children is 1.5 to 2 mg/kg.

PEDIATRIC SEDATION

A. Sedation can facilitate procedures in the ED and minimize the psychologic trauma to the child as well as to the ED staff and the parents.

B. Sedation requirements.

1. Need good monitoring including 0_2 saturation, pulse, BP if possible, respirations, and level of consciousness.

The child should be closely monitored until he or she has returned to functional baseline value.
2. Sedation does not equal pain relief. Give medications that relax the child and medications that provide pain relief.
3. The traditional DPT (demerol, phenergan, and thorazine) AKA Kiddy Cocktail/Lytic Cocktail is fraught with problems and cannot be recommended.
4. Benzodiazepines have the advantage of causing amnesia especially midazolam.
5. Despite drug company literature, there is no significant difference in the recovery times of diazepam and midazolam when used as a single dose for sedation in the ED. In fact, the recovery time was faster with diazepam in most studies.
6. Postsedation discharge requires:
    a. Return to baseline verbal skills if appropriate
    b. Return to baseline muscular control
    c. Return to baseline mental status
    d. Parent or responsible person can understand instructions
7. Drugs for sedation and pain control in children (Table 1-4). Note: *Sedative doses are for conscious sedation, which requires constant monitoring.* See Chapter 20 for doses for other indications!

COMA

I. WHAT TO DO FIRST IN COMA

A. ABCs including cervical spine immobilization if *any* possibility of trauma.
1. If hypertension with associated bradycardia, consider increased intracranial pressure.
2. Intubate to protect airway if no gag reflex.

B. Check finger-stick glucose and rapidly administer:
1. *Thiamine* 100 mg IV prevents Wernicke-Korsakoff encephalopathy.
    a. Do not withold glucose if thiamine not available. A single dose of glucose will not induce Wernicke-Korsakoff encephalopathy.
2. *Glucose* 25 to 50 g IV treats hypoglycemia.
3. *Naloxone* 2 to 4 ampules of 0.4 mg treats narcotic overdose.
    a. Some will start with 2 mg and then 4 mg if no response.
    b. Make sure to restrain the patient if suspect will precipitate narcotic withdrawal. Recently the routine use of naloxone has been questioned in those patients without evidence of narcotic intoxication. However, it should be considered for use in all patients.
4. If suspect benzodiazapine overdose (valium, alprazolam, and others).

TABLE 1-4
Medications for sedation and pain control in children

Medication	Route	Dose (mg/kg)	Maximum dose	Side effects and comments
PAIN MEDICATIONS				
Meperidine (Demerol)	IV/IM	1.0 to 2.0 mg/kg	100 mg	Reversible with naloxone (Watch for respiratory depression) (May cause hypotension)
Morphine	IV/IM	0.1 to 0.2 mg/kg	10 mg	Same as above
Codeine	PO	1.0 mg/kg	60 mg	Same as above
SEDATIVES				
Diazepam (Valium and others)	IV	0.05 to 0.2 mg/kg	10 mg	Watch for respiratory depression Reversible with flumazanil
	PR	0.5 mg/kg		
Midazolam (Versed)	IV/IM	0.01 to 0.08 mg/kg (some have used up to 0.2 mg/kg)	4 mg	Titrate to effect; precautions as above
	PO/IN/PR	0.3 to 0.7 mg/kg		As above
Chloral hydrate	PO	25 to 100 mg/kg	1000 mg, though some will go to 2000 mg	Cannot reverse Less likely to be effective in head injured or neurologically impaired patients

IM, Intramuscular; *IO*, intranasal; *IV*, intravenous; *PO*, per os, by mouth; *PR*, per rectum.

- *Flumazenil* (Romazicon) 0.2 mg up to 5 mg IV. Do not use flumazenil if suspect concurrent tricyclic overdose or chronic benzodiazapine use. It may precipitate status epilepticus. This should not be routinely administered to the unconscious patient unless there is a clear indication and no contraindication.

II. DIFFERENTIAL DIAGNOSIS OF COMA

A. Coma with no localizing CNS signs can be caused by:

1. Metabolic insults including hypoglycemia, uremia, nonketotic hyperosmolar coma, Addision's disease, diabetic ketoacidosis, hypothyroidism, hepatic coma.
   - Children and young adults will often get hypoglycemic and may present with coma after alcohol ingestion including mouthwash!
2. Respiratory including hypoxia, hypercapnia.
3. Intoxication including barbiturates, alcohol, opiates, carbon monoxide poisoning, benzodiazepines.
4. Infections (severe systemic) including sepsis, pneumonia, typhoid fever.
5. Shock including hypovolemic, cardiogenic, septic, anaphylactic.
6. Epilepsy.
7. Hypertensive encephalopathy.
8. Hyperthermia (heat stroke), hypothermia.

B. Coma with meningeal irritation without localizing signs can be caused by meningitis, subarachnoid hemorrhage from ruptured aneurysm, AV malformation.

C. If focal brainstem or lateralizing signs, can be caused by pontine hemorrhage, CVA, brain abscess, subdural-epidural hemorrhage.

D. If appear awake but unresponsive:

1. ***Abulic state.*** Frontal lobe function depressed and so may take several minutes to answer question.
2. ***Locked-in syndrome.*** Destruction of pontine motor tracts. Is able to look upward.
3. ***Psychogenic state.*** Unresponsiveness.

III. PATHOPHYSIOLOGY OF COMA

Coma can be caused only by:

A. Bilateral cortical disease.

B. Reticular activating system compromise.

IV. TO DIFFERENTIATE BETWEEN CORTICAL AND BRAINSTEM LESIONS

A. Use calorics–ice water in each ear. Nystagmus refers to the fast return phase. Four possible responses:

1. Both eyes deviate toward side cold water instilled and have good nystagmus. Patient not comatose.

2. Both eyes deviate toward cold water; no fast return phase. Brainstem function intact. Coma is caused by cortical problem.
3. No eye movement despite cold stimuli to both sides, thus no brainstem function (same as absent oculocephalic reflex, or "doll's eyes").
   - Not necessarily a permanent lesion; may be caused by severe hypothermia or drug overdose.
4. Movement of only one eye ipsilateral to stimulus, thus intranuclear lesion, which almost always indicates brainstem damage and demands rapid evaluation to determine if a correctable lesion is present.

B. Pupils.

1. Generally resistant to metabolic insult.
2. Remember that a dilated eye may be secondary to topical or systemic drugs.
3. A dilated pupil in an alert person is not likely attributable to increased intracranial pressure and herniation.
   - *A dilated pupil in an unconscious patient may herald imminent uncal herniation.*
4. ***Small reactive pupils.*** Generally metabolic or diencephalic lesion.
5. ***Unilateral, dilated, fixed.*** Third nerve lesion or uncal lesion.
6. ***Bilateral pinpoint pupils.*** Pontine lesion.
7. ***Midposition, fixed.*** Midbrain lesion.
8. ***Bilateral large, fixed.*** Tectal lesion.
9. Propoxyphene (Darvon and others) can cause coma without pinpoint pupils.
10. Eyes will deviate toward side of physiologically inactive lesion (CVA) and away from an active lesion (seizure).
11. 5% of the normal population will have anisocoria (asymmetric pupils).

V. LABORATORY WORK-UP OF COMA

A. CBC, electrolytes, BUN, creatinine, glucose, calcium, magnesium, arterial blood gas, toxic screen, carboxyhemoglobin, liver enzymes.

B. CT scan and LP.

- If suspect meningitis, do not withhold antibiotics while waiting to do an LP. Antibiotics should be started before the patient goes to the CT scanner. Your culture results will not be affected.

HEAD TRAUMA

See also evaluation of coma above.

A. Frequently associated with other severe trauma.

1. ***ABCs take priority.*** Saving only the head will not save the patient.

2. Hypotension in adults is never caused by an isolated head injury except near death. Look for other injuries including cord injuries.
3. Physical exam includes complete neurologic exam as well as inspection for evidence of basilar skull fracture (CSF rhinorrhea, Battle's sign, raccoon eyes, hemotympanum), etc.

B. Low-risk injuries.

1. ***Criteria.***
   a. Minor trauma, scalp wounds.
   b. No signs of intracranial injury, loss of consciousness.
2. ***Treatment.*** Observation for any sign or symptom of brain injury. Must discharge to a reliable observer who will continue observation at home.

C. Moderate-risk injuries.

1. ***Criteria.***
   a. Symptoms consistent with intracranial injury including vomiting, transient loss of consciousness, severe headache, posttraumatic seizures, amnesia, evidence of basilar skull fracture (CSF rhinorrhea, Battle's sign, raccoon eyes, hemotympanum).
   b. *Nonfocal neurologic exam.*
2. ***Treatment.*** Observation and "neuro checks"; consider CT; use clinical judgment.
3. Admit for observation and monitoring.

D. High-risk injuries.

1. ***Criteria.*** Depressed level of consciousness, focal neurologic signs, penetrating injury of skull or palpable depressed skull fractures.
2. ***Approach.*** Immediate CT, neurosurgical consultation.
3. Support while awaiting definitive neurosurgical care.
   a. Intubation. Pretreatment with lidocaine 1 mg/kg IV may prevent rise in intracranial pressure (ICP). See also rapid sequence intubation (RSI), p. 31.
   b. Hyperventilation to maintain P_{O_2} >90 torrs, P_{CO_2} 25 to 30 torrs.
      (1) Maintains adequate oxygenation and reduces intracranial pressure.
      (2) PEEP relatively contraindicated because reduces cerebral blood flow.
      (3) Avoid tight cervical collars. Any pressure on the external jugular veins will increase the ICP.
   c. Maintain normal cardiac output.
      (1) If hypotensive from other cause such as multitrauma, hypertonic saline (3% *or* 7.5%; see section on shock, p. 48) may be best *IV fluid* because stabilizes BP, improves cerebral blood flow, prevents increase in ICP from edema.
      (2) If hypertensive, consider labetalol or nitroprusside. Vasodilator such as nitroprusside will increase

cerebral blood flow and ICP (see section on hypertensive emergencies for dosing, p. 46).

d. Treating increased ICP.
   (1) Hyperventilation as above.
   (2) Mannitol 1 g/kg IV over 20 minutes induces osmotic diuresis. (Controversial if patient not herniating. Consult your neurosurgeon.)
   (3) Some suggest furosemide (Lasix and others) 20 mg IV.
   (4) Elevate head of bed 30 degrees.
   (5) Steroids ineffective in controlling ICP in the trauma setting.

E. Glasgow coma scale (Table 1-5).

- Useful in a general sense, but 18% of those with a GCS score of 15 have an abnormal CT scan, and 5% of those with a GCS score of 15 require neurosurgical intervention. The GCS score is especially unreliable in children.

F. Skull radiographs. Head CT with bone windows generally preferable.

1. Generally not indicated in adults unless one suspects depressed fracture and cannot palpate skull because of hematoma, etc.
   - Can have intracranial injury without a skull fracture and vice versa.

TABLE 1-5.
Glasgow coma scale

Parameter	Response	Score
Eye opening	Spontaneous	4
	To voice	3
	To pain	2
	None	1
Verbal response	Oriented	5
	Confused	4
	Inappropriate	3
	Incomprehensible sounds	2
	None	1
Motor response	Localizes pain	5
	Withdraws to pain	4
	Flexion response to pain	3
	Extension response to pain	2
	None	1

Coma score is most useful in triage and in following status. Initial score of <7 indicates a poor prognosis if a cause other than trauma cannot be found and corrected quickly. Assessment should be done frequently and recorded accurately on a flow sheet with times documented.

2. May be useful in those up to 7 years of age because a skull fracture can lead to nonunion because of rapid head growth. Use clinical judgment as to severity of injury.

G. Postconcussive syndrome.

1. May occur with minor trauma.
2. Characterized by headache, memory difficulty, attention deficit, personality changes, negative CT (may represent disruption of axonal support structures, axonal stretching).
3. May have findings on formal neuropsychologic testing.
4. May last for a year or more.
5. Treat headache with nonnarcotic analgesia and depression as per Chapter 15.

TRAUMA: MULTIPLE TRAUMA AND GENERAL PRINCIPLES

I. STABILIZATION AND PRIMARY SURVEY

Remember ABCDE: Airway, Breathing, Circulation, Drugs/Disability/Allergies and Eating/Exposure

A. Airway. If depressed level of consciousness or upper airway bleeding, intubate *without moving neck.*

1. Intubation safe even with neck fracture, but avoid Sellick maneuver.
2. Confirm placement with a radiograph and by auscultation.

B. Breathing. Ventilate with 100% O_2.

- Check breath sounds and place chest tubes as needed for hemothorax, pneumothorax, tension pneumothorax.

C. Circulation. For "all" multiple trauma victims:

1. Stop obvious bleeding with pressure,
   - Consider the chest and abdomen to be sights of potential blood loss in the hypotensive patient.
2. Two large-bore peripheral IV lines (14 to 16 gage). The short catheters allow more rapid volume replacement than longer central lines.
3. Run NS or LR wide open if tachycardic or hypotensive. Using warmed fluids will decrease mortality and help preserve hemostatic mechanisms.
   a. As a rule of thumb, if more than 2 liters of isotonic fluid are needed in a trauma setting, the patient will need blood.
   b. Can also use 7.5% saline (250 ml over 1 to 5 minutes) if unable to infuse large volumes, and although not standard, use of 7.5% saline is associated with an increased survival in those with head trauma.
   c. *For children,* use 20 ml/kg IV and repeat to a total of 60 ml/kg. Consider blood at this point if child still hypotensive from hypovolemia.
      - In pediatric septic shock there is evidence that the administration of at least 60 ml/kg of fluid in the first hour is associated with an increased survival.

d. There is no advantage to colloids in this setting.
e. Not all people in shock are tachycardic. Use clinical judgment.
f. Hypotension is not caused by isolated brain injury in adults except near death.

D. Drugs, allergies, disability. Document functional status for a baseline examination.

E. Eating and exposure. Time of last meal. Uncover the patient including visualizing the back.

F. A Foley catheter should be inserted after ruling out GU trauma (see section on urologic trauma, p. 45). Urine output is a good indication of adequate perfusion. Try to maintain output at 30 to 60 ml/hour in adults or 0.5 to 1 ml/kg/hour in children.

II. LABORATORY AND X-RAY EVALUATION OF THE MULTIPLE TRAUMA PATIENT

A. CBC, electrolytes, BUN, creatinine, glucose, coagulation studies, liver enzymes, amylase, lipase, urinalysis, pregnancy test, ABG. Not all patients need all tests; use clinical judgment. (CBC, complete blood count often indicates an anemia with acute blood loss but may not reflect the true magnitude of the problem until blood equilibrates with infused fluids.)

B. If patient known to be hypotensive in the field, get two units of type O-negative blood ready.

C. Radiographs. Cross-table C-spine, CXR, AP pelvis.

D. Remember antibiotics as indicated, CT as indicated, full spine series when stable, tetanus prophylaxis, etc.

III. SECONDARY SURVEY TO SET FURTHER PRIORITIES

Stabilize patient first.

A. Complete head-to-toe examination.

B. Pass NG tube if no contraindication such as basilar skull fracture. Can pass oral gastric tube if midface trauma, etc.

C. Identify possible internal injuries. See specific sections below. Any head-injured multitrauma patient should have the abdomen evaluated by CT or DPL (diagnostic peritoneal lavage) because of an inability to report pain accurately.

D. Splint bones, etc.

E. A comment on MAST (military antishock trousers, pneumatic antishock garment). They are contraindicated in penetrating cardiac trauma, cardiogenic shock, impaled objects/evisceration, diaphragmatic injury. Head injury is NOT a contraindication. Seem to help in intra-abdominal bleeding from the spleen and aorta. Overall benefit probably less than previously believed. Useful when stabilizing pelvic and femur fractures.

F. There is growing evidence that a prophylactic vena cava filter can reduce mortality in major trauma. This is still an evolving area.

NECK TRAUMA

A. Initial treatment. Must immobilize neck and restrain chest if want to immobilize cervical spine.

1. Sand bags not a good idea because, if want to turn patient on backboard, may fall against neck causing further injury.
2. If strongly suspect C-spine injury and unable to restrain patient, consider paralysis (see section on rapid sequence intubation, p. 31).
3. Neutral position differs in adults and children.
   a. Children <8 years of age may require elevation of shoulders and back to approximate a neutral position.
   b. Adults and older children may require padding under the head to approximate a neutral position.
4. Prolonged immobilization (even <30 minutes) on a backboard will cause most individuals to have occipital headache and lumbosacral pain regardless of underlying trauma.

B. Blunt injury including falls and motor vehicle accidents:

1. Have effectively ruled out a C-spine fracture if:
   a. Patient is not having neck pain.
   b. Does not have neck tenderness on exam.
   c. Has a normal mental status without loss of consciousness or use of drugs or alcohol on board.
   d. AND does not have another confusing variable such as severe pain elsewhere (such as an ankle fracture).
   e. To clinically clear the C-spine, all the above conditions must be met. All others require clearance of the C-spine by radiograph. These criteria have not been adequately tested in children.
2. ***X-ray approach.***
   a. Need five views, which include C7 to T1 to effectively rule out a C-spine fracture. The most common cause of missed C-spine injuries is an inadequate C-spine series.
   b. In ambiguous radiographic findings, CT may be helpful.
   c. Those with one spinal fracture have about a 10% chance of having another, noncontiguous, spine fracture and should have a full spine series.

C. Cord injuries.

1. Look for paralysis, other signs of cord injury including priapism, urinary retention, fecal incontinence, paralytic ileus, immediate loss of all sensation, and reflex activity below the level of the injury.
2. Spinal neurogenic shock leads to vasomotor instability from loss of autonomic tone, may lead to hypotension or temperature instability.
3. May get hypoxia, hypoventilation if above C5; consider intubation.
4. "Spinal shock" is a separate, neurologic entity occurring as a result of cord injury, which presents with flaccid paralysis and usually recovers in hours to weeks.

- Frequently occurs in children without associated C-spine fractures SCIWORA syndrome = spinal cord injury without radiologic abnormality).

5. Any person with a spinal cord injury should receive methylprednisolone 30 mg/kg bolus followed by 5.4 mg/kg/hr IV over the next 23 hours. This should be started within 8 hours of the injury.

D. Penetrating neck trauma. Although management still controversial, "all" should be explored in OR. Do NOT remove foreign body until patient in OR. Consider CT/angiography if foreign body close to arterial blood supply.

E. Airway injuries.

1. ***Clinical signs.*** Stridor, hoarseness, dyspnea, subcutaneous emphysema.
2. ***Management.*** ENT consultation, intubation orally if possible and if indicated. Avoid causing further trauma.

CHEST TRAUMA

A. Flail Chest. Paradoxical chest wall motion secondary to multiple fractured ribs.

- ***Treatment*** by intubation and chest tube on affected side. Positive-pressure ventilation may lead to a tension pneumothorax.

B. Tension pneumothorax. Air under pressure in the pleural space.

1. Decreased breath sounds, shifted heart sounds, dyspnea, trachea shift from midline, hyperresonance on percussion, distended neck veins, chest pain, hypotension.
2. ***Treatment.*** Needle thoracostomy followed by a chest tube. See p. 670.

C. Simple pneumothorax-hemothorax from deceleration or penetrating trauma (pneumothorax may also occur spontaneously).

1. Symptoms as above but without midline shift, may have hypotension from blood loss in hemothorax.
2. Best to do expiratory chest radiograph. CT scanning is more sensitive, but the clinical significance of pneumothorax-hemothorax found only on CT scan is unknown. Some suggest the placing of a chest tube if the patient has rib fractures and is going to have positive-pressure ventilation.
3. ***Treatment.*** Tube thoracostomy (chest tube) (see Chapter 17).
   - If small pneumothorax (<15%), can observe.

D. Cardiac tamponade

1. ***Clinically.*** Note hypotension, juglar venous distension, muffled heart sounds, pulsus paradoxus.
   - Pulsus paradoxus. Normally, systolic pressure drops less than 10 mm Hg on inspiration. Decide on systolic

pressure when patient has exhaled. Next have the patient inhale and determine the difference between the two systolic pressures. If this number is >10, "pulsus paradoxus" is present.

2. ***Treatment*** is rapid fluid infusion, pericardiocentesis.

E. Myocardial contusion defined as blunt trauma to the heart.
1. 33% to 88% will have abnormal ECG.
2. Many have normal CPK-MB, and there is no correlation between the CPK-MB and the degree of injury.
3. Best diagnostic tests are echocardiography, first-pass biventricular angiography.
4. Best approach is to simply monitor the hemodynamically stable patient. Specific intervention is seldom needed, and the stable patient does not require diagnostic imaging studies to "prove" the presence of cardiac contusion. Usually the only clinical problem is episodes of PSVT or self-limited ventricular tachycardia.

F. Aortic disruption.
1. From deceleration injury.
2. Look for widened mediastinum on chest radiograph, blurred and enlarged aortic knob, esophageal deviation to right (look at NG tube), apical cap (blood collected at the upper apex of the lungs), chest pain, hypotension. Definitive diagnosis by CT or angiogram. More recently transesophageal echocardiogram has been used with success. Accuracy depends on experience in a particular institution.
3. Open emergency thoracotomy is not indicated for blunt chest trauma. It is almost never successful. A stab wound to the heart or aorta may be amendable to emergency department intervention. Do this only if trained in the technique and with the blessing of the surgeon who will manage the case in the OR unless patient is obviously terminal if not treated immediately.

ABDOMINAL TRAUMA IN THE MAJOR TRAUMA VICTIM
(including assault and abuse in children)

A. Diagnosis. Possible intra-abdominal injury indicated by:
1. Systolic blood pressure less than 100 *or* hematocrit <29.
   • No criterion is absolute; so use clinical judgment.
2. "Lap-belt ecchymosis" in children is associated with hollow organ injury, lumbar spine fracture, solid organ (liver/spleen) injury.
3. Elevated ALT and AST may indicate liver injury.
4. Physical exam only about 65% accurate.
5. Associated with the presence of chest injuries.
6. Associated with the presence of pelvic fractures.

B. *Penetrating trauma* of the abdomen requires exploration if penetrates the peritoneum.

- Some centers are doing CT only but not yet universally accepted as standard of care.

C. Blunt trauma of the abdomen.

1. If hemodynamically *unstable* and have acute abdomen, need laparotomy. Do not wait for CT or diagnostic peritoneal lavage (DPL) before consulting surgery.
2. If hemodynamically *stable* and patient is complaining of abdominal pain or is intoxicated or head injured, or there is an associated injury noted above, proceed with CT or DPL. Both CT and DPL have strengths and weaknesses.

EXTREMITY TRAUMA

See orthopedic section for fracture and dislocation management in Chapter 6.

I. ARTERIAL INJURY

A. Can be caused by blunt or sharp injury.

- Blunt may be more dangerous because less obvious.

B. Absolute indications for arteriogram. Pain, pallor, paralysis, paresthesia, pulselessness, hemorrhage, expanding hematoma, bruits.

C. Penetrating trauma in proximity to a vessel is not necessarily an indication for arteriogram.

1. *Arterial pressure index* (arterial pressure in injured limb divided by arterial pressure in unaffected limb). Good screening: if >0.90, can safely observe in the absence of other indications for arteriography.
2. *Shotgun injuries* are a high-risk category and should be studied with arteriography.

II. COMPARTMENT SYNDROME

A. Caused especially by crush injuries, electrical burns, circumferential scars, tight casts, hematoma in compartment, snake bites, and anything else that can increase pressure in a compartment.

B. Can result in muscle, nerve, and vessel necrosis from hypoperfusion.

C. ***Clinical presentation.***

1. Severe, constant pain in affected limb.
2. Pain on muscle palpation, passive stretch, active contraction.
3. Paresthesia and loss of distal pulses are late signs and herald poor outcome.
4. Compartment may be tense, but a normal turgor does not rule out compartment syndrome. Can diagnose by manometry:
   a. Normal tissue pressure less than 10 mg Hg.
   b. Capillary blood flow compromised at 20 mm Hg.

c. At risk ischemic necrosis above 30 mm Hg.

D. Treatment is by fasciotomy and requires surgical consultation immediately.

III. AMPUTATIONS

A. Control bleeding with direct pressure. Avoid clamping vessels.

B. Place severed part in saline-soaked gauze, place in plastic bag, and put in cooler with ice. *Avoid freezing part.*

C. Refer to plastic or orthopedic surgery.

UROLOGIC TRAUMA

I. KIDNEY TRAUMA

A. Blunt.

1. Serious injury *rare* with microscopic hematuria <30 RBC per HPF if the patient is hemodynamically stable.
    a. IVP or CT not required in these patients unless have other indications of urologic trauma such as pelvic fractures, lower rib fractures, localized hematoma, since it is unlikely there will be a surgically correctable lesion.
    b. Management. Frequent monitoring of vital signs and repeat urinalysis at about 4 hours.
2. In those with >30 RBC/HPF, gross hematuria, or <30 RBC/HPF and shock, IVP or CT is indicated.
    a. IVP has a 30% false-negative rate in those with renal pedicle injuries. 36% of those with pedicle injuries will *not* have hematuria. However, they will usually have a deceleration mechanism suggestive of this injury and other associated injuries.
        (1) Renal pedicle injuries represent 2% of all renal injuries.
        (2) IVP will show a nonfunctioning kidney.
    b. CT scanning is an acceptable alternative and may actually be better at defining renal and other intra-abdominal trauma.
    c. Most renal contusions, tears, and hematomas can be managed conservatively.
    d. Renal pelvis rupture rare and will be high fever, increasing abdominal pain, tenderness. Diagnosed by retrograde pyelogram.

B. Penetrating. All penetrating trauma to the kidney warrants investigation including IVP or CT if other injury is clinically suspected. Some would argue for surgical exploration in all these patients.

II. URETHRAL TRAUMA

A. Heralded by blood at the meatus, high-riding prostate in males.

B. Requires retrograde urethrogram *before* catheterization or other manipulation of the urethra.

C. Obtain urology consultation.

III. BLADDER TRAUMA

A. In adults, usually related to pelvic fracture.
B. Cystogram shows extravasation of urine into abdomen.
C. Exploration of abdomen and surgical repair indicated.

HYPERTENSIVE CRISIS

I. *Clinically* hypertensive emergency must have end-organ damage or dysfunction including CHF, renal failure, hypertensive encephalopathy, hematuria, retinal hemorrhage, etc. This is not based on the absolute level of blood pressure.

A. Goal is to reduce blood pressure by 30% in 30 minutes.
B. Individuals with chronic hypertension may not tolerate a "normal" blood pressure.
C. **Drugs**
1. ***Nitroprusside.*** Mix 50 mg of Nipride in 500 ml D_5W (100 μg/ml) and start infusion at 0.5 μg/kg/min. Titrate until desired blood pressure reduction is obtained. Average dose is 0.5 to 10 μg/kg/min.
   a. Very potent arterial and venous dilator.
   b. Can be used in all hypertensive emergencies though it is not the drug of choice for preeclampsia (see Chapter 8).
   c. Its use with clonidine has caused MIs.
2. ***Nitroglycerin.*** Mix 25 mg in 250 ml and start infusion at 10 μg/min (6 ml/hr). Titrate by 10 to 20 μg/min until desired effect is obtained.
   a. Venous and arterial dilator with maximum affect on capacitance vessels.
3. ***Labetalol*** (Normodyne, Trandate). Give by bolus, 20 to 40 mg IV. May repeat in 10 minutes. Usual effective dose is 50 to 200 mg, *or* continuous infusion of 2 mg/min (mix 200 mg in 160 ml D_5W = 200 ml = 2 ml/min. Stop the infusion when blood pressure control is achieved. Could combine by giving initial bolus and then infusion.
   a. Combined alpha-blocker and beta-blocker though primarily a beta-blocker.
   b. Does not change cerebral blood flow. Probably drug of choice in hypertension secondary to increased intracranial pressure.
   c. Especially useful in catecholamine-mediated hypertension such as a pheochromocytoma, discontinuation of clonidine.
   d. Avoids reflex tachycardia.
   e. Onset is in 5 minutes, maximum response in 10 minutes. Duration about 8 hours.

NOTE: The use of oral or sublingual medications in hypertensive emergencies is not indicated.

II. HYPERTENSIVE URGENCY INCLUDES DIASTOLIC PRESSURE OF GREATER THAN 115 mm Hg WITHOUT EVIDENCE OF END-ORGAN DAMAGE

A. Goal is to reduce blood pressure to "normal" within 24 to 48 hours. If possible, start the patient on a drug that he or she will be able to continue to use as part of antihypertensive regimen.

B. There is no evidence that an elevated diastolic pressure of 115 or less is a risk factor for an acute event (stroke, MI) unless there is evidence of end-organ damage (see above). This requires follow-up care but does not require emergency treatment.

C. *Never* make the diagnosis of new onset, mild, hypertension in an emergency department setting. The BP elevation may be attributable to pain or may be situational.

D. Treatment.

1. In most patients, simple observation and time is *as effective as* pharmacologic intervention.
2. If want to treat:
   a. Nifedipine 10 to 20 mg orally.
      (1) No advantage to sublingual administration, since absorbed by gastric mucosa. Have patients swallow capsule. The use of nifedipine in this setting has fallen out of favor.
   b. Captopril 25 mg PO or SL.
      (1) Absorbed in 30 minutes with peak effect 50 to 90 minutes.
      (2) Beneficial effect in CHF.
      (3) Helps cardiac ischemia.
   c. Labetalol 200 mg PO.

AORTIC DISSECTION (THORACIC)

A. Characterized by a severe tearing pain in the chest, back, epigastrium, and flanks. Have high index of suspicion in those with unexplainable chest pain.

B. Pain generally of short duration, very intense.

C. Only 16% have loss of peripheral pulses.

D. Diagnosis is by:

1. Radiograph to demonstrate a wide mediastinum, blurred and enlarged aortic knob, esophageal deviation to right (look at NG tube), apical cap (blood collected at the upper apex of the lungs).
2. Extension of aortic wall beyond calcific border.
3. Transesophageal ultrasonography and CT are gaining in popularity but aortogram remains the gold standard.

E. Treatment.

1. Control blood pressure with a combination of
   a. Nitroprusside (see previous hypertensive emergencies for dose) and a beta-blocker to prevent shear forces caused by reflex tachycardia.

b. Propranolol (Inderal) 0.5 to 1 mg IV Q2–5 min to control heart rate. Avoid exceeding 3 mg IV.
or
c. Esmolol. Mix 5 mg in 500 ml to give concentration of 10 mg/ml. Give loading dose of 500 µg/kg (0.5 mg/kg) over 1 minute and start infusion of 50 µg/kg/min for 4 minutes. If no response, reinfuse bolus and increase drip to 100 µg/kg/min for 4 minutes. Continue this procedure increasing the drip by 50 µg/kg/min until have achieved desired results or get a total of 200 µg/kg/min, since will not get added benefit.
   • Has advantage of short, 9-minute, half-life.

2. Surgical consultation is mandatory for consideration of repair.

SHOCK

I. CHARACTERIZED BY INADEQUATE TISSUE PERFUSION AND CELLULAR HYPOFUNCTION

II. CLASSIFIED BY ETIOLOGY

A. **Hypovolemic shock,** based on dehydration, blood loss, burns.
B. **Distributive shock,** based on loss of vascular tone (anaphylactic, septic, toxic shock).
C. **Cardiogenic shock,** based on pump failure.

III. DIAGNOSIS

A. **Hypotension.** Orthostatic vital signs may be normal in hypovolemic individuals, *or* normal individuals may exhibit orthostatic changes; so use clinical judgment. Additionally, alcohol ingestion, a meal, or increased age may cause orthostatic changes in BP and pulse.
   1. An orthostatic diastolic decrease of 10 to 20 mm Hg *or* increase in pulse of 15 beats/min is considered "significant."
   2. Take orthostatic vital signs recumbent and after standing for 1 to 2 minutes.

B. **Tachycardia** usually present but may not be especially in the presence of diaphragmatic irritation, which causes vagal stimulation.
C. **Hypoperfusion** including decreased urine output, decreased mentation, cool extremities, mottling, etc.
   • Goal of resuscitation is to maintain urine output between 30 and 60 ml/hr.

IV. TREATMENT

Remember to keep patient warn and in Trendelenburg (contraindicated in CHF, though). Remember the ABCs.

A. **Hypovolemic shock.** See Trauma section p. 39.
B. **Septic shock.** See Chapter 18.

C. Anaphylactic shock (applies also to acute urticaria).

1. Systemic allergic reaction characterized by urticaria, itching, angioedema, dyspnea/cough/wheezing, hypotension/syncope.
2. Caused by IgE-mediated hypersensitivity.
3. Anaphylactic shock has about a 3% mortality.
4. Common causes include foods, insect venoms especially Hymenoptera stings, drugs including aspirin and penicillins, radiocontrast materials (about 5% of patients are allergic).
5. Management of anaphylaxis.
   a. Epinephrine.
      (1) *If stable:* Epinephrine 0.3 to 0.5 ml of 1:1000 subcutaneous (0.01 ml/kg in children). May repeat Q10-15 min × 3.
      (2) *If hypotensive or unstable:* Epinephrine 0.1 mg or more IV in boluses or can infuse at 1 to 4 µg/min (in adults) or 0.1 µg/kg/min in children.

   All patients should also get:

   b. *Diphenhydramine* 25 to 50 mg PO for mild or up to 2 mg/kg IV for serious reactions (1 to 1.5 mg/kg/dose in children Q6h). This is a $histamine_1$-blocker.

   AND

   c. *Cimetidine* 300 mg IV (5 to 10 mg/kg Q6-12h in children, maximum 300 mg/dose), or *Ranitidine* 50 mg IV (0.33 to 0.66 mg/kg IV Q8h in children, maximum 50 mg/dose).
      (1) Has been shown to be more effective than diphenhydramine with less sedation.
      (2) Is an H_2-blocker.
      (3) Should use concurrently with diphenhydramine.
   d. *Corticosteroids* will not help stabilize the patient with anaphylactic shock. They are useful in preventing recurrence and in blocking late-phase reactants. Administer hydrocortisone succinate 100 mg IV to block late-phase reactants. Other options are methylprednisolone 60 to 125 mg IV (1 to 2 mg/kg in children) or oral prednisone.
   e. *For discharge.* Need to continue diphenhydramine or hydroxyzine 25 to 50 mg PO Q6h and cimetidine 300 mg Q6h *or* ranitidine 150 mg PO BID for 72 hours. Can also continue on prednisone 40 mg QD if desired for 5 to 7 days. This will reduce itching and urticaria. See Chapter 20 for pediatric dosages.
      - Can have return of anaphylaxis because of late-phase reactants.

D. Staphylococcal toxic shock syndrome.

1. Characterized by high fever, vomiting, diarrhea, confusion, severe myalgias, conjunctivitis, pharyngitis, sandpaper-like diffuse maculosquamous rash (sunburn like) with desquamation for palms and soles, hypotension or shock. Differentiate from Kawasaki's disease, streptococcal

toxic shock (have skin bullae), Rocky Mountain spotted fever, etc.
2. Renal dysfunction (decreased urinary output, elevated BUN/creatinine), leukocytosis, early thrombocytopenia followed by thrombocytosis.
3. Associated with tampon use, other staphylococcal infections (20%) including postoperative type, ingrown nails, etc.
4. *Treatment* includes a beta-lactamase–resistant pencillin (such as nafcillin), fluids, and pressors as noted in septic shock (see Chapter 18).

E. Cardiogenic shock. See Chapter 2 for acute pulmonary edema, p. 95.

HICCUPS

Hiccups are caused by an involuntary contraction of the muscles of respiration, especially the diaphragm. Most episodes are brief and self-limited, but occasionally hiccups can last for hours, days, or even more.

A. Common causes. Diaphragmatic irritation as with an abscess, gastric distension (outlet obstruction, gastric paresis), cholelithiasis, carcinoma. May also be caused by drugs such as alcohol and steroids.

B. Treatment.
1. Relieve gastric distension with NG tube or drugs that help gastric emptying (cisapride, erythromycin).
2. Vagal stimulation such as Valsalva maneuver, pressure on the eyeballs, carotid massage may be helpful.
3. Medications that may be helpful include baclofen 5 to 10 mg PO TID, haloperidol 2 to 10 mg IM, metoclopramide 5 to 10 mg TID-QID.

OVERDOSE AND TOXINDROMES

I. GENERAL APPROACH

A. Remember ABCs (see section on ACLS, p. 1; shock, p. 48).
B. Remember to decontaminate gut, clothing, skin, and environment.
C. If unconscious, see section on coma, p. 33.
D. Determine to best of ability what was ingested. All overdose patients should have serum acetaminophen levels drawn (see acetaminophen below).
E. Contact your closest poison control center for further information about the particular toxin in question.
G. Poisoning in a child may indicate neglect.
- Can also be associated with pica and lead toxicity.

II. GUT DECONTAMINATION

A. Ipecac is not very useful. Only partially effective in emptying gastric contents and may propel pills beyond pylorus.

1. Ipecac contraindicated in obtunded patients, those unable to protect airway. *Do not use ipecac in tricyclic overdoses, theophylline overdoses, or any other overdose that may cause a change in mental status because of the risk of aspiration!*
2. Contraindicated in caustic ingestions or petroleum distillates.
3. Inhibits retention of charcoal; delays charcoal administration.
4. ***Dose.*** Ipecac 15 or 30 ml in children 1 to 12 years of age and adults respectively; follow with water.

B. Gastric lavage.

1. May empty more stomach contents than ipecac. Not effective beyond 1½ hours after ingestion but may want to try in severely ill patients.
2. Use largest NG tube available or orogastric tube.
3. Most effective if give charcoal 20 to 30 minutes before lavage. Repeat charcoal when finished with lavage.
4. Should have airway protection (patient should be alert or intubated).
5. Instill 300 ml aliquots of saline and remove until clear or have irrigated with 5 liters of fluid.
6. Lavage alone is not adequate for gastric emptying and delays administration of charcoal.

C. Activated charcoal.

1. Treatment of choice in most ingestions.
   - Does not work for metals such as iron and lithium.
2. Administer 10 to 25 g in children, 50 to 100 g in adults (1 g/kg)
   - A sorbitol mixture reduces transit times but should be used only with the first dose if are going to use multiple doses of charcoal.
3. Administer by NG tube or if will drink this is OK.
4. 30% will vomit it. Can readminister if needed.
5. Multiple-dose charcoal still controversial.
   - May be indicated for theophylline, tricyclics, phenobarbital, phenytoin, digitalis.

D. Whole bowel irrigation (WBI).

1. May be useful after the ingestion of enteric-coated and time-release medications. Also useful in "body packers," etc. Reduces bowel transit time. Use in other ingestions may be helpful, but data are sparse. Do not delay charcoal administration to use WBI.
2. Use polyethylene glycol (that is, Go-Litely) 1 to 2 L/hr in adults, 500 ml/hr in children to a total of 3 to 8 liters.

III. TOXINDROMES. Symptom complexes associated with a toxin.

A. Cholinergics.

1. Cholinergics include organophosphates, carbamates, pilocarpine, and in some mushrooms.

2. Toxindrome diaphoresis, salivation, lacrimation, defecation, urination, miosis, mental status changes, weakness (blind as a mole, moist as a slug, weak as a kitten).
   a. Mostly farmers and other industrial workers.
   b. Manifestations are cholinergic including nausea, sweating, diarrhea, salivation, headache, fatigue, convulsions, muscle weakness, and cardiovascular collapse.
   c. Cholinergic effects divided into:
      (1) Muscarinic. Sweating, constricted pupils, lacrimation, salivation, diarrhea, incontinence.
      (2) Nicotinic. Striated muscle problems including fasciculations, collapse.
   d. Death usually occurs from respiratory muscle depression and excessive secretions or bronchospasm.
3. ***Treatment.***
   a. Decontaminate. Decontamination including washing with alkaline soap and then ethanol (increased solubility). Decontaminate GI tract if needed including lavage and multiple-dose charcoal. Watch for ileus secondary to atropine.
   b. Atropine 2 mg IV every 15 to 20 minutes using the drying of secretions or evidence of toxicity as an end point. For children use dose of 0.05 mg/kg. Atropine will treat the muscarinic effects only.
   c. Pralidoxime (2-PAM). Adults 1 g IV over 15 to 20 minutes, children 20 to 40 mg/kg over 15 to 20 minutes. Can repeat in 1 to 2 hours.
      (1) Should be reserved for those who are symptomatic.
      (2) 2-PAM regenerates acetylcholine esterase.
      (3) The organophosphate-enzyme complex becomes irreversible after 24 to 36 hours.
   d. Morphine and aminophylline contraindicated.
4. ***Sequelae.***
   a. Intermediate syndrome recently described. Occurs 24 to 96 hours after treatment of initial insult and presents with rapidly developing respiratory failure, cranial nerve palsy, and proximal upper limb girdle weakness. Treatment is supportive only and does not respond to pharmacologic therapy.
   b. Long-term sequelae include impairment of auditory attention, visual memory, visuomotor speed, sequencing, and problem solving, motor steadiness, reaction time, and dexterity. No increase in depression, other psychologic problems.
   c. May also have a delayed peripheral neuropathy starting at 1 to 5 weeks that may progress for 3 months but will eventually resolve.

B. Anticholinergics.

1. ***Anticholinergics.*** Atropine, scopolamine, belladonna alkaloids, antihistamines, antipsychotics, plants (Jimsonweed and others), tricyclics, mushrooms (*Amanita* species).
2. ***Toxindrome.*** "Dry as a bone, red as a beet, mad as a hatter." Mydriasis, dry mucous membranes, urinary retention, cutaneous flushing, mental status changes.
3. ***Treatment.*** Conservative therapy with decontamination. Treat seizures, arrhythmias (avoid class la agents), hyperpyrexia, and hypertension as in any other patient. Treat agitation with benzodiazepines (avoid phenothiazines that have anticholinergic properties). Physostigmine 0.5 to 2 mg IV in adults and 0.02 mg/kg in children may be used if severe symptoms that cannot be controlled otherwise (malignant hypertension, coma with respiratory depression, seizures unresponsive to conventional therapy, for example. *Reserve for severe problems, may induce seizures and arrhythmias. Do not use in tricyclic overdose!*

C. Opiate poisoning.

1. By heroin, morphine, clonidine, codeine, diphenoxylate (Lomotil), others.
2. ***Toxindrome.*** Sedation, hypotension, bradycardia, respiratory depression, usually pinpoint pupils (may not be present with mixed overdose or propoxyphene [Darvon and others]).
3. ***Treatment.*** Use these drugs with caution in those who are narcotic addicts. May precipitate acute opiate withdrawal. Can intubate and support until narcotic wears off if this is a concern. *Always observe the patient until there is no chance of further respiratory depression. This is especially important with naloxone, which has a relatively short half-life.*
   a. Naloxone 5 µg/kg IV (usually start with 0.4 to 2 mg in adults) up to 20 mg and may repeat if needed. Short acting; half-life is 1.1 hours. *May have recurrent narcotization when naloxone wears off.*
   b. Nalmefene. Long acting, half-life is 10.8 hours. However, still should observe patient until certain no possibility of recurrent sedation. Methadone has a longer half-life.
      (1) For non–opiate dependent patients start with 0.5 mg/70 kg and follow with another 1.0 mg/70 kg in 2 to 5 minutes. If total dose of 1.5 mg/70 kg does not work, no further drug is indicated.
      (2) For opiate-dependent patients, use a test dose of 0.1 mg/70 kg, and if there is no withdrawal in 3 to 5 minutes, follow above guidelines.

IV. SPECIFIC INGESTIONS

Read general guidelines for decontamination first.

A. Petroleum distillates (gasoline, fuel oil, airplane glue).

1. Main toxicity is pulmonary from inhalation.
2. Do not perform lavage or induce vomiting if swallowed.
3. CXR (ARDS, infiltrates), ABG, and follow clinical course.
4. If no symptoms within 6 hours, no need for further observation.

B. Tricyclic antidepressants.

1. ***Main toxicity.*** Cardiac arrhythmias, anticholinergic effects (see toxindrome above), vomiting, hypotension, confusion, seizures.
2. Avoid emesis. May aspirate.
3. Charcoal/lavage (see above) mainstay of treatment.
4. May appear fine and rapidly deteriorate. Need to be admitted to a monitored unit. *Be prepared to intubate the patient.* If are asymptomatic 6 hours after ingestion, no need to admit to monitored bed but may still require psychiatric admission.
5. ***Cardiac complications.*** Prolonged QRS, QT interval, torsade, other arrhythmias.
   a. Sodium bicarbonate to maintain blood pH above 7.45 (1 to 2 mEq/kg bolus until QRS <100 msec narrows, QT shortens, 2 amps in 1 liter of D_5W as a drip to maintain alkalinization). Helps prevent the development of arrhythmias. Recent data indicates that hyperventilation may also be effective.
   b. IV magnesium sulfate can be used to control torsades de pointes: 2 g of magnesium sulfate IV over 5 to 10 minutes depending on acuity (see section on ACLS, p. 1).
   c. Lidocaine can be used for arrhythmias as well. Avoid class IA and IC antiarrhythmics, beta-blockers, calcium-channel blockers, phenytoin.
5. ***Neurologic complications.*** Agitation, seizures.
   a. Diazepam 5 to 10 mg IV titrating to control agitation.
   b. Seizures are usually brief and self-limited. Treat as per seizure section, p. 24. Avoid phenytoin!
7. ***Hypotension.***
   a. Treat initially with fluids and sodium bicarbonate IV (see above).
   b. Norepinephrine is the vasopressor of choice. Dopamine may give a paradoxical hypotension.
8. Physostigmine, the mainstay of therapy in the past, is now controversial (see anticholinergic toxindrome, p. 51) and should not be used unless patient is agitated and cannot otherwise be controlled and there is a narrow QRS complex *and* there are other peripheral signs of anticholinergic toxicity (dilated pupils, fever, etc.; see above).

C. Salicylates (aspirin).

1. ***Main toxicity.*** Tinnitus, nausea, vomiting, hyperventilation (primary respiratory alkalosis), metabolic acidosis, fever, hypokalemia, hypoglycemia, seizures, coma.

- Many are misdiagnosed as sepsis or gastroenteritis on initial presentation (fever, acidosis, vomiting, etc.). This misdiagnosis is particularly common in the elderly.

2. ***Toxic dose*** 150 mg/kg with 300 mg/kg being very toxic.
3. ***Treatment.***
   a. Includes IV normal saline to maintain BP.
   b. Urine alkalinization (promotes excretion of salicylates). Use IV sodium bicarbonate (1 to 2 mEq/kg bolus, 2 amps in 1 liter of D_5W as drip). Must have adequate K^+ otherwise will get potassium reabsorption in exchange for hydrogen ions. Therefore will not alkalinize the urine.
   c. Hemodialysis for severe toxicity.
4. Follow clinically and with serum salicylate levels. The Dome nomogram is not accurate unless there was only a single ingestion without previous ingestion in the last 24 hours and no enteric-coated ASA.

D. Acetaminophen (Tylenol and others).

1. ***Main toxicity*** is hepatic, which occurs 24 to 72 hours after ingestion. May also manifest vomiting, nausea.
   - If patient is vomiting and unable to keep down charcoal, consider metoclopramide. Ondansetron has also been particularly effective.
2. Toxic ingestion is 140 mg/kg or >10 g in adults. In alcoholics the toxic dose is often much less, even as little as 4 g/day.
3. *Check acetaminophen level at least 4 hours after ingestion.*
4. Compare to Rumack-Matthew nomogram to determine risk (Fig. 1-9).
5. If in toxic range, treat with *N*-acetylcysteine 140 mg/kg orally or by NG tube and then 17 doses of 70 mg/kg every 4 hours.
   a. Repeat any doses vomited within 1 hour of administration.
   b. The same doses have been given IV in Europe, but this is not standard of care or an improved usage in the United States.
   c. Do not withhold *N*-acetylcysteine even if 24 to 26 hours from ingestion. Late *N*-acetylcysteine, though not so effective as early type, still reduces mortality.
6. Charcoal is all right in acetaminophen overdose and only minimally interferes with *N*-acetylcysteine. Additionally, should be giving charcoal early and *N*-acetylcysteine at least 4 hours later.

E. Caustic ingestion including alkaline (drain cleaner), bleach, battery acid, etc. Household bleach usually not bad except for superficial burns.

1. ***Main toxicity.*** Local tissue necrosis of esophagus with alkali and of stomach with acids; respiratory distress. May have obvious facial, oral burns and emesis. Have hoarseness and stridor reflecting epiglottic edema. This especially true in acids.

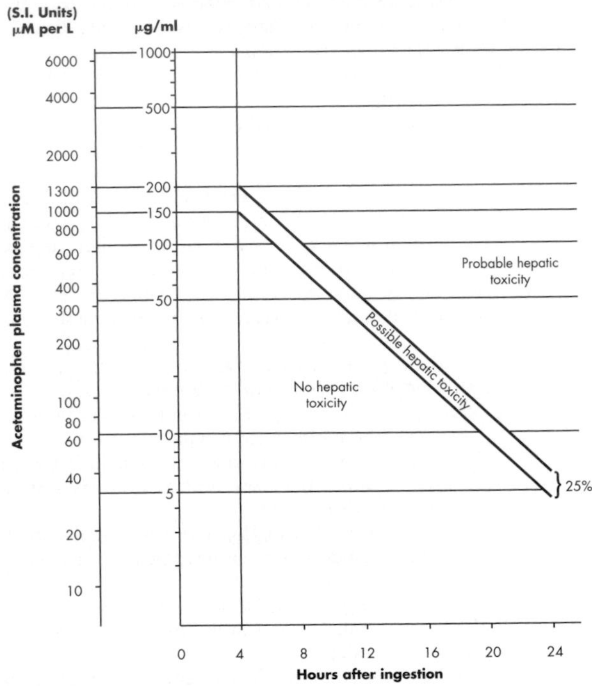

FIG. 1-9 Rumack-Matthew nomogram for single acute acetaminophen poisoning. Semilogarithmic plot of plasma acetaminophen levels versus time. Cautions for use of this chart: (1) The time coordinates refer to time of ingestion. (2) Serum levels drawn before 4 hours may not represent peak levels. (3) The graph should be used only in relation to a single acute ingestion. (4) The lower solid line 25% below the standard nomogram is included to allow for possible errors in acetaminophen plasma assays and estimated time from ingestion of an overdose. (Adapted from Rumack BH, Matthew H: *Pediatrics* 55:871-876, 1975.)

2. ***Treatment.*** Do not induce emesis or lavage patient. Charcoal is not indicated. If have visible burns, have a 50% chance of lower burns of significance. However, the absence of visible lesions does not rule out significant injury (10% to 30% will have burns beyond the mucosa), and all ingestions need to have EGD.

F. Digoxin.

1. ***Main toxicity.*** Any cardiac arrhythmia is possible with digoxin intoxication. Hypokalemia predisposes to digoxin toxicity (but digoxin toxicity causes hyperkalemia).

2. ***Manifested by*** anorexia, nausea, confusion, blurred vision, altered color perception (yellow tinge but occurs only in a minority).
3. ***Laboratory.*** Hyperkalemia, elevated serum digoxin level.
4. ***Treatment.***
   a. Treat arrhythmias as in ACLS section, p. 1 (magnesium sulfate particularly effective for digoxin-induced arrhythmias).
   b. Digoxin-specific antibody fragments indicated for:
      (1) Hyperkalemia >5.5; life-threatening arrhythmias; ingestion of >10 mg in adults, 0.1 mg/kg in children; serum level >5 mg/dl with signs of toxicity.
      (2) Calculate Fab dose: 1 vial of Fab (40 mg) will bind 0.6 mg of digoxin.
      (3) Calculate total body digoxin load: Total body dose dig = (Serum dig level × 5.6 L/kg × Wt in kg)/1000 × 0.8 (bioavailability).
      (4) Vials Fab = Total body dig/0.6.
      (5) If dose unknown and cannot get digoxin level, give 10 to 20 vials. If more likely a chronic toxicity, give 4 or 5 vials to start.
      (6) Serum digoxin level useless after digoxin Fab given. Will measure both bound and unbound digoxin. Serum digoxin level may increase tenfold to twentyfold after digoxin Fab.
      (7) Watch for hypokalemia (reverse digoxin-induced hyperkalemia).
   c. Reverse hyperkalemia (see hyperkalemia, p. 213); avoid calcium because increases binding digoxin. Avoid hypokalemia.

G. Carbon monoxide.

1. ***Main toxicity.*** Central nervous system including confusion, coma, seizures, headache, fatigue, nausea. May have arrhythmias, cardiac ischemia.
2. ***Diagnosis*** is by clinical background (exposure to furnace, car exhaust [especially in children in the back of pickup trucks, etc.]), carboxyhemoglobin level. Venous carboxyhemoglobin level just as good as arterial. Oxygen saturation is frequently normal.
3. ***Treatment.*** Administration of 100% oxygen (displaces carbon monoxide from hemoglobin). Hyperbaric oxygen is recommended for any patient with evidence of myocardial ischemia, carboxyhemoglobin level >30% (some say >15% to 18%) at exposure time zero, any impairment of CNS function. Even if the patient seems well when seen or is recovering from the CNS insult, hyperbaric oxygen has been shown to reduce long-term sequelae.

H. Cocaine.

1. ***Major toxicity.*** Seizures, hypertension, tachycardia, paranoid behavior or other alteration in mentation, rhabdomyolysis, myocardial infarction, CVA.
2. ***Treatment.*** Cocaine has a relatively short half-life, and so most symptoms are self-limited.
   a. Beta-blockade (esmolol, propranolol, others) *IS CONTRAINDICATED* in the treatment of cocaine-induced hypertension, tachycardia, and coronary spasm. Unopposed alpha-adrenergics may worsen problems.
   b. For coronary vasospasm, hypertension, or tachycardia, observation is probably adequate, since cocaine has short half-life.
   c. If treatment urgent, phentolamine 5 to 10 mg IV probably the drug of choice.
      (1) Treat as would any MI; thrombolytics are safe.
      (2) MI and CVA may occur up to 72 hours after cocaine use.
      (3) Concurrent use of alcohol increases the likelihood of cardiac vasospasm.
      (4) All chest pain is not MI. Think of pneumomediastinum in crack use, bronchospasm.
   d. Seizures. Generally self-limited but will respond to normal seizure treatment (see section on seizures, p. 24).
   e. CNS symptoms such as agitation and paranoia can be treated by diazepam.

BITES

I. ANIMAL BITES

The main morbidity from animal bites is infection or scarring. Rabies must be considered in any warm-blooded animal bite but is almost nonexistent in the domestic animal population of the United States. It is present in the wild, mainly in bats, raccoons, and skunks or dogs from Mexico or Latin America, Asia, or Africa. Rabies is very rarely found in rodents (such as squirrels, rats, or mice).

A. Gather data on what species of animal was involved and whether it has a current vaccination, whether the attack was provoked or unprovoked, the extent of wounds, and whether the animal is available for examination.

B. Management.

1. Cleanse the wounds thoroughly with soap and water.
2. Contact the local police. Domestic, unvaccinated animals should be observed by a veterinarian for 10 days or killed and the heads refrigerated and sent to an appropriate lab for testing, generally the state lab. All wild animals captured or killed should have the head sent for testing.
3. Check tetanus status and give booster if >5 years.

4. Treat wound like any other wound with irrigation and débridement. Do not close puncture wounds or human bites because of high incidence of infection. Consider consultation for extensive damage or facial wound. Dog bites especially cause a lot of soft-tissue damage with pain and surrounding bruising.
5. Antibiotics for bites
   a. *Human bites.* Antibiotics should be given prophylactically for all human bites: amoxicillin/clavulanate 20 to 40 mg/kg/day divided TID; cefixime is an alternative. Consider IV antibiotics if infection has already occurred, especially on the hand.
   b. *Cat bites.* Antibodies are routinely given for cat bites. The drug of choice is amoxicillin/clavulanate 20 to 40 mg/kg/day divided TID × 7 days. Doxycycline or ceftriaxone are acceptable alternatives.
   c. *Dog bites.* Only 5% become infected, and routine prophylaxis is not recommended. If need to treat, amoxicillin/clavulanate is the drug of choice with clindamycin, plus a fluoroquinolone or TMP/SMX, being good alternatives.
6. Rabies prophylaxis should be instituted for all wild carnivore bites (such as skunk, fox, raccoon, cat, dog, or bat) unless animal available for study.
   a. Rabies immunoglobulin in persons not previously immunized 20 IU/kg, one half of the dose infiltrated around the wound and one half given IM.
   b. Human diploid cell rabies vaccine, 1.0 ml IM on days 0, 3, 7, 14, and 28.

II. TICK BITES

Tick bites can be from a variety of different species, the deer tick *Ixodes dammini* (Lyme disease carrier) and wood tick and dog tick, which are carriers of Rocky Mountain spotted fever, are most well known. Tick bites can also cause tick paralysis, an ascending motor paralysis caused by a neurotoxin secreted in the tick's saliva.

1. Ticks should be looked for especially on ankles or scalp after any exposure to woods or tall grass. Removal is accomplished by steady traction with forceps grasping tick as close to skin as possible to avoid leaving the head behind. Do not use hot matches or other home remedies because they often kill the tick leaving the head embedded and may cause the tick to regurgitate, increasing the risk of infection.
2. Prevention is best accomplished with covering exposed skin and wearing insect repellent when exposed to tick-infested areas. Prompt removal of ticks can prevent transmission of disease.
3. See Chapter 18 for information on Rocky Mountain spotted fever, Lyme disease, and other tick-borne illnesses.

Prophylactic antibiotics after an *Ixodes* tick bite is recommended in endemic areas.

III. SPIDER BITES

Spider bites are usually not serious unless there is an allergic reaction. Treatment with ice, cleansing, and acetaminophen is usually adequate. Black widow and brown recluse spiders can cause more severe reactions and occasionally death. Specific discussion is beyond the scope of this manual.

ENVIRONMENTAL ILLNESS AND BURNS

I. SUNBURN

Sunburn occurs after exposure to sun and presents within 24 hours of sun exposure. Generally peaks at 72 hours and may have erythema, blistering, and pain.

A. Best therapy is prevention with the wearing of clothing or sun block; avoid sun exposure at peak day (10:00 A.M. to 3:00 P.M.).

B. Cool compresses and pain medications may produce symptomatic relief.

C. Topical steroids (such as betamethasone) and oral NSAIDs (such as indomethacin) may be of benefit and seem to be additive.

D. Oral prednisone 20 to 30 mg/day in adults may decrease symptoms.

II HYPERTHERMIA

Hypothermia results from an imbalance in heat production, dissipation. Predisposing factors include dehydration, chronic illness, old age, alcohol, alteration in skin function (scleroderma etc.)., drugs including anticholinergics, phenothiazines, tricyclic antidepressants, MAO inhibitors, amphetamines, succinylcholine. *Think of thyroid storm.*

A. Malignant hyperthermia.

1. ***Cause.*** 1:20,000 in response to a muscle-relaxing agent such as succinylcholine) or an inhaled anesthetic (such as halothane). Is hereditary. May also be secondary to physical or emotional stress.
2. ***Characteristics.*** Hyperthermia, muscle rigidity, tachycardia, acidosis, shock, coma, rhabdomyolysis.
3. ***Treatment*** includes IV dantrolene 1 to 10 mg/kg IV titrated to effect, management of acidosis and shock, peripheral cooling (see management of heat stroke, next page).

B. Neuroleptic malignant syndrome.

1. ***Cause.*** Neuroleptics (phenothiazines, etc.)
2. ***Characteristics.*** Same symptoms as malignant hyperthermia but generally develops over days instead of minutes.
3. ***Treatment.*** As per malignant hyperthermia.

C. Serotonin syndrome.

1. ***Cause.*** Serotonin excess. Generally secondary to combination of MAO and SSRI.
2. ***Characteristics.*** Rapid development of fever, hypertension, muscle rigidity, decreased mental status. Much for rapid onset than neuroleptic malignant.
3. ***Treatment.*** Treat like malignant hyperthermia. Also diazepam in 5 mg aliquots IV for muscle spasm, intubation as needed, cooling blankets, acetaminophen. Treat hypertension as per malignant hypertension.

D. Heat cramps.

1. ***Cause.*** Strenuous physical activity.
2. ***Characteristics.*** Skeletal muscle cramps, profuse sweating, hyponatremia secondary to free water intake, normal body temperature.
3. ***Treatment.*** Rest, oral rehydration.

E. Heat exhaustion.

1. ***Cause.*** Secondary to sweating, volume depletion, tissue hypoperfusion.
2. ***Characteristics.*** Fatigue, light-headedness, nausea, vomiting, headache, tachycardia, hyperventilation, hypotension, normal or slightly elevated temperature, profuse sweating.
3. ***Treatment.*** Rest, rapid IV fluid replacement (1 to 2 liters of NS or more).

F. Heat stroke.

1. ***Cause.*** Volume depletion, sweating, etc.
2. ***Characteristics.*** Hyperpyrexia (often >40° C [106° F]), sweating or may be dry, loss of consciousness or alteration in mental status (hallucinations, bizarre behavior, status epilepticus, other neurologic symptoms).
3. ***Treatment.*** *This is a true emergency.* Check and follow labs including electrolytes, CBC-complete BID count, liver enzymes, CPK, and clotting studies. Remove clothing; apply water to skin and fan to promote evaporative heat loss. (Avoid inducing shivering and peripheral vasoconstriction with ice. Shivering can be controlled with diazepam IV or chlorpromazine.) Treat with fluids (but many do not have significant fluid deficits; be cautious), cooling blanket.

BURNS, COLD, AND THERMAL INJURY

I. ASSESSMENT OF BURNS

A. Surface area (see Fig. 1-10).

B. Depth. It is frequently impossible to tell the final depth of a burn at the initial evaluation. All burns should be serially examined over days and followed closely.

1. ***Superficial (first degree).*** Epidermis only, painful and erythematous.
2. ***Superficial partial thickness.*** Epidermis and outer half of dermis with sparing of hairs.

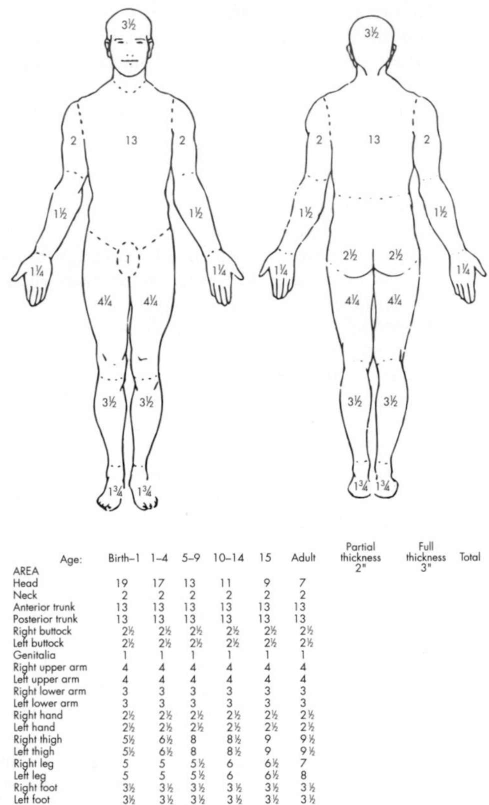

AREA / Age:	Birth–1	1–4	5–9	10–14	15	Adult	Partial thickness 2°	Full thickness 3°	Total
Head	19	17	13	11	9	7			
Neck	2	2	2	2	2	2			
Anterior trunk	13	13	13	13	13	13			
Posterior trunk	13	13	13	13	13	13			
Right buttock	2½	2½	2½	2½	2½	2½			
Left buttock	2½	2½	2½	2½	2½	2½			
Genitalia	1	1	1	1	1	1			
Right upper arm	4	4	4	4	4	4			
Left upper arm	4	4	4	4	4	4			
Right lower arm	3	3	3	3	3	3			
Left lower arm	3	3	3	3	3	3			
Right hand	2½	2½	2½	2½	2½	2½			
Left hand	2½	2½	2½	2½	2½	2½			
Right thigh	5½	6½	8	8½	9	9½			
Left thigh	5½	6½	8	8½	9	9½			
Right leg	5	5	5½	6	6½	7			
Left leg	5	5	5½	6	6½	8			
Right foot	3½	3½	3½	3½	3½	3½			
Left foot	3½	3½	3½	3½	3½	3½			

FIG. 1-10 Estimating surface area in burns. (Adapted from Nussbaum MS, editor: *The Mont Reid handbook,* St. Louis, 1987, Mosby.)

3. ***Deep partial thickness.*** Epidermis and destruction of reticular dermis. Can easily convert to full thickness if secondary infection, mechanical trauma, or progressive thrombosis. (Partial-thickness burns previously classified as second-degree burns.)
4. ***Full thickness.*** Dry, pearly white, charred, leathery. Heals by epithelial migration from the periphery and by contracture. May involve adipose, fascia, muscle, or bone.

(Full-thickness burns previously classified as third-degree burns.)

C. Severity.

1. *Minor burn* defined as first degree and partial thickness <15% body surface area (BSA) in adults and <10% BSA in children <6 years of age; full thickness <2% BSA in adults.
2. *Moderate burn* defined as partial-thickness 15% to 25% BSA in adults and 10% to 20% in children; full-thickness burns <10% BSA.
3. *Major burn* (requiring burn unit or burn center care) defined as partial-thickness burns >20% to 25% BSA in adults and >20% in children; full-thickness burns >10% BSA; burns of hands, face, eyes, ears, feet, perineum; inhalation burns; electrical burns; burns complicated by fracture or major trauma; all burns in infants or elderly, patients at poor risk secondary to prior medical conditions.

D. Causes of burns.

1. ***Thermal.***
   a. Flame, especially with clothing, tends to be full thickness.
   b. Molten metal, tars, or melted synthetics lead to prolonged skin contact, should be cooled as rapidly as possible. See p. 64 for tar removal.
   c. Liquid burns should be cooled rapidly and any clothing in contact with the area rapidly removed to decrease the contact time.
2. ***Electrical.*** Similar to crush injuries: get muscle necrosis, rhabdomyolysis, myoglobinuria.
   a. Watch for cardiac arrhythmias. Cardiac monitoring essential for 24 hours if significant exposure.
   b. Place in cervical collar; look for long bone fractures secondary to muscle contraction.
   c. In children with lip burns from electrical cords, watch for bleeding from the labial artery 3 or 4 days after injury.
   d. Follow CBC count, electrolytes, ECG, urine myoglobin, cardiac enzymes, ABG.
   e. Can cause thrombosis of any vessel in the body. Injury usually much more than visible on the skin. Be cautious and observe these patients closely.
3. ***Chemical agents.***
   a. Strong acids are quickly neutralized or quickly absorbed. Rinse off skin and call Poison Control Center for specific instructions.
   b. Alkalis cause liquefaction necrosis and can penetrate deeply, leading to progressive necrosis up to several hours after contact.
4. ***Radiation burns.***

a. Initially appear hyperemic and may later resemble third-degree burns. Changes can extend deeply into the tissue.
b. Sunburns are of this type and involve moderate superficial pain.

II. TREATMENT OF BURNS

Always watch for renal failure from rhabdomyolysis and sepsis in severe burns.

A. Emergency department. Cover wounds with normal saline–soaked gauze for pain control and use intravenous narcotics for pain. Tetanus immunization status should be checked and the patient treated accordingly.

1. Clean with bland soap and water.
2. Débride loose and foreign material. May leave blister intact if relatively small and patient is reliable.
3. Rinse well with normal saline.
4. Wound-dressing choices:
   a. Nonadherent inner layer of water-soluble porous material followed by soft bulky absorbent gauze and covered with semielastic outer layer.
   b. Topical antibacterial agents such as 1% silver sulfadiazine or bacitracin are applied and then covered with gauze pads. Dressings should be done once to twice daily with washing to remove old cream. Absolute contraindications to silver sulfadiazine: term pregnancy, premature infants, or less than 1 month old, hypersensitivity, G6PD deficiency. Relative: possible cross-sensitivity to other sulfonamides, pregnancy.
   c. Fluids. Initiate if >15% to 20% body surface area burns in adults, >10% in children.

      Fluids in first 24 hours = 2.4 ml × % of percentage of body surface area burned

      Give 1/2 in first 8 hours and 1/2 in next 16 hours (see Fig. 1-9). Colloids are not indicated in this setting. Maintain urine output at 1 mg/kg/hr in children, about 30 to 60 ml/hr in adults.
   d. Heterograft, allograft, or xerograft dressings can be used on an inpatient basis for partial-thickness wounds. These should be examined daily and débrided as needed or removed if signs of infection develop.
5. Chemical burns should be washed with tap water at least 15 and preferably 30 minutes in duration *after powders are removed by brushing.* This should be started at the scene if possible. Alkali burns should be irrigated for 1 to 2 hours after injury. Chemical binding may be required for certain burns.
6. Tar burns need cooling, gentle cleaning, and application of a petrolatum-based antibacterial ointment. Polysporin

and other petroleum-based products or household shortening can be used to soften the tar for removal. Butter-soaked gauze has also been used with success. Avoid chemical solvents, which may cause additional burns. After 24 hours the tar can be washed away and treated as a thermal burn.

7. Electrical burns should be cleaned as in thermal burns with a topical antibacterial agent applied (see above for further information about electrical burns).

B. Follow-up care.

1. Daily to twice daily dressing changes should be performed. Mild soap can be used for cleaning. Necrotic debris and eschar may require débridement as healing occurs. Tub soaks can help loosen coagulum and speed separation of necrotic debris. Absolute sterility is not mandatory for dressing changes; however cleanliness and thorough cleaning of hands, sinks, tubs, and any instruments used must be emphasized. 0.25% acetic acid can be applied for pseudomonal prophylaxis.
2. Contractures may not be apparent for weeks to months. Therefore range-of-motion exercises should be started during the early healing period. Any person with burns across joints should practice range-of-motion exercises frequently. If the hands are involved extensively, early excision and autografting may decrease the scarring of deep partial-thickness and full-thickness burns. Splinting and prolonged physical therapy may be required for rehabilitation. If the patient is prone to keloids, special garments may be used to reduce this scarring.
3. Analgesics should be given as needed and especially before dressing changes. Codeine or hydrocodone is normally adequate after the initial ED visit. If the dose is taken a half hour before the dressing change, it will facilitate cleaning and débridement.
4. All burns should be seen within 24 hours of initial treatment, and if any signs of infection develop, cultures should be performed and hospitalization considered.
5. Prophylactic antibiotics should rarely be required but may be considered for immunocompromised hosts, patients at high risk of endocarditis, or patients with artificial joints. Broad-spectrum coverage with first-generation cephalosporin or with a penicillinase-resistant penicillin plus an aminoglycoside may be used if necessary. Vancomycin may be needed depending on your institution.
6. In circumferential burns, extensive extremity burns, or electrical burns, watch for vascular or neurologic compromise, indicating a developing compartment syndrome. Immediate escharotomy is then required. Extremities should be elevated to minimize swelling.

7. In extensive burns, nutritional support is extremely important. Metabolic rate may be increased 100% to 200% above normal. Electrolytes must be frequently checked to replace maintenance needs, loss through the burn wound, and loss secondary to elevated body temperature. Intravenous hyperalimentation may be required until the gastrointestinal tract is functioning.

III. COLD INJURY

A. Without tissue freezing.

1. ***Chilblain.*** Peripheral cold injury without freezing of tissue.
   a. *Cause.* Prolonged dry exposure at temperatures above freezing.
   b. *Clinically.* Areas are pruritic, reddish-blue, maybe swollen, may have blisters or superficial ulcerations.
   c. *Treatment.* Rewarm as for frostbite.
   d. Areas may be more temperature sensitive in future; no permanent injury. Pain medication should be provided.
2. ***Trench foot and immersion injury.***
   a. *Cause.* Prolonged wet exposure at temperatures above freezing.
   b. *Clinically* may have tissue destruction resembling partial-thickness burns including blisters, pain, hypersensitivity to cold. Temperature sensitivity may be permanent.
   c. *Treatment.* Rewarm as for frostbite.

B. With tissue freezing: frostbite.

1. ***Cause.*** Freezing of the tissue with ice crystal formation.
2. ***Classification.***
   a. Frostnip. Superficial, skin changes reversible.
      (1) *Clinically.* Skin blanched, numb, loss of sensation.
      (2) *Treatment.* As below.
   b. Superficial frostbite tissue below skin pliable, soft.
      (1) *Clinically.* Blisters in 24 to 48 hours, fluid resorbs, develops hard, blackened eschar generally superficial, remains sensitive to heat, cold.
      (2) *Treatment.* As below. Treat conservatively. Generally resolves without surgical intervention in 3 to 4 weeks.
   c. Deep frostbite. Feels woody under skin; affects muscles, tendons, etc.
      (1) *Clinically.* Extremity cool, deep purple or red, with dark, hemorrhagic, blisters, loss of distal function.
      (2) *Treatment.* As below. May take several months to determine extend of injury. Frozen tissue will eventually slough.
      (3) *Treatment. Rapid* rewarming of part by immersion in 42° C water. Do not rub. Slow rewarming is not so good! If in field, do not thaw extremity until assured will not refreeze.

(a) Pruritus and burning sensation increase with rewarming. May require narcotic analgesia for severe injury.
(b) Nonsteroidal anti-inflammatory agents and topical aloe may help minimize tissue injury.
(c) Débridement of clear blisters.
(d) Local wound care, whirlpools, topical antibiotics, etc.
(e) Delay surgical intervention. Generally looks much worse than it is.

IV. HYPOTHERMIA

A. Defined as core temperature less than 35° C (95° F). Need to use a hypothermia thermometer, since most thermometers will not read low enough.

B. Risks. Chronic illness, altered state of consciousness, elderly, neonates, drugs such as alcohol and barbiturates.

C. Causes. Exposure to cold, metabolic (Addison's disease, hypothyroidism, hypopituitarism, hypoglycemia), CNS dysfunction, sepsis, alcohol, barbiturates, Wernicke's encephalopathy.

D. Clinically. All changes are progressive and more pronounced with a greater degree of hypothermia.

1. *Presentation* is of progressive decrease in mental status including confusion, lethargy, coma with areflexia, shivering or may have loss of shivering reflex, bradycardia, hypotension; have cold diuresis; may be hypovolemic.
2. *Cardiac irritability.* Usually bradycardia to ventribular fibrillation. Do not roughly handle the hypothermic patient. This may induce arrhythmias. ECG may show J wave (Osborne wave).

E. Treatment.

1. Remove wet clothing and move to a warm environment.
2. Examine the patient for a full minute (or have on monitor) before beginning CPR, since pulse may be very difficult to detect in the bradycardic or hypothermic patient.
3. Use blankets, heating blankets, warm-water immersion, radiant heat.
4. Use heated IV fluids; warm, humidified, oxygen.
5. Use heated gastric or colonic lavage, bladder irrigation, peritoneal or pleural lavage.
6. Mediastinal irrigation, heated hymodialysis, cardiopulmonary bypass.
7. Peripheral rewarming can be associated with shock, acidosis, hyperkalemia when cold, acidotic peripheral blood is returned centrally. Central body rewarming is preferred with the extremities left for last.

F. No one is dead unless that person is warm and dead.

1. If have ventricular fibrillation, defibrillate twice and then continue CPR and rewarm to 30° C. The heart is relatively

resistant to drug therapy when cold. Try debrillation periodically during rewarming.

2. Based on the clinical situation, consider administration of thiamine 100 mg IV, glucose 50 ml of $D_{50}W$, hydrocortisone succinate 100 mg IV, thyroid hormone replacement.

V. COLD WATER DROWNING

A. Diving reflex is protective.

B. May survive intact after 40 minutes of cold water drowning. However this is the exception rather than the rule. Warm patient to at least 86° or 90° F before abandoning resuscitation.

BIBLIOGRAPHY

Albano A et al: Rectal diazepam in pediatric status epilepticus, *Am J Emerg Med* 7(2):168, 1989.

Allen BJ et al: Magnesium sulfate therapy for sustained monomorphic ventricular tachycardia, *Am J Cardiol* 64 (18):1202, 1989.

Angeli P et al: Comparison of sublingual captopril and nifedipine in immediate treatment of hypertensive emergencies: a randomized, single-blind clinical trial, *Arch Intern Med* 151(4):678, 1991.

Ariano RE et al: Comparison of sedative recovery time after midazolam versus diazepam administration, *Crit Care Med* 22(9):1492, 1994.

Bakker AJ et al: Troponin T And myoglobin at admission: value of early diagnosis of acute myocardial infarction, *Heart J* 15(1):45, 1994.

Baraff L et al: Orthostatic vital signs: variation with age, specificity, and sensitivity in detecting a 450 ml blood loss, *Am J Emerg Med* 10(2):99, 1992.

Barnett JC et al: Short-term control of supraventricular tachycardia with verapamil infusion and calcium pretreatment, *Chest* 97(5):1106, 1990.

Barone MA, editor: *The Harriet Lane Handbook: a manual for pediatric house officers,* ed 14, St. Louis, 1996, Mosby.

Bentur L et al: Controlled trial of nebulized albuterol in children younger than 2 years of age with acute asthma, *Pediatrics* 89(1):133, 1992.

Berg AT et al: Predictors of recurrent febrile seizures: a metaanalytic review, *J Pediatr* 116(3):329, 1990.

Better OS et al: Early management of shock and prophylaxis of acute renal failure in traumatic rhabdomyolysis, *N Engl J Med* 322(12):825, 1990.

Bissoni RS et al: Colloids versus crystalloids in fluid resuscitation: an analysis of randomized controlled trials, *J Fam Pract* 32(4):387, 1991.

Bosse GM: Conservative management of patients with moderately elevated serum iron levels, *J Toxicol Clin Toxicol* 33(2):135-140, 1995.

Bracken ME et al: Methylprednisolone or naloxone treatment after acute spinal cord injury: 1-year follow-up data, *J Neurosurg* 76(1):23, 1992.

Bridges KG et al: CT detection of occult pneumothorax in multiple trauma patients, *J Emerg Med* 11(2):179, 1993.

Buckley N et al: Slow-release verapamil poisoning: use of polyethylene glycol whole-bowel lavage and high-dose calcium, *Med J Aust* 158(3):202, 1993.

Bukata R et al: Rapid sequence intubation, *Emerg Med Abstr,* vol 14, no 8, Aug 1988.

Burkhart KK et al: The rise in the total iron-binding capacity after iron overdose, *Ann Emerg Med* 20(5):532, 1991.

Buss CS et al: The diagnosis of abdominal injuries in comatose patients, *S Afr J Surg* 28(4):137, 1990.

Casesprevitera C et al: Predictive value of visible lesions (cheeks, lips, oropharynx) in suspected caustic ingestion: May endoscopy reasonably be omitted in completely negative pediatric patients? *Pediatr Emerg Care* 6(3):176, 1990.

Chan D et al: The effect of spinal immobilization on healthy volunteers, *Ann Emerg Med* 23(1):48, 1994.

Chiulli DA et al: The influence of diazepam or lorazepam on the frequency of endotracheal intubation in childhood status epilepticus, *J Emerg Med* 9:13, 1991.

Clark RF: Clinical presentation and treatment of black widow spider envenomation: a review of 163 cases, *Ann Emerg Med* 21(7):782, 1992.

Committee on Drugs: Reappraisal of lytic cocktail/Demerol, Phenergan, and Thorazine (DPT) for the sedation of children, *Pediatrics* 95(4):598, 1995.

Cummins RO et al: The frequency of "occult" ventricular fibrillation masquerading as a flat line in prehospital cardiac arrest, *Ann Emerg Med* 17(8):813, 1988.

De Bleecker J et al: The intermediate syndrome in organophosphate poisoning: presentation of a case and review of the literature, *Clin Toxicol* 30(3):321, 1992.

Dieckmann RA et al: High-dose epinephrine in pediatric out-of-hospital cardiopulmonary arrest, *Pediatrics* 95(6):901, 1995.

Dolan DL: intravenous calcium before verapamil to prevent hypotension, *Ann Emerg Med* 20(5):588, 1991.

Engel T et al: Glucocorticosteroid therapy in acute severe asthma: a critical review, *Eur Respir J* 4(7):881, 1991.

Fabian TC et al: A prospective evaluation of myocardial contusion. correlation of significant arrhythmias and cardiac output with CPK-MB measurements, *J Trauma* 31(5):653, 1991.

Farwell JR et al: Phenobarbital for febrile seizures: effects on intelligence and on seizure recurrence, *N Engl J Med* 322(6):364, 1990.

Ferguson RK et al: How urgent is "urgent" hypertension? *Arch Intern Med* 149(2):257, 1989.

Finkelstein Y et al: Antidotal therapy of severe organophosphate poisoning: multiple hospital study, *Neurotoxicol Teratol* 11:593, 1989.

Frabetti L et al: Intravenous dilitiazem in patients with paroxysmal re-entrant supraventricular tachycardia, *Int J Cardiol* 23:215, 1989.

Francis H et al: Vascular proximity: Is it valid indication for arteriography in asymptomatic patients? *J Trauma* 31(4):512, 1991.

Frykberg ER et al: The reliability of physical examination in the evaluation of penetrating extremity trauma for vascular injury: results at one year, *J Trauma* 31(4):502, 1991.

Gobel, EJAM et al: Randomised, double-blind trial of intravenous dilitiazem versus glyceryl trinitrate for unstable angina pectoris, *Lancet* 346:1653, 1995

Goetting MG et al: High-dose epinephrine improves outcome from pediatric cardiac arrest, *Ann Emerg Med* 20(1):22, 1991.

Graber MA, Hoehns B, Perry P: Sertraline-Phenelzine drug interaction: a serotonin syndrome reaction, *Ann Pharmacother* 28(6):732-735, 1994.

Grigorian Greene M: *The Harriet Lane handbook: a manual for pediatric house officers,* ed 12, St. Louis, 1996, Mosby.

Gunnar WP et al: The utility of cardiac evaluation in the hemodynamically stable patient with suspected myocardial contusion, *Am Surg* 57(6):373, 1991.

Hackshaw KV et al: Naloxone in septic shock, *Crit Care Med* 18(1):47, 1990.

Harrison PM et al: Improved outcome of paracetamol-induced fulminant hepatic failure by late administration of acetylcysteine, *Lancet* 335:1572, 1990.

Haude M et al: Sublingual administration of captopril inpatients with acute myocardial ischemia, *Clin Cardiol* 14(6):463, 1991.

Helmers S et al: Cholinesterase risk for Iowa farmers, *Iowa Med,* 80(2):73-76, 1990.

Heywood JT et al: Effects of intravenous diltiazem on rapid atrial fibrillation accompanied by congestive heart failure, *Am J Cardiol* 67(113):1150, 1991.

Hoffman, RS et al: The poisoned patient with altered consciousness: controversies in the use of a "coma cocktail," *JAMA* 274(7):562, 1995.
Holland RW et al: Grand mal seizures temporally related to cocaine use: clinical and diagnostic features, *Ann Emerg Med* 21(7):772, 1992.
Hollander JE, et al: Cocaine-induced myocardial infarction: an analysis and review of the literature, *J Emerg Med* 10:169, 1992.
Honigman B et al: The role of the pneumatic antishock garment in penetrating cardiac wounds, *JAMA* 266(17):2398, 1991.
Hughes, GS et al: Synergistic effects of oral nonsteroidal drugs and topical corticosteroids in the therapy of sunburn in humans, *Dermatology* 184(1):54, 1992.
Johansen K et al: Non-invasive vascular test reliably exclude occult arterial trauma in injured extremities, *J Trauma* 31(4):515, 1991.
Joint Working Group of the Research Unit of the Royal College of Physicians and the British Paediatric Association: *Guidelines for the management of convulsions with fever: Br Med J* 303(6803):634, 1991.
Kastor JA: Multifocal atrial tachycardia, *N Engl J Med* 322(24):1713, 1990.
Katz RW et al: Safety of continuous nebulized albuterol for bronchospasm in infants and children, *Pediatrics* 92(5):666, 1993.
Kaulesar Sukul DMKS et al: sixty-three cases of traumatic injury of the diaphragm, *Injury* 22(4):303, 1991.
Keenen TL et al: Non-contiguous spinal fractures, *J Trauma* 30(4):489, 1990.
Keren A et al: Magnesium therapy in ventricular arrhythmias, *Pace* 13(7):937, 1990.
Khansarinia S et al: Prophylactic Greenfield Filter placement in selected high-risk trauma patients, *Vasc Surg* 22(3):231-235; discussion 235-236, 1995.
Klein S et al: Hematuria following blunt abdominal trauma: the utility of intravenous pyelography, *Arch Surg* 123(9):1173, 1988.
Klein-Schwartz W et al: Assessment of management guidelines: acute iron ingestion, *Clin Pediatr* 29(6):316, 1990.
Kornberg AE et al: Pediatric ingestions: charcoal alone versus ipecac and charcoal, *Ann Emerg Med* 20(6):648, 1991.
Lange RA et al: Potentiation of cocaine-induced coronary vasoconstriction by beta-adrenergic blockade, *Ann Intern Med* 112(2):897, 1990.
Lebby T et al: Blood pressure decrease prior to initiating pharmacological therapy in nonemergent hypertension, *Am J Emerg Med* 8(1):27, 1990.
Levine SR et al: Cerebrovascular complications of the use of the "crack" form of alkaloidal cocaine, *N Engl J Med* 323(11):699, 1990.
Lin RY et al: Continuous versus intermittent albuterol nebulization in the treatment of acute asthma, *Ann Emerg Med* 22(12):1847, 1993.
Ling LJ et al: Absorption of iron after experimental overdose of chewable vitamins, *Am J Emerg Med* 9:24, 1991.
Litovitz T et al: Ingestion of cylindrical and button batteries: an analysis of 2382 cases, *Pediatrics* 89(4):747, 1992.
Mackersie RC et al: Intra-abdominal injury following blunt trauma: identifying the high-risk patient using objective risk factors, *Arch Surg* 124(7):809, 1989.
McNamara RM et al: Cervical spine injury and radiography in alert, high-risk patients, *J Emerg Med* 8(2):177, 1990.
McNamara RM et al: Efficacy of charcoal cathartic versus ipecac in reducing serum acetaminophen in a simulated overdose, *Ann Emerg Med* 18(9):934, 1989.
Merigian KS et al: Prospective evaluation of gastric emptying in the self-poisoned patient, *Am J Emerg Med* 8(6):479, 1990.
Mitchell WG et al: Lorazepam is the treatment of choice for status epilepticus, *J Epilepsy* 3(1):7, 1990.
Mohindra SK et al: Intravenous esmolol in acute aortic dissection, *Ann Pharmacother* 25:735, 1991.

Moscati RM et al: Comparison of cimetidine and diphenhydramine in the treatment of acute urticaria, *Am Emerg Med* 19(1):12, 1990.
Murata GH et al: Intravenous and oral corticosteroids for the prevention of relapse after treatment of decompensated COPD: effect on patients with a history of multiple relapses, *Chest* 98(4):845, 1990.
Nasraway SA et al: Inotropic response to digoxin and dopamine in patients with severe sepsis, cardiac failure, and systemic hypoperfusion, *Chest* 95(3):612, 1989.
Nypaver M et al: Neutral cervical spine positioning in children, *Ann Emerg Med* 23(2):208, 1994
Okayama H et al: Treatment of status asthmaticus with intravenous magnesium sulfate, *J Asthma* 28(1):11, 1991.
Olsen KM et al: Comparison of fluid volumes with whole bowel irrigation in a simulated overdose of ibuprofen, *Ann Pharmacother* 29(3):246-250, 1995.
Olsen KM et al: Low-volume whole bowel irrigation and salicylate absorption: a comparison with ipecac-charcoal, *Pharmacotherapy* 13(3):229, 1993.
Pang D et al: Spinal cord injury without radiographic abnormality in children–the *SCIWORA* syndrome, *J Trauma* 29(5):654, 1989.
Papo MC et al: A prospective, randomized study of continuous versus intermittent nebulized albuterol for severe status asthmaticus in children, *Crit Care Med* 21(10):1479, 1993.
Parent JM et al: Treatment of refractory generalized status epilepticus with continuous infusion of midazolam, *Neurology* 44(10):1837, 1994.
Plum F, Posner PD: *Diagnosis of stupor and coma,* Philadelphia, 1977, FA Davis.
Pollack CV et al: Outpatient management of acute urticaria: the role of prednisone, *Ann Emerg Med* 26(5):547, 1995.
Potter PC et al: Hydration in severe acute asthma, *Arch Dis Child* 66(2):216, 1991.
Raphael JH et al: Effects of the cervical collar on cerebrospinal fluid pressure, *Anaesthesia* 49(5):437, 1994.
Ravkilde J et al: Diagnostic performance and prognostic value of serum troponin T in suspected acute myocardial infarction, *Scand J Clin Lab Invest* 53(7):677, 1993.
Reed MD et al: Ondansetron for treating nausea and vomiting in the poisoned patient, *Ann Pharmacother* 28(3):331, 1994.
Rees RS et al: Brown recluse spider bites: a comparison of early surgical excision versus dapsone and delayed surgical excision, *Ann Surg* 202(5):659, 1985.
Rhee KJ et al: Oral intubation in the multiply injured patient: the risk of exacerbating spinal cord damage, *Ann Emerg Med* 19(5):511, 1990.
Roden DM: Magnesium treatment of ventricular arrhythmias, *Am J Cardiol* 63(14):43G, 1989.
Roelofse JA et al: Preanesthetic medication with rectal midazolam in children undergoing dental extractions, *J Oral Maxillofac Surg* 48(8):791, 1990.
Rosenstock L et al: Chronic central nervous system effects of acute organophosphate pesticide intoxication, *Lancet* 338:223-227, 1991.
Rosman NP et al: A controlled trial of diazepam administered during febrile illnesses to prevent recurrence of febrile seizures, *N Engl J Med* 329(2):79, 1993.
Rossing TH.: Methylxanthines in 1989, *Ann Intern Med* 110(7):502, 1989.
Rudnitsky GS et al: Comparison of intermittent and continuously nebulized albuterol for treatment of asthma in an urban emergency department, *Ann Emerg Med* 22(12):1842, 1993
Rumm PD et al: Efficacy of sedation of children with chloral hydrate, *South Med J* 83(9):1040, 1990.
Sacchetti A et al: Pediatric analgesia and sedation, *Ann Emerg Med* 23:237-250, 1994.
Saddison D et al: Clinical indications for cervical spine radiographs in alert trauma patients, *Am Surg* 57(5):366, 1991.

Saetta JP et al: Gastric emptying procedures in the self-poisoned patient: Are we forcing gastric content beyond the pylorus? *J R Soc Med* 84(5):274, 1991.

Sager, SM: Neuroleptic malignant syndrome: a diagnostic dilemma, *J R Soc Med* 84 (8):500, 1991.

Sahdev P et al: Evaluation of liver function tests in screening for intra-abdominal injuries, *Ann Emerg Med* 20(8):838, 1991.

Salerno DM et al: Efficacy and safety of intravenous diltiazem for treatment of atrial fibrillation and atrial flutter, *Am J Cardiol* 63(15):1046, 1989.

Sand IC et al: Experience with esmolol for the treatment of cocaine-associated cadiovascular complications, *Am J Emerg Med* 9(2):161, 1991.

Sanford JP: *A guide to antimicrobial therapy,* Dallas, 1996, Antimicrobial Therapy, Inc.

Scarfone RJ et al: Nebulized dexamethasone versus oral prednisone in the emergency treatment of asthmatic children, *Ann Emerg Med* 26(4):480, 1995.

Schneider SM: Neuroleptic malignant syndrome: controversies in treatment, *Am J Emerg Med* 9(4):360, 1991.

Schriger D: Spinal immobilization on a flat backboard: Does it result in neutral position of the cervical spine? *Ann Emerg Med* 20(8):878, 1991.

Schuh S et al: High-versus low-dose frequently administered, nebulized albuterol in children with severe, acute asthma, *Pediatrics* 83(4):513, 1989.

Schuh S et al: Nebulized albuterol in acute childhood asthma: comparison of two doses, *Pediatrics* 86(4):509, 1990.

Seraj MA et al: Are heat stroke patients fluid depleted? Importance of monitoring central venous pressure as a simple guideline for fluid therapy, *Resuscitation* 21(1): 33, 1991.

Sinert R et al: Exercise-induced rhabdomyolysis, *Am Emerg Med* 23(6):1301, 1994.

Smilkstein MJ et al: Acetaminophen overdose: a 48-hour intravenous *N*-acetylcysteine treatment protocol, *Ann Emerg Med* 20(10):1058, 1991.

Smith SW, Ling LJ, Halstenson CE: Whole-bowel irrigation as a treatment for acute lithium overdose, *Ann Emerg Med* 20(5):536-539, 1991.

Snyder HS et al: Lack of tachycardiac response to hypotension in penetrating abdominal injuries, *J Emerg Med* 7:335, 1989.

Snyder HS: Lack of tachycardiac response to hypotension with ruptured ectopic pregnancy, *Am J Emerg Med* 8(1):23, 1990.

Stalker HP et al: The significance of hematuria in children after blunt abdominal trauma, *Am J Roengenol* 154(3):569, 1990.

Tenenbein M: Multiple doses of activated charcoal: Time for reappraisal? *Ann Emerg Med* 20(5):529, 1991.

Tenenbein M et al: The total iron-binding capacity in iron poisoning: Is it useful? *Am J Dis Child* 145(4):437, 1991.

Terndrup TE et al: Intramuscular meperidine, promethazine, and chlorpromazine: analysis of use and complications in 487 pediatric emergency department patients, *Ann Emerg Med* 18(5):528, 1989.

Thom SR et al: Delayed neuropsychologic sequelae after carbon monoxide poisoning: prevention by treatment with hyperbaric oxygen, *Ann Emerg Med* 25(4):474, 1995.

Thomason RB et al: Microscopic hematuria after blunt trauma: Is pyelography necessary? *Am Surg* 55(3):145, 1989.

Tiernan E et al: Butter in the initial treatment of hot tar burns, *Burns* 19(5):437, 1993.

Tintinalli JE et al: *Emergency medicine, a comprehensive study guide,* New York, 1996, McGraw-Hill.

Tomaszewski C et al: Effect of acute ethanol ingestion on orthostatic vital signs, *Ann Emerg Med* 25(5):636, 1995.

Touger M, Gallagher EJ, Tyrell J: Relationship between venous and arterial carboxyhemoglobin levels in patients with suspected carbon monoxide poisoning, *Ann Emerg Med* 25(4):481-483, 1995.

Vassar MJ et al: 7.5% sodium chloride/dextran for resuscitation of trauma patients undergoing helicopter transport, *Arch Surg* 126(9): 1065, 1991.
Vassar MJ et al: Analysis of potential risks associated with 7.5% sodium chloride resuscitation of traumatic shock, *Arch Surg* 125(10):1309, 1990.
Verbeek PR et al: Nontapering versus tapering prednisone in acute exacerbations of asthma: a pilot trial, *J Emerg Med* 13(5):715, 1995.
Viskin S et al: Aminophylline for bradyasystolic cardiac arrest refractory to atropine and epinephrine, *Ann Intern Med* 118(4):279, 1993.
Vukmir RB: Torsades de pointes: a review, *Am J Emerg Med* 9(3):250, 1991.
Weaver FA et al: Is arterial proximity a valid indication for arteriography in penetrating extremity trauma? *Arch Surg* 125:1256, 1990.
Welch RD et al: Incidence of cocaine-associated rhabdomyolysis, *Ann Emerg Med* 20(2):154, 1991.
Werkman HA et al: Urinary tract injuries in multiply-injured patients: a rational guideline for the initial assessment, *Injury* 22(6):471, 1991.
Wisner DH et al: Suspected myocardial contusion: triage and indications for monitoring, *Ann Surg* 212(1):82, 1990.
Wright SW et al: Cervical spine injuries in blunt trauma patients requiring emergent endotracheal intubation, *Am J Emerg Med* 10(2):104, 1992.
Yarbrough JA et al: Cimetidine in the treatment of refractory anaphylaxis, *Ann Allergy* 63(3):235, 1989.

2

Cardiology

PETER P. TOTH

ISCHEMIC HEART DISEASE

Angina pectoris is a symptom of myocardial ischemia caused by an imbalance between myocardial oxygen supply and demand.

I. ETIOLOGY

Ischemia is secondary to coronary artery disease in 95% of patients. A decreased oxygen supply from anemia, hypotension, vasospasm, or arrhythmias or an increase in oxygen demand secondary to exercise, emotional stress, CHF, hypertension, tachycardia, and sepsis can lead to a worsening of symptoms. Ischemia can occur in patients with normal coronary arteries in the setting of LV hypertrophy, aortic insufficiency, hypertrophic cardiomyopathy, coronary vasospasm, or cocaine abuse.

II. TYPES OF ANGINA

A. **Stable.** Intensity, character, and frequency of episodes can be predicted, and angina occurs in response to a known amount of exercise or other stress.

B. **Unstable.** Intensity, frequency, or duration of episodes is changed and can no longer be predicted. Pain is precipitated by less exercise or is of longer duration. This includes angina at rest and new-onset angina.

C. **Variant.** Pain, which may occur at rest, is secondary to vasospasm of coronary arteries.

III. DIAGNOSIS

A. **History.** Classically described as substernal chest pressure or heaviness radiating to the left shoulder and arm, neck, or jaw, associated with nausea, diaphoresis, and shortness of breath. It is usually brought on and exacerbated by exercise and stress and alleviated with rest or sublingual nitroglycerin. Typically lasts 2 to 10 minutes and rarely >30 minutes. Atypical presentations may include epigastric pain, indigestion, right arm pain, light-headedness, nausea, or shortness of breath alone (anginal equivalents). In the elderly other symptoms (such as confusion, pallor) maybe suggestive of ischemia. Ambulatory ECG monitoring demonstrates that at least 25% of anginal episodes are silent even in patients with a history of typical angina.

B. Physical exam. An S_4 gallop may be transiently present during an episode, and the patient may be dyspneic or diaphoretic or have a new heart murmur. High-risk features of angina include heart failure and hypotension. A complete physical exam is crucial in making an assessment of risk.

C. Evaluation of patients with angina.

1. ***ECG.*** During an episode of pain, the ECG may show ST-segment depression, T-wave inversions, or it may be normal. The absence of ECG changes during an episode of angina does not rule out cardiac ischemia because the circumflex and posterolateral distributions can be electrically silent. Increasing use is being made of echocardiography and thallium studies (see below) to evaluate patients with continuing symptoms in the absence of ECG changes. Coronary artery disease is suggested if there is evidence of an old MI.
2. ***Graded exercise stress test or treadmill (GXT).*** The predictive value of a positive test depends on the prevalence of disease in the population being tested. Specificity is high in particular groups of symptomatic individuals but is generally <50% in asymptomatic individuals. Compared with men, women (especially young women) have higher rates of false-positive GXT. An early positive GXT may be indicative of left main disease or three-vessel disease. Absolute contraindications to GXT include CHF, acute MI, active myocarditis, unstable angina, recent embolism, dissecting aneurysm, acute illness, thrombophlebitis, and moderate to severe aortic stenosis. Relative contraindications include severe hypertension, mild to moderate aortic stenosis, hypertrophic obstructive cardiomyopathy, frequent ectopy, and many other conditions that may increase the risk of a GXT.
3. ***Thallium dipyridamole scan, or thallium GXT.*** Thallium dipyridamole scans can be useful for patients who cannot tolerate the physical demands of the GXT (because of arthritis, COPD). During the test, thallium is taken up by viable, well-perfused myocardium. Areas of myocardial infarction are indicated by fixed perfusion defects with no uptake during rest or exercise. During the thallium-GXT, areas that are hypoperfused (that is, ischemic) demonstrate thallium uptake only during the postexercise "resting" images. Adenosine, dipyridamole, and dobutamine may be used to augment the perfusion of normal myocardium

and shunt blood flow away from areas of relative ischemia. These agents are used in patients who have a contraindication to exercise or are unlikely to attain target heart rates.

4. ***Echocardiography.*** The stress echocardiogram is a widely performed test used to assess patients for coronary disease. Baseline echocardiographic images are obtained at rest. These are used to evaluate left ventricular function, wall motion, and valve function. Images are then acquired during peak stress (that is, during a GXT or with dobutamine) and compared with those at rest. Regional wall-motion abnormalities with stress indicate areas of hypoperfusion or ischemia. Echocardiography is now used routinely to assess CAD in women because of their high false-positive rate on GXT. It is also gaining increased usage among patients with an abnormal baseline ECG (that is, LBBB), those receiving digoxin, and after CABG or PTCA. Transesophageal echocardiography is more sensitive at identifying abnormalities such as valvular vegetations or atrial and ventricular thrombi.
5. ***Coronary angiography.*** Used to identify foci of coronary disease. It is the evaluation of choice in patients with angina that is (1) poorly responsive to medication, or (2) unstable. It is also indicated in patients with test results consistent with a high risk for CAD.

IV. TREATMENT OF ANGINA

A. Medical. May use two- or three-drug combination to maximize benefit while minimizing side effects.

1. ***Aspirin.*** Daily aspirin (325 mg) unless contraindicated to inhibit platelet aggregation.
2. ***Beta-blockers*** (metoprolol, atenolol, nadolol, propranolol, and others). Decrease myocardial oxygen demand by decreasing heart rate, systolic blood pressure, and contractility. Because they prolong diastole, beta-blockers also increase O_2 supply by increasing myocardial perfusion time. Some beta-blockers (those without intrinsic sympathomimetic activity [ISA] activity, especially lipophilic ones [see below]) prolong life when given for the first year after an MI. This benefit extends into subsequent years in those with a complicated course. Lipophilic beta-blockers (timolol, metoprolol, and propranolol) decrease the incidence of postinfarction ventricular fibrillation and sudden death in both men and women by increasing the electrical stability of myocardium. They are also useful in patients whose angina is regularly provoked by exercise though they may limit exercise tolerance. Start with a low dose and increase until symptoms are controlled or the resting heart rate is 50 to 60 beats/min. Side effects can include bradycardia, bronchospasm, fatigue, GI upset, symptoms

of LV failure, and orthostatic hypotension. Impotence, depression, and Raynaud's phenomenon can occur. Do not discontinue beta-blockers abruptly, since rebound tachycardia can occur.

3. ***Calcium-channel blockers*** (verapamil, diltiazem, nifedipine, and others). These drugs act by blocking the influx of calcium through slow channels into vascular smooth muscle and myocardial cells. They promote peripheral arterial vasodilatation, which decreases oxygen demand by decreasing afterload. Calcium-channel blockers also decrease coronary vasospasm and improve collateral flow. Diastolic relaxation of the LV is enhanced, and coronary perfusion is increased with those agents that slow heart rate. Verapamil and diltiazem decrease conduction through the AV node and can be useful to abolish SVT or to slow the ventricular response in atrial fibrillation and atrial flutter. Heart block or asystole can develop in patients with AV node or sinus node disease. First-generation calcium-channel blockers have negative inotropic effects, which can lead to CHF in patients with impaired LV function. Other common side effects of calcium-channel blockers include headache, ankle swelling, GI upset, and constipation. Diltiazem and verapamil are relatively contraindicated after MI in those with CHF and should be avoided. Recent information suggests that nifedipine may increase mortality in some patients (probably as a result of reflex tachycardia).
4. ***Nitrates*** (nitropaste, nitropatches, isosorbide dinitrate, others). Effects include venous and arteriolar vasodilatation, which decreases oxygen demand. The resulting coronary artery vasodilatation increases coronary oxygen supply. Tolerance can develop but can be overcome by providing an 8-hour nitrate-free interval each day. Preparations include oral, transdermal patches, ointment, sublingual tablets, or spray. A common side effect is headache, which usually responds to aspirin or acetaminophen and tends to improve with continued use. Sublingual nitroglycerin tablets (0.4 mg PRN) or spray are used for acute episodes of angina and may be repeated at 5-minute intervals for up to 3 doses. Patients should be instructed to go to the emergency department if angina is not relieved after 3 doses of nitroglycerin.
5. ***ACE inhibitors,*** though not traditionally indicated for angina, may be useful in the patient whose symptoms are difficult to control. ACE inhibitors reduce afterload and directly dilate coronary arteries.

B. Revascularization.

1. ***Coronary artery bypass grafting*** (CABG). Primary indication is angina refractory to medical therapy or lesions that are more amenable to surgery than to angioplasty.

CABG has been shown to prolong survival in patients with left main disease (>50% luminal narrowing) and in three-vessel CAD with LV dysfunction (ejection fraction >50%). Surgery *may* prolong survival in three-vessel disease with normal LV function and in two-vessel disease with significant proximal stenosis of LAD (if not anatomically suited for PTCA).

Contraindications. Advanced age with pronounced debility, absence of ischemia, or ungraftable coronary arteries. Advanced age in and of itself is not a contraindication. In one sample of patients 80 years and older, coronary revascularization by either CABG or PTCA (see below) was associated with a high likelihood of attaining a good or excellent quality of life and of a patient being able to care for himself or herself subsequent to an MI.

2. ***PTCA*** (percutaneous transluminal coronary angioplasty). Can be useful for significant (<50% luminal narrowing) single-vessel CAD when lesions are amenable to the procedure. PTCA does not prevent MI or prolong life. Randomized clinical trails comparing medical therapy with PTCA in single-vessel disease have not shown any significant advantage to using PTCA. Several controlled clinical trials have shown that PTCA can be used as an alternative to CABG in two- and three-vessel CAD when lesions are amenable to PTCA. There was general agreement among these trials that the procedures provide equal improvement in angina. The PTCA groups generally have a higher frequency of antianginal use after 1 year and are more likely to require additional intervention (CABG or repeat PTCA) compared to patients who undergo CABG. PTCA is an acceptable alternative to repeat CABG if lesions are amenable to dilatation (single-vessel stenosis, or easily accessible two-vessel stenoses). Diabetics have a particularly poor long-term result with PTCA. Intracoronary stenting may be preferred in these patients.
3. ***Intracoronary stenting.*** Controlled clinical trials have demonstrated that intracoronary stenting reduces restenosis rates after PTCA from a range of 40% to 50% to a range of 15% to 25%. Recently developed stent deployment techniques using high-pressure balloon inflation and combinations of aspirin and ticlodipine have reduced the abrupt closure rate for stents to <1% and reduced hospital stays to 1 or 2 days.

ISCHEMIC HEART DISEASE: INPATIENT

Inpatient treatment is indicated for (1) unstable angina, (2) prolonged anginal episode, which might represent an infarction, and (3) myocardial infarction. See section on acute treatment of chest pain (p. 13).

I. UNSTABLE ANGINA

A. Management.

1. The decision to admit is based on the history, since 50% of patients with acute MI will have no acute ECG changes and cardiac enzymes will not be positive for up to 6 hours after an infarction. If ECG changes indicate MI, or if enzymes are positive, treat as per MI section below.
2. Admit to ICU. Bed rest, continuous cardiac monitoring, oxygen, and IV access. Obtain screening *lab* tests, including CBC count, glucose, BUN, creatinine, UA, enzymes, SMA-23 now or A.M., PT/PTT if planning to anticoagulate.
3. Obtain serial cardiac enzyme levels. A common protocol is creatine kinase (CPK) Q8h × 3 (not counting initial set). Obtain MB isoenzyme level if the total CPK is elevated. The CPK will rise by 6 to 8 hours and peak at 24 hours while the AST will rise by 8 to 12 hours and peak by 18 to 36 hours. If the patient is >1 day since chest pain, the LDH-1 might be helpful because it rises at 24 hours and peaks at 3 to 6 days. Cardiac troponin I is a protein that is highly sensitive and specific for myocardial injury. Levels of troponin I remain elevated for 4 to 7 days after an MI. Laboratory assays for this marker of cardiac injury are becoming increasingly available.
4. Serial ECGs with intervals depending on circumstances.
5. Increase antianginals. Topical, oral, or SL nitrates; calcium-channel blockers, or beta-blockers. May need IV nitroglycerin. Morphine (2 to 5 mg Q10-20 min) may be given for analgesia, preload reduction, and anxiety; however, these uses must be weighed against the fact that ongoing ischemia may be masked. *Ongoing chest pain that does not respond to standard anti-ischemic regimens (aspirin, heparin, beta-blockers, IV nitroglycerin, and diltiazem) is a cardiac emergency and should prompt consideration of referral to a center equipped with a catheterization laboratory.*
6. Sedation may be of benefit in certain patients.
7. Acetaminophen and a stool softener may be given for headache and preventing the need to strain, respectively.
8. With few exceptions, aspirin should be given to anyone with unstable angina or an evolving MI. Four large trials using aspirin in patients hospitalized with unstable angina have shown a reduction in MI and death. Aspirin should be continued indefinitely. Those patients who appear particularly unstable or who have recurrent ischema are likely to benefit from adding heparin (APTT 1.5 to 2 times normal) to aspirin for the duration of the period of the unstable angina. If coronary artery bypass surgery is planned, aspirin should be started preoperatively because it increases postoperative graft-patency rates.

9. For patients not anticoagulated, heparin 5000 units subcutaneously Q12h should be given for DVT prophylaxis.
10. If cardiac enzymes become positive, treat the patient for MI. If the patient is ruled out for an MI, the patient will still need some assessment of myocardium at risk (such as GXT on increased medications, a thallium study, or cardiac catheterization).

II. MYOCARDIAL INFARCTION

Modalities begun for acute angina (see p. 13) should be continued. Thrombolysis should be used as an additional measure.

A. Defined by ECG changes or serum cardiac enzyme changes. 50% of patients with an acute MI will have a normal initial ECG, and so the decision to admit should be made on the basis of the history.

1. ***ECG patterns.***
   a. Ischemia indicated by ST-segment depression, nonspecific ST-T–segment changes, and T-wave inversion. These may also accompany a non–Q wave infarction.
   b. Injury indicated by ST-segment elevation. Tall peaked T waves (>10 mV) are suggestive of hyperacute injury.
   c. Infarct indicated by the development of Q waves.
2. Infarct location by ECG (Table 2-1).

B. Management. For acute management of chest pain, see p. 13.

1. Orders similar to unstable angina. Unless contraindication, all patients should have aspirin.
2. Hypokalemia and hypomagnesemia are risk factors for arrhythmias and should be corrected if present.

TABLE 2-1
Infarct Location by ECG

ECG changes	Location of injury	Coronary artery involved
II, III, aV_F	Inferior wall (may be associated with RV injury, consider right precordial leads)	RCA or dominant distal left circumflex
V_{1-3}	Anteroseptal	LAD
V_{3-5}	Anterior wall	LAD
V_6, I, aV_L	Lateral	Marginal branch off circumflex or diagonal off LAD
ST depression in V_{1-2} with large R wave.	Posterior	RCA

3. Some small studies have suggested that magnesium is helpful in the patient with an acute MI because it may decrease mortality and the incidence of arrhythmias. However, the Fourth International Study of Infarct Survival (ISIS 4) did not support these conclusions in a large prospective controlled clinical trial. Rather, this study found that magnesium conferred no survival advantage.
4. ***Thrombolytics.*** It is recommended that every patient with an evolving MI be *considered* for thrombolytic therapy, which reduces both in-hospital and 1-year mortality by 25%. Evolving MI is defined as at least 30 minutes of ischemic cardiac pain and at least 1 mm of ST-segment elevation in at least two adjacent limb leads or at least 1 to 2 mm of ST-segment elevation in at least two adjacent precordial leads. (These criteria indicate a high likelihood of evolving MI.) The presence of a complete bundle branch block in addition to characteristic pain is suggestive that the patient may also benefit from thrombolysis. Patients with only ST-segment depression do not benefit, nor do patients with normal ECGs. There is evidence that patients who receive thrombolytics from 6 to 12 hours after onset of acute MI may still benefit, though the benefit is less than that for patients who present less than 6 hours after onset of pain.
   a. *Absolute contraindications* to thrombolytic therapy include recent (<6 weeks) surgery or biopsy of a noncompressible site, recent stroke, *any history of hemorrhagic stroke,* intracranial neoplasm, recent head trauma, pregnancy, or prolonged or traumatic CPR, aortic dissection, acute pericarditis, active bleeding, and antibodies to streptokinase (substitute tissue-type plasminogen activator [TPA] if the patient has antibodies to streptokinase). If there has been a previous allergic reaction to streptokinase or anistreplase (APSAC), use TPA. Also use TPA if streptokinase (SK) or APSAC has been given in the past 12 months.
   b. *Relative contraindications* to thrombolysis. Potential hemorrhagic focus, GI or GU hemorrhage, proliferative diabetic retinopathy, severe uncontrolled hypertension (SBP >200 and DPB >120), history of a bleeding diathesis, cancer, or hepatic dysfunction. Neither age nor menstruation are contraindications for thrombolysis.
   c. *Thrombolytic therapy and administration.* TPA yields a greater decrease in mortality than streptokinase does. In general, if there are no contraindications, streptokinase is preferred by some because of its lower cost. However, an exhaustive analysis has shown that, despite its expense, the use of TPA is cost effective,

particularly in patients with anterior infarctions, and may reduce mortality.

(1) *Streptokinase* 1.5 million IU given IV over 1 hour *or*

(2) TPA 100 mg of single-chain preparation. Give 60 mg in first hour and 20 mg each in hours 2 and 3. The accelerated dose regimen consists in giving two thirds of the dose during the first half hour and the remainder over an additional hour and is now preferred.

5. ***Heparin and aspirin.*** It is recommended that every patient who receives thrombolytic therapy be considered for adjuvant anticoagulation therapy for approximately 48 hours (heparin to keep APTT 1.5 to 2 times control). Adjuvant heparin is normally used in patients who receive TPA to maintain arterial patency. The GUSTO trial showed that there was no advantage to using IV heparin over SQ heparin in patients treated with SK. Several other studies have suggested that heparin is not necessary as an adjunct to SK or TPA. However, many hospital protocols still call for the use of IV heparin with SK. *Discontinuing heparin after 72 hours or so may result in rebound angina because of a relatively hypercoagulable state from anti–thrombin III deficiency.* Long-term aspirin therapy (160 to 325 mg QD) should be considered for all patients who can tolerate it, since ISIS-2 demonstrated that it significantly reduces the incidence of stroke, reinfarction, and death during the first month of recovery.
6. ***Beta-blockers.*** Beta-blockers are indicated for most patients early (within 6 or 7 hours) during the evolution of an MI. A beta-blocker such as metoprolol 15 mg can be given in 5 mg aliquots Q5min. This should be followed by oral beta-blocker therapy in patients with acute MI to reduce long-term mortality. The Beta-Blocker in Heart Attack Trial demonstrated that patients who have a high-risk clinical course (that is, recurrent ischemia, congestive heart failure, arrhythmias, or severe comorbidity) experience a 43% decline in mortality after 1 year if they are treated with long-term beta-blocker therapy. Patients who are seen in the first 4 to 6 hours of onset of an MI or who present with hypertension or sinus tachycardia and are not in heart failure are considered to be good candidates for beta-blockade.
   a. Beta-blockers should be used in patients without contraindications whose MI is complicated by persistent or recurrent pain, progressive or recurrent serum enzyme elevations indicating the extension of an infarct, and tachyarrhythmias that do not respond to lidocaine or procainamide.
   b. Some of the contraindications to beta-blocker use include lengthening of the PR interval >0.24 second,

second- or third-degree AV block, bradycardia with pulse <50, systolic blood pressure <90 mm Hg, pulmonary artery wedge pressure greater than a range of 20 to 24 mm Hg, rales audible in greater than one third of the lung fields, wheezing or history of asthma or bronchospasm, and recent use of IV calcium-channel blockers.

7. ***Angiotensin-converting enzyme (ACE) inhibitors.*** There are several large prospective controlled clinical trials demonstrating the efficacy of ACE inhibitors both acutely and chronically in patients who have sustained an MI (Acute Infarction Ramipril Efficacy Trial, GISSI-3 and ISIS-4, Survival and Ventricular Enlargement Trial). Starting an ACE inhibitor within 24 hours of an MI (enalapril 2.5 mg PO BID titrated to 10 mg PO BID) reduces mortality. Additionally, ACE inhibitors (captopril titrated to 50 mg PO TID or ramipril given at a dose of 5 mg PO BID) continued after an MI in those with CHF or an ejection fraction <45% will decrease mortality (including sudden death), increase exercise capacity, reduce CHF, enable ventricular remodeling, etc.
8. ***Angiography.*** Post-MI coronary angiography and revascularization are indicated for patients with continuing ischemia. Whether asymptomatic patients without any inducible angina who *could* have persistently occluded coronary arteries would benefit from PTCA requires further study.
9. ***Ambulatory monitoring.*** Ambulatory monitoring after an MI adds information and may be an alternative to stress testing in determining which patient continues to have asymptomatic ischemia.
10. ***Prophylactic lidocaine*** is no longer routinely used for patients with suspected acute MI. Lidocaine is still the drug of choice for the treatment of malignant ventricular arrhythmias in patients with acute MI. Many patients with ventricular tachycardias or ventricular fibrillation will not have a warning arrhythmia (see below). The dose should be reduced in elderly patients and in those with CHF or hepatic dysfunction.

COMPLICATIONS OF ACUTE MYOCARDIAL INFARCTION

I. LEFT VENTRICULAR DYSFUNCTION

(See also under section on pulmonary edema, p. 95.)

A. The extent of LV dysfunction in the days after an acute MI provides prognostic information.

B. Treatment of LV dysfunction (CHF) depends on severity but may include:

1. Avoiding medications that exacerbate heart failure.

2. A low-sodium diet and a diuretic to prevent fluid overload (such as furosemide).
3. Increase FiO_2 and provide ventilatory support if required.
4. If the patient is in cardiogenic shock, IV inotropic agents such as dopamine 2 to 20 μg/kg/min or dobutamine 2.5 to 15 μg/kg/min may help to improve LV function. Hemodynamic monitoring and a urinary catheter may be required to manage fluid status. A PCWP <10 mm Hg is suggestive of the need for additional fluid volume, whereas a PCWP >20-25 mm Hg is suggestive of fluid overload.
5. If the cardiogenic shock is secondary to ischemic "stunned" myocardium, then intra-aortic balloon counterpulsation, cardiac catheterization, or emergency revascularization may be warranted.

II. RIGHT VENTRICULAR DYSFUNCTION

A. Especially prominent with an inferior wall MI secondary to right ventricular infarction. Pronounced hypotension in response to nitrates should be suggestive of this diagnosis.

B. The triad of clear lung fields, hypotension, and jugular venous distension (JVD) in a patient with an inferior infarction is highly suggestive of a right ventricular infarction. JVD has a sensitivity of 88% and a specificity of 69% for right ventricular infarction. Kussmaul's venous sign (distension of the jugular vein during inspiration) is also highly sensitive and specific for this condition. The patient may also present with tricuspid regurgitation, right ventricular gallops, and atrioventricular dissociation.

C. An ECG with right-sided chest leads can be done to confirm right ventricular myocardial infarction (RVMI). A 1 mm ST-segment elevation in the right precordial lead CR4R is highly predictive for an RVMI (sensitivity 70%, specificity 100%). Other ECG findings include right bundle branch block and complete heart block.

D. Echocardiography may reveal right ventricular wall dyskinesia and dilatation. There may be abnormal interventricular septal motion because of a reversal in the transseptal pressure gradient secondary to increased right ventricular end-diastolic pressure.

E. In addition to conduction deficits, patients with RVMI may develop right ventricular mural thrombi (placing them at high risk for pulmonary embolism), tricuspid regurgitation, and pericarditis.

F. The following are important components of a treatment regimen for right ventricular infarction:

1. Maintain right ventricular preload with volume loading as indicated. The infusion of IV normal saline frequently corrects hypotension and increases cardiac output.
2. The use of nitrates, diuretics, and morphine sulfate are all relatively contraindicated, since these medications decrease preload.

3. Reduce right ventricular afterload if there is concomitant left ventricular dysfunction.
4. Initiate inotropic support with dobutamine if the patient is not stabilized hemodynamically with a saline infusion.
5. Begin sequential atrioventricular pacing if the patient develops complete heart block.
6. Initiate thrombolytic therapy or perform angioplasty as indicated.

G. Among patients who survive a right ventricular infarction, right ventricular function returns to nearly normal levels over time.

III. TACHYARRHYTHMIAS COMPLICATING ACUTE MI

A. Premature ventricular complexes (PVCs).

1. Common in first 72 hours after an MI.
2. Usually do not require treatment unless they are:
   a. Frequent (>10/min).
   b. Multiform.
   c. Occurring close to preceding T-wave (R-on-T phenomenon), or
   d. Occurring in pairs, triplets, or short runs.
3. Usually treated with a lidocaine bolus followed by infusion. (See ACLS protocols, p. 1.)

B. Ventricular tachycardia or fibrillation. See ACLS protocols, p. 1.

C. Supraventricular tachycardias including PSVT and atrial fibrillation or flutter. See ACLS protocols, p. 1.

1. Tachycardia increases O_2 demand; so treat promptly.
2. Rule out reversible underlying causes (such as electrolyte abnormalities such as hypokalemia or hypomagnesemia and hypoxia).

IV. ATRIOVENTRICULAR BLOCK

A. Mobitz I (Wenckebach).

1. Common in acute inferior infarction.
2. See ACLS treatment protocols, p. 1.
3. A permanent pacemaker is rarely required, since Wenckebach block usually resolves within days.

B. Mobitz II.

1. Usually occurs in patients with acute anterior MIs.
2. In the setting of an acute MI, with Mobitz II AV block, a temporary pacemaker should be placed. Often the block is permanent, and a permanent pacemaker should be placed if the block persists for 1 week or more.

C. Third-degree AV block.

1. Third-degree AV block is often transient in the setting of an acute inferior MI.
2. When associated with an anterior MI, it often represents necrosis of the conducting tissue below the AV node and may be permanent, requiring permanent pacemaker implantation.

D. Bundle branch block.

1. A left bundle branch block is the most common bundle branch block seen with an MI. The combination of a right bundle branch block and a left anterior hemiblock is also frequently seen.
2. When a bundle branch block occurs, the site of the infarction is usually anteroseptal, and the infarct is often large.
3. If the patient is known to have an old bundle branch or fascicular block. a temporary pacemaker is not necessarily indicated unless dictated by the patient's symptoms and hemodynamic status.
4. If the patient has a *new* left bundle branch block or bifascicular block associated with an MI, a temporary pacemaker is indicated. A bifascicular block is defined as the combination of a right BBB and a left anterior or posterior hemiblock.

V. LEFT VENTRICULAR ANEURYSM

A. Incidence 7% to 15%, suggested by persistent ST elevations weeks to months after an MI.

B. May lead to CHF, systemic emboli (caused by mural thrombus formation), and recurrent arrhythmias.

C. Can be demonstrated on echocardiogram or radionuclide ventriculogram.

D. Some authors recommend long-term anticoagulation to reduce the risk of embolization. Surgical resection may be indicated for refractory LV failure, recurrent emboli despite anticoagulation, or medically refractory ventricular arrhythmias if electrophysiology studies indicate that the aneurysm may be the focus of the arrhythmia.

VI. RECURRENT CHEST PAIN

A. Extension of MI.

1. Occurs in 10% to 15%.
2. Characterized by reelevation of cardiac enzymes and additional ECG changes.
3. Patients with non–Q wave infarcts are at higher risk of extension of infarct in the 12 months after an MI than patients with transmural infarcts.

B. Angina. For treatment and diagnosis, see section above. If post-MI angina is refractory to medical therapy, cardiac catheterization may be indicated to define anatomy and suitability for revascularization or to perform PTCA.

C. Pericarditis. May occur after an MI, as the result of a viral infection (especially coxsackievirus), or secondary to uremia.

1. In the setting of an infarction, pericarditis usually occurs after a large transmural infarct.
2. Physical exam may reveal an audible friction rub.

3. Pleuritic pain, exacerbated by lying supine, relieved by sitting forward, may be present. The pain tends to radiate to the shoulder and be worse on inspiration.
4. ECG may show diffuse ST-segment elevations, and echocardiogram frequently reveals the presence of a pericardial effusion.
5. Treatment. NSAIDs, especially indomethacin. Steroids may be used for viral pericarditis but should be avoided in an acute MI. *Avoid* anticoagulation because of the risk of converting the effusion into a hemorrhagic one with risk of cardiac tamponade.

D. **Pulmonary embolism.** Post-MI patients should be maintained on prophylactic doses of SQ heparin (5000 units Q12h) until fully mobile.

E. **Pneumonia.**

VII. DRESSLER'S SYNDROME

A. **Cause.** Pleuropericarditis occurring usually 2 to 4 weeks after an MI. Possibly represents an autoimmune inflammatory reaction.

B. **Symptoms.** Pericardial and pleural pain.

C. **Signs.** Fever, pericardial friction rub (may be intermittent), and perhaps decreased breath sounds at lung bases and a pleural rub. Chest radiograph may show enlarged cardiac silhouette because of pericardial effusion. ECG may show diffuse ST-segment elevations, decreased R-wave voltage, and occasionally electrical alternans. An echocardiogram may show pericardial effusion.

D. **Treatment.** Usually self-limited. NSAIDs; glucocorticoids if NSAIDs not effective. *Avoid* anticoagulation for reasons stated above.

CARDIAC ARRHTHYMIAS

For outpatient assessment, an "event monitor" that is worn for a prolonged period and activated when patient has symptoms is more sensitive than a 24- to 28-hour "Holter" monitor and is the preferred modality.

A. **Atrial fibrillation.** Gives rise to the loss of atrial contraction and an irregular ventricular rate. Clinically recognized by an irregularly irregular heart rate. Causes include hyperthyroidism, acute pulmonary embolism, CHF, valvular disease (especially mitral regurgitation), acute alcohol use ("holiday heart").

1. See ACLS protocols, p. 1, for acute management of atrial fibrillation with a rapid ventricular response.
2. *Rate control.* Long-term usage must control ventricular rate with agents that increase the refractory period of the AV node (digoxin, verapamil, or beta-blockers). The ventricular rate should be decreased to a range of 80 to 100

beats/min. Generally, verapamil or diltiazem are the drugs of choice. Digoxin is most effective in rate control in those with CHF or at bed rest but may not be sufficient in those who are ambulatory. Additionally, it may increase incidence of A Fib in those with paroxysmal A Fib.

3. *Long-term anticoagulation* with warfarin (INR 2.0 to 3.0) is indicated for those in A Fib who are older than 60 years of age or have valvular disease, underlying heart disease, hypertension, diabetes, or previous evidence of embolism (CVA, TIA). Those with "lone" A Fib (<60, no above risk factors, no cardiovascular disease) have a low incidence of complications and need not be anticoagulated. Aspirin is second best and should be reserved for those in whom anticoagulation is not an option.
4. Many of those with A Fib will convert back to sinus rhythm spontaneously. May attempt to convert back to a sinus rhythm with either class I drugs (quinidine or procainamide), flecainide, or cardioversion. *However, these patients should be anticoagulated for 3 weeks before cardioversion unless A Fib has been present for less than 48 hours.* Anticoagulation should be continued for 2 weeks after conversion.
5. Although quinidine and procainamide may help to maintain sinus rhythm, the Stroke Prevention in Atrial Fibrillation Trial showed that these drugs are associated with a 2.5-fold higher incidence of mortality probably because of an increased development of torsades de pointes or other arrhythmias. Recently both sotalol and low-dose amiodarone have been used to maintain sinus rhythm and were not associated with an increase in mortality. However, further data are needed before their use in the primary care setting can be suggested.

B. Paroxysmal supraventricular tachycardia. Most commonly caused by atrioventricular node reentry with 1:1 atrioventricular conduction, though may also be caused by sinus node reentry, atrial ectopy, or an accessory pathway. Commonly associated with Wolff-Parkinson-White syndrome.

1. Must be distinguished from a ventricular tachycardia.
2. See ACLS treatment protocol, p. 1.
3. Chronically may be suppressed with calcium-channel blockers (verapamil and diltiazem). However, radioablation of the accessory pathway is both safe and effective.

C. Ventricular tachycardia. With this arrhythmia, ventricular rate is generally 150 to 180 beats/min. Rhythm tends to be regular, and AV dissociation is a common feature. By definition it is characterized by three or more consecutive complexes arising inferior to the bifurcation of the bundle of His at a rate that exceeds 100 beats/min.

1. May be caused by heart disease, electrolyte imbalances, hypoxia, and drug toxicity. The most frequent cause of

sustained ventricular tachycardia is reentry along the margin of old infarcted myocardium.

2. See Figs. 1-1 and 1-5 for acute treatment.
3. Since recurrence rates are high, long-term antiarrhythmic therapy or the implantation of a cardioverter-defribrillator may be indicated *for those with sustained or symptomatic ventricular tachycardia.* Traditional antiarrhythmic agents actually increase mortality. The Cardiac Arrhythmia Suppression Trial demonstrated that when post-MI patients were treated with either flecainide or encainide for asymptomatic ventricular ectopy, their mortality was twofold to threefold higher than patients receiving placebo. Sotalol and amiodarone are showing promise in the treatment of these patients. Beta-blockers (such as metoprolol, propranolol) may be useful in treating this arrhythmia. Generally a cardiology consult should be obtained to determine the best approach to chronic suppression of this arrhythmia.

D. Sick sinus syndrome.

1. Episodes of bradycardia interspersed with episodic tachycardia from sinus tachycardia or atrial fibrillation. May cause syncope.
2. Generally a disease of the elderly.
3. Treatment generally requires pacemaker to prevent bradycardia as well as medications such as digoxin or verapamil to control tachycardia.

RHEUMATIC FEVER AND RHEUMATIC CARDITIS

A. Etiology and present significance. Acute rheumatic fever (ARF) and rheumatic carditis represent the clinical sequelae of infection with group A streptococci. Peak age of incidence is 5 to 15 years. Primary and recurrent illness occurs in adulthood as well, especially in those with established rheumatic heart disease. The risk of ARF is increased in those with large increases in antistreptolysin O (ASO) titers or persistent pharyngeal colonization.

B. Clinical signs and symptoms.

1. The development of rheumatic fever requires an antecedent streptococcal infection (as evidenced by streptococcal pharyngitis or scarlet fever). If there is uncertainty regarding recent streptococcal infection, streptococcal antibody tests may be performed. If titers for two antibodies are obtained (ASO and either antihyaluronidase or anti-DNAase B), an elevation in the titer of at least one will be found in 90% of ARF cases.
2. The revised Jones criteria account for both major and minor manifestations of the disease. The development of two major criteria or one major and two minor criteria are suggestive of a high probability of rheumatic fever.

a. Major manifestations.
   (1) Polyarthritis. May have any degree of arthritis; generally migratory and in large joints. Resolves in about 1 month.
   (2) Carditis. See below.
   (3) Sydenham's chorea ("St. Vitus's dance")
   (4) Erythema marginatum
   (5) Subcutaneous (Aschoff) nodules (painless subcutaneous nodules over bony surfaces)
b. Minor manifestations.
   (1) Previous episode of ARF or rheumatic heart disease
   (2) Arthralgia
   (3) Fever
   (4) Elevations in acute-phase reactants (ESR, C-reactive protein)
   (5) Leukocytosis
   (6) Prolonged PR interval on ECG

C. Cardiac manifestations. 40% to 60% of patients develop carditis during the initial episode of ARF. To be diagnosed with carditis a patient must have one of the following diagnoses:
- Cardiomegaly
- Heart murmur
- Pericarditis
- Congestive heart failure

A murmur usually develops in response to rheumatic carditis. Auscultation may reveal the apical holosystolic murmur of mitral regurgitation, the diastolic murmur of aortic regurgitation, an apical middiastolic murmur (Carey-Coombs murmur), a pericardial friction rub, or muffled heart sounds secondary to a pericardial effusion. Chest radiography may reveal cardiomegaly as well as evidence of CHF (pulmonary edema, pleural effusion, Kerley B lines, and pulmonary vascular engorgement). Tachycardia is a frequent finding. With pericarditis, ST segments may be elevated. Supraventricular and ventricular tachyarrhythmias may also develop. The evolution of valvular disease typically requires 10 to 30 years. Among patients with rheumatic heart disease the incidence of valvular disease is as follows: mitral valve 85%, aortic valve 44%, tricuspid valve 10% to 16%, whereas the pulmonic valve is affected very infrequently.

D. Treatment and prophylaxis. Antibiotics (such as benzathine penicillin G) are given to eradicate tonsillar and pharyngeal rheumatogenic group A streptococci but do not affect the course of ARF or the later development of carditis or valvular disease. Aspirin is used to treat the acute polyarthritis. Corticosteroids (such as prednisone) are used to treat carditis and are administered for 3 to 6 weeks. Congestive heart failure developing in patients with carditis is managed as described in the section on congestive heart failure below. Primary prevention is achieved by treatment of streptococcal pharyngitis with appropriate antibiotics (such as penicillin VK 500 mg TID for 10 days, or erythromycin 333 mg PO TID for 10 days). Secondary prevention consists in the chronic administration of antibiotics to patients who have already sustained significant damage from rheumatic carditis to prevent further cardiac injury. Secondary prophylaxis is not generally given to patients after only a single episode of ARF. In patients in whom it is warranted, a monthly IM injection of 1.2 million units of penicillin G benzathine appears to provide optimal prophylaxis. Prophylaxis in these patients should be lifelong.

VALVULAR HEART DISEASE: MITRAL VALVE PROLAPSE

A. **Definition.** MVP may result from leaflet billowing, progressive expansion of the mitral annulus, or valve-leaflet myxomatous degeneration. Most patients with MVP are asymptomatic and will have a benign clinical course. Symptoms may include palpitations, fatigue, dyspnea, syncope, atypical chest pain, and episodes of supraventricular tachycardia. A small proportion of patients experience CVAs, TIAs, seizures, or episodes of amaurosis fugax. Patients with severe myxomatous change and thickened leaflets are at greatest risk of embolic events. It is estimated that 4000 patients die from MVP-associated sudden death per year. Men and patients over 45 years of age are at increased risk for complications such as infective endocarditis and severe mitral regurgitation. 15% of patients with MVP will go on to develop mitral regurgitation with heart failure and may need to undergo surgical valve replacement.

B. **Auscultatory findings.** MVP is associated with a midsystolic click, which may be intermittent. If there is mitral regurgitation, the aforementioned click will be followed by a midsystolic to late systolic murmur.

C. **Diagnosis.** Diagnosis may be confirmed with the use of echocardiography.

D. **Endocarditis prophylaxis.** Antibiotic prophylaxis should be used for patients with MVP who have regurgitation or are symptomatic from their illness.

CONGESTIVE HEART FAILURE

I. CAUSES

Two thirds caused by coronary artery disease. The second most common cause is dilated cardiomyopathy, which can be idiopathic or may result from toxins (alcohol, doxorubicin), infection (often viral), or collagen vascular disease. Other causes include chronic hypertension (diastolic dysfunction), valvular heart disease, hypertrophic cardiomyopathy, and restrictive cardiomyopathy (amyloidosis, sarcoidosis, and hemochromatosis).

II. EVALUATION

A. **History.** Typical symptoms include fatigue, dyspnea, orthopnea, paroxysmal nocturnal dyspnea, nocturia, or chronic cough.

B. **Physical exam.** JVD, hepatojugular reflux, S_3 gallop, rales, and peripheral edema. However, these are not present in all those with CHF.

C. **Studies.** Baseline CXR and ECG. An echocardiogram may be indicated to evaluate LV and RV ejection fractions, movement of chamber walls and valves, and chamber sizes. In systolic dysfunction, ejection fraction is decreased. Electrolytes, BUN, creatinine, ABG, CBC count, and serum digoxin level if indicated.

III. TREATMENT OF CHF SECONDARY TO PUMP WEAKNESS (THAT IS, SYSTOLIC DYSFUNCTION)

A. **Nonpharmacologic therapy.** Avoid excessive physical stress, reduce dietary salt, consider compressive stockings if needed to reduce risk of DVT (consider SQ heparin if inpatient), and weight loss if obese.

B. **Pharmacologic therapy.**

1. ***Diuretics.*** In mild heart failure, a thiazide diuretic may be sufficient. With moderate to severe failure or evidence of volume overload, a loop diuretic (usually furosemide) is required. Some patients develop resistance to loop diuretics after chronic usage. A single dose of metolazone (5 to 20 mg QD) will often result in significant diuresis in such patients. Patients with heart failure who are receiving diuretics should have potassium and magnesium levels monitored. Supplementation should be provided if necessary, since hypokalemia and hypomagnesemia are risk factors for the development of arrhythmias.
2. ***ACE inhibitors.*** These agents function primarily as afterload reducers and have been shown to reduce morbidity (CHF progression, MI, need for hospitalization) and mortality in several large trials of patients with CHF (SOLVD, CONCENSUS I, and SAVE). ACE inhibitors have also been shown to improve hemodynamics and increase exercise tolerance in heart failure patients. Up to now only captopril, enalapril, lisinopril, and ramipril have been shown to be efficacious in large controlled clinical trials. Begin therapy at low doses such as enalapril 2.5 mg PO BID and titrate to 10 mg PO BID gradually. Observe the patient for hypotension or persistent cough. Monitor electrolytes and renal function because ACE inhibitors can cause elevation of serum potassium and can cause a reversible decrease in renal

function in some patients. Patients at high risk for adverse effects from ACE inhibitors include those with connective tissue diseases, preexisting renal insufficiency, or bilateral renal artery stenosis. Contraindications to their use include a history of hypersensitivity to ACE inhibitors, serum potassium greater than 5.5 mEq/L (consider evaluation for hypoaldosteronism or Addison's disease), or a previous episode of angioedema during their use. Relative contraindications include renal failure and hypotension. However, ACE inhibitors actually protect renal function in those with chronic renal failure (see Chapter 11 for details). In the latter two patient groups, the ACE inhibitor therapy should be initiated at half the usual starting dose and titrated to desired effect. In patients who tolerate them, ACE inhibitors should supplant diuretics as first-line therapy for CHF.

3. ***Other vasodilators.*** The V-HEFT II Trial demonstrated enalapril therapy to increase survival in heart failure patients over that seen with combination hydralazine and isosorbide therapy during the first 2 years of therapy. However, in patients unable to tolerate ACE inhibitors, a combination of hydralazine and isosorbide dinitrate may be used. If the major problem is decreased cardiac output, hydralazine may be given to decrease afterload. If the patient is dyspneic, the addition of isosorbide dinitrate will decrease pulmonary capillary wedge pressure and pulmonary congestion. In patients receiving combination digoxin-diuretic ACE inhibitor therapy who are not hemodynamically stable, hydralazine and isosorbide dinitrate may be added to the regimen, and consideration should be given to cardiac transplantation.
4. ***Digoxin.*** Shown to improve symptoms in severe heart failure and in cases where atrial fibrillation is a complication of CHF. Rapid digitalization is not necessary in patients with chronic CHF. The half-life of digoxin is $1\frac{1}{2}$ to 2 days in patients with normal renal function. The usual starting dose is 0.25 mg/day. Decrease the dose in small or elderly patients and in those receiving other drugs (such as quinidine, amiodarone, verapamil) that raise digoxin levels. Decrease the dose in patients with impaired renal function. Monitor levels, especially after dose adjustments or after changes in other medications that may affect digoxin levels (such as quinidine, verapamil, oral azole antifungals). The effect of digoxin on mortality in CHF has not been proved, but large scale trials are underway. *Avoid digoxin in patients with IHSS (idiopathic hypertrophic subaortic stenosis) and those with diastolic dysfunction.* Watch potassium levels closely; hypokalemia renders the heart more sensitive to digoxin and will predispose to digoxin toxicity.

5. ***Dobutamine.*** Dobutamine is the parenteral inotropic agent of choice in acute, severe CHF. Onset of action is immediate and stops quickly when the infusion is discontinued. It should not be used in patients with IHSS. May cause tachycardia, angina, and ventricular arrhythmias.
6. ***Calcium-channel blockers.*** Some calcium-channel blockers, especially verapamil and diltiazem, are relatively potent negative inotropic agents and should generally be avoided in patients with poor LV function. In patients with CHF and hypertension, amlodipine (a second-generation dihydropyridine calcium-channel blocker with no negative inotropicity) has been shown to be efficacious.
7. ***Beta-blockers.*** The use of beta-blockers in patients with CHF caused by systolic dysfunction is gaining favor but is not yet standard of care. These agents appear to confer myocardial protection by inhibiting a variety of damaging neurohumoral effects activated by CHF.
8. ***Antithrombotic therapy.*** Patients with a previous history of embolism or atrial fibrillation are at high risk for thromboembolic complications and should be considered for warfarin therapy, unless a contraindication exists. Titrate the dose to an INR of 2.0 to 3.0 (prothrombin time not more than 1.5 times normal) to avoid increased risk of bleeding complications. If warfarin cannot be used, consider aspirin for the antiplatelet effect (80 to 300 mg/day).

DIASTOLIC DYSFUNCTION

A. General. Diastolic dysfunction refers to congestive heart failure with a normal or increased ejection fraction but decreased cardiac output caused by a stiff, noncompliant ventricle and small chamber size secondary to muscle hypertrophy. Depending on the population studied, diastolic dysfunction is found in up to 40% of the patients presenting with symptoms of congestive heart failure. Generally found in the elderly, those with long-standing hypertension, those on dialysis. May be secondary to cardiac fibrosis, hypertension, valvular disease, other underlying illness.

B. Clinically. May be indistinguishable from CHF secondary to systolic dysfunction. However, echocardiogram or gated pool study demonstrate good ejection fraction, hypertrophy of ventricle wall.

C. Treatment.

1. ***Verapamil*** is useful in patients with IHSS and diastolic dysfunction (reduced ventricular compliance). Start low dose and increase slowly and only if desired clinical effect and no evidence of increase in CHF.
2. ***Beta-blockers*** are indicated for the treatment of CHF induced by diastolic dysfunction. They do not promote

myocardial relaxation. However, beta-blockers are believed to exert benefit by reducing myocardial oxygen demands, slowing the heart rate, controlling hypertension, and promoting the regression of left ventricular hypertrophy (thereby restoring the ventricle's elasticity and normalizing end-diastolic pressure and volume). Again, start with a low dose and work up.

3. ***Digoxin and afterload reducers*** may be detrimental in these patients and should be used with caution.
4. ***Diuretics*** may be helpful in acute dyspnea. However, preload reduction may also reduce cardiac output, and so diuretics must be used with caution.
5. ***ACE inhibitors*** may allow for left ventricular remodeling and may have a direct effect on myocardium that is beneficial in diastolic dysfunction.

ACUTE PULMONARY EDEMA

I. CAUSES

A. Altered capillary permeability. Infections, inhaled toxins such as chlorine or ammonia, circulating toxins (endotoxic shock), vasoactive substances (histamine, kinins), disseminated intravascular coagulation, immunologic reaction, uremia, near-drowning, aspiration, smoke inhalation, ARDS.

B. Increased pulmonary venous pressure. LV failure, mitral stenosis, subacute bacterial endocarditis, pulmonary venous disease or malformation, fluid overload.

C. Decreased plasma oncotic pressure. Hypoalbuminemia from any cause.

D. Miscellaneous. Lymphatic insufficiency, high altitude, neurogenic (CNS trauma), heroin overdose, eclampsia, others.

E. Precipitators of acute pulmonary edema (in a previously compensated patient). Poor compliance with medical or diet therapy, increased metabolic demands (infection, pregnancy, anemia, hyperthyroidism), progression of underlying heart disease, arrhythmias, drug effect (beta-blockers, calcium-channel blockers, other negative inotropes), silent MI, pulmonary embolism.

II. DIAGNOSIS

The diagnosis of pulmonary edema is usually made initially by physical exam and confirmed by CXR. Treatment may have to be started before one obtains a detailed history, etc. However, once the patient is stable, a careful work-up should be undertaken to determine underlying causes and precipitating factors.

A. History. Past history of cardiac and pulmonary disease or hypertension. History of shortness of breath, orthopnea, dyspnea on exertion, faintness, chest pain. Recent weight gain, edema. Recent infection, exposure to toxic inhalants, smoke, possible aspiration. Current medication regimen, compliance with diet and medications.

B. Physical exam. Tachypnea, tachycardia, often BP is elevated. If patient has fever, suspect concurrent infection, which may increase metabolic demand and lead to CHF. Cyanosis, diaphoresis, retractions, use of accessory muscles of respiration, wheezing ("cardiac asthma"), and rales on lung auscultation. Cough may be productive of pink, frothy sputum. Listen for S_3 gallop or murmurs, which might indicate preexisting valvular disease. Peripheral edema and positive hepatojugular reflux are suggestive of CHF, and bruits may be a clue to underlying vascular disease.

C. Diagnostic tests.

1. ***Lab tests.*** Electrolytes, BUN, creatinine, cardiac enzymes, serum protein and albumin, urinalysis, differential CBC count, and ABG.
2. ***CXR.*** Initially will show interstitial edema as well as thickening and loss of definition of the shadows of pulmonary vasculature. Fluid in septal planes and interlobular fissures cause the characteristic appearance of Kerley A and B lines. Eventually, pleural effusions and perihilar alveolar edema may develop in the classic "butterfly" pattern. CXR findings may lag behind the clinical presentation by up to 12 hours and may take 4 days to clear after clinical improvement in the patient.
3. ***ECG.*** Evaluate for evidence of MI and arrhythmia. The sudden onset of atrial fibrillation or PSVT may cause acute decompensation in previously stable chronic CHF. LVH may signal underlying aortic stenosis, hypertension, or cardiomyopathy.
4. ***Echocardiography.*** Not imperative acutely. In work-up for underlying cause, it is useful to evaluate for valvular disease, valvular vegetations, wall-motion abnormalities, LV function, and cardiomyopathy.

III. TREATMENT

A. Oxygen. Usually provide oxygen by nasal cannula or mask. May require endotracheal intubation if unable to adequately oxygenate despite use of 100% oxygen by nonrebreather mask. Mask continuous positive airway pressure (CPAP) has been shown in numerous studies to reduce the need for intubation and is an excellent alternative.

B. Other general measures. Elevate head of bed 30 degrees. May need Swan-Ganz catheter for hemodynamic monitoring if the patient becomes hypotensive. However, Swan-Ganz catheters may have an adverse effect on mortality and should be used only after careful consideration. Place a Foley catheter for fluid management.

C. Medications.

1. ***Furosemide and other diuretics.*** If the patient has never been treated with furosemide, may start with 20 mg IV and observe response. Titrate dose upward until adequate diuresis is established. If the patient is receiving furosemide over a long term give 1 to 2 times the usual daily dose by slow (over 1 to 2 minutes) IV bolus. Larger doses (up to 1 g) may be needed in those patients receiving large doses or with a history of renal disease. Alternatively, a furosemide drip can be established for higher doses. Give 20% of the dose as a bolus (that is, 200 mg) and infuse the rest over 8 hours. This has a greater efficacy than a single, large bolus does. Up to 2 g has been safely administered in this fashion. Ethacrynic acid 25 to 100 mg IV may be needed if the patient does not respond to furosemide. Bumetanide (0.5 to 1.0 mg IV) and metolazone (5 to 20 mg) may also be used. Furosemide may transiently increase afterload unless the patient has already been treated with afterload and preload reducers. Some authors would consider phlebotomy if diuretics are ineffective and patient has a high HCT.
2. ***Vasodilators*** act by decreasing afterload and thereby decreasing LV work. May also reverse myocardial ischemia. Vasodilators are the initial treatment of choice for CHF. IV nitroglycerin is commonly used especially if there is concern that ischemia is an underlying or precipitating factor. Start at 10 to 20 μg/min and increase by increments of 10 to 20 μg/min every 5 minutes until the desired effect is achieved. Sublingual nitroglycerin 0.4 mg repeated Q5 min PRN can also be used acutely as topical nitrate pastes can be used. Nitroprusside is an alternative (start at 0.5 μg/kg/min and increase by 0.5 μg/kg/min every 5 minutes). Most patients respond to less than 10 μg/kg/min but titrate to effect. Nitroprusside is more likely to cause hypotension than is IV nitroglycerin. A fluid bolus may help to reverse nitrate-induced hypotension.
3. ***Digoxin.*** Check ECG, serum potassium, BUN, and creatinine first before loading with digoxin. After digoxin loading, it may be difficult to distinguish ischemic changes on ECG from digoxin effect. Inquire about previous use of digoxin and any adverse reactions. Determine if patient has any history of renal, pulmonary, liver, or thyroid disease. Be aware of other medications that the patient takes that might affect digoxin levels such as amiodarone, flecainide, quinidine, and verapamil. Decrease digoxin dose if the patient has renal disease. The aim is to achieve serum levels of 1.0 to 1.5 ng/ml.

DIGOXIN LOADING DOSE

Oral: Total oral loading dose = Body weight (kg) × 0.015 mg/kg digoxin. Give in 3 or 4 divided doses over 24 hours

IV: Total loading dose = 0.01 mg/kg given in divided doses over 24 hours.

4. *Morphine* acts as a venodilator and decreases anxiety. Start with 1 to 2 mg IV. Titrate carefully in COPD and CHF, since narcotics can decrease respiratory drive.
5. *ACE inhibitors* can be used acutely in the management of CHF. Captopril 12.5 to 25 mg SL or IV at 0.16 mg/min increased by 0.08 mg/min every 5 minutes until have desired effect.
6. *Dobutamine* (2.5 to 15 µg/kg/min) or dopamine (2 to 20 µg/kg/min) may be needed for pressure support or as a positive inotrope. These drugs are effective immediately; however, although dopamine increases renal perfusion, may not increase GFR.

D. Surgery may be indicated under rare conditions such as valvular heart disease or rupture of ventricular septum after an MI. In severe LV failure, an intra-aortic balloon pump may be beneficial as a temporizing measure.

IV. FOLLOW-UP

Once the acute episode of pulmonary edema is under control, a careful search for the underlying cause must be undertaken. Further work-up might include echocardiography to evaluate valve function and chamber size, radionuclide studies to evaluate LV and RV ejection fraction and wall motion, and cardiac catheterization. See sections concerning LV dysfunction after an MI, p. 86, and chronic CHF, p. 91.

HYPERTENSION

I. OVERVIEW

Hypertension is defined as a sustained systolic blood pressure of greater than or equal to 140 mm Hg or a sustained diastolic blood pressure of greater than or equal to 90 mm Hg. Before diagnosing an individual as hypertensive, one should document an elevated blood pressure on at least three occasions over a 2-week period. The patient should be free of stress at the time of the exam including being free of pain and anxiety (such as white coat hypertension). Use a cuff of the proper size (small size gives falsely elevated readings) and arm should be resting comfortably on armrest. If results are still inconclusive, consider 24-hour ambulatory monitoring. Treatment of hypertension can reduce many of the complications of chronic hypertension, such as CHF, nephropathy, and cerebrovascular events, which are consequences of hypertensive arteriolar disease.

II. CAUSES

A. Essential hypertension is the most common form of hypertension in all age groups except children. The cause of essential hypertension is not completely understood.

B. Secondary hypertension is the result of some identifiable pathologic process, usually related to renal physiology. Causes of secondary hypertension include renal artery stenosis (or other cause of increased plasma renin), renal parenchymal disease (glomerulonephritis, diabetic nephropathy, polycystic disease, obstructive uropathy), drugs (oral contraceptives, steroids), increased levels of catecholamines (pheochromocytoma), glucocorticoids (Cushing's syndrome), or mineralocorticoids (hypoaldosteronism).

III. EVALUATION

A. Initial evaluation of the patient with newly detected mild to moderately elevated blood pressure should include the following:

1. Through history regarding diabetes, hypertension (HTN), and cardiovascular disease in the family, personal history of cardiovascular symptoms, drug and alcohol use, level of physical activity, and diet.
2. A physical examination to include weight, funduscopic exam for evidence of retinopathy, cardiac examination, auscultation of abdomen and neck for bruits, and palpation of kidneys.
3. Laboratory evaluation may be postponed until follow-up visits have established the diagnosis of HTN.
4. Recommended salt restriction, increased exercise, weight reduction if indicated, and follow-up exam in 2 to 4 weeks for blood pressure recheck.

B. Evaluation of the patient with HTN should include:

1. Urine analysis and serum creatinine to evaluate for renal disease; ECG; cholesterol and triglycerides (as part of coronary artery disease risk factor assessment); electrolytes and uric acid as baseline for determining appropriate medications; and serum glucose to evaluate for diabetes.
2. Other tests may be indicated by physical exam or laboratory results that indicate a possible cause of secondary hypertension. IVP, renal arteriography, captopril renal scan, and urinary catecholamine evaluation may be indicated in certain patients. Routine use of these studies is not suggested unless additional factors support the presence of a secondary cause.

IV. TREATMENT

A. Education. All patients with HTN should be counseled regarding the nature of the disorder and the importance of long-term compliance with particular treatment regimens. Home blood pressure monitoring should be taught.

B. Lifestyle interventions. Exercise, salt restriction, and weight reduction are appropriate for many patients with HTN but may be of limited efficacy. Smoking cessation should be encouraged. If the patient abuses alcohol or other substances; appropriate treatment should be encouraged and arranged. Increased intake of calcium and magnesium should be encouraged to help reduce blood pressure unless a contraindication is present.

C. **Medications.** Numerous medications are available for the pharmacologic treatment of HTN. The widely varying side-effects, costs, and dosing schedules allow tailoring of the medications to the particular needs of each patient. Pharmacologic intervention is indicated in the mildly to moderately hypertensive individual when the above-mentioned measures have not produced adequate control. A stepped-care regimen has been advocated in the past; however, some studies have suggested that monotherapy with more potent agents may be as or more effective in preventing sequelae of HTN. Individualized therapy is recommended with consideration for factors such as demographics (race and age, which may affect response to certain antihypertensive agents), quality of life (related to side effects), and concomitant medical disease and cardiovascular risk factors, which may influence choice of therapy.

1. ***Diuretics.*** Thiazide diuretics are effective alone and are useful in offsetting the fluid retention caused by other agents. Loop diuretics are more effective in patients with impaired renal function. Examples of thiazides are hydrochlorothiazide and chlorothiazide. The dosing range of HCTZ is 6.25 to 50 mg PO QD. *Advantages:* safe, inexpensive. *Disadvantages:* may result in hypokalemia, impaired glucose tolerance (usually not clinically significant); increased uric acid levels and risk of gout, and increased plasma lipids. Some evidence indicates that when used alone the non–potassium sparing thiazides may increase mortality. Dyazide and Maxzide are combinations of HCTZ and triamterene and are potassium sparing. Long term, the potassium-sparing diuretics are less expensive, since they do not require potassium monitoring and replacement.
2. ***Beta-blockers*** (nadalol, atenolol, metoprolol, propranolol, and others) reduce cardiac output (negative inotropic and chronotropic effects) but increase peripheral resistance. Also useful to treat angina and arrhythmias and as prophylaxis against migraines. Generally felt to be most effective in the younger patient with a "hyperdynamic" cardiovascular system as evidenced by elevated resting pulse (high normal or tachycardic) and excessive response of blood pressure to exercise. *Advantages:* many are relatively inexpensive and effective. *Disadvantages:* relatively contraindicated in CHF, may cause significant bradycardia or AV block, sedation, fatigue, bronchospasm in patients with asthma,

erectile dysfunction, impaired glucose tolerance, possibly elevated uric acid and plasma lipids (except those with ISA activity). May mask symptoms of hypoglycemia in diabetics. Should not be withdrawn abruptly, especially in patients with coronary artery disease, because rebound tachycardia and hypertension may occur. Labetalol is a unique agent that provides both alpha-blockade and (predominantly) beta-blockade. It tends to cause less bradycardia than other agents do and has a direct peripheral vasodilating effect.

3. ***Central sympatholytics.*** Methyldopa, clonidine, guanabenz, and guanfacine. Sedation and fatigue may occur. A withdrawal syndrome may occur with abrupt cessation (especially clonidine).
4. ***Alpha-blockers.*** Prazosin and terazosin. Severe orthostatic hypotension may occur with first dose. Fluid retention may occur. Sedation and headache are commonly seen early during treatment but tend to diminish with time. These drugs are good choices in elderly men who have hypertension and benign prostatic hypertrophy.
5. ***Arterial vasodilators.*** Hydralazine and minoxidil. Both are potent vasodilators and may cause reflex tachycardia and fluid retention. Should be used only with a diuretic and sympathetic inhibitor (such as a beta-blocker). Should not be used in patients with angina. Minoxidil is usually reserved for severe hypertension. A lupuslike syndrome has been seen with hydralazine.
6. ***Calcium-channel blockers.*** Verapamil, diltiazem, nicardipine, nifedipine, amlodipine, and others. Verapamil and diltiazem both slow AV nodal conduction. Both also have some negative inotropic effect (especially verapamil) and peripheral vasodilatory effects. Calcium-channel blockers generally do not adversely affect glucose tolerance or plasma lipids. They may be especially appropriate in the patient who needs both antianginal and an antihypertensive drug. Mild edema and constipation are frequent side effects of calcium-channel blockers. Orthostatic hypotension and reflex tachycardia can occur, particularly with nifedipine. There is some concern that nifedipine may increase cardiac mortality. This remains to be confirmed.
7. ***ACE inhibitors*** (angiotensin-converting enzyme inhibitors). Captopril, enalapril, lisinopril, and others. All are effective for HTN and have been used in CHF. Captopril requires more frequent dosing. All may contribute to hyperkalemia and cause reversible decreased renal function. Side effects tend to be minimal with no significant sedation, fatigue, or exercise intolerance in most patients. Occasional patients may have trouble with persistent cough; aspirin 325 mg PO QD may decrease cough as may

indomethacin or inhaled cromolyn. However, switching to another ACE inhibitor does not improve the cough caused by these agents. Angioedema occurs in a small subset of patients taking ACE inhibitors and may be life threatening. Patients should be warned about this possibility. Patients at high risk for adverse renal effects include those with connective tissue disease, bilateral renal artery stenosis, or preexisting renal insufficiency. ACE inhibitors may have a favorable effect in preserving renal function or in slowing the progression of proteinuria in chronic renal failure. They also facilitate cardiac remodeling.

8. ***Angiotensin II type 1 receptor antagonists.*** If ACE inhibitors are poorly tolerated by a patient, consideration should be given to losartan (Cozaar), a member of this new drug class. Losartan antagonizes the action of angiotensin II by displacing it from its receptor. It thereby inhibits angiotensin II–induced vascular smooth muscle contraction, aldosterone release, and adrenal and presynaptic catecholamine release, among other effects. Losartan does not stimulate cough and has been shown to be as effective as enalapril in controlling hypertension. It does not adversely affect lipid parameters or glucose levels. Because of its uricosuric activity it reduces serum uric acid levels.

D. **Follow-up study.** Initially patients should be scheduled for frequent office visits until blood pressure is adequately controlled and potential side-effects are evaluated. Thereafter, visits may be scheduled every 3 to 6 months. Laboratory evaluation should include those indicated by the medications they are using (such as K^+ level if receiving diuretics).

SYNCOPE

I. DEFINITION

Be sure to differentiate between near syncope and vertigo. The differential diagnosis is different. See Chapter 14 for work-up and differential of vertigo.

A. **Syncope** is a sudden, brief loss of consciousness (LOC) and, strictly speaking, is related to abrupt cerebral hypoperfusion.

B. **Near syncope** is a sense of impending LOC or weakness, occurs more frequently, and provides valuable diagnostic clues, since the patient usually has better recollection of the event.

C. **Frequency of causes.** 55% vasovagal, 10% cardiac, 10% neurologic, 5% metabolic or drug-induced, 5% "other," and 10% undiagnosed causes.

II. CAUSES OF SYNCOPE AND NEAR SYNCOPE

A. **Cardiac and circulatory.**

1. ***Vasodepressor syncope*** (vasovagal syncope) is the most common cause and tends to be familial. It occurs when a

susceptible person is confronted with a stressful situation. *Prodromal symptoms:* restlessness, pallor, weakness, sighing, yawning, diaphoresis, and nausea. These symptoms may be followed by light-headedness, blurred vision, collapse, and LOC. Occasionally, mild clonic seizures occur, but a seizure work-up is not indicated unless other signs point in this direction. Spells are brief in duration with prompt recovery on recumbency. These episodes may be recurrent.

2. ***Orthostatic hypotension*** is a fall in BP when one is assuming an upright position. It is seen in a variety of settings:
   a. Hypovolemia (hemorrhage, vomiting, diarrhea, diuretics).
   b. Interference with normal reflexes (nitrates, vasodilators, calcium-channel blockers, neuroleptics).
   c. Autonomic failure. Primary or secondary. Diabetes most common form of secondary autonomic neuropathy, whereas advanced age is a common cause of primary autonomic failure. Also consider Shy-Dragger syndrome (autonomic failure with CNS symptoms).
3. ***Outflow obstruction.*** IHSS, aortic stenosis, mitral stenosis, pulmonic stenosis, and subclavian steal syndrome. These patients may present with exertional syncope. Mechanical valve malfunction may also cause outflow obstruction.
4. ***Myocardial ischemia or infarction.***
5. ***Arrhythmias.***
   a. Bradyarrhythmias: sick sinus syndrome, AV-node blocks, etc.
   b. Tachyarrhythmias: PSVT, Wolf-Parkinson-White syndrome, ventricular tachycardia, etc.
6. ***Carotid sinus hypersensitivity.*** Syncope may occur with shaving or wearing a tight collar. Rarely the cartoid sinus may be stimulated by tumor.

B. Metabolic causes. Episodes are usually amplified by exertion but may occur when patient is supine. The onset and resolution are usually prolonged.

1. Hypoxia, as with shunting in congenital heart disease.
2. Hyperventilation. Results in cerebral vasoconstriction with symptoms of breathlessness, anxiety, circumoral tingling, paresthesias of hands or feet, carpopedal spasm, and, occasionally, unilateral or bilateral chest pain. Patients can reproduce these spells by hyperventilating in a controlled environment.
3. Hypoglycemia.
4. Alcohol intoxication.

C. Neurologic causes. Transient ischemic attacks (TIAs) rarely if ever cause syncope. To do so the reticular activating system must be involved. When this occurs, there are "always" other neurologic manifestations such as cranial nerve abnormalities.

1. Migraine. Second most common cause in adolescents. LOC is followed by headache.
2. Seizure. Usually easily differentiated by aura, history of tonic-clonic movements, and postictal state.
3. Abrupt rise of intracranial pressure as seen with subarachnoid hemorrhage or obstructive colloid cyst of the third ventricle.

D. **Reflex syncope** results from impaired right-sided heart filling and global cerebral hypoperfusion. The patient is usually standing upright before an episode because gravitational pooling of blood plays a role in its cause. Potential causes include pulmonary embolism or infarction, pericardial tamponade, pulmonary hypertension, a pregnant uterus as it compresses the inferior vena cava, and coughing, which decreases preload by increasing intrathoracic pressure.

E. **Miscellaneous**

1. Cough syncope.
2. Postmicturition syncope.
3. Psychogenic.
4. Severe visceral or ligamentous pain.
5. May also occur subsequent to severe vertigo.

III. EVALUATION

A. **History** is the most important part of evaluation. The patient and witnesses should be questioned as to precipitating circumstances, prodromal symptoms, time course of onset and recovery, and medication history.

B. **Physical exam.**

1. BP and pulse supine and standing.
2. Auscultation of subclavian and carotid arteries.
3. Cardiac exam with attention to murmurs, extra heart sounds. Provocative maneuvers (Valsalva) as indicated.
4. Careful neurologic exam.

C. **Laboratory studies** should be directed by history and physical exam but are not all inclusive! May include blood glucose, blood gases, electrolytes, and hematocrit.

D. **ECG/Holter Ambulatory Monitoring/Event monitor.** Event monitors that are worn for a month and activated when patient has a feeling of palpations or near syncope are more cost effective and sensitive than 24 to 48 hours of ambulatory monitoring.

E. Signal-averaged ECG may be helpful in patients suspected of having ventricular arrhythmias.

F. **Echocardiography.** Useful in evaluating valvular and myocardial disease.

G. **EEG.** Obtain if seizure disorder is suspected; however, may be falsely negative in 50% of cases. Nasopharyngeal leads, sleep deprivation, and hyperventilation may all increase yield.

H. Electrophysiologic invasive cardiac studies may be indicated in patients with structural heart disease and unexplained syncope, or a history that is suggestive of an arrhythmia.

I. The tilt test is not helpful because of its low specificity.

IV. TREATMENT. Dependent on cause.

A. No treatment is indicated for vasovagal syncope except avoiding stimuli that trigger syncope. The frequency of cough syncope might be reduced by antitussives.

B. Medical. See appropriate section based on diagnosis. Antiepileptics, antiarrhythmics, mineralocorticoids (for chronic orthostatic hypotension), or migraine prophylaxis will all be useful in selected cases.

C. Surgical. For critical aortic stenosis, carotid artery disease, etc.

DYSLIPIDEMIAS

I. CLASSIFICATION

A. May be grouped on the basis of serum lipid concentrations and electrophoretic patterns, genotype, or by pathophysiologic features (Table 2-2).

B. May be classified as primary, which includes familial hyperlipidemia.

C. Secondary causes.

1. ***Exogenous.*** Alcohol, oral contraceptives, estrogens, androgens, corticosteroids, diuretics (thiazides), beta-blockers, obesity, and high-cholesterol diet.
2. ***Endocrine and metabolic.*** Diabetes, hypothyroidism, Cushing's or Addison's diseases, hepatic disease, nephrotic syndrome.
3. ***Miscellaneous.*** Pregnancy, pancreatitis, SLE.

II. EVALUATION AND INITIAL THERAPY

Recommendations of the American Heart Association and the American College of Physicians differ.

A. Initial classification is based on total cholesterol.

1. <200 desirable, repeat every 5 years.
2. 200 to 240 borderline.
3. >240 high.

B. If, on repeat testing, cholesterol is >240 or 200 to 240 and the patient has CHD or two CHD risk factors (age [men >45, women >55], family history of premature CHD in first-degree relative [men <55, women <65], premature menopause without estrogen replacement, smoking, HTN, HDL <35, diabetes, obesity, history of cerebral or peripheral vascular disease), *then* obtain full lipid profile after a 12 to 14-hour fast. When risk factors are being evaluated, if

TABLE 2-2

Classification of Lipoprotein Disorders by Phenotypes, Genotypes, and Corresponding Clinical Manifestations

	Plasma lipid levels					
Phenotype	Cholesterol	Triglyceride	Lipoprotein in excess	Genotype	Xanthomas	Other clinical manifestations
I	Normal or ↑	↑ Lipemia	Chylomicrons	Familial lipoprotein lipase deficiency. Apo C-II deficiency	Eruptive, tuberoeruptive	Recurrent abdominal pain, other gastroin-testinal symptoms, hepatosplenomegaly
IIA	Normal	↑	LDL	FHC, familial combined hyperlipidemia–polygenic and sporadic hypercholesterolemia	Tendinous, xanthelasma, tuberous; planar (homozygous)	Premature CAD, arcus corneae, aortic stenosis (homozy-gous FHC), arthritic symptoms
IIB	↑	↑	LDL + VLDL	Familial combined hyper-lipidemia, FHC		
III	↑	↑	VLDL + LDL	Familial dysbetalipoprotein-emia	Planar (especially palmar), tuberous	Premature CAD and peripheral vascular disease, male > female, obesity, abnormal glucose tolerance, hyper-uricemia, aggravated by hypothyroidism, good response to therapy

IV	Normal or ↑	↑	VLDL	Familial hypertriglyceridemia, familial combined hyperlipidemia, sporadic hypertriglyceridemia	Usually none; rarely eruptive or tuberoeruptive	CAD and peripheral vascular disease, obesity, abnormal glucose tolerance, hyperturicemia, arthritic symptoms, gallbladder disease
V	Normal or ↑	↑	Chylomicrons + VLDL	Homozygous FHC	Eruptive, tuberoeruptive	Recurrent abdominal pain, other gastrointestinal symptoms, hepatosplenomegaly, peripheral paresthesia

CAD, Coronary artery disease; *FHC,* familial hypercholesterolemia; *IDL,* intermediate-density lipoprotein; *LDL,* low-density lipoprotein; *VLDL,* very-low-density lipoprotein.

the patient has HDL >60, one risk factor may be subtracted from the total.

C. If total cholesterol is borderline and <2 risk factors, initiate step-1 diet.

D. Can also classify on the basis of LDL level.

1. *LDL calculation.* LDL = Total chol − (TG/5) − HDL
2. <130 desirable. Repeat every 5 years.
   a. If the patient has <2 risk factors and no CHD, then:
      (1) Step-1 diet if >160 mg/dl.
      (2) Diet and medication if >190 mg/dl.
      (3) The goal for these patients is an LDL <160 mg/dl. Repeat lipid profile annually to monitor LDL level.
   b. If the patients has >2 risk factors and no CHD, then:
      (1) Diet if >130 mg/dl.
      (2) Diet and medication if >160 mg/dl.
      (3) The goal of therapy is an LDL <130 mg/dl.
   c. If the patient has coronary artery disease (patients with angina, survivors of MI), then:
      (1) Diet if LDL >100 mg/dl.
      (2) Diet and medication if LDL >130 mg/dl.
      (3) The goal of therapy is LDL <100 mg/dl.
      (4) In patients who do not reach target LDL level, may change drugs or add a second agent to regimen.

E. Initiation of step-1 diet. Reduce total fat to <30%, saturated fat to <10% of calories, reduce cholesterol to <300 mg/day.

F. Check cholesterol in 6 weeks and 3 months. If no improvement, refer to dietitian for retrial of step-1 diet, or advance to step-2 diet: Reduce saturated fat to <7%, reduce cholesterol to <200 mg/day.

G. Exercise, weight loss, and smoking cessation should also be part of the program.

H. Administer above for 3- to 6-month trial. If no improvement, consider pharmacologic therapy.

I. Triglyceride levels. A triglyceride level of <250 mg/dl is desirable. The risk for CHD may begin to increase at >250 mg/dl.

1. If the triglyceride level is >250 mg/dl, then recommend weight loss, a low-fat diet (<10% fat), exercise, and reduced alcohol consumption.
2. If the TG level is >1000, the patient has an increased risk of pancreatitis.

J. American College of Physicians recommends the following as screening guidelines:

1. Total cholesterol screening is not to be performed in men younger than 35 or women younger than 45 unless:
   a. There is suspicion of a lipoprotein disorder by either history or physical examination.
   b. The patient has at least two other CHD risk factors.

2. Cholesterol screening for the primary prevention of CHD is appropriate but not mandatory for 35- to 65-year-old men and 45- to 65-year-old women.
3. There is insufficient evidence to recommend or discourage screening for the primary prevention of CHD in patients 65 to 75 years of age.
4. Screening is not recommended for patient >75 years of age.
5. All patients with CHD or peripheral vascular or cerebrovascular disease should undergo periodic lipid evaluation.

III. PHARMACOLOGIC THERAPY

A. **Bile acid sequestrants and resins** (colestipol, cholestyramine) decrease total and LDL cholesterol by 20% to 40%. Considered drugs of choice for isolated LDL elevation because of low incidence of systemic side effects. Start at 4 g BID and increase to 16 to 24 g/day. Constipation and GI upset are frequent side effects, which may be alleviated somewhat by increasing dietary fiber and adding psyllium laxatives. Resins may increase TG and should be used with caution in patients with elevated TG. Often used with other agents such as niacin, lovastatin, or gemfibrozil. May affect the GI absorption of other drugs; other medications should be taken 1 to 2 hours before or 4 hours after resin dose. Levels of concurrent medications (such as digoxin or PT/INR for patients receiving warfarin) should be monitored.

B. **Nicotinic acid (niacin)** decreases both LDL and TG, increases HDL. Also lowers lipoprotein A blood levels. Common side effects include skin flushing, GI upset, elevation in serum glucose, elevated liver enzymes, and elevated uric acid. Rare side effects can include headaches, worsening of peptic ulcer disease, cardiac dysrhythmias, and elevations in serum muscle enzymes. Tolerance to minor side effects (flushing, nausea) can be improved if one starts with low doses (100 mg BID-TID) and takes with meals. The maximum dose is 3 g QD. Taking 325 mg of aspirin 30 to 60 minutes before niacin decreases flushing. The sustained-release preparations of niacin are hepatotoxic and should not be used.

C. **HMG CoA reductase inhibitors** (lovastatin, simvastatin, pravastatin, atorvastatin) inhibit HMG CoA reductase, which is the rate-limiting enzyme in the production of cholesterol by the liver. These agents reduce total cholesterol and LDL. A slight to moderate decrease in TG and an increase in HDL may occur, especially with atorvastatin. Side effects are rare and include elevated liver function test results, elevated muscle creatinine phosphokinase secondary to myopathy, and rarely rhabdomyolysis. The Scandinavian Simvastatin Survival Study demonstrated improved survival in both male and female patients treated with the aforementioned drug. A metanalysis of pravastatin therapy showed it to reduce the incidence of MI by 62% after 1 year. Pravastatin has also been shown angiographically to reduce the rate of atherosclerotic plaque progression compared to placebo. The starting dose of simvastatin is 5 to 10 mg PO QP.M. and can be titrated up to a maximum dose of 40 mg PO QP.M. Pravastatin is started at 10 to 20 mg PO QHS and can be titrated to 40 mg PO QHS. Repeat fasting serum lipid levels can be obtained at 4- to 6-week intervals until the desired adjustments are achieved.

D. **Fibric acid derivatives** (gemfibrozil, clofibrate). Use of clofibrate has declined because of one large trial showing an increase in GI cancers and increased overall mortality. Gemfibrozil is still used to decrease VLDL synthesis and lower fasting TG. It may increase HDL and has a variable effect on LDL. GI side effects common. Rare side effects: myalgias, increase in liver or muscle enzymes, headache, gallstones, arrhythmias, hypokalemia, anemia, and leukopenia. Can potentiate oral hypoglycemics and warfarin.

E. **Probucol.** Originally developed as an antioxidant. Decreases total and LDL cholesterol. Also decreases HDL. Commonly causes QT prolongation on ECG.

F. **Fish oils** (omega-3 fatty acids) decrease VLDL synthesis, may decrease chylomicrons (and therefore TG). May reduce risk of acute pancreatitis in patients with severe hypertriglyceridemia. Clinical trials underway regarding role of fish oils in slowing progression of CAD.

PROPHYLAXIS AGAINST BACTERIAL ENDOCARDITIS

I. GENERAL COMMENTS

Endocarditis can occur from transient bacteremia. Because a variety of health care procedures can result in bacteremia, prophylaxis against bacteria that can adhere to endocardium is recommended, particularly in patients at high risk for endocarditis. The frequency of bacteremia is highest subsequent to oral and dental procedures (because of the abundant oral flora), intermediate for genitourinary procedures, and lowest for diagnostic procedures of the gastrointestinal tract. It is important to give prophylactic antibiotics before a procedure because bacterial adhesion can occur within minutes after bacteremia develops.

II. ENDOCARDITIS PROPHYLAXIS RECOMMENDED

A. Cardiac conditions.

1. Prosthetic cardiac valves (including bioprosthetic, homograft, and mechanical).
2. Previous episode of bacterial endocarditis.
3. Most congenital cardiac defects (especially cyanotic congenital heart disease, patent ductus arteriosus, ventricular septal defects, and surgically repaired intracar-

diac defects with residual hemodynamic abnormalities).

4. Valvular heart disease resulting from rheumatic or other disease (aortic regurgitation and stenosis, mitral regurgitation and stenosis).
5. Hypertrophic cardiomyopathy.
6. Mitral valve prolapse with regurgitation.

B. Dental or surgical procedures.

1. Dental or surgical procedures that cause gingival or mucosal bleeding, including mechanical dental hygienic procedures.
2. Tonsillectomy or adenoidectomy.
3. Surgical procedures involving upper respiratory or gastrointestinal mucosa.
4. Rigid bronchoscopy.
5. Sclerotherapy of esophageal varices.
6. Esophageal dilatation.
7. Gallbladder surgery.
8. Urethral catheterization or urinary tract surgery if infection present.
9. Prostate surgery.
10. I & D of infected tissue.
11. Vaginal hysterectomy.
12. Vaginal delivery in the presence of infection (chorioamnionitis, etc.)

III. ENDOCARDITIS PROPHYLAXIS NOT RECOMMENDED

A. Cardiac conditions.

1. Previous coronary artery bypass surgery.
2. Mitral valve prolapse without regurgitation. (If MPV is associated with thickening or redundancy of valve leaflets, may have increased risk of endocarditis, especially in men >45 years of age).
3. Functional or innocuous heart murmurs.
4. Cardiac pacemakers and implantable defibrillators.
5. Isolated secundum atrial septal defect.
6. 6 months or more status after surgical repair of PDA, VSD without residua.
7. Previous rheumatic heart disease or Kawasaki disease without valve dysfunction.

B. Dental or surgical procedures.

1. Dental procedures not likely to cause gingival bleeding such as fillings above the gum line, adjustment of orthodontic appliances.
2. Injection of intraoral anesthetics.
3. Shedding of primary teeth.
4. Tympanostomy tube insertion.
5. Endotracheal intubation, flexible bronchoscopy with or without biopsy specimens.

6. Cardiac catheterization.
7. Endoscopy with or without biopsy.
8. In absence of infection, urethral catheterization, D&C, uncomplicated vaginal delivery, abortion, sterilization procedures, insertion or removal of an IUD, or laparoscopy.

IV. STANDARD REGIMENS

A. Dental, oral, upper respiratory tract.

1. *For adults.* Amoxicillin 3.0 g PO 1 hour before procedure, then 1.5 g 6 hours later.
2. *In penicillin-allergic patients.* Erythromycin ethylsuccinate 800 mg, or erythromycin stearate 1.0 g PO 2 hours before procedure, then 1/2 dose 6 hours after initial dose. Clindamycin 300 mg 1 hour before procedure and 150 mg 6 hours after initial dose is another alternative.
3. *If unable to take oral medications.* Ampicillin 2.0 g IV or IM 30 minutes before procedure, then 1.0 g IV or IM 6 hours after initial dose. Alternative: clindamycin 300 mg IV 30 minutes before procedure, then 150 mg IV or PO 6 hours later.
4. *In the high-risk, penicillin-allergic patient.* Vancomycin 1.0 g IV over 1 hour, starting 1 hour before surgery. A repeat dose is not necessary.

B. GI or GU procedures.

1. Ampicillin 2.0 g IV + Gentamicin 1.5 mg/kg IV (not to exceed 80 mg) 30 minutes before procedure, then amoxicillin 1.5 g PO 6 hours later, or repeat IV regimen 8 hours after first dose.
2. In pencillin-allergic patients. Vancomycin 1.0 g IV (over 1 hour) starting 1 hour before procedure + Gentamicin 1.5 mg/kg IV (not to exceed 80 mg) 1 hour before. May be repeated 8 hours later.
3. Low risk. Amoxicillin 3.0 g 1 hour before and 1.5 g 6 hours after procedure.

C. Pediatric dosages (initial).

1. Amoxicillin-ampicillin 50 mg/kg.
2. Erythromycin ethylsuccinate or stearate 20 mg/kg.
3. Clindamycin 10 mg/kg.
4. Gentamicin 2.0 mg/kg.
5. Vancomycin 20 mg/kg.

Total pediatric dose should not exceed adult dose. Follow-up dose is 1/2 initial dose.

BIBLIOGRAPHY

Acute Infarction Ramipril Efficacy (AIRE) Study Investigators: Effect of ramipril on mortality and morbidity of survivors of acute myocardial infarction with clinical evidence of heart failure, *Lancet* 342:821, 1993.

Adams JE et al: Diagnosis of perioperative myocardial infarction with measurement of cardiac troponin I, *N Engl J Med* 330:670, 1994.

Alpert JS, Rippe JM: *Manual of cardiovascular diagnosis and therapy*, ed 3, Boston, 1991, Little, Brown & Co.

Baker DW, Wright RF: Management of heart failure, IV. Anticoagulation for patients with heart failure due to left ventricular systolic dysfunction, *JAMA* 272:1614, 1994.

Baker DW et al: Management of heart failure, III. The role of revascularization in the treatment of patients with moderate or severe left ventricular systolic dysfunction, *JAMA* 272:1528, 1994.

Baker DW et al: Management of heart failure, *JAMA* 272:1361, 1994.

Barnett JC et al: Sublingual captopril in the treatment of acute heart failure, *Curr Therap Res* 49(2):274, 1991.

Bean LC: Cardiac imaging after acute myocardial infarction, *Postgrad Med* 92:8, 1992.

Bellandi F et al: Propafenone and sotalol in the prevention of paroxysmal atrial fibrillation: long-term safety and efficacy study, *Curr Therap Res* 56(11):1154, 1995.

Bisno AL: Rheumatic fever. In Wyngaarden JB et al, editors: *Cecil textbook of medicine,* Philadelphia, 1992, Saunders.

Bonow RO, Udelson JE: Left ventricular diastolic dysfunction as a cause of congestive heart failure, *Ann Intern Med* 117: 502, 1992.

Bovill EG et al: Hemorrhagic events during therapy with recombinant tissue-type plasminogen activator, heparin, and aspirin for acute myocardial infarction, *Ann Intern Med* 115:256, 1991.

Byington RP et al: Reduction in cardiovascular events during pravastatin therapy: pooled analysis of clinical events of the Pravastatin Atherosclerosis Intervention Program, *Circulation* 92:2419, 1995.

Cairns JA et al: Antithrombotic agents in coronary artery disease, *Chest* 102:4, 1992.

Cairns JA et al: Coronary thrombolysis, *Chest* 102:4, 1992.

Cannegeiter SC et al: Optimal oral anticoagulant therapy in patients with mechanical heart valves, *N Engl J Med* 333:11, 1995.

Chatterjee K: Use of angiotensin converting enzyme inhibitors, *Heart Disease and Stroke* 1:3, 1992.

Chun SH et al: Long-term efficacy of amiodarone for the maintenance of normal sinus rhythm in patients with refractory atrial fibrillation or flutter, *Am J Cardiol* 76(16):47, 1995.

Cody RJ: Comparing angiotensin-converting enzyme inhibitor trial results in patients with acute myocardial infarction, *Arch Intern Med* 154:2029-2036, 1994.

Cohn JN et al: A comparison of enalapril with hydralazine–isosorbide dinitrate in the treatment of chronic congestive heart failure, *N Engl J Med* 325:303, 1991.

Dalal JN, Jain AC: Chronic stable angina pectoris: risk factor stratification and treatment, *Postgrad Med* 91:4, 1992.

Devereux RB: Diagnosis and prognosis of mitral-valve prolapse, *N Engl J Med* 320:1077, 1989.

Dormans T et al: Diuretic efficacy of high dose furosemide in severe heart failure bolus injection vs. continuous infusion, *J Am Coll Cardiol* 28(2):376, 1996.

Durack DT: Prevention of infective endocarditis, *N Engl J Med* 332:38, 1995. Emergency Cardiac Care Committee and Subcommittees, American Heart Association: Guidelines for cardiopulmonary resuscitation and emergency cardiac care, *JAMA* 268:16, 1992.

Falk RH et al: Digoxin for atrial fibrillation: a drug whose time has gone? *Ann Intern Med* 114(7):573, 1991.

Garg R, Yusuf S: Overview of randomized trials of angiotensin-converting enzyme inhibitors on mortality and morbidity in patients with heart failure, *JAMA* 273:1450, 1995.

Gilkson M, Espinosa RE, Hayes DL: Expanding indications for permanent pacemakers, *Ann Intern Med* 123:443, 1995.

Gilligan DM et al: A double-blind, placebo-controlled crossover trial of nadolol and verapamil in mild and moderately symptomatic hypertrophic cardiomyopathy, *J Am Coll Cardiol* 21:1672-1679, 1993.

Hamm CW et al: A randomized study of coronary angioplasty compared with bypass surgery in patients with symptomatic multivessel coronary disease, *N Engl J Med* 331:1037, 1994.

Harper KJ: Antihypertensive therapy: current issues and challenges, *Postgrad Med* 91:6, 1992.

Hillis DL et al: *Manual of clinical problems in cardiology,* Boston, 1988, Little, Brown & Co.

Hopson JR, Kienzle MG: Evaluation of patients with syncope, *Postgrad Med* 91:5, 1992.

ISIS-2 Collaborative Group: Randomised trial of intravenous streptokinase, oral aspirin, or neither among 17,187 cases of suspected acute myocardial infarction: ISIS-2, *Lancet* 2:349, 1988.

ISIS-3 Collaborative Group: ISIS-3: a randomised comparison of streptokinase vs tissue plasminogen activator vs anistreplase and of aspirin plus heparin vs aspirin alone among 41,299 cases of suspected acute myocardial infarction, *Lancet* 339:753, 1992.

ISIS-4 Collaborative Group: ISIS-4: a randomised factorial trial assessing early oral captopril, oral mononitrate, and intravenous magnesium sulphate in 58,050 patients with suspected acute myocardial infarction, *Lancet* 345:669, 1995.

Jaffe AS: Prophylactic lidocaine for acute myocardial infarction: an update, *Heart Disease and Stroke* 1:4, 1992.

Karon BL: Diagnosis and outpatient management of congestive heart failure, *Mayo Clin Proc* 70:1080, 1995.

Kendall MJ et al: Beta-blockers and sudden cardiac death, *Ann Intern Med* 123(5):358, 1995.

Kienzle MG: Syncope: pursuing the common and prognostically important causes, *Heart Disease and Stroke* 1:3, 1992.

Kinch JW, Ryan TJ: Right ventricular infarction, *N Engl J Med* 330:1211, 1994.

King SB et al: A randomized trial comparing coronary angioplasty with coronary bypass surgery, *N Engl J Med* 331:1044, 1994.

King SB et al: A randomized trial comparing coronary angioplasty with coronary bypass surgery, *N Engl J Med* 331:1044-1050, 1994.

Kirklin JW et al: Coronary bypass: it's status today, *Patient Care* 25:12, 1991.

Kirshenbaum JM: Therapy for acute myocardial infarction: an update, *Heart Disease and Stroke* 1:4, 1992.

Krumholz HM et al: Coronary revascularization after myocardial infarction in the very elderly: outcomes and long-term follow-up, *Ann Intern Med* 119:1084, 1993.

Kulick DL, Rahimtoola SH: Selection of patients for cardiac valve replacement: an update for Braunwald E, editor: *Heart disease,* Philadelphia, 1992, Saunders.

Langes K et al: Efficacy and safety of intravenous captopril in congestive heart failure, *Curr Therap Res* 53(2):167, 1993.

Lee KL et al: Holding GUSTO up to the light, *Ann Intern Med* 120:876-881, 1994.

Lewis EJ et al: The effect of angiotensin-converting-enzyme inhibition on diabetic nephropathy, *N Engl J Med* 329:1456-1462, 1993.

Mamby SA, Kloner RA: Valvular heart disease, *Cardiovasc Rep Res*, pp 27-47, 1991.

Mark DB et al: Cost effectiveness of thrombolytic therapy with tissue plasminogen activator as compared with streptokinase for acute myocardial infarction, *N Engl J Med* 332:1418, 1995.

McCarthy BD et al: Missed diagnosis of acute myocardial infarction in the emergency department: results from a multicenter study, *Ann Emerg Med* 22:579, 1993.

Parmley WW, McBride PE: Congestive heart failure, *American Familyu Physician* monograph, 1992.

Paspa PA, Mavahed A: Thrombolytic therapy in acute myocardial infarction, *Am Fam Phys* 45:2, 1992.

Pasternak RC et al: Acute myocardial infarction. In Braunwald E, editor: *Heart disease,* Philadelphia, 1992, Saunders.

Pfeffer MA: Effect of captopril on mortality and morbidity in patients with left ventricular dysfunction after myocardial infarction: results of the Survival and Ventricular Enlargement Trial, *N Engl J Med* 327:669-677, 1992.

Pitt B et al: Pravastatin limitation of atherosclerosis in the coronary arteries (PLAC 1): reduction in atherosclerosis progression and clinical events, *J Am Coll Cardiol* 26:1133-1139, 1995.

Roden DM: Risks and benefits of antiarrhythmic therapy, *N Engl J Med* 331:785, 1994.

Sackner-Bernstein JD, Mancini DM: Rationale for treatment of patients with chronic heart failure with adrenergic blockade, *JAMA* 274:1462, 1995.

Sanford JP et al: *Guide to antimicrobial therapy,* Dallas, 1995, Antimicrobial Therapy, Inc.

Scandinavian Simvastatin Survival Group: Randomised trial of cholesterol lowering in 4444 patients with coronary heart disease: the Scandinavian Simvastatin Survival Study, *Lancet* 344:1383: 1994.

Selzer A: Changing aspects of the natural history of valvular aortic stenosis, *N Engl J Med* 317:91-97, 1987.

Serneri GG et al: Randomised comparison of subcutaneous heparin, intravenous heparin, and aspirin in unstable angina, *Lancet* 345:1201, 1995.

Sigurdsson E et al: Unrecognized myocardial infarction: epidemiology, clinical characteristics, and the prognostic role of angina pectoris, *Ann Intern Med* 122:96, 1995.

Smith LK: Medical treatment after myocardial infarction, *Postgrad Med* 92:8, 1992.

Stevenson LW et al: the limited reliability of physical signs for estimating hemodynamics in chronic heart failure, *JAMA* 261(6):884, 1989.

The GUSTO Investigators: An international randomized trial comparing four thrombolytic strategies for acute myocardial infarction, *N Engl J Med* 329:673, 1993.

The International Collaborative Study Group: Reduction of infarct size with the early use of timolol in acute myocardial infarction, *N Engl J Med* 311:218, 1984.

The MIAMI Trial Research Group: Metoprolol in acute myocardial infarction (MIAMI): a randomized placebo-controlled international trial, *Eur Heart J* 6:199, 1985.

The SOLVD Investigators: Effect of enalapril on survival in patients with reduced left ventricular ejection fractions and congestive heart failure, *N Engl J Med* 325:293, 1991.

Thomson SP et al: Incremental value of the leukocyte differential and the rapid creatine kinase-MB isoenzyme for the early diagnosis of myocardial infarction, *Ann Intern Med* 122:335-341, 1995.

Villella A et al: Prognostic significance of maximal exercise testing after myocardial infarction treated with thrombolytic agents: the GISSI-2 database, *Lancet* 346:523-529, 1995.

Viscoli CM et al: Beta-blockers after myocardial infarction: influence of first-year clinical course on long-term effectiveness, *Ann Intern Med* 118:99-105, 1993.

Woods KL et al: Intravenous magnesium sulphate in suspected acute myocardial infarction: results of the second Leicester Intravenous Magnesium Intervention Trial (LIMIT 2), *Lancet* 339(8809):1553, 1992.

3

Pulmonary Medicine

Mark A. Graber

PULMONARY EMBOLISM AND DEEP VENOUS THROMBOSIS

I. DEEP VENOUS THROMBOSIS (DVT)

A. Characterized by unilateral swelling and tenderness of the calf and thigh. May be erythematous and warm. These physical findings are present in only 23% to 50% of patients with a DVT.

B. May also have upper-extremity DVT especially in active individuals with repetitive upper arm motions or sports activities.
- May present up to several weeks out from clot formation.

C. Homan's sign (dorsiflexion of the foot causing calf pain) is unreliable.

D. DVTs in the calf rarely embolize; those in thigh and pelvis do. However, serial Doppler studies should be done to follow a calf DVT for propagation into the thigh or pelvis.

E. DVT predisposed to by:
1. Smoking, prior DVT, recent lower extremity surgery or trauma, stasis such as with bed rest (such as MI) or long trips, even as short as 2 hours.
2. Hypercoagulable states including lupus (may have paradoxically elevated PTT), protein C and protein S deficiency, antithrombin III deficiency, estrogen use, cancer, anticardiolipin antibodies, nephrotic syndrome, etc.
3. Recently, a mutation of factor V, factor V Leyden, has been shown to be the most common cause of familial thrombosis.
4. One third of patients with homocystinuria will develop deep venous thrombosis, and elevated levels of homocysteine have been linked to an increased risk of DVT in the elderly. Folate and pyridoxine supplementation can minimize this risk.

F. Diagnosis.
1. Venogram is the standard but is painful, requires a dye load, and may induce DVT formation in a normal extremity.
2. Venous Doppler studies excellent for clots above knee (those with risk of embolization) but not reliable in pelvis or lower leg.
3. Impedance plethysmography is not sensitive.

G. Treatment of DVT.

1. ***Anticoagulate.*** Traditionally, heparin has been dosed as a bolus of 5000 U of heparin and drip at 1000 U/hr in 70 kg adult. *More recently, weight-based nomograms that are more likely to result in a therapeutic anticoagulation have been developed. Start with a bolus of 80 U/kg followed by a drip of 18 U/kg/hr.* Check PTT in 4 hours and adjust heparin drip to keep PTT about 1½ to 2 times normal. Simultaneously, should start warfarin (Coumadin) 5 to 10 mg QHS × 2 or 3 days. Should check PT/PTT Q A.M. Want to maintain an INR of 2.0 to 3.0 (PT 1½ times normal) and should continue patient on warfarin (Coumadin) for at least 3 months. An INR of 3.0 to 4.5 may be appropriate for recurrent disease.
2. Subcutaneous low-molecular-weight heparins are safer and more effective than IV heparin and are generally preferable. They do not affect the PTT, and laboratory monitoring of the PTT is not required. There is also a lower incidence of bleeding and thrombocytopenia than with unfractionated heparin. The best studied up to now and the currently available LMW heparin is enoxaparin, which is dosed at 1 mg/kg SQ Q12h for anticoagulation for DVT or PE. However, *this is not an FDA approved use of this drug* (see below for DVT prophylaxis dose, which is different). Although not standard of care, recent evidence indicates that the subcutaneous administration of enoxaparin at home for DVT may be both safe and effective and may preclude the need for hospital admission.

H. DVT Prophylaxis After Surgery. See p. 399.

II. PULMONARY EMBOLISM

A. Characterized by dyspnea (78%), pleuritic chest pain (59%), cough (43%), tachycardia (30%), tachypnea (73%), rales (55%), syncope (13%), and hypoxia. These symptoms and signs are relatively nonspecific for PE but can help to raise your level of suspicion. Any sign or symptom may be missing in a patient and the absence of one or more symptoms or signs cannot be used to rule out PE.

B. Look for predisposing factors for DVT, which increase likelihood of PE.

C. Look for ventilation-perfusion mismatch by calculating the alveolar (A)–arterial (a) gradient. An elevated A/a gradient is present in 80% to 90% of those with PE.

PAO_2 (alveolar) $= 150 - 1.2(PaCO_2)$

A/a gradient $=$ PaO_2 (alveolar) $-$ PaO_2 (arterial)

Normal:
Age less than 20: 3-4
Age 20 to 60: 4-6
Age >60: 6-8

D. Testing for pulmonary embolism.

1. Angiography is the gold standard and is safe.
2. A chest radiograph and ECG should be done to rule out other causes of dyspnea and tachypnea but are not sensitive or specific enough to rule out PE if normal.
3. O_2 saturation and ABG may be normal or abnormal and cannot be used to differentiate between those with or without PE although they do change your pretest probability.
4. ***Ventilation-perfusion scanning*** (V/Q scanning).
   a. Must use caution with interpretation.
   b. Isolated perfusion scanning probably as good as V/Q scanning if it is entirely normal.
   c. Possible V/Q scan outcomes:
      (1) High-probability scan in patient with high clinical suspicion has a 96% probability of having PE.
      (2) Low-probability scan in patient with low clinical suspicion still has 4% possibility of having PE.
      (3) Normal V/Q scan with low clinical suspicion still has 2% possibility of PE.
      (4) Those with medium- and low-probability scans with a moderate clinical suspicion have 33% and 12% rate of angiographically proved PE and are therefore not adequate to rule out PE.
      (5) Intermediate V/Q scans or any other combination other than what is listed above is not clinically useful.
      (6) Spiral CT is useful to demonstrate central PE but is less sensitive for subsegmental PE than V/Q scanning is.
   d. If a patient has swollen leg and symptoms are suggestive of PE, consider examination of the extremity for DVT first, since will need to anticoagulate anyway. However, 30% of patients with angiographically proved PE will not have an obvious source on Doppler scanning and venogram.
   e. D-dimer, a marker for thrombosis and fibrinolysis, can be useful in the exclusion of PE. In those with non–high probability scans and a history suggestive of PE, a D-dimer of less than 300 ng/ml has an approximately 100% sensitivity and a negative predicative value for PE. If a latex agglutination test is used, the cutoff is 500 ng/ml. Contact your lab about their cutoff value. However, specificity is only 26%. Most people without PE have an elevated D-dimer.
5. ***Treatment.***
   a. Treat as for any respiratory distress including O_2, monitoring hospitalization, fluid resuscitation for secondary right-sided heart failure, dopamine, etc. (See Chapter 1 for treatment of shock, p. 48.)
   b. Anticoagulate per DVT above.

- Heparin prevents PE-induced pulmonary vasoconstriction and V/Q shunt.

c. If patient is hypoxic or hemodynamically unstable and has not responded to stabilization measures including heparin, aggressive fluids, intubation, and 100% O_2, can consider use of thrombolytics if have documented PE.
   (1) Regimens approved by FDA include:
      (a) Streptokinase 250,000 IU over 30 minutes followed by 100,000 IU/hr for 24 to 72 hours.
      (b) TPA 100 mg as continuous infusion over 2 hours.
   (2) Still require heparin anticoagulation. Low-molecular-weight heparin, though not approved for this indication, is more effective than unfractionated heparin and has fewer side effects. See treatment of DVT above.
   (3) Menustration is not a contraindication to the use of thrombolytics or heparin if they are needed to treat PE. Data are anecdotal, but up to now there have been no bleeding problems.

d. Continue using anticoagulation (warfarin) for at least 3 months (see above).

e. In those in whom anticoagulation is contraindicated either acutely or for chronic use or is ineffective, consider vena cava interruption with a filter such as the Greenfield filter.

PLEURAL EFFUSION (HYDROTHORAX)

A. Definition. An abnormal accumulation of fluid in the pleural space.

B. Three categories based on underlying illness.

1. Transudates from vessels leaking into the pleural space secondary to increased hydrostatic pressure (such as CHF) or decreased intravascular oncotic pressure (such as hypoproteinemia or anasarca).
   - Differential diagnosis includes cardiac, renal, or hepatic failure; hyponatremia; superior vena cava obstruction; hypoalbuminemia.
2. Exudates of an inflammatory nature.
   - Differential diagnosis includes rheumatoid arthritis, SLE, sarcoidosis, TB, pancreatitis, esophageal rupture.
3. Illnesses that can cause exudates or transudates include trauma, neoplasms, infection, pulmonary embolism, idiopathic.

C. Clinically.

1. Generally have dyspnea, tachycardia, and orthopnea. The course of symptom onset is variable and may be either abrupt or gradual.

2. Will have decreased breath sounds and increased dullness to percussion if effusion >300 ml.

D. Diagnosis.

1. ***Chest radiograph shows effusion.*** Will layer out on recumbency if not loculated. May have fluid in fissures, blunting of the costophrenic angles.
2. ***Pleurocentesis.*** Send fluid for specific gravity, pH, glucose, cell count, differential diagnosis, amylase, total protein, LDH, culture for aerobes, anaerobes and mycobacteria, Gram stain, AFB stain, cytologic analysis, CEA as indicated.
3. Laboratory differentiation.
   - ***Specific gravity.*** Under 1.016 is suggestive of a transudate.
   - ***Protein.*** Less than 3 g/dl is suggestive of a transudate.
   - ***Pleural fluid protein–to–serum protein ratio.*** <0.5 is suggestive of a transudate.
   - ***Pleural fluid LDH–to–serum LDH ratio.*** <0.6 is suggestive of a transudate.
4. ***Work-up.*** Can include chest CT, bronchoscopy, pleural biopsy (for TB, mesothelioma) depending on clinical presentation. Consider abdominal CT if suspect lymphoma.
5. ***Management.***
   a. Treat underlying disease.
   b. An empyema or effusion should be drained by repeated needle aspirations or a chest tube.
   c. Intrapleural urokinase can be helpful in treating loculated fluid if used early.

HEMOPTYSIS

A. Definition. Expectoration of blood or bloody sputum.

B. Divided into two categories based on whether the problem is a primary pulmonary abnormality or has an extrapulmonary cause.

1. ***Intrapulmonary source.***
   a. Infectious including bronchitis, TB, pneumonia, abscess, fungal infections.
   b. Structural including arteriovenous malformation, tumor, infarction (as from PE), foreign body.
   c. Vascular including Goodpasture's syndrome, pulmonary vasculitis, traumatic vessel disruption.
   d. Cardiac including CHF, mitral stenosis.
2. ***Extrapulmonary sources.***
   a. GI including hematemesis (aspirated blood).
   b. Extrapulmonary structural including epistaxis, oronasopharyngeal lesions.
   c. Systemic coagulopathies including DIC.

C. Diagnosis.

1. History of concomitant illness, presence of shock, presence of vomiting, other bleeding sites, etc.
2. CBC, platelet count, PT/PTT, fibrinogen, fibrin-degradation products, sputum for culture, Gram stain, and AFB stain. Sputum for cytologic analysis is also indicated.
3. A CXR should be done and a chest CT or angiogram may be indicated depending on the clinical situation.

D. Management.

1. In general, treat the underlying disease state.
2. Massive hemoptysis should be treated as per the section on hypovolemic shock, p. 48. Surgery and pulmonary consults should be obtained in the event acute intervention is required to stop the bleeding.
3. Maintain airway and ventilation.
4. Use clinical judgment in making decisions about the need for admission and imminent work-up. If the bleeding is minor and from a self-limited cause (such as bronchitis), patients may be followed as outpatients.

CHRONIC OBSTRUCTIVE PULMONARY DISEASE (COPD)

I. DEFINITION

A generalized increased resistance to airflow during expiration and includes chronic bronchitis, emphysema, chronic asthma, and bronchiolitis. COPD occurs in 10% to 15% of cigarette smokers.

II. CHRONIC BRONCHITIS

A. Characterized by chronic cough productive of mucus for at least 3 months in each of last 2 years.

B. Results from prolonged exposure to pulmonary irritants including cigarettes and allergens, pollution, recurrent infections.

C. Have inflammatory changes in bronchial mucosa.

III. EMPHYSEMA

A. Characterized by destruction of the lung parenchyma beyond the terminal bronchioles with coalescence of alveoli.

B. Divided into:

1. Panlobular, which is the result of alpha$_1$-antitrypsinase deficiency.
2. Centrilobular, which is the result of smoking and of chronic bronchitis.

C. Clinical synopsis. Rarely have pure emphysema or chronic bronchitis. Most patients will have both processes present (Table 3-1).

IV. LABORATORY DATA

A. With acute exacerbations, CBC count, ABG, CXR, and ECG are indicated depending on the clinical situation.

TABLE 3-1
Characteristics of Emphysema Versus Chronic Bronchitis

Characteristic	Emphysema (pink puffer)	Chronic bronchitis (blue bloater)
Body habitus	Thin	Edematous
Age at diagnosis	55 to 75	45 to 65
Smoking history	Common	Common
Cough	Little	Common
Sputum	Little	Very mucoid/mucopurulent
Ronchi	Little	Common
Breath sounds	Decreased	May have wheezing that clears with cough, may have reversible episodes of bronchospasm
Infections (pulmonary)	Infrequent	Frequent
Hypoxia		
At rest	End stage only	Common early
With exertion	May have early	Common early
CO_2 retention	Late only	Common earlier
Diffusing capacity	Reduced	May be normal
Compliance (lung)	Increased	Normal
Spirometry	Obstructive pattern	Obstructive pattern
X-ray film	Decreased markings, hyperinflation, bullae present	Increased markings
Cor pulmonale	Present late in disease	Common
Hematocrit	Normal	May be >55%

1. Hypercapnia with acidosis is suggestive of acute decompensation.
2. A high CO_2 level with a normal pH is suggestive of a compensated chronic state.

B. ECG may show multifocal atrial tachycardia, and if it is present, one should be aware of the possibility of theophylline toxicity.

C. Bedside peak flows can document response to treatment.

V. ACUTE TREATMENT OF COPD

A. See p. 27.

B. Treat any underlying infection as per pneumonia section, p. 136.

C. Hospitalize if clinically indicated (worsening tachypnea, falling O_2, acidosis, increasing CO_2.

D. *Beware if the patient seems too calm. It may indicate CO_2 retention with CO_2 narcosis. This can occur as the result of giving high-flow O_2 to a patient with chronic COPD. However, do not withhold oxygen from a dyspneic patient.*

VI. LONG-TERM MANAGEMENT OF COPD

A. All patients with COPD should have a Pneumovax and yearly flu shot.

B. Patients should be educated about their disease and should be taught that if they start having difficulties with breathing they should contact their health care professional.

C. Low-flow O_2 has been shown to be useful in reducing pulmonary arterial resistance, which, if uncontrolled, leads to cor pulmonale.

1. Use continuous oxygen in those with either a Po_2 <55 mm Hg, an O_2 saturation of <89%, or a Po_2 <59 mm Hg with evidence of cor pulmonale (peripheral edema, HCT >55, P pulmonale on ECG).
2. O_2 saturation should be kept above 90% (Po_2 of 60 to 80 mm Hg).
3. Usually can be accomplished with 2 L/min O_2 but titrate to patient's needs.
4. Survival significantly enhanced with oxygen use 24 hours a day. Patients should be encouraged to use oxygen at least 15 hours a day.

D. **Inhaled bronchodilators.** The use of these medications is predicted on instruction of the patient in their proper use. A spacer should be used with most metered dose inhalers. Additionally patients should be given instructions about what to do if they notice a need for increased amounts of medication to remain symptom free or if their symptoms persist despite the use of normal doses of bronchodilators. Since response varies over time, even those with a poor response on post-bronchodilators PFTs should be given a long-term trial of inhaled bronchodilators.

1. *Beta-adrenergic agonists* (such as albuterol, metaproterenol) to be used PRN for symptoms.
   a. PRN usage seems to provide better control than scheduled use.
   b. Many of those with COPD are resistant to beta-agonists and will respond better to inhaled anticholinergics (below).
   c. *Dose.* One nebulizer of albuterol (2.5 mg) is equal to about 6 to 8 puffs of an MDI via spacer. Patients can use 4 to 8 puffs every 3 to 4 hours as needed but should be instructed on what to do (such as start steroids by mouth) if their need for albuterol increases.
   d. Long-acting beta-agonists such as salmeterol may be used to prevent nocturnal symptoms and to control symptoms during the day. However, salmeterol is not useful for the control of acute symptoms.
2. An *anticholinergic agent* (such as ipratropium) is the bronchodilator of choice in COPD to be used on a PRN basis. Its effect is additive to the inhaled beta-agonists. Normal dose is 2 puffs every 6 hours. Also available for nebulization.
3. Inhaled *steroids* (such as beclomethasone) should be used in almost all with COPD who require more than an occasional use of beta-agonists. Generally, those who are responsive to inhaled bronchodilators and have acute attacks of dyspnea will be responsive to steroids. Oral steroids (such as prednisone) are all helpful but have many side effects and should be reserved for acute exacerbations and for those who do not respond to inhaled steroids.
4. *Theophylline.* Some authors recommend the use of theophylline preparations, but these have a low therapeutic window, and blood levels should be kept between 10 and 15 µg/ml (because of frequent side effects, the FDA has changed the previous recommendation of 10 to 20 µg/ml). Theophylline seems to be a major cause of multifocal atrial tachycardia in those with COPD and is falling out of favor.
5. Long-term antibiotics are not helpful but should be used to treat acute purulent exacerbations. Amoxicillin or amoxicillin/clavulanate 500 mg TID, trimethoprim-sulfamethoxazole (Septra DS) 1 PO BID, or doxycycline 100 mg PO BID are recommended.
6. Pulmonary rehabilitation including conditioning and breathing techniques is helpful.

BRONCHIECTASIS

A. Definition. Bronchiectasis is a chronic dilatation and inflammation of medium-sized bronchi. Clinically it looks similar to chronic bronchitis with chronic mucopurulent sputum production. However, sputum production is often copious and may contain *Pseudomonas* organisms.

B. It occurs mostly in the left lower lobe followed by the lingula and the right middle lobe.

C. Predisposed to by recurrent pneumonia, granulomatous disease, carcinoma, or any process that can lead to a sequestered lobe.

D. There may be hemoptysis and recurrent pneumonia in a single lobe.

E. CT scanning will demonstrate areas of bronchiectasis, but bronchography is the current standard.

F. Treat as with COPD. In addition treat with long-term, alternating antibiotics to prevent resistance. Patients with bronchiectasis may benefit from a course of antibiotics for the first 10 days of every month (such as TMP/SMX or doxycycline).

G. Surgical resection of the affected lobe is an alternative treatment if antibiotics fail.

PULMONARY FUNCTION TESTS

I. LUNG VOLUMES AND CAPACITIES

A. Diagram (Fig. 3-1).

- *Normal.* Values may vary in the normal individual about 20% predicted. Values will change with position, age, sex, height, effort, and altitude.

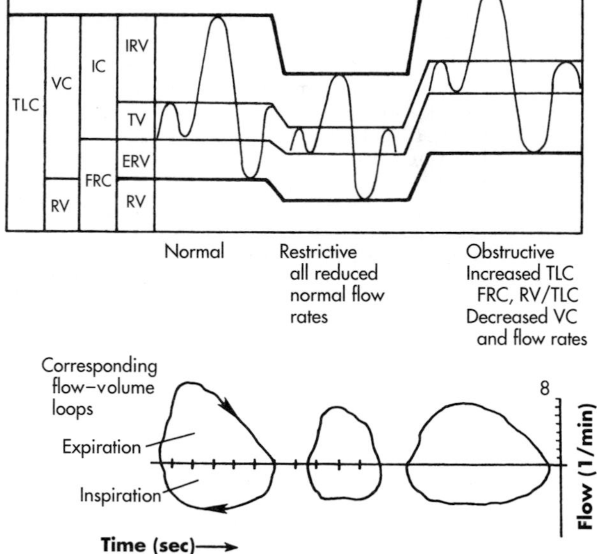

FIG. 3-1 Pulmonary function tests.

- *Restrictive.* Most volumes are decreased, but flow rates are normal or increased.
- *Obstructicve.* Increase in TLC, FRC, RV/TLC, decrease in VC, flow rates (see below for acronyms).

B. Definitions.

1. ***TV.*** Tidal volume is the volume inspired and expired during normal respirations.
2. ***IRV.*** Inspiratory reserve volume is the additional volume that can be inspired with maximum effort after a normal inspiration. (Inspiratory capacity − Tidal volume).
3. ***IC.*** Inspiratory capacity is the maximum volume that can be inspired after a normal, nonforced, expiration (IRV + TV).
4. ***ERV.*** Expiratory reserve volume is the additional volume that can be expired with maximum effort after a normal expiration (approximately 25% of VC).
5. ***RV.*** Residual volume is the volume left in the lungs after a maximal expiration.
6. ***FRC.*** Functional residual capacity is the volume left in the lungs after a normal expiration level (ERV + RV).
7. ***VC.*** Vital capacity is the maximum volume that can be expired after a maximal inspiration.
8. ***TLC.*** Total lung capacity is the volume in lungs at the end of a maximal inspiration.

C. Average values.

1. ***Vital capacity (predicted).***
   - Women = (21.78 − [0.101 × Age in years]) × Height in cm.
   - Men = (27.63 − [0.112 × Age in years]) × Height in cm.
2. ***Tidal volume.***
   - *Child:* 7.5 ml/kg.
   - *Adult female:* 6.6 ml/kg.
   - *Adult male:* 7.8 ml/kg.

II. SPIROMETRY

A. Diagram (Fig. 3-2).

B. Definitions.

1. ***FVC.*** Forced vital capacity is the maximum volume of gas that can be expired forcefully after a maximum inspiration.
2. ***FEV_1.*** Forced expired volume is the volume of gas expired during the first second of a FVC maneuver.
3. ***FEF 25% to 75%.*** Forced expiratory flow is less dependent on effort, more dependent on compliance of airways. Normal = 2 to 4 L/sec. It becomes abnormal earlier in obstructive disease than the FEV_1.

III. DIFFUSION

A. Alterations in the character of the alveolar membrane affects the diffusion of oxygen across the membrane.

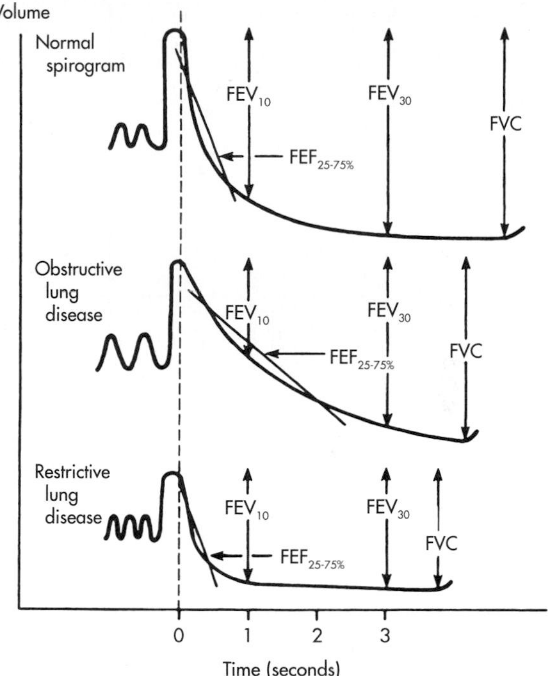

FIG. 3-2 Spirometry.

B. The total surface area of the alveolar membrane also affects diffusion. A decrease in the surface area (as in pneumonectomy, emphysema) will decrease diffusion.

C. Causes of low DLCO (diffusion of carbon monoxide, usually 25 to 30 ml of CO/mm Hg/min).

1. Alveolar wall thickening (as with fibrosis).
2. Alveolar wall destruction (as with emphysema).
3. Anemia (fewer RBCs to accept oxygen).

IV. INTERPRETING PATTERNS OF ABNORMAL PULMONARY FUNCTION TESTS (PFT)

- Patterns of abnormal PFTs
    1. ***Obstructive disorders.*** Emphysema, chronic bronchitis, asthma (Table 3-2).
    2. ***Restrictive disorders.***
        a. *Interstitial lung disorders.* Sarcoidosis, environmental disease, interstitial pneumonias, connective tissue disorders, pulmonary vascular diseases.

TABLE 3-2
Pulmonary Function Tests in Various Disease States

Condition	VC	FEV_1	RV	TLC	DLCO
Normal	75% to 100% predicted	2.5 L	1000 to 1200 ml	75% to 100% predicted	25 to 30 ml of CO/mm Hg/min
Asthma	Decreased	Decreased	Increased	Increased	Normal
Chronic bronchitis	Usually decreased	Decreased	Decreased	Normal or decreased	Normal or slightly decreased
Emphysema	Normal or slightly decreased	Decreased	Increased	Increased	Increased
Pulmonary fibrosis	Decreased	Normal or slightly decreased	Normal or decreased	Decreased	Decreased

b. *Impairment of ventilation mechanics (bellows disorders).* Obesity, kyphoscoliosis, status post surgery, paralysis, ascites, pleuritis, pleural effusion.

VENTILATORS AND OXYGEN THERAPY

Respiratory failure is defined as the inability of the lungs to meet the metabolic demands of the body. This can involve failure of tissue oxygenation or failure of CO_2 homeostasis, or both. Acute respiratory failure is a medical emergency requiring prompt diagnosis and management and should be suspected when a patient breathing room air has a Po_2 <60 mm Hg or a Pco_2 >50 mm Hg with a pH <7.3.

I. OXYGEN THERAPY

A. Oxygen-delivery systems (Table 3-3).

B. Complications of oxygen therapy.

1. Pulmonary oxygen toxicity including mucosal drying, mucociliary dysfunction, atelectasis, interstitial and alveolar edema, and alveolar hemorrhage.
2. Decreased respiratory drive, carbon dioxide retention, and respiratory failure in patients with chronic hypoxemia, who have a respiratory drive based on hypoxia (as in those with COPD).
3. Retrolental fibroplasia in neonates of low birth weight or gestational age <34 weeks.
4. Bronchopulmonary dysplasia in infants who require mechanical ventilation after birth.
5. Risk of fire and explosion.

II. VENTILATORS

A. Indications for mechanical ventilation.

1. ***Hypercapnia*** (increased Pco_2 with inability to maintain adequate alveolar ventilation. Seek treatable causes of hypercapnia (such as narcotics). Some patients with chronic lung disease will tolerate an increased $PAco_2$, remaining awake and comfortable. However, an arterial pH below 7.1 is considered an indication for mechanical ventilation.
2. ***Raised intracranial pressure.*** Deliberate hypocapnia by intermittent positive-pressure ventilation may be indicated to lower intracranial pressure in certain situations.
3. ***Hypoxemia.*** PAo_2 will usually be improved by IPPV. Specific criteria for instituting mechanical ventilation are (a) PAo_2 <40 torrs on maximal inspired O_2, (b) increasing obtundation, (c) rapidly progressing respiratory disease, (d) increased work of breathing (as with intercostal retractions during inspiration), (e) elevation of $PAco_2$.

TABLE 3-3
Oxygen-delivery Systems

Type	O_2 flow (L/min)	% O_2 delivered	Comments
LOW-FLOW SYSTEMS			
1. Nasal cannula	0.25 to 8	22 to 45	Precise regulation of FiO_2 not possible
			Comfortable but limited to low flow rate <4 L/min
			Nasal mucosa drying common
2. Simple mask	6 to 10	35 to 55	Offers little over nasal cannula
			Less comfortable, hot; skin irritation
			Not low enough FiO_2 for COPD
			O_2 rates must be at least 5 L/min to clear CO_2
3. Reservoir masks	12 to 15	90 to 95	High FiO_2 delivered; reservoir fills during expiration, which provides increased volume of O_2
a. Nonrebreathing	8 to 12	50 to 80	
b. Partial rebreathing			Flow must be sufficient to keep reservoir bag from deflating upon inspiration

HIGH-FLOW SYSTEMS			
1. Venturi mask	4 to 12	21 to 100	Exact FiO_2 can be delivered Poor humidification Uncomfortable
2. Nebulizer with:			
a. Aerosol mask, face tent	0 to 12	30 to 100	Used to deliver precise FiO_2 or aerosol, or both Can provide controlled temperature of gas May need 2 or 3 setups to meet inspirational flows for FiO_2 >0.5 Aerosol may induce bronchospasm, fluid overload, overmobilization of secretions, or contamination
b. Mask CPAP and BiPAP	0 to 12	Up to 100	Useful in COPD and CHF but not in asthma. May prevent intubation and decrease hospital stays.
c. T-tube	0 to 12	30 to 100	For spontaneous breathing through endotracheal tube Flow rates should be 2 or 3 times minute ventilation

B. Modes of mechanical ventilation.

1. ***Controlled ventilation.*** The ventilator is initiating all breaths at a preselected rate and volume. There are few indications for this use.
2. ***Assist-control (AC).*** A fixed minimum rate and volume is delivered by the machine, but each of the patient's spontaneous breaths triggers the ventilator to deliver a selected volume. This mode allows the patient to adjust respirations to changing metabolic status. It is the mode most commonly used.
3. ***Intermittent mandatory ventilation (IMV).*** The ventilator delivers a minimum fixed number of breaths per minute. However, the patient's spontaneous breaths are taken into account and do not trigger machine ventilations. For example, if the minimum number of ventilations required is 12 and the patient initiates 10, the ventilator will deliver 2 breaths. Ventilator breaths are either intermittent (IMV) or synchronized (SIMV) to the patient's spontaneous breaths. This can be used as a weaning method, allowing the patient to gradually assume more of the work of breathing.
4. ***Continuous positive airway pressure (CPAP).*** The ventilator supplies a continuous source of positive airway pressure and oxygen. The patient ventilates on his own.

C. Ventilator management.

1. Recent data indicate that allowing a ventilated patient's CO_2 to rise may actually reduce mortality from ventilator-related causes such as barotrauma *as long as the patient is oxygenating well.* Although the teaching in the past has been to adjust ventilations to keep the CO_2 about 35 to 40 mm Hg, more recent data indicate that "permissive hypercapnia," with associated decreases in pH, is acceptable as along as oxygenation is maintained and circulation is not compromised.
2. ***Minute ventilation.*** The produce of tidal volume and rate, generally it is approximately 5 to 10 L/min or 100 ml/kg/min.
3. ***Tidal volume (Vt).*** Initial volume is 10 to 12 ml/kg. A large Vt improves gas exchange and prevents atelectasis. However, it may decrease venous return. A smaller tidal volume may be required if PEEP is added. Consider a lower Vt in patients with chronic lung disease or asthma because hyperinflation and greatly increased pleural pressures may develop, leading to pneumothorax or other barotrauma. *Allowing the CO_2 to rise will allow the limiting of the tidal volume and reduce the risk of hyperinflation.*
4. ***Inspiratory waveform.*** Adjust inspired flow rate to maintain a ratio of inhalation time to exhalation time of 1 to 1.5.

5. ***Rate.*** After the Vt is chosen, the rate can be determined by the equation:

   Rate = Minute ventilation/Tidal volume

   Generally a slower rate and larger tidal volume will reduce intrathoracic pressures and improve compliance. Usually a rate of 8 to 14 breaths per minute is a reasonable starting point for adults. Adjust the rate to keep PCO_2 approximately 35 torrs (see above note at II C 1).
6. Positive end-expiratory pressure (PEEP). Usually increases compliance and decreases the work of breathing, atelectasis, and shunting, often allowing a decrease in FiO_2. It is usually begun at 3 to 5 cm H_2O and increased in small increments. High levels may result in decreased venous return, overventilation, and barotrauma. Cardiac output should be measured because it may increase or decrease with increased PEEP.
7. ***FiO_2 (% oxygen delivered).*** The goal is to maintain a PO_2 of 60 to 100 torrs with an FiO_2 <60%, since toxicity is seen earlier when the FiO_2 >60%. Start with a high FiO_2 and adjust in 5% to 10% increments. Check ABGs or oxygen saturations 30 minutes after each change in ventilator settings. If the only change is in the FiO_2, oxygen saturations are adequate. However, ABGs should be obtained if an adjustment is expected to change the PCO_2 (increased ventilation rate, increase Vt).
8. ***Peak airway pressure.*** This reflects the pressure required to overcome airway resistance and is the peak pressure during the inspiratory cycle. The alarm limit should be set 10 cm H_2O above this. If the peak inspiratory pressure increases, you need to consider obstruction in the ET tube, bronchospasm, decreased lung compliance, or a pneumothorax from barotrauma.
9. ***Sedation and neuromuscular paralysis.***
   a. Sedation allows better patient compliance with the ventilator as well as rest and anxiety control. Initial therapy includes midazolam 1 to 2 mg IV titrating up in 1 mg increments, or diazepam 5 to 10 mg IV. Dosages should be titrated to desired effect, with monitoring of hemodynamic and respiratory status.
   b. Neuromuscular paralysis is occasionally necessary if sedation fails, *but patients should still be sedated.* Monitoring alarms must be functioning because ventilator malfunction is rapidly fatal if the patient is paralyzed. Short-term paralysis (3 to 7 minutes) can be achieved with succinylcholine 1 mg/kg IV. For long-term paralysis use vecuronium (Norcuron) 0.1 mg/kg IV initially followed by maintenance infusion starting at 1 µg/kg/min with the average dose being 0.8 to

1.2 μg/kg/min (1 ml of 10 mg of vecuronium in 100 ml = 0.1 mg/ml). Start 20 to 40 minutes after bolus when there is evidence of spontaneous recovery from bolus. If necessary, a neostigmine-atropine combination can be used to reverse its effects. Sedation should be provided for paralyzed patients.

D. Prevention of respirator-associated complications.

1. Continuous subglottic aspiration of secretions reduces the incidence of nosocomial pneumonia.
2. Data indicates but does not prove that H_2-blockers are less effective than sucralfate at preventing "stress ulcers" and that there may be a higher incidence of nosocomial pneumonia and death in those who are using H_2-blockers versus sucralfate.

E. Withdrawal of mechanical ventilation.

1. ***Guidelines for weaning from mechanical ventilation.***
   a. An awake, alert patient.
   b. PO_2 >60 torrs, with an FiO_2 <50%.
   c. PCO_2 acceptable and a pH in normal range.
   d. PEEP <5 cm H_2O.
   e. Vital capacity >12 ml/kg.
   f. Patient is able to generate maximum voluntary ventilation without retractions.
   g. Patient is able to generate a peak negative inspiratory pressure of at least 20 cm H_2O.
2. ***Weaning from the ventilator.***
   a. Explain the process to the patient and encourage cooperation.
   b. Begin during the daytime; allow the patient to rest at night.
   c. Place the patient in an upright position.
   d. Discontinue weaning if:
      - pH <7.3, PCO_2 >50 torrs, PO_2 <60 torrs.
      - Patient becomes anxious or fatigued or demonstrates increasing respiratory distress or develops significant arrhythmias or hemodynamic deterioration.
   e. T-tube method. (A T-tube allows the patient to breathe through an endotracheal tube without assistance from the ventilator.) Have the patient use a T-tube with humidified oxygen. If the patient tolerates this for 1 to 4 hours as demonstrated by above parameters, discontinue mechanical ventilation. If the patient fails the attempt, resume mechanical ventilation and consider IMV method (below) for weaning.
   f. IMV method. Gradually decrease the number of assisted respirations in 1 or 2 breath increments over 30- to 90-minute intervals. Monitor ABGs and vital signs. When an assisted rate of <4 breaths/min is achieved, consider a brief T-tube trial. If the patient remains stable, discontinue mechanical ventilation. If the trial fails, increase

assisted rate until patient stabilizes. Repeat attempt the following day with a more gradual decrease in the rate of assisted breaths.

VIRAL UPPER RESPIRATORY TRACT INFECTIONS

Approximately 80% of acute respiratory illnesses result from viral infections. These are usually self-limited syndromes caused by a variety of viruses: rhinovirus, adenovirus, echovirus, coxsackievirus, influenza and parainfluenza viruses. Occasionally pneumonia may complicate these infections, either primary viral pneumonia, or secondary bacterial pneumonia. In the compromised host less common pathogens, such as varicellavirus, measles virus (paramyxovirus), CMV, and herpes simplex virus can result in life-threatening infections.

I. THE COMMON COLD

- **A. Causes.** Rhinovirus, adenovirus, echovirus, and coxsackievirus, respiratory syncytial virus (RSV).
- **B. Clinical presentation.** Chief complaints include congestion, sneezing, clear to mucopurulent nasal discharge, dry sore throat, low-grade fever, and cough. Physical exam reveals erythematous nasal and oropharyngeal mucosa, and there is a normal chest exam.
- **C. Management.** Treatment is primarily symptomatic. Rest, hydration, decongestants such as pseudoephedrine for comfort, acetaminophen for analgesia and fever. Antihistamines have no proved benefit.
- **D.** Ipratropium nasal spray is now available for symptomatic treatment of the cold. Use the 0.06% spray, 2 puffs per nostril BID or TID.
- **E.** Zinc gluconate lozenges (13.3 mg) every 2 hours while awake has been shown to hasten cold resolution (4.4 days versus 7.6 days for placebo group) if started with 24 hours of symptoms.

II. INFLUENZA

A. Overview.

Influenza is a systemic illness resulting from infection with an influenza virus, which are orthomyxovirus types A, B, or rarely C. These viruses can change their envelope proteins as their host population develops immunity, thereby maintaining the ability to cause recurrent infection in a single host population. Influenza vaccinations for the predicted virulent strains are available in the fall months and are generally effective in preventing or decreasing the intensity and duration of infection.

B. Clinical presentation.

There is usually an abrupt onset of high fever, chills, dry cough, headache, myalgia, and prostration. Physical exam is usually unremarkable with the exception of bibasilar rales in some patients. Chest radiograph is usually normal.

Occasionally, perihilar prominence and increased markings can be present. The development of infiltrates is suggestive of a complicating pneumonia, either viral or bacterial.

C. Management.

The illness is usually self-limited, lasting 4 to 7 days. Rest, hydration, and acetaminophen are recommended. For influenza type A, amantadine hydrochloride 100 mg PO BID for 10 days given early in the course can reduce symptoms and can be used for prophylaxis in compromised close contacts of infected individuals. Rimantadine 100 mg PO BID may also be used and has a lower incidence of side effects. Reduce dosage of both drugs for renal or liver impairment, for the elderly, and in the presence of a seizure disorder.

D. Complications.

Myocarditis, myositis (including rhabdomyolysis), pericarditis, Reye's syndrome, and Guillain-Barré have been reported as complications of influenza. Additionally, secondary bacterial pneumonia may occur. This should be considered if a patient is getting better and develops worsening symptoms of cough, dyspnea, fever.

III. BRONCHITIS

A. Characterized by cough with purulent sputum, rhonchi, and sometimes fever. Mostly viral in cause, but also consider *Haemophilus influenzae, Streptococcus pneumoniae, Moraxella.*

B. Treatment. There is little evidence that antibiotics are useful in nonsmokers. Cough suppression and inhaled beta-agonists are the mainstay of treatment. Erythromycin, doxycycline, and TMP/SMX are good antibiotic choices if antibiotics are indicated. Benzonatate 100 mg PO Q6h will suppress cough as will codeine (such as acetaminophen and codeine). Albuterol and other beta-agonists are excellent for cough suppression in the patient with bronchitis.

PNEUMONIA

I. DIFFERENTIAL DIAGNOSIS OF PULMONARY INFILTRATES

Bacterial, viral, and fungal (coccidioidomycosis, aspergillosis) pneumonia (including atypical organisms such as *Mycoplasma, Legionella,* and *Rickettsia*), CHF, pulmonary infiltrates with eosinophilia; pulmonary hemorrhage, TB, Goodpasture's syndrome, pulmonary embolism, neoplastic disease (especially lymphoma and alveolar cell carcinoma), radiation injury, inhalation of mineral oil or other lipoid substances, pulmonary contusion, bronchiolitis obliterans with organizing pneumonia (BOOP), Wegener's granulomatosis, collagen-vascular disorders (including rheumatoid lung disease, lupus, scleroderma), amyloidosis, and sarcoidosis. Consider also interstitial pneumonitis from antigens (farmers, bird breeders), drugs including hydrochlorothiazide, asbestos, silicosis. This list is not inclusive, and your patient may have an illness not listed here.

II. GENERAL

A. Symptoms that may be present include fever, cough, chills, dyspnea, mental status changes (especially in elderly), sputum production, pleuritic chest pain, and shock.

B. X-ray resolution may lag behind clinical improvement. X-ray resolution will be evident in 73% at 6 weeks and 94% at 24 weeks. In the presence of clinical response, this delay is not concerning. However if the patient is still ill, consider the possibility of a resistant organism or underlying pulmonary disease, such as TB, foreign body, or cystic fibrosis.

C. Some pneumonococci are penicillin resistant. This is a drug-binding phenomenon, and therefore clavulanate does not help.

D. *Haemophilus influenzae* is often beta-lactamase producing and is not covered by erythromycin. It requires broad-spectrum coverage (as with cefuroxime, TMP/SMX, amoxicillin-clavulanate).

E. Consider amantadine or rimantadine during an influenza A epidemic.

F. Treat bacterial pneumonia for 7 to 14 days depending on severity. Change to oral antibiotics in those hospitalized after stable and afebrile for 24 to 48 hours.

G. In children, pneumonia frequently presents with only fever and tachypnea; rales may not be present on exam. Physical exam may reveal clear lungs in up to 50% of children who have pneumonia present on CXR.

III. NEONATES (See Table 3-4 for organisms and treatment.)

A. Congenital pneumonia. Caused by transplacental agents.

B. Perinatally acquired. Associated with inhalation of infected amniotic fluid (often with prolonged rupture of membranes) or hematogenous seeding of lungs.

C. Pneumonia acquired after birth, usually caused by exposure to infected nursery personnel other infants, infected equipment.

D. Evaluation.

1. ***History.*** Maternal fever, preterm delivery, prolonged rupture of membranes, foul-smelling amniotic fluid all increase suspicion.
2. ***Physical exam.*** Fever, lethargy, tachypnea, grunting, flaring of nasal alae, retractions, irregular breathing, apnea, cyanosis, rales. It is rare for newborn to exhibit cough or mucus production associated with pneumonia. Neonates may present with nonspecific symptoms such as poor feeding or irritability.
3. ***Lab results.*** CBC with differential, CXR, gastric aspirate for Gram stain and culture. Cultures and Gram stain of blood, urine, CSF, tracheal aspirate, and blood gas. Pleural tap may be done if pleural effusions are present.

TABLE 3-4
Pneumonia in Children

Age	Predominant organisms	Treatment
Neonatal (<5 days of age at onset); perinatally or prenatally acquired	Caused by maternal vaginal flora, such as group A, B, or G streptococci; *Escherichia coli; Chlamydia trachomatis* May also have TORCHS organisms *Treponema pallidum* (congenital syphilis), *Listeria,* TB, genital *Mycoplasma,* CMV	Treat specific organism if identified and as per neonatal sepsis, such as ampicillin and gentamicin or third-generation cephalosporin with antipseudomonal activity (such as ceftazidime)
Infant 5 days to less than 1 month	Group A or B streptococci, *Staphulococcus, Escherichia coli, Pseudomonas, Chlamydia, Pneumocystis*	Penicillinase-resistant synthetic penicillin (such as nafcillin) with gentamicin Consider vancomycin if methicillin-resistant *Staphylococcus* is prevalent (see Chapter 10) If *Chlamydia* by clinical exam (conjunctivitis) and titers, add erythromycin (see Chapter 10)
Children (1 month to 5 years)	Mild to moderate usually viral (80%), such as RSV, parainfluenza, influenza, adenovirus. Bacterial causes include *Streptococcus pneumoniae, Haemophilus influenzae, Chlamydia, Mycoplasma*	Mild viral conditions may not need treatment Clarithromycin or amoxicillin is a good choice for the nontoxic outpatient, or consider ceftriaxone, cefotaxime or penicillinase-resistant synthetic penicillin (such as nafcillin) with antipseudomonal aminoglycoside (such as gentamicin) for those hospitalized

TABLE 3-4
Pneumonia in Children—cont'd

Age	Predominant organisms	Treatment
Children (>5 years)	Pneumococcus, *Mycoplasma pneumoniae* In immunocompromised children: gram-negative enteric bacteria *Pneumocystis carinii,* CMV, fungus, anaerobes from aspiration, viral infection, bacterial superinfection after viral with *Staphylococcus aureus,* group A streptococcus or *Streptococcus pneumoniae,* TB	If viral, antibiotics not indicated If require hospitalization, initiate antibiotics Oral erythromycin can be used in a dose of 30 to 50 mg/kg/day, divided QID, for 10 days Clarithromycin, which is more expensive but has fewer side effects, can be given in a dose of 15 mg/kg/24 hours divided Q12h Reevaluate if child fails to respond to therapy

E. Treatment. General supportive measures: electrolyte, acid-base balance, maintain HCT, blood volume, blood pressure, nutrition, temperature control. Respiratory support, including O_2 as needed, respiratory therapy, intermittent positive-pressure ventilation if indicated. Drainage of pleural fluid if present. See Table 3-4 for organisms and treatment.

IV. INFANTS AND CHILDREN (1 MONTH TO 5 YEARS), OLDER CHILDREN

A. In children 1 month to 5 years, most pneumonias are viral. *Chlamydia trachomatis* can present as an afebrile pneumonia in infants 3 to 16 weeks of age. 50% will have an associated conjunctivitis, and peripheral eosinophilia is common. CXR shows hyperinflation and diffuse interstitial or patchy infiltrates. Nasal washings used for diagnosis. Treated with macrolide or sulfisoxazole.

B. Treatment and organisms. See Table 3-4.

V. CHILDREN 5 YEARS OLD AND OLDER

A. Evaluation. CBC with differential CBC count, CXR (PA and LAT), TB skin test, sputum or tracheal aspirate for Gram stain and culture. Culture or fluorescent antibody techniques for respiratory viruses sometimes useful. Obtain blood cultures if patient appears toxic.

B. See Table 3-5 for atypical pneumonia.

TABLE 3-5
Common Atypical Pneumonias

Organism or disease	Clinical presentation	Diagnosis and treatment
Chlamydia pneumoniae (TWAR)	10% of all pneumonias in U.S.A., hoarseness may be present Clinically similar to mycoplasma pneumonia without neurologic and GI symptoms May also cause bronchitis and asthma	WBC usually normal; IgG antibody test available; self-limited but may use tetracyclines or macrolide
Fungal pneumonias (coccidioidomycosis/ blastomycosis/histoplasmosis)	Occur in a geographical distribution Coccidioidomycosis in Southwest and California Blastomycosis in southeastern and south central U.S.A. Histoplasmosis in eastern U.S.A. to Midwest All cause an influenza-like illness with pneumonia	Coccidioidomycosis: find spores in sputum, positive skin test, IgG antibody Prescribe fluconazole, itraconazole, or amphotericin B Blastomycosis culture from sputum (4 weeks!); KOH exam of sputum Prescribe itraconazole, ketoconazole, amphotericin B Histoplasmosis organism culture; skin test (not specific); identification of polysaccharide in urine and blood (with disseminated disease) Prescribe itraconazole but amphotericin B if moderately or severely ill

Hantavirus	Mice and rats are vectors, occurs throughout the U.S.A. (most common in Southwest) Myalgias, fever, headache, abdominal pain, cough, rapid onset of respiratory failure, ARDS	Hemoconcentration, thrombocytopenia, hypoxia gM and IgG antibody tests available Ribavirin may be useful; contact the CDC
Legionnaires' disease (*Legionella pneumophila*)	1- or 2-day prodrome of headache , myalgias, then fever, chills, tachypnea, dry cough May become obtunded; associated vomiting, diarrhea	WBC mildly elevated (8000 to 10,000); cold agglutinins negative; sputum immunofluorescent antibody available; look for *Legionella* antigen in urine (90% sensitive but only for one serotype); serum antibody titers available Treatment is erythromycin (500 mg Q6h), clarithromycin, or azithromycin
Pneumocystis pneumonia	See Chapter 16	See Chapter 16
Mycoplasma pneumoniae	Occurs in epidemics, has associated pharyngitis, fever, headache Dry cough, may have clear exam but infiltrate on radiograph May have cold agglutinin-medicated hemolysis, meningeal signs, cranial nerve deficits, nausea, vomiting, diarrhea	WBC usually normal (<25% elevated 10,000 to 20,000; cold agglutinin titer 1:128 (other pneumonias may have lower titers) IgG and IgM antibodies Polymerase chain reaction testing available Treat with erythromycin, azithromycin, clarithromycin

Continued

TABLE 3-5
Common Atypical Pneumonias—cont'd

Organism or disease	Clinical presentation	Diagnosis and treatment
Psittacosis (*Chlamydia psittaci*)	Especially in bird owners Headache, high fever, dry cough, myalgias, chest pain, perhaps vomiting and diarrhea Splenomegaly common and suggestive of the diagnosis, hepatomegaly, myocarditis may occur	WBC usually normal but may be up or down Antibody titers diagnostic Treat with doxycycline 100 mg BID Radiograph may not clear for 6 weeks
Q fever (*Coxiella burnetii*)	Especially in dairy and abattoir workers and those with livestock contact, have fever, cough, headache, malaise, hepatitis, endocarditis	Antibody titers against *Chlamydia burnetii* diagnostic Treat with tetracycline 500 mg Q6h
Tularemia (*Francisella tularensis*)	From rabbits (are nonpulmonary variants as well) Have tracheitis, pneumonia, cough, dyspnea, hemoptysis	Antibody titers and culture to diagnose Treatment is streptomycin
Viral diseases (influenza viruses, parainfluenza viruses, RSV, adenovirus)	Varies by virus	Generally normal WBC unless secondary infection

C. Therapy and organisms. See Table 3-4.

VI. ADULTS TO 60 YEARS OF AGE, COMMUNITY ACQUIRED, NO UNDERLYING DISEASE, OUTPATIENT TREATMENT

A. Common pathogens. *Streptococcus pneumoniae,* group A streptococci, *Haemophilus influenzae, Mycoplasma* (less common in this age group), *Legionella,* influenzaviruses.

B. Antibiotics. For outpatient treatment, a macrolide such as erythromycin, clarithromycin, or azithromycin is the best choice. Doxycycline is an acceptable alternative in those >8 years old.

VII. AGE OVER 60 OR UNDERLYING DISEASE (SUCH AS ALCOHOL ABUSE, DIABETES, CHF, DEBILITATION), OUTPATIENT THERAPY

A. Pathogens. In addition to usual pathogens discussed above, also must consider *Klebsiella,* Enterobacteriaceae, *Legionella, Chlamydia, Staphylococcus aureus.*

B. Antibiotics. Macrolide (erythromycin, clarithromycin, or azithromycin) plus one of the following: TMP/SMX, amoxicillin-clavulanate, cefixime, or cefuroxime.

C. Consider amantadine if influenza A epidemic.

VIII. ADULT, HOSPITALIZED, COMMUNITY-ACQUIRED, NONSEVERE PNEUMONIA

A. Most common organisms. *Streptococcus pneumoniae, H. influenzae, Legionella,* polymicrobial organisms, anaerobes, gram-negative bacilli, viruses, and chlamydias.

B. Antiobiotic choices include erythromycin 15 to 20 mg/kg IV QD or an extended-spectrum macrolide (clarithromycin, azithromycin) plus an IV second- or third-generation cephalosporin (that is, third = ceftriaxone, ceftazidime; second = cefoxitin, cefamandole). Alternatives include ampicillin-sulbactam, ticarcillin-clavulonate, and imipenem.

IX. ADULT, HOSPITALIZED, SEVERE, COMMUNITY-ACQUIRED PNEUMONIA

A. Organisms. As above.

B. Antiobiotic choices. Ceftriaxone or vancomycin plus erythromycin. Alternatives include imipenem, or ticarcillin-clavulanate.

X. ADULT, HOSPITALIZED, NOSOCOMIALLY ACQUIRED PNEUMONIA

A. Organisms. Enterobacteriaceae *(Enterobacter, Citrobacter, Acinetobacter), Pseudomonas, Legionella.*

B. Need to cover usual community-acquired pathogens and enteric gram-negative rods, *Staphylococcus aureus.*

C. **Antiobiotics.** Imipenem-cilastatin, ticarcillin-clavulanate, ceftazidime and clindamycin. For *Pseudomonas,* coverage must add an aminoglycoside to the above regimens. Add erythromycin for coverage of atypical organisms.

XI. FOR NEUTROPENIC FEVER, see Chapter 18.

XII. ATYPICAL PNEUMONIA SYNDROME

A. Cough may be nonproductive and often has associated pleuritic pain, URI symptoms, fever, headache, myalgia. Symptoms are usually milder than with bacterial pneumonia.
B. Common in school-aged children and young adults.
C. Usually pleuropneumonia *(Mycoplasma)*; others can include TWAR *(Chlamydia pneumoniae)*, Q fever *(Coxiella burnetii)*, psittacosis *(Chlamydia psittaci,* especially in bird owners), influenza A and B, diseases caused by adenovirus and RSV, Legionnaires' disease, *Pneumocystis* pneumonia (PCP), etc. in the immunocompromised (see also differential diagnosis of pulmonary infiltrates, p. 136, Table 3-5, and Chapter 16).
D. Erythromycin, clarithromycin, or azithromycin are appropriate and cover mycoplasmas as well as pneumococci. Clarithromycin and azithromycin have the advantage of fewer side effects than erythromycin and an extended spectrum, which includes *Haemophilus influenzae.* Consider adding TMP/SMX to cover PCP if indicated.
E. Clinical synopsis of selected atypical pneumonias (by no means all inclusive; see also Chapter 16 and Table 3-5).

ASTHMA

I. OVERVIEW AND DEFINITION

According to the National Asthma Education Program, asthma is a lung disease with the following characteristics:

A. Airway obstruction or airway narrowing that is reversible either spontaneously or with treatment. May not have complete resolution of narrowing in some patients.
B. Airway inflammation.
C. Airway hyperresponsiveness to a variety of stimuli.

II. EVALUATION

A. History.

1. Symptoms might include cough, wheezing, shortness of breath, chest tightness.
2. Ask about associated conditions: rhinitis, sinusitis, nasal polyps, atopic dermatitis.
3. Precipitating factors include viral URIs, allergens, irritants, emotions, drugs, food additives, cold air, exercise. Reflux esophagitis is a common precipitant for asthma especially if primarily nocturnal symptoms.

4. Age at onset, progresssion of the disease.
5. Previous work-up, treatments, response to treatment.
6. Present management, including the plan for exacerbations.
7. Prior ER visits, hospitalizations, intubation, ICU admits.
8. Days missed from school or work.
9. Nocturnal symptoms.
10. Effect on lifestyle, growth, school, work.
11. Smoking, exposure to passive smoke, occupational exposure.
12. Family history of asthma or atopy.

B. Physical exam.

1. Breath sounds, wheezing, evidence of hyperinflation, retractions.
2. Evidence of associated conditions such as rhinitis, sinusitis, nasal polyps.

C. Additional tests.

1. Consider CBC; sputum and nasal secretion Gram stain for eosinophils.
2. CXR can rule out other causes of airway obstruction but no need for CXR with exacerbations unless indicated by fever, rales, or other symptoms.
3. Pulmonary function tests. Spirometry should be done to provide an objective measure in all patients in whom the diagnosis of asthma is considered. Complete pulmonary function tests may be indicated in some patients.
4. Allergy testing in some cases.
5. Rhinoscopy, sinus radiographs, pH probe to evaluate for gastroesophageal reflux (which can exacerbate asthma) if indicated.
6. Bronchoprovocation with methacholine, histamine, or exercise challenge may be used to establish diagnosis in some patients.

D. Differential diagnosis.

1. ***Children.*** Foreign-body obstruction in large airways, vascular rings, mass (tumor lymph nodes), tracheomalacia, viral bronchiolitis, cystic fibrosis, chlamydial infection, bronchopulmonary dysplasia, aspiration, pulmonary edema.
2. ***Adults.*** Foreign body or other mechanical obstruction of airways, laryngeal dysfunction, emphysema or chronic bronchitis, CHF, pulmonary embolus, pulmonary infiltrate, drug-induced cough (such as ACE inhibitors).

III. MEDICATIONS

A. Anti-inflammatory agents.

1. ***Corticosteroids.***
   a. Oral. Use early in exacerbation prevents progression, reduces ED visits and hospitalizations, decreases morbidity. Onset of action about 3 hours, peak 6 to

12 hours. Adverse effects include hyperglycemia, increased appetite, fluid retention, mood changes, hypertension, peptic ulcers, aseptic necrosis of the bone (most common head of femur, spine). Long-term effects can include osteoporosis, Cushing syndrome, cataracts, adrenal suppression, impaired immune function. Because of the side effects of orally administered corticosteroids, attempts should be made to reduce dependence on oral steroids by using inhaled corticosteroids, at high doses if necessary. It may be necessary to use two to four times the usual daily dose of inhaled steroids initially when trying to wean down on oral corticosteroids.

b. Inhaled corticosteroids are safe and effective and are the primary therapy for moderate and severe asthma. Concentrations per inhalation vary among the formulations (beclomethasone, triamcinolone, flunisolide). Systemic adverse effects are rare. Local adverse effects can include candidiasis, or upper airway irritation from the aerosol.

2. Cromolyn sodium and nedocromil are believed to work by stabilizing and preventing mediator release from mast cells. The patient may need a 4- to 6-week trial to determine whether he or she will respond. They have very few side effects (bad taste, cough, pharyngitis). Useful as a prophylactic medication to prevent early- and late-phase allergen-induced airway narrowing. Not useful in acute attack.

B. Bronchodilators.

1. ***Beta-agonists.*** Beta$_2$-adrenegic agonists (albuterol, metaproterenol) relax airway smooth muscle. Inhaled beta$_2$-agonists are the treatment of choice for acute asthma exacerbations and exercise-induced asthma. Using a spacer device with a metered-dose inhaler increases efficacy. *The use of beta-agonists PRN tends to control disease better than around-the-clock use.* There have been reports of diminished response to beta-agonists with chronic use, especially overuse. Inhaled beta-agonists give better bronchodilatation with less systemic side effects than oral preparations have. Salmeterol, a long-acting beta-agonist can be used for baseline control twice daily. However, it is not useful in treating an acute attack of asthma.
2. ***Methylxanthines.*** Methylxanthines are falling out of favor and should be third-line agents after inhaled beta-agonists and inhaled steroids. Theophylline has a long duration of action when given as the sustained-release preparation. May produce additional bronchodilatation when used in combination with a beta-agonist. IV aminophylline is not recommended in the emergency treatment of acute asthma. Dose should be adjusted by serum levels. The therapeutic

range is 10 to 15 μg/ml (the FDA has recently changed the recommended serum level from 10-20 to 10-15 μg/ml). Many conditions may alter theophylline clearance; fever, liver disease, heart failure, and certain drugs can predispose to toxicity. Monitor levels carefully if using in combination with cimetidine, quinolones, erythromycin, other drugs. GI symptoms, seizures, CNS stimulation, tachycardia, arrhythmias can occur with toxicity.

3. ***Anticholinergics (such as ipratropium).*** Produce bronchodilatation by reducing vagal tone to airways. Useful in COPD. Some reports have shown usefulness in acute asthma when used along with beta-agonists in nebulized form.
4. ***Leukotriene inhibitors (zafirlukast, Accolate) and others.*** Reserve for patients unresponsive to conventional therapy. Place in therapy not yet well defined. Will not abort acute attacks. For chronic use only.

IV. GENERAL PRINCIPLES OF TREATMENT

A. Treat asthma triggers and associated conditions.

1. Reduce exposure to allergens and irritants such as cigarette smoke.
2. Viral upper respiratory infections often lead to acute exacerbations, especially in children. Asthma regimen may need to be intensified during URI to avoid deterioration of asthma control. Some authors recommend prophylactic steroids during URIs in those children known to have a URI trigger for asthma.
3. Treat bacterial otitis media or sinusitis if present.
4. Treat reflux esophagitis if present.
5. Encourage influenza and pneumococcal vaccines in patients with moderate or severe asthma.
6. Treat allergic rhinitis if it coexists with asthma. Antihistamines, nasal corticosteroids, and cromolyn sodium nasal sprays may be effective.
7. If exposure to a know trigger is unavoidable, such as exercise, pretreat with an inhaled beta-agonist or cromolyn sodium before exposure.
8. Although not entirely proved, an increasing amount of evidence indicates that at least some asthma is related to infection with *Chlamydia pneumoniae* and may respond to treatment with doxycycline (100 mg BID) or a macrolide antibiotic (azithromycin 1000 mg PO every week; erythromycin 1000 mg/day) for 4 weeks.

V. TREATMENT PROTOCOLS IN ADULTS

A. Mild asthma with intermittent symptoms.

1. Symptoms are usually controlled with inhaled beta-agonists, and pulmonary function normalizes between episodes of wheezing.

2. If inhaled beta-agonists are needed daily, additional treatment may be indicated.

B. Moderate asthma.

1. Symptoms are not controlled by PRN beta-agonists, exacerbations occur more than twice a week, or pulmonary functions do not normalize with treatment. The FEV_1 or PEFR may decrease to a range of 60% to 80% of predicted (or patient's personal best value) when the patient is symptomatic. Exacerbations may affect sleep or activity level and exacerbations may last several days.
2. ***Treatment.*** PRN inhaled beta-agonists must be available for acute exacerbations. Inhaled corticosteroids or cromolyn sodium should be used as primary maintenance therapy. Bursts of oral corticosteroids are indicated when asthma is not controlled by a combination of bronchodilators and cromolyn sodium or inhaled corticosteroids. Usually prednisone is given at about 40 mg PO per day for 5 days. Most patients can simply stop the prednisone at this point without a tapering down. If the patient's symptoms cannot be controlled by a short burst of prednisone, if the bursts are effective for less than 2 or 3 weeks, or if bursts have to be repeated frequently, the patient has severe asthma and needs additional measures. If the patient has mostly nocturnal symptoms, salmeterol can be used for overnight control. Alternatively but less desirable, an evening dose of a sustained-release theophylline preparation or long-acting oral beta-agonist may help control symptoms.

C. Severe asthma. May need systemic corticosteroids on a routine basis. The lowest possible alternate-day or single daily dose should be used, and the patient must be monitored carefully for adverse effects of chronic corticosteroids. Administration of high doses of inhaled corticosteroids may allow the dose of oral steroids to be reduced.

D. Monitoring asthma.

1. Teaching patients to recognize their symptoms early and to intervene with beta-agonists and steroids can reduce emergency department visits and hospital admissions.
2. Peak flowmeters may be a useful adjunct in patients with moderate to severe asthma. However, the patient training in symptom recognition and response seems to be more important than the meter itself.

VI. ASTHMA IN CHILDREN

A. Mild asthma. PRN inhaled beta-agonists are a first-line therapy. Metered-dose inhalers can usually be used for children over 5 years of age, especially if used with a spacer device. Children under 5 years may be able to use an MDI with a spacer or an alternative preparation such as albuterol

Rotacaps. If the patient is unable to cooperate with these modalities, he or she may need either oral or nebulized medications. Nebulized beta-agonists are more effective and have less systemic side effects than oral preparations do but are expensive and bulky to transport.

B. Moderate asthma. Maintenance therapy: cromolyn sodium, inhaled corticosteroid, or sustained-release theophylline. Theophylline in oral dose to achieve serum lever of 5 to 15 μg/ml. Beta-agonist via a metered-dose inhaler or nebulizer as needed for symptom relief. Cromolyn and inhaled steroids are preferred over theophylline.

C. Severe asthma. Inhaled beta-agonist TID or QID PRN, plus inhaled corticosteroid or cromolyn sodium. May need to add an oral sustained-release theophylline. Oral corticosteroids may be needed in younger children, who usually cannot use inhalers effectively. If oral corticosteroids are required on a chronic basis, the lowest possible dose should be used, and the dose should be given as a single, alternate-day dose if possible.

VII. EMERGENCY DEPARTMENT MANAGEMENT OF ASTHMA EXACERBATIONS IN ADULTS AND CHILDREN

See Chapter 1.

EVALUATION OF THE CHRONIC COUGH

A. Most common causes in order of frequency. Postnasal drip/chronic sinusitis, asthma, including postviral reactive airways, GE reflux disease. Consider also medication (ACE inhibitors), CHF, pertussis, TB. Pertussis in adults may present only with chronic cough and may be present despite childhood immunization and represent 21% of those with chronic cough in one series (check acute and convalescent titers).

B. One approach.

1. Treat with antihistamine or decongestant empirically. Consider course of antibiotics for sinusitis if appropriate.
2. If this fails, do bronchoprovocation testing for asthma and treat patients with positive results with beta-agonists and prednisone (if fail, beta-agonists alone).
3. If cough continues or bronchoprovocation negative, do CXR and sinus CT. Treat positives.
4. Evaluate negatives for GE reflux and give trial of H_2-blocker.
5. If patient still coughing, consider bronchoscopy.
6. This approach leads to successful treatment in 96% (though there are recurrences).
7. If positive titer for pertussis, treat with erythromycin or other macrolide.

OBSTRUCTIVE SLEEP APNEA

Affects 2% to 4% of the population

A. Clinically complain of:

1. Daytime sleepiness, snoring, headache, personality changes, intellectual deterioration, sexual dysfunction. Partners may complain of restless sleep, periods of apnea. Daytime sleepiness, depression, unrefreshing sleep, etc. are not specific and may occur with other sleep disorders, depression.
2. 40% of women with sleep apnea have amenorrhea or dysmenorrhea that resolves with treatment.
3. May have secondary hypertension, right- and left-sided heart failure, dysrhythmias, MI, CVA, increased risk of motor vehicle accident (sevenfold increase!).
4. Only 50% are obese. Women with obstructive sleep apnea may be thin and have small neck circumference. Menstrual irregularities are common.

B. Diagnosis by:

1. ***Polysomnography (sleep study).*** Expensive and time consuming but is the gold standard. Criteria include:
   a. Cessation of air flow for 10 seconds even though maintain respiratory effort.
   b. 5 or more episodes of apnea per hour.
   c. Decrease in oxygen saturation of at least 4% during episodes.
2. ***Continuous nocturnal oxygen saturation measurement at home.*** Using 10 desaturations per hour as the cutoff, it has a 98% sensitivity but only a 48% specificity with a positive predictive value of 61% and a negative predictive value of 97% in those with a history suggestive of sleep apnea.
   a. Not valid in those receiving oxygen therapy.
   b. Can use to screen before ordering sleep study, since it has a high negative predictive value and is inexpensive.
3. ***Treatment.***
   a. Relieve nasal obstruction including polyps, allergic causes, structural abnormalities (such as septal deviation).
   b. Avoid sedatives, androgens, alcohol.
   c. Weight loss.
   d. Drugs including medroxyprogesterone, protriptyline, and fluoxetine have some benefit but only in mild cases.
      (1) Oxygen alone can be used if mild desaturation or not able to tolerate other modalities.
      (2) Treat hypothyroidism if present.
      (3) Mask or nasal CPAP (continuous positive airway pressure) is the treatment of choice.
         (a) Need to customize positive pressure by observing result in a sleep study.
         (b) Only 46% will have adequate compliance.
   e. Surgical therapy including:

(1) Tonsillectomy, uvulopalatopharyngoplasty (efficacy only 30% to 50% but no good controlled studies).
(2) Tracheostomy.

SARCOID

A diffuse inflammatory process of unknown cause leading to the formation of noncaseating granulomas, which may form in any organ. The lungs are the primary site of involvement with chest radiograph findings in 95% of those with sarcoid.

A. Clinically.

1. Generally affects those 20 to 40 years of age but may occur at any age.
2. Much more common in African-Americans. Also tends to be more severe in this group.
3. Must differentiate from tuberculosis and fungal illnesses (histoplasmosis etc.), which may have a similar clinical appearance. Also must exclude carcinoma and lymphoma.
4. Symptoms and signs related to organ involved.
   a. Pulmonary manifestations include bilateral hilar adenopathy, dyspnea, reduced vital capacity, and reduced diffusion capacity. May have dyspnea and cough, pleural effusion.
   b. Systemic manifestations include fever, erythema nodosum, infiltrative skin lesions, ocular involvement with uveitis (causes about 4% of uveitis).
   c. CNS involvement may present as meningitis, seizure disorder, cranial nerve abnormality.
   d. Endocrine including hypercalcemia and hypercalciuria, pituitary dysfunction secondary to mass lesions.
   e. Cardiac involvement with arrhythmias, heart block, sudden death.
   f. Bone and joint involvement with pain, arthritis, etc.
   g. Liver and pancreas involvement are common.

B. Diagnosis. Demonstration of noncaseating granulomas by biopsy.

1. Transbronchial biopsy or mediastinal biopsy generally diagnostic.
2. May biopsy skin lesions, peripheral adenopathy, if present.
3. Classically, elevated levels of angiotensin-converting enzyme (ACE) have been used to make the diagnosis of sarcoid. However, this is nonspecific, and ACE levels may be elevated in miliary TB, silicosis, asbestosis, and other conditions. However, once diagnosis is made, can follow ACE levels as measure of disease activity though this is generally not needed.

C. Treatment of sarcoidosis.

1. Corticosteroids are the mainstay of treatment. Generally will respond to relatively low dose steroids (10 to 15 mg/day of prednisone). May use higher doses to help control acutely (60 mg QD for 1 to 2 weeks).

2. Methotrexate and chlorambucil have also been used.
3. Many go into remission spontaneously; so should withdraw steroids after 1 year to see if disease still active.

WEGENER'S GRANULOMATOSIS

Wegener's granulomatosis is a systemic illness that primarily affects the nasal and sinus mucosa, the lung, and the kidney. Necrotizing granulomas are found in the perivascular areas. Generally occurs in middle-aged adults but may occur in younger patients (mean age 40 years).

A. Clinical symptoms.

1. Pulmonary symptoms such as cough, recurrent pneumonia, hemoptysis.
2. Renal symptoms including hematuria, pyuria, renal failure from glomerulonephritis.
3. Recurrent sinusitis.
4. Systemic symptoms including fever, arthralgias, and polyarthritis, weight loss.

B. Diagnosis.

1. c-ANCA (central antineutrophil cytoplasmic antibody) is 85% sensitive. Only other vasculitides will give a false-positive c-ANCA result.
2. Multiple plumonary nodules (may be cavitary) or infiltrates on chest radiograph (90%).
3. Biopsy specimen that shows classic granulomas.
4. May have anemia, elevated sedimentation rate, leukocytosis, pyuria, and hematuria.
5 Complement levels are normal, and the ANA is negative.

C. Treatment and course.

1. Has a 90% mortality within 1 to 2 years if not treated.
2. Steroids have been used for treatment but are not particularly effective.
3. Cyclophosphamide is the treatment of choice early in the disease before there is frank renal failure. This should be initiated after consultation with rheumatology and immunology staff.
4. Trimethoprim-sulfamethoxazole has been used with some success 1 DS tablet PO BID) in those with isolated sinus disease.
5. Methotrexate has been used with some success as have other immunosuppressive agents.
6. *However, it is suggested that a consultation be obtained before you initiate the treatment of Wegener's granulomatosis.*

BIBLIOGRAPHY

American Academy of Allergy and Immunology: *Advances in asthma care: participant workbook,* New York, 1991, SCP Communications, Inc.

Berk JL, Sampliner JE, editors: *Handbook of critical care,* ed 3, Boston, 1990, Little, Brown & Co.

Bidani A et al: Permissive hypercapnia in acute respiratory failure, *JAMA* 272(12):957, 1994.

Bittar G et al: The arrhythmogenicity of theophylline: a multivariate analysis of clinical determinants, *Chest* 99(6):1415, 1991.

Breiman RF et al: Emergence of drug-resistant pneumococcal infections in the United States, *JAMA* 271(23):1831, 1994.

Bukata R: Warfarin therapy, *FP/IM Database Essays,* vol 2, no 3, March 1993.

Conti CR: Is menstruation a contraindication to thrombolytic therapy? *Clin Cardiol* 15:625, 1992.

Dale DC, Federman DD, editors: *Scientific American Medicine,* New York, 1996, Scientific American, Inc.

Dalton AM: A review of radiological abnormalities in 135 patients presenting with acute asthma, *Arch Emerg Med* 8(1):36, 1991.

Den Jeijer M et al: Hyperhomocysteinemia as a risk factor for deep-vein thrombosis, *N Engl J Med* 334 (12):759, 1996.

Drummond N et al: Effectiveness of routine self monitoring of peak flow in patients with asthma, *Br Med J* 308(6928):564, 1994.

Dunagan WC, Ridner ML editors: *Manual of medical therapeutics,* ed 26, Boston, 1989, Little, Brown & Co.

Dunmira S: Pulmonary embolism, *Emerg Med Clin North Am* 7(2):339, 1989.

Ebell MH: *C. pneumoniae* in adult asthma, *J Fam Pract* 41:405-406, 1995.

Emre U et al: The association of *Chlamydia pneumoniae* infection and reactive airway disease in children, *Arch Pediatr Adolesc Med* 148(7):727-732, 1994.

Ginsberg JS et al: D-dimer in patients with clinically suspected pulmonary embolism, *Chest* 104(6): 1679-1684, 1993.

Goldhaber SZ: Recent advances in the diagnosis and lytic therapy of pulmonary embolism, *Chest* 99(4):173S, 1991.

Graef JW, editor: *Manual of pediatric therapeutics,* ed 4, Boston, 1988, Little, Brown & Co.

Guilleminault C et al: Upper airway sleep-disordered breathing in women, *Ann Intern Med* 122(7):493-501, 1995.

Hahn DI: Treatment of *Chlamydia pneumoniae* infection in adult asthma: a before and after trial, *J Fam Pract* 41:345-351, 1995.

Hatoum HT: Meta-analysis of controlled trials of drug therapy in mild chronic asthma: the role of inhaled corticosteroids, *Ann Pharmacother* 28(11):1285, 1994.

Hickling KG et al: Low mortality rate in adult respiratory distress syndrome using low-volume, pressure-limited ventilation with permissive hypercapnia: a prospective study, *Crit Care Med* 22(10):1568, 1994.

Hudgel DW: Pharmacologic treatment of obstructive sleep apnea, *J Lab Clin Med* 126(1):13-18, 1995.

Hull RD et al: Subcutaneous low-molecular-weight heparin compared with continuous intravenous heparin in the treatment of proximal vein thrombosis, *N Engl J Med* 326(15):975, 1992.

Imperiale TF et al: A meta-analysis of methods to prevent venous thromboembolism following total hip replacement, *JAMA* 271(22):1780, 1994.

Kastor JA: Multifocal atrial tachycardia, *N Engl J Med* 322(24):1713, 1990.

Koopman MMW et al: Treatment of venous thrombosis with intravenous unfractionated heparin administered in the hospital compared with subcutaneous low-molecular-weight heparin administered at home, *N Engl J Med* 334(11):682, 1996.

Lanter PL et al: Safety of thrombolytic therapy in normally menstruating women with acute myocardial infarction, *Am J Cardiol* 74(2):179, 1994.

Lee HN et al: Inadequacy of intravenous heparin therapy in the initial management of venous thromboembolism, *J Gen Intern Med* 10(6):342, 1995.

Levine M et al: A comparison of low-molecular-weight heparin administered primarily at home with unfractionated heparin administered in the hospital for proximal deep-vein thrombosis, *N Engl J Med* 334(11):677, 1996.

Mandel H, Brenner B et al: Coexistence of hereditary homocystinuria and factor V Leiden: effect on thrombosis, *N Engl J Med* 334(12):763, 1996.
Mandell GL et al: *Handbook of antimicrobial therapy 1992*, New York, 1992, Churchill Livingstone.
Maneker AJ et al: Contribution of routine pulse oximetry to evaluation and management of patients with respiratory illness in a pediatric emergency department, *Ann Emerg Med* 25(1):36, 1995.
Mittl RL et al: Radiographic resolution of community-acquired pneumonia, *Am J Resp Crit Care Med* 149(3):630, 1994.
Molina E: Need for emergency treatment in subclavian vein effort thrombosis, *J Am Coll Surg* 181:414-420, 1995.
Mossad SB et al: Zinc gluconate lozenges for treating the common cold, *Ann Intern Med* 125:81-88, 1996.
Odens MI, Fox CH: Adult sleep apnea syndromes, *Am Fam Physician* 52(3)859-866, 871-872, 1995.
Pratter MR et al: An algorithmic approach to chronic cough, *Ann Intern Med* 119(10):977, 1993.
Raschke RA et al: The weight-based heparin dosing nomogram compared with a "standard care" nomogram, *Ann Intern Med* 119(9):874, 1993.
Sanders RJ, Cooper MA: Surgical management of subclavian vein obstruction including six cases of subclavian vein bypass, *Surgery* 118:856-863, 1995.
Sandford JP: A guide to antimicrobial therapy, Dallas, 1996, Antimicrobial Therapy, Inc.
Schachter J: The association Of *Chlamydia pneumoniae* infection and reactive airway disease in children, *Arch Pediatr Adolescent Med* 148(7):727-732, 1994.
Sériès F, Marc I, Cormier Y, La Forge J: Utility of nocturnal home oximetry for case finding in patients with suspected sleep apnea hypopnea syndrome, *Ann Intern Med* 119:449-453, 1993.
Simonneau G et al: Subcutaneous low-molecular-weight heparin compared with continuous intravenous unfractionated heparin in the treatment of proximal deep vein thrombosis, *Arch Intern Med* 153(13):1541, 1993.
Stein PD et al: Clinical characteristics of patients with acute pulmonary embolism, *Am J Cardiol* 68:1724, 1991.
Stein PD et al: Complications and validity of pulmonary angiography in acute pulmonary embolism, *Circulation* 85(2):462, 1992.
Stein PD et al: Values of ventilation/perfusion scans versus perfusion scans alone in acute pulmonary embolism, *Am J Cardiol* 69(14):1239, 1992.
Strollo PJ Jr, Rogers RM: Obstructive sleep apnea, *N Engl J Med* 334(2):99, 1996.
Taylor DR et al: Regular inhaled beta agonist in asthma: effects on exacerbations and lung function, *Thorax* 48(2):134, 1993.
Tintinalli JE et al: *Emergency medicine: a comprehensive study guide*, New York, 1995, McGraw Hill.
Tryba M: Prophylaxis of stress ulcer bleeding: a meta-analysis, *J Clin Gastroenterol* 13 (suppl 2):S44-S55, 1991.
Vallés J, Artigas A, Rello J et al: Continuous aspiration of subglottic secretions in preventing ventilator-associated pneumonia, *Ann Intern Med* 122:179-186, 1995.
Van Schayck CP et al: Bronchodilator treatment in moderate asthma or chronic bronchitis: continuous or on demand? A randomised controlled study, *Br Med J* 303(6815):1426, 1991.
Wells PS et al: Graduated compression stockings in the prevention of postoperative venous thromboembolism: a meta-analysis, *Arch Intern Med* 154:67, 1994.
Wright SW et al: Pertussis infection in adults with persistent cough, *JAMA*, 273(13):1044, 1995.

4

Gastroenterology

Peter P. Toth

ACUTE DIARRHEA

I. DEFINITION

A. Abnormally increased frequency or decreased consistency of stools for less than 2 to 3 weeks in duration.

B. Pathophysiologic mechanisms.

1. ***Osmotic.*** Caused by ingestion of poorly absorbed solute (carbohydrate malabsorption: ingestion of mannitol, sorbitol, lactulose; generalized malabsorption; ingestion of magnesium-containing antacids).
2. ***Secretory diarrhea.*** Increased small intestinal secretion or reduced absorption. This may result from bacterial enterotoxins, hormonal secretagogues, gastric hypersecretion, laxatives, pancreatic insufficiency, or small intestinal mucosal disease. Usually large-volume, watery stools without blood or white cells.
3. ***Exudative diarrhea.*** Inflammatory states such as inflammatory bowel disease; infection with invasive organisms; cytotoxins, ischemia, or vasculitis. The intestinal mucosa is inflamed, causing mucus, blood, and pus to leak into the lumen.
4. ***Motility disturbance.*** Diarrhea associated with hyperthyroidism, carcinoid, or postgastrectomy dumping syndrome.

II. CAUSES OF ACUTE DIARRHEA

A. Infectious. Although water is an obvious reservoir, contaminated food is the most frequent source of organisms causing diarrhea.

1. ***Bacteria.*** *Campylobacter,* enterotoxigenic *Escherichia coli, Salmonella, Shigella, Clostridium, Yersinia enterocolitica, Vibrio cholerae, Aeromonas, Plesiomonas shigelloides,* and noncholera vibrios.
2. ***Viruses.*** Rotavirus, Norwalk agent, enterovirus, hepatitis-associated virus.

3. ***Fungi.*** *Candida, Actinomyces, Histoplasma.*
4. ***Parasites.*** *Giardia lamblia* (mountainous areas of Russia and North America), *Entamoeba histolytica, Cryptosporidium, Strongyloides.*

B. Toxin.

1. ***Bacterial toxins.*** *Staphylococcus* (food poisoning), *Clostridium perfringens, C. botulinum, C. difficile, Cryptosporidium, E. coli.*
2. ***Chemical poisons.*** Heavy metals, mushroom poisoning.

C. Dietary. Nonabsorbable sugar substitutes (sorbitol), food intolerance or allergy, irritating foods, excessive caffeine.

D. Drugs. Laxatives, magnesium-containing antacids, colchicine, antibiotics, cholinergic agents, lactulose, quinidine.

E. Visceral causes. Appendicitis, diverticulitis, GI hemorrhage, fecal impaction, ischemic colitis, pseudomembranous colitis.

III. DIAGNOSIS

A. Acute diarrhea is often self-limited, and the diagnosis can be made by history and physical examination.

B. If the patient develops systemic toxicity, severe pain, dehydration, or bloody stools, or if symptoms persist more than 24 hours without improvement, then consider:

1. CBC with differential.
2. Stool studies, including ova and parasites, fecal leukocytes, and occult blood.
3. *Clostridium difficile* toxin if recent antibiotic use.
4. Serum electrolytes if needed to manage dehydration.
5. ***Sigmoidoscopy.*** Consider in patients with bloody diarrhea. Can also be useful in diagnosing inflammatory bowel disease, Shigellosis, and amebic dysentery.
6. ***Abdominal, radiographs, flat and upright.*** Obtain if there is bloating, severe pain, obstructive symptoms, or suspected perforation.

IV. TREATMENT

A. Rehydration. (See also Chapter 10.)

1. ***Oral*** (clear liquids, sodium- and glucose-containing oral rehydration solutions).
2. ***Intravenous*** (normal saline or lactated Ringer's solution, especially if severely dehydrated or patient has intractable vomiting).

B. Absorbents (Kaopectate, aluminum hydroxide). These do not alter the course of the disease or reduce fluid loss but allow the patient more control over the timing of defecation. Other medications should be taken ½ hour before or 2 hours after absorbents are used.

C. Antisecretory agents such as bismuth subsalicylate (Pepto-Bismol). Usual dose is 30 ml every 30 minutes for 8 doses.

D. Antiperistaltics, such as opiate derivatives. Do not use in patients with fever, systemic toxicity, or bloody diarrhea. Discontinue if no improvement or if patient deteriorates.

1. ***Diphenoxylate with atropine (Lomotil).*** Available in tablets (2.5 mg of diphenoxylate) and liquid (2.5 mg of diphenoxylate/5 ml). The initial dose for adults is two tablets QID (20 mg/day). For children the dose is 0.1 mg/kg/dose QID. The dose is tapered as diarrhea improves. It is not indicated for diarrhea caused by pseudomembranous colitis or enterotoxin-producing or invasive bacteria. Lomotil should not be used in ulcerative colitis or in children under 2 years of age.
2. ***Loperamide (Imodium).*** Available over the counter in 2 mg capsules and liquid (1 mg/5 ml). It increases the intestinal absorption of electrolytes and water and decreases intestinal motility and secretion. The dose in adults is 4 mg initially, followed by 2 mg after each diarrhea stool, not to exceed 16 mg in one 24-hour period. In children the dose is based on age, with 2 to 5 year olds receiving 1 mg TID 6 to 8 year olds 2 mg BID, and 9 to 12 year olds 2 mg TID on the first day of treatment. Thereafter 0.1 mg/kg is administered after each diarrhea stool, not to exceed the total daily dose recommended for the first day of therapy. Loperamide is safe and decreases the number of unformed stools and the duration of diarrhea in patients with *Shigella*-induced dysentery who are treated with ciprofloxacin.

E. Antibiotics. Not necessary for most episodes of diarrhea but should be directed against known or strongly suspected pathogens. Once cultures are done, empiric with an agent that covers *Shigella* and *Campylobacter* is reasonable in those with severe diarrhea with systemic signs. A 3-day course of a fluoroquinolone (ciprofloxacin 500 mg PO BID or norfloxacin 400 mg PO BID) is the first-line therapy. TMP/SMX (Bactrim DS 1 tab PO QD) is an alternative therapy, but resistant organisms are common in the tropics. If the diarrhea is caused by seafood ingestion, infection with either *Vibrio cholerae* or *Vibrio parahaemolyticus* is possible and can be treated with either a fluoroquinolone or with doxycycline 100 mg PO BID.

F. Traveler's diarrhea. Prophylaxis not routinely recommended because of the risk of adverse effects from the drugs (rash, anaphylaxis, vaginal candidiasis) and the development of resistant gut flora. Possible regimens for prophylaxis include bismuth subsalicylate (Pepto-Bismol) 524 mg PO QID with meals and QHS, doxycycline 100 mg PO QD (resistance documented in many areas of the world), TMP/SMX 160 mg/800 mg (1 double-strength tablet) PO QD, or norfloxacin 400 mg PO QD (fluoroquinolones should not be prescribed to children or pregnant women). No significant resistance to the fluoroquinolones has yet been reported in high-risk areas, and they are the most effective antibiotics in regions where susceptibilities are not known. Loperamide can be added to the fluoroquinolones or TMP/SMX when treating traveler's diarrhea. These medications should be continued for 1 or 2 days after patient returns home.

G. **Fluid repletion.** A simple oral rehydration solution may be composed of 1 level teaspoon of salt and 4 heaping teaspoons of sugar added to 1Liter of water. Bottled flavored mineral water with saltine crackers is an acceptable alternative. See Chapter 10 for further details of preparation.

CHRONIC DIARRHEA

I. DEFINITION

Diarrhea persisting for more than 4 weeks.

II. ETIOLOGY

A. **Infection.** Giardiasis, amebiasis, *Clostridium difficile, Cryptosporidium* (see also Chapter 16).

B. **Inflammation.** Ulcerative colitis, Crohn's disease, ischemic colitis, diverticulitis, AIDS-related chronic diarrhea, collagenous colitis (very common in middle-aged and elderly women), microscopic (lymphocytic) colitis.

C. **Drugs.** Laxatives, antibiotics, NSAIDs, magnesium-containing antacids, alcohol.

D. **Malabsorption.** Short bowel syndrome, celiac sprue, carbohydrate malabsorption, pancreatic insufficiency, bacterial overgrowth.

E. **Endocrine.** Hyperthyroidism, diabetes, adrenal insufficiency, hypoparathyroidism, Zollinger-Ellison syndrome.

F. **Motility disorders.** Irritable bowel syndrome, dumping syndrome.

G. **Infiltrative disorders.** Amyloidosis, diffuse intestinal lymphoma, scleroderma.

H. **Hormone-producing tumors.** VIPoma, carcinoid tumor, pheochromocytoma, ganglioneuroma.

III. EVALUATION

A. **History.** Inquire about diurnal variation, relationship to meals, weight loss, and character of stools (such as, foul-smelling or greasy stools characteristic of malabsorption, chronic bloody stools with abdominal pain, tenesmus suggestive of inflammatory bowel disease or tumor).

B. **Physical examination.** Look for abdominal tenderness, distension, organomegaly, anal fistulas, rectal mass, and hyperactive bowel sounds.

C. **Laboratory analyses.**

1. ***CBC with differential.*** Anemia is suggestive of chronic blood loss, infection, malabsorption, or neoplasm. Eosinophilia may be secondary to parasitic disease or allergic

reaction. Megaloblastic anemia may result from vitamin B_{12} or folate malabsorption.

2. ***ESR.*** If elevated, may indicate chronic inflammation.
3. ***Serum electrolytes, magnesium, iron, renal function, albumin, cholesterol.*** Calcium, phosphate, and alkaline phosphatase levels to evaluate for parathyroid disease. A fasting or 2-hour postprandial glucose can be used to screen for diabetes. Carotene levels may be low because of fat malabsorption. PT/PTT may be abnormal because of decreased vitamin K absorption. Thyroid function abnormalities should be ruled out.
4. ***Stool exam for occult blood, leukocytes, and ova and parasites.*** A stool specimen should be sent for culture and sensitivity. Stool antigen test (sensitivity 92%, specificity 98%) is available for *Giardia* organisms and is more sensitive than an "O & P."

D. Special tests.

1. 72-hour fecal fat quantitation or Sudan staining of stool if steatorrhea is suspected.
2. D-Xylose absorption (decreased in disorders of proximal small intestine).
3. A stool pH <5.3 is diagnostic of a carbohydrate intolerance. Breath hydrogen test for lactase deficiency. Can also check for reducing substances in stool or therapeutic trial of lactose-free diet.
4. Small intestinal biopsy (useful for Whipple's disease, celiac sprue, collagenous colitis, regional enteritis, some parasitic infestations).
5. Serum IgA antigliadin and smooth muscle endomysial antibody titers may be positive in celiac sprue/gluten insensitivity.
6. Small bowel culture for bacterial overgrowth.
7. Stool test with phenolphthalein (test for factitious laxative abuse). Bring stool pH to 8.0. If the specimen turns maroon in color, this indicates the presence of phenolphthalein, a common ingredient in over-the-counter laxative products. Urine tests are available to detect aloes, senna alkaloids, and bisacodyl.
8. Sigmoidoscopy should be done to detect inflammation of the colon or rectum, neoplasms, and parasites.
9. ***Radiographic studies.*** Plain abdominal radiography and barium studies of the upper GI tract, small intestine, and colon.

IV. TREATMENT

A. Should be directed toward underlying cause of the chronic diarrhea.

B. Occasionally, when a definitive diagnosis cannot be made, one might empirically try:

1. Restricting lactose, gluten, or long-chain fatty acids in the diet. Restrictions should be done systematically so that if symptoms improve, the restricted factor can be identified and removed permanently from the diet. Lactase replacement (such as Lactaid caplets) is available over the counter for those patients found to be intolerant to lactose.
2. Pancreatic enzyme supplementation (Creon [pancrelipase] capsules) for suspected pancreatic exocrine deficiency (such as cystic fibrosis, chronic pancreatitis).
3. Increase dietary or supplemental fiber.
4. Cholestyramine, which tends to have a constipating effect.
5. Antimicrobials (such as metronidazole).
6. Judicious use of antidiarrheal medication (opiate derivatives) may be useful for symptomatic relief in some patients. See acute diarrhea section for dosages and cautions, p. 155.
7. Many patients with chronic watery diarrhea accompanied by abdominal pain will not have a diagnosable cause for their diarrhea. These patients typically have a form of irritable bowel syndrome.

IRRITABLE BOWEL SYNDROME

I. GENERAL FEATURES

A. History. Patients often describe a long history of chronic or intermittent diarrhea, which usually starts before 50 years of age and is exacerbated by anxiety or stress. Diarrhea is often worse in the morning and after meals. These patients often complain of a sensation of incomplete evacuation, distension, passage of mucus, with or without associated abdominal, pelvic, and back pain. Pain is relieved by evacuation. Alternating constipation, diarrhea, and bloating is typical of irritable bowel syndrome. Diarrhea is not bloody unless accompanied by an anorectal lesion such as hemorrhoids or a fissure. There are no systemic symptoms or weight loss, and nutritional status is not compromised.

B. Etiology. The following factors are believed to play a mechanistic role in irritable bowel syndrome, and more than one may operate in a given individual: (1) abnormal motility, (2) abnormal visceral perception, (3) psychologic factors, (4) luminal compounds (lactose, short-chain fatty acids, food allergens, and bile acids), which may irritate the bowel.

C. Physical examination is usually normal.

D. A work-up should be done to exclude other causes. Stool will usually be negative for occult blood. Sigmoidoscopy and barium enema are also usually normal.

E. Associated symptoms and signs that increase the likelihood of organic disease include blood in stools, nocturnal diarrhea, recent onset, weight loss, painless diarrhea, positive HIV status. The absence of the above supports the diagnosis of functional bowel disease.

F. Treatment.

1. ***Supportive.*** Stress reduction, reassurance.
2. ***Diet and fiber therapy.*** Avoid foods that the patient notices increase symptoms. High-fiber diet or fiber supplements are helpful in some patients.
3. ***Antispasmodics.*** Dicyclomine 10 to 20 mg QID may be helpful, but frequency of side-effects may limit use.
4. Eliminate laxatives.
5. Patients with diarrhea may have some relief with low doses of diphenoxylate or loperamide PRN (see section on acute diarrhea, p. 155).
6. Long-term follow-up studies indicate that most symptoms may resolve with time and the survival of these patients is unaffected by irritable bowel syndrome. Maintaining a positive, sympathetic physician-patient relationship, addressing patient concerns and expectations, setting limits, and involving the patient in treatment decisions contribute to better results and fewer follow-up visits.

CONSTIPATION AND FECAL IMPACTION

See Chapter 10 for pediatric considerations.

I. CONSTIPATION: ETIOLOGY AND DIFFERENTIAL DIAGNOSIS

A. Drugs. Aluminum-containing antacids, calcium supplements, iron supplements, opiates, antihypertensives (calcium-channel blockers, clonidine), anticholinergic agents (antidepressants, neuroleptics, antihistamines), some antiparkinsonian drugs, antispasmodics, estrogen and progestins, among many others.

B. Dietary. Inadequate fluid and fiber intake.

C. Lack of exercise.

D. Metabolic. Hypothyroidism, hypercalcemia, Addison's disease, Cushing's syndrome, other electrolyte abnormalities.

E. Neurogenic. Multiple sclerosis, Parkinson's disease, spinal cord disease, autonomic neuropathy.

F. Colonic disease. Tumors, diverticular disease, irritable bowel syndrome, inflammatory strictures.

G. Other. Anal fissure (pain), withholding, dementia, many others.

II. EVALUATION

A. Infants and young adults usually need minimal work-up. Exceptions would be suspected Hirschsprung's disease or chronic refractory constipation. See Chapter 10.

B. In older adults the extent of the evaluation depends on the nature and duration of symptoms. A more detailed evaluation may be indicated if there is a history of severe straining, incomplete evacuation, or presence of anemia. Blood in the stool (occult or frank) merits a work-up for colon cancer in older adults with constipation. In this case colonoscopy is more cost effective than barium enema because polypectomy and mucosal biopsy can be concomitantly performed with optimal visualization of the bowel lumen.

C. **Studies.** Consider serum electrolytes, calcium, glucose, thyroid function tests, sigmoidoscopy, and barium enema.

III. MANAGEMENT

A. **Patient education.** Avoid irritant and combination laxatives. Allow adequate time and a relaxed environment to have a bowel movement. Increase exercise.

B. **Fluid and fiber.** Soluble fiber is more important than insoluble in treating constipation. Soluble fiber is found in grains and legumes, as well as in commercial psyllium preparations (Metamucil). Increase fluid intake to several glasses per day.

C. **Stool softeners and lubricants.** Avoid products that combine stool softeners with irritant laxatives unless specifically indicated. An example of a stool softener is docusate (usual dose 100 mg BID). Mineral oil is an alternative that works as a lubricant. Usual starting dose is 1 tablespoon QHS and the dose can be increased as needed to a maximum of 4 tablespoons per day. Mineral oil may interfere with the absorption of fat-soluble vitamins. Be cautious in the elderly or those with swallowing problems because of the danger of aspiration.

D. **Hyperosmotic preparations.** Mainstay of therapy for chronic constipation. Examples include nonabsorbable sugars such as lactulose or sorbitol. These agents work by increasing the water content of stools. The usual dose of lactulose is 1 or 2 tablespoons up to qid; start with a low dose and titrate to desired effect. 70% sorbitol is less expensive and also effective.

E. **Local agents (enemas, suppositories).** Initiate reflex evacuation by distending or irritating colon and rectum. Common enema solutions include soap suds, water, and saline. Bisacodyl and glycerin suppositories work as local irritants.

F. Misoprostol is an effective agent for treating constipation but is expensive.

G. Surgical treatment may be required in certain circumstances (Hirschsprung's disease, idiopathic megacolon, and pseudo-obstruction).

H. Psychosocial issues concerning defecation (embarrassment, aversion, anxiety, depression) may also have to be explored.

IV. FECAL IMPACTION

Firm, immobile mass of stool, most often in the rectum but may also occur in sigmoid or descending colon. Most common in elderly, inactive patients. Differential diagnosis is similar to that for constipation. Impaction may present with involuntary leakage of stool around the impaction, which may be mistaken for diarrhea. May have fever, symptoms of acute abdomen, or mental status changes. Treatment involves manual disimpaction or enemas (warm water, saline, or mineral oil). Mineral oil can be given orally if there is no danger of aspiration.

DIVERTICULAR DISEASE

I. DEFINITIONS

A. **Diverticulum (plural, diverticula).** Outpocketing from bowel wall. The most common colonic diverticula are pseudodiverticula, which are herniations of mucosa and submucosa through the muscularis at sites of penetration of nutrient arteries. Most occur in the sigmoid and descending colon.

B. **Diverticulosis.** Presence of mulitple diverticula. Does not imply a pathologic condition.

C. **Diverticulitis.** Inflammation and infection in one or more diverticula.

II. SYMPTOMATIC DIVERTICULOSIS

A. **Symptoms.** Most patients with colonic diverticula are asymptomatic. Some will have chronic or intermittent left lower quadrant abdominal pain and constipation or diarrhea. The symptoms overlap with those of irritable bowel syndrome.

B. **Physical exam.** Possibly tenderness, firm feces-filled sigmoid colon in the left lower abdomen. Rectal exam may reveal firm, guaiac-negative stool.

C. Studies may not be indicated if symptoms are mild and the patient is otherwise healthy. If symptoms are more severe or if the patient has occult blood in stool, weight loss, or other symptoms of concern, one should obtain a CBC, UA, and perform a flexible sigmoidoscopy and barium enema or colonoscopy.

D. **Differential diagnosis.** Irritable bowel syndrome, diverticulitis, colon cancer, inflammatory bowel disease, or a urologic or gynecologic disorder.

E. **Treatment.** Similar to irritable bowel syndrome. Recommend high-fiber diet. Antispasmodics such as dicyclomine may help with cramping. Avoid cathartic laxatives.

III. DIVERTICULITIS

A. **Symptoms.** When full blown, may have acute abdominal pain, fever, chills, and tachycardia. May present acutely, but more often develops over hours to days with left lower quadrant pain, anorexia, fever, nausea, vomiting.

B. **Physical examination.** Abdominal tenderness to palpation with possible rebound tenderness. A palpable mass may be present, representing an abscess or inflammatory phlegmon. Bowel sounds may be active if there is partial obstruction; hypoactive or absent if peritonitis has developed. A rectal exam may help localize the abscess or inflammatory mass.

C. **Diagnostic studies.** Differential CBC and UA. Abdominal pain films (flat and upright) to evaluate for ileus, obstruction, and free air (perforation). Ultrasonography of the abdomen and pelvis may be helpful in identifying an inflammatory mass or abscess, but a CT scan is the imaging procedure of choice. Sigmoidoscopy may be performed cautiously if there is no evidence of perforation and if necessary for diagnosis. However, sigmoidoscopy and barium enema are both best delayed until after acute symptoms resolve.

D. **Differential diagnosis.** Appendicitis, inflammatory bowel disease, ischemic colitis, colon cancer, other causes of bowel obstruction, urologic or gynecologic disorders.

E. **Treatment.** Keep NPO, place nasogastric tube, and maintain hydration with IV fluids. Broad-spectrum antibiotics such as ampicillin/gentamycin/clindamycin or cefoxitin alone should be used for inpatients. TMP/SMX (DS 1 tab PO BID) and metronidazole 500 mg PO QID is a good regimen for outpatients. Antibiotics should be continued for 7 to 10 days. Abscess may require percutaneous drainage under ultrasound or CT guidance. Surgery may be required if there is peritonitis, with or without evidence of perforation, unresolved obstruction, or development of a colovesical fistula. Other indications for surgical intervention are failure to improve after several days of medical treatment or recurrence after successful treatment.

ANORECTAL DISEASES

I. HEMORRHOIDS

A. **Definition.** Dilated vein within the anal canal and distal area of rectum. Internal hemorrhoids are derived from the internal hemorrhoidal plexus above the dentate line and are covered by rectal mucosa. External hemorrhoids are derived from the external hemorrhoidal plexus below the dentate line and are covered by stratified squamous epithelium.

B. **Causes.** Increased abdominal pressure secondary to straining during bowel movements, heavy lifting, childbirth, and benign prostatic hypertrophy.

C. **Classification.**

1. ***First degree.*** No prolapse.

2. ***Second degree.*** Condition prolapses but reduces spontaneously.
3. ***Third degree.*** Reduces with manual reduction.
4. ***Fourth degree.*** Permanently prolapsed, will not reduce.

D. Symptoms. Bright red bleeding with defecation, external protrusion, tenderness (severe pain unusual unless thrombosed), itching.

E. Treatment.

1. ***General principles.*** High-fiber diet, stool softeners; avoid straining during bowel movements; avoid heavy lifting. Warm sitz baths BID and lubrication with glycerin suppositories may help to reduce symptoms. Medicated suppositories such as Anusol HC (contains hydrocortisone) may help to decrease inflammation. Limit steroid-containing medications to less than 2 weeks of continuous use to avoid atrophy of anal tissues.
2. ***Thrombosed external hemorrhoids.*** Often can be treated nonsurgically. However, if a patient presents within 48 to 72 hours of onset, excision of thrombus often provides dramatic relief of pain. Incision and drainage is not adequate; the entire thrombus should be excised.
3. Infrared photocoagulation is probably the treatment of choice for first-degree hemorrhoids that cannot be managed with the conservative measures outlined above.
4. Rubber band ligation is useful for second-degree and small third-degree hemorrhoids. Limit treatment to two hemorrhoidal areas at one time. Subsequent treatments can be performed at 4 to 6 week intervals. Consider surgical referral if symptoms persist after 3 or 4 treatments.
5. ***Work-up for bleeding presumed to be from hemorrhoids.*** Digital rectal exam and anoscopy is the minimum work-up for the patient who presents with rectal bleeding. If the bleeding source is not apparent or if the history is not consistent with hemorrhoids as the source, then do sigmoidoscopy. If the patient is >40 years of age, do sigmoidoscopy as part of the initial evaluation of rectal bleeding. A barium enema (in addition to sigmoidoscopy) or colonoscopy should be done in patients over 50 with rectal bleeding, or in patients whose stools remain guaiac positive after treatment of their hemorrhoids.

II. ANAL FISSURES

A. Definition. Superficial tear in the distal lining of the anal canal, usually posteriorly in the midline. Consider inflammatory bowel disease, leukemia, syphilis, and TB as possible secondary causes of lesions located outside the midline.

B. History. Usually acute onset of sharp anal pain brought on by a bowel movement. The pain lasts several minutes to hours. A small amount of bleeding may be present.

C. Treatment. Bulk laxatives, stool softeners, sitz baths. Usually heal in 2 to 4 weeks. Glyceryl trinitrate ointment applied BID promotes healing and can obviate the need for surgery. Botulinum toxin injections have been used with some success. If the fissure does not heal, the patient may require sphincterotomy. Chronic fissures are characterized by a deeper fissure, exposed underlying sphincter muscle, a skin tag at the distal end of the tear, and hypertrophy of the anal papilla at the proximal end. Chronic fissures may require sphincterotomy to heal.

III. ANORECTAL ABSCESS

A. Cause. Obstruction of the anal glands, leading to infection and abscess formation.

B. Locations. Perianal (40% to 50%), ischiorectal (20% to 30%), intersphincteric (20% to 25%), supralevator (5% to 7%).

C. Signs and symptoms. Pain, swelling, and redness for superficial abscesses. Deeper abscesses may present only with systemic symptoms such as fever, malaise, and an elevated white blood cell count. Examination will reveal fullness or a tender mass.

D. Treatment. Incision and drainage. Antibiotic therapy is usually not needed if external drainage is adequate. However, antibiotics may be necessary for patients with significant surrounding cellulitis and in diabetic patients. If there is substantial soft-tissue inflammation, hospitalization, IV antibiotics, drainage and débridement, and surgical referral may be warranted. Intersphincteric and supralevator abscesses are treated by internal drainage into the rectum, performed under anesthesia. The patient should be warned that fistulas develop in approximately 25% of cases, usually occurring several weeks after the abscess is drained.

GASTROINTESTINAL BLEEDING

I. TYPES

A. Hematemesis. Vomiting of blood.

1. May be bright red blood or coffee grounds–like material.
2. Usually from bleeding proximal to the ligament of Treitz.
3. ***Sources.***
   a. Peptic ulcer disease may be asymptomatic until first bleed especially in patients taking NSAID.
   b. Gastritis, especially from alcohol.
   c. Mallory-Weiss tear occurs after prolonged vomiting or retching and is generally a self-limited bleed. Look for mediastinal air on CXR.
   d. Esophageal varices from portal hypertension especially secondary to chronic alcohol consumption.
   e. Swallowed blood from epistaxis or other source of bleeding.

B. Melena. Passage of black, tarry stools secondary to GI bleeding with intestinal transit time allowing for the digestion of hemoglobin.

1. May be of upper or lower GI origin (Table 4-1).
2. Black, tarry stools can be the result of ingested iron, licorice, or bismuth, but the stool will be guaiac negative.

C. Hematochezia. Bright red blood per rectum.

1. Can be secondary to anal disease (hemorrhoids, rectal fissure).
2. May be secondary to bleeding diverticulum, other colonic disease such as angiodysplasia, Crohn's disease, ulcerative colitis, carcinoma (very rarely causes gross bleeding), dysentery (especially amebiasis, *Campylobacter, Shigella,* or other invasive organisms).
3. Ingestion of beets may simulate hematochezia.

II. EVALUATION OF THE GI BLEED

A. Laboratory studies should include CBC and platelets, PT/PTT, electrolytes, BUN/creatinine (GI bleeders will frequently have elevated BUN secondary to the increased ingestion of nitrogen from digested blood). The patient should be typed and crossed for at least 2 units of packed red blood cells.

B. Physical examination often reveals hyperactive bowel sounds secondary to intraluminal blood. If an acute abdomen is present, consider CXR and an upright abdominal film to look for free air.

C. Endoscopy may be done acutely for upper GI bleeding to help define the source and treat endoscopically if able.

D. Angiography or nuclear medicine studies can be useful to localize lower GI bleeding.

TABLE 4-1
Etiology of GI Bleeding

Category	Upper GI bleed	Lower GI bleed
Inflammatory	Peptic ulcer	Ulcerative colitis
	Esophagitis	Crohn's disease
	Gastritis	Diverticulitis
	Stress ulcer	Enterocolitis
Mechanical	Mallory-Weiss tear	Anal fissure
	Hiatal hernia	Diverticulosis
Vascular	Esophageal varices	Hemorrhoids
		Hemorrhoids and AV malformations
		Angiodysplasia
Neoplastic	Carcinoma	Carcinoma and polyps
Systemic	Blood dyscrasias	Blood dyscrasias

III. MANAGEMENT OF THE ACUTE GI BLEED

A. Upper GI bleeding.

1. Start IV fluid resuscitation and manage shock as per Chapter 1.
2. An NG tube should be placed to document the source and relative rate of bleeding (blood is usually present in the NG aspirate during an upper GI bleed). The NG tube may be removed after the diagnosis is made unless it is needed to prevent nausea and vomiting. *Ice saline lavage does not serve a useful purpose.*
3. H_2-antagonist therapy with either cimetidine (300 mg) or ranitidine (50 mg) can be given IV but will *not* act to slow current bleeding.
4. Transfuse as needed.
5. Endoscopy and endoscopic therapy is the treatment of choice if possible.
6. ***Esophageal varices.***
   a. Vasopressin has been shown to be no more effective than placebo in controlling bleeding from esophageal varices or other upper GI sources. There is no difference in the need for transfusion or surgery, nor is there any difference in mortality when vasopressin is compared to placebo.
   b. The combination of sclerotherapy and octreotide (a synthetic somatostatin analog, 25 μg/hour) is superior to sclerotherapy alone in controlling acute variceal bleeding in patients with cirrhosis. However, a recent metanalysis indicates that octreotide alone may not have any advantage over placebo. If used, the dose is 250 μg as a bolus and continuous infusion of 250 μg of somatostatin per hour for 24 hours. Maybe most useful as adjunct to banding.
   c. A method gaining increasing attention and use is the transjugular intrahepatic portosystemic shunt (TIPS). This is regarded as a safe and established means of treating variceal hemorrhage in patients with portal hypertension who fail sclerotherapy. The shunt decreases the portal venous pressure gradient by an average of 57% and helps to prevent variceal rebleeding in 92% and 82% of patients at 6 and 12 months after therapy respectively.
   d. Prophylactic banding of varices before a bleed occurs does not seem to confer any advantage over treatment after hemorrhage.
   e. The combined use of a beta-blocker and nitrate (nadalol and isosorbide mononitrate) has been shown to reduce portal pressure and decrease variceal bleeding. This combination may be superior to sclerotherapy. However, neither agent alone is beneficial.

B. Lower GI bleeding.

1. Start IV fluid resuscitation and manage shock as per p. 48.
2. Work-up may include colonoscopy, barium enema, selective angiography, and radionuclide bleeding studies.
3. A surgical consultation should be obtained in case operative intervention is needed.
4. Most causes of lower GI bleeding are initially self-limited.

DYSPEPSIA AND PEPTIC ULCER DISEASE

I. GENERAL

Predisposing factors for both duodenal and gastric ulcers include alcohol, tobacco, aspirin and other NSAIDS, and physiologic stress such as multiple trauma, sepsis, neurosurgical problems, other ICU stresses.

II. DUODENAL ULCER

A. Clinically. Patient will usually report gnawing or burning midepigastric or right upper quadrant pain that is worse several hours after meals and relieved with food or antacids. Pain may awaken the patient at night. Up to 10% of the U.S. population may be affected at some time in their lives. *However, many ulcers, especially those that are NSAID related, may be painless and may initially present with an upper GI bleed.*

B. Physical exam. May reveal midepigastric or RUQ tenderness. Rectal examination should be done to rule out bleeding.

C. Laboratory exam. Should include a CBC count if the patient's stool is guaiac positive (see previous section on acute bleeding for work-up of unstable patient).

D. Who needs a study to visualize the upper GI tract? Those over 65 years of age or with other symptoms suggestive of malignancy such as fever, weight loss, early satiety, or vomiting should be evaluated on presentation. Others can be treated presumptively but should be worked up if have recurrent disease or disease that is difficult to control. Work-up can be either a barium upper GI study or endoscopy. Endoscopy is a superior test for diagnosis but is more costly and has less patient acceptance.

E. The role of *Helicobacter pylori*. Excluding patients with Zollinger-Ellison syndrome and NSAID-induced ulcer disease, *Helicobacter pylori* (a urease-producing flagellated bacterium) infection has been proved to play an etiologic role in up to 95% of duodenal ulcers and greater than 80% of gastric ulcers. There is also evidence that *H. pylori* infection is highly correlated with atrophic gastritis, intestinal metaplasia, gastric carcinoma, gastric non-Hodgkin's lymphoma, and mucosa-associated lymphoid tissue lymphomas of the stomach. Treating for *H. pylori* increases healing and decreases relapse rate.

1. ***Testing for Helicobacter pylori.*** If the patient is not receiving an NSAID, consider presumptive treatment for *H. pylori* without a work-up. Presumptive treatment has been shown to be clinically cost effective. Patients receiving an NSAID should have this stopped, and if symptoms or ulceration resolves, there is no need to treat for *H. pylori.*
2. Several antibiotic regimens are effective in treating *H. pylori.* Current data indicate that optimal treatment requires 2 weeks of therapy with a combination of an acid inhibitor and antibiotics. Both options below have a >90% cure rate. Options include:
   a. Bismuth (Pepto-Bismol, 1 tablet PO QID) with tetracycline (500 mg PO QID) and metronidazole (250 mg PO TID). Amoxicillin (1 g BID) or clarithromycin may be substituted if patient has recently taken metronidazole. Adding an H_2 blocker or proton pump inhibitor increases success. Many do not successfully complete this regimen.
   b. Clarithromycin 500 mg PO TID and omeprazole 40 mg PO QD × 14 days.
3. If symptoms persist or patient does not respond to treatment, further evaluation is indicated. *H. pylori* can be detected by both invasive and noninvasvive tests.
   a. Invasive. Endoscopy and biopsy can be done with either histologic confirmation of infection, demonstration of urease activity in specimen, or direct culture of *H. pylori.*
   b. Noninvasive (sensitivity and specificity >95%). Serologic test for *H. pylori*–directed IgG, breath test for urease activity with orally administered radioactive carbon–labeled urea.

F. The role of acid-control measures. All the following have been shown to be effective for treating duodenal ulcers when given for 6 to 8 weeks. *However, be sure to address* H. pylori *infection as noted above. Using acid control measures alone is inadequate.*

1. H_2-blockers.
   a. Cimetidine (Tagamet) 800 mg QHS. There is no good evidence that BID dosing is superior. Maintenance is 400 mg PO QHS. Will cause increased theophylline levels, affects the metabolism of warfarin, phenytoin, and some tricyclic antidepressants. May cause confusion in the elderly.
   b. Famotidine (Pepcid) 40 mg PO QHS. Does not cause CNS side effects; does not inhibit hepatic metabolism of drugs. Safety beyond 8 weeks of therapy is not established. A negative inotropic effect of famotidine has been noted in healthy subjects and in patients with CHF.

c. Ranitidine (Zantac) 300 mg PO QHS and 150 mg PO QHS for maintenance. Has similar drug interactions to cimetidine but only about 10% of that seen with cimetidine.

d. Nizatidine (Axid) 300 mg PO QHS and 150 mg PO QHS for maintenance. Does not have drug interactions as encountered with cimetidine. Rare mental confusion reported but no increased incidence in the elderly.

2. ***H^+/ATPase inhibitors (omeprazole and lansoprazole).*** Omeprazole 20 mg PO QD for 4 to 8 weeks. May prolong elimination of diazepam, warfarin, and phenytoin. Should also monitor theophylline levels and may change the activity of propranolol. May be used for chronic suppression.
3. ***Sucralfate.*** Indicated for therapy of duodenal ulcers (1 g PO ½ hour before meals and QHS for 6 to 8 weeks). Effective and no systemic side effects but difficult to maintain regimen. 1 g PO BID can be used as maintenance therapy.

G. Role of lifestyle factors. To be successful at treating ulcer disease, it is important that the patient be advised to avoid factors that predispose to ulceration including alcohol, NSAIDs and aspirin, and tobacco use.

H. Preventing recurrence. Continue maintenance for 2 additional weeks after 6 to 8 weeks of treatment and consider long-term suppression in those at high risk of recurrence (smokers, alcohol abusers) and in those with a high risk of bleeding. Treating for *H. pylori* is effective at preventing recurrence.

I. Recurrent duodenal ulcers.

1. Should have full work-up including upper GI or endoscopy, or both, and formal evaluation for *H. pylori.*
2. Consider surgical consult for vagotomy and antrectomy.
3. Measure fasting plasma gastrin to rule out Zollinger-Ellison syndrome (multiple recurrent ulcers secondary to increased gastrin secretion).
4. Consider causes such as carcinoma. In the immunosuppressed, cytomegalovirus should be considered a potential cause.

J. Complications of duodenal ulcer disease.

1. Gastric outlet obstruction with early satiety and reflux symptoms.
2. Perforation. Usually occurs posteriorly and presents as an acute abdomen.
3. GI bleeding. See section on gastrointestinal bleeding, p. 166.

III. GASTRIC ULCERS

A. Clinically. Patients are generally older (>40), and pain is made worse by food.

B. Examination. Same as for duodenal ulcer.

C. Laboratory studies. Same as for duodenal ulcer.

D. Radiograph. An upper GI should be done if history consistent with gastric ulcer.

E. Endoscopy. All lesions found by radiography should be biopsied to rule out gastric carcinoma. Several samples should be taken of each ulcer as well as brushings for cytologic examination.

F. Treatment. Same as for duodenal ulcers. *Resolution of symptoms and healing of ulcer with treatment do not ensure that it is not a carcinoma. All gastric ulcers require biopsy.*

IV. NSAID-INDUCED GASTRODUODENAL ULCERS

A. General. NSAIDs are the most widely prescribed drugs in the world. They are potent cyclo-oxygenase inhibitors and prevent the gastric synthesis of prostaglandins, which are necessary for the production of gastric protective mucus and bicarbonate. *NSAID-induced ulcers are not related to infection with* H. pylori *and therefore will not respond to antibiotic therapy.*

B. Presentation. Many NSAID-related ulcers are painless because NSAIDs are such potent pain relievers. Dyspeptic symptoms do not correlate well with NSAID-induced ulcers. Those with symptoms frequently do not have ulcers and those without symptoms frequently do.

C. Treatment.

1. Stop offending drug and use acetaminophen for pain control if possible. If not, choose one of the NSAIDs with lower GI side effects such as ibuprofen, salsalate, or nabumetone (Relafen). The first two are much less expensive.
2. Antacids (Maalox or Mylanta 30 ml PO QHS and 3 hours after meals), and sucralfate (1 g PO ½ hour before meals and QHS) may all be used to promote ucler healing and *prevent a duodenal ulcer but not a gastric ulcer.*
3. H_2-blockers (see duodenal ulcer above) may be used as a treatment for NSAID-induced ulcers and most will *prevent duodenal ulcers but not gastric ulcers.* High-dose famotidine (40 mg BID) can reduce the incidence of gastric ulcers from 20% to 8%.
4. Misoprostol (Cytotec, a prostaglandin E_1 analog) can be used to prevent gastric ulcer development and recurrence in patients receiving NSAID and aspirin therapy. *However, misoprostol does not reliably prevent duodenal ulcers.* Side effects such as diarrhea and abdominal pain can be reduced by a prescription of misoprostol 200 µg BID or TID rather than QID; there is a small decrease in effectiveness at the lower doses. Because it is an abortifacient it should never be given to women who are or might be pregnant.
5. ***Summary.*** Both an H_2-blocker and misoprostol need to be used together to protect from both gastric and duodenal ulcers.

ESOPHAGEAL DISEASES

I. DYSPHAGIA

The sensation of difficulty in swallowing and feeling as though food is getting stuck in the esophagus. This is a common presenting complaint with many esophageal diseases just as "cardiac"-like chest pain is.

A. Consider esophagitis (as from *Candida,* herpes simplex virus) in the appropriate setting.

B. Always consider espohageal malignancy when dysphagia is present.

C. See also specific disease entities below.

II. ESOPHAGEAL FOREIGN BODIES

A. Clinically. Presents as inability to swallow without regurgitation including the inability to swallow saliva.

1. Usually occurs after eating a large bolus of meat.
2. May have a previous history of esophageal obstruction.

B. Diagnosis can be made clinically. Barium swallow can define the area of obstruction though generally is not indicated, since endoscopy may be needed.

C. Treatment. Should not allow impaction to remain for >12 hours because of the risk of perforation.

1. Glucagon 1 mg IV followed in 20 minutes by another 2 mg.
2. IV diazepam may be helpful to relax the patient.
3. Nifedipine or SL NTG have been used with some success.
4. ***Endoscopy.*** Treatment of choice if the above are not successful.
5. Proteolytic enzymes (such as Adolf's meat tenderizer) have been associated with esophageal perforation and are therefore not recommended.

D. Evaluation. All patients should be evaluated for esophageal rings and strictures after the foreign body is removed.

III. SWALLOWED FOREIGN BODIES (EXCLUDING FOOD)

A. Coin ingestion.

1. 35% of children or more are asymptomatic.
2. An esophageal coin is visible as a disk on AP radiograph, whereas one in the trachea tends to be on edge.
3. If has been over 24 hours, consider passing a Foley catheter under fluoroscopy; inflate Foley and pull out coin. The airway must be protected.
4. Endoscopy still treatment of choice. If in the stomach, no need for retrieval.

B. Button battery ingestion.

1. *A true emergency! May have perforation in 4 hours!*
2. *Requires endoscopic retrieval if lodged in esophagus.*
3. If in stomach, may watch for 24 to 48 hours to see if it passes. If not, must be removed endoscopically.

4. Call the National Button Battery Ingestion Hotline with questions: (202)-625-3333.

C. Ingestion of sharp objects.

1. If longer than 5 cm or wider than 2 cm, it may not pass through stomach and should be removed.
2. Remove sharp objects such as razor blades and safety pins, if possible.
3. If not, document passage with serial radiographs.
4. If symptomatic, obtain surgical consultation.

IV. ACHALASIA

Motility disorder of the esophagus in which there is aperistalsis of the esophageal body, failure of the lower esophageal sphincter (LES) to relax with swallowing, and elevated LES pressures.

A. Clinically. Dysphagia, regurgitation, chest pain.

1. Presenting age is 20 to 40 years.
2. There is about a 5% chance of developing esophageal carcinoma.

B. Diagnosis. Barium swallow will demonstrate narrowing of the distal area of esophagus (bird beaking) and dilatation of the proximal area of esophagus.

C. Cause. Loss of Auerbach's neural plexus.

D. Treatment.

1. Nitroglycerin 0.4 mg SL ½ hour before meals and at bedtime.
2. Isosorbide dinitrate 10 to 30 mg PO ½ hour before meals.
3. Calcium-channel blockers such as nifedipine 10 to 30 mg SL ½ hour before meals.
4. Esophageal dilatation with a bougienage may be helpful.
5. Surgical myotomy may be required.

V. DIFFUSE ESOPHAGEAL SPASM

Motor disorder with large-amplitude, long-duration, repetitive contractions of esophageal smooth muscle with the absence of coordinated peristalsis.

A. Clinically patient may have chest pain and dysphagia.

- May be precipitated by stress, cold liquids.

B. Diagnosis.

1. Barium swallow shows diffuse esophageal spasm.
2. Manometry shows normal LES pressures and uncoordinated contraction but some normal peristaltic activity.

C. Treatment. With medications as noted under the discussion of achalasia above.

VI. ZENKER'S DIVERTICULUM

A. Generally. Presents after 60 years of age but patients may have years of symptoms.

B. Clinically.

1. Regurgitation of undigested food when patient bends over or lies down.
2. May lead to aspiration pneumonia.

C. Diagnosis. By barium swallow.

D. Treatment. By surgical resection.

VII. SCLERODERMA

A. Clinically. Dysphagia and acid reflux secondary to lower esophageal sphincter incompetence. Have predisposition to Barrett's metaplasia and stricture of the esophagus. Also predisposed to esophageal adenocarcinoma.

B. Diagnosis.

1. Barium swallow shows dilatation of the lower espohagus with poor sphincter tone.
2. Manometry shows low pressures especially at LES.

C. Treatment is symptomatic as for reflux esophagitis (below).

VIII. GASTROESOPHAGEAL REFLUX AND REFLUX ESOPHAGITIS

Reflux of gastric contents (including acid, pepsin, and bile salts) into the esophagus resulting in mucosal damage. Caused by transient relaxation of the lower esophageal sphincter muscle. These episodes of relaxation are more common after meals and are stimulated by fat in the duodenum.

A. Clinically.

1. Presents as heartburn, dysphagia.
2. Frequently found in asthmatics.
3. ***Predisposing factors.*** Increased gastric volume (from meals, pyloric obstruction, diabetic gastroparesis), increased abdominal pressure as with obesity, pregnancy, ascites, hiatal hernia, smoking, caffeine, alcohol, chocolate, fats.

B. Diagnosis.

1. By history.
2. Esophagoscopy will show esophagitis.
3. Barium swallow may show reflux from stomach to esophagus.
4. Manometry will show decreased LES pressure.
5. ***Bernstein test.*** Solution of 0.1 M HCl is dripped into the distal esophagus at 8 ml/hour. A positive test reproduces the patients symptoms. Saline should be used as a control.
6. 24-hour esophageal pH monitoring.

C. Treatment.

1. Eliminate precipitating factors (see above).
2. Elevate head of bed on block (adding pillows does not work).
3. Histamine-receptor antagonists) cimetidine, ranitidine, nizatidine, and famotidine) and H^+/ATPase inhibitors (omeprazole, lansoprazole) are the only agents known to heal erosive

esophagitis. The H^+/ATPase inhibitors are more expensive and should be reserved for those patients unresponsive to an H_2-blocker. For long-term control, omeprazole (20 mg PO QD) has been shown to be superior at 1 year compared to cisapride (10 mg PO TID) or ranitidine (150 mg PO TID).

4. ***Agents that increase LES tone.***
   a. Metoclopramide (Reglan) 5 to 10 mg PO ½ hour before meals and QHS. Generally needs to be used with an H_2-antagonist, and side effects are relatively frequent.
   b. Omeprazole (Prilosec) 20 mg PO QD for 4 to 8 weeks. This agent acts both by suppressing acid formation and increasing LES tone.
   c. Cisapride (Propulsid) 10 to 20 mg PO ½ hour before meals. This is effective as single-agent therapy but is synergistic with acid-suppressive drugs. Decreases reflux by increasing cholinergic stimulation at lower esophageal myenteric plexus and promotes gastric emptying.
5. Surgical fundoplication for incapacitating disease.

D. Complications. Aspiration pneumonia, acid laryngitis, asthma, pulmonary fibrosis. Barrett's esophagus, stricture formation, and predisposition to carcinoma if chronic.

ACUTE PANCREATITIS

Should be in the differential diagnosis of any acute abdomen.

I. ETIOLOGY

A. Cholelithiasis is the most common cause in the United States, Western Europe, and Asia (45% of cases).

B. Chronic alcohol ingestion is the second leading cause (35% of cases).

C. "Traumatic" causes including *postoperative stress,* ERCP, direct trauma, manometry of the sphincter of Oddi, endoscopic sphincterotomy, and perforation of a duodenal ulcer.

D. Metabolic insults including hypertriglyceridemia (>1000 mg/dl as in type V hyperlipoproteinemia), hypercalcemia (as from hyperparathyroidism), and renal failure.

E. Drugs including DDI (dideoxycytosine), DDC (dideoxyinosine), azathioprine, mercaptopurine, valproic acid, acetaminophen, and others.

F. Infectious causes including viruses (paramyxovirus [mumps], togavirus [rubella], cytomegalovirus, adenovirus, HIV, coxsackievirus B), bacteria *(Mycoplasma, Campylobacter, Legionella, Mycobacterium tuberculosis, M. avium* complex), and parasites (*Ascaris* [ascariasis], *Opisthorchis* [clonorchiasis]).

G. Connective-tissue disorders (SLE, polyarteritis nodosa, sarcoidosis) and idiopathic causes.

II. CLINICAL PRESENTATION

Generally have abdominal pain in midepigastric region radiating to the back, nausea, vomiting, Depending on severity may have low-grade fever and signs of shock. However, patients may be pain free and manifest only shock. Patients may also have evidence of intra-abdominal bleeding (Cullen's sign, Grey Turner's sign). Complications include:

1. Multisystem organ failure (ARDS, renal failure from ATN), shock, DIC and hemorrhage.
2. Pleural effusions, pneumonia, and atelectasis.
3. Formation of pancreatic fluid collections (pseudocysts and abscesses) account for 70% to 80% of mortality.
4. Ileus, colonic obstruction, CNS hypoperfusion with confusion, etc.

III. DIAGNOSIS

A. Amylase and lipase levels should be determined. Amylase is elevated in 80% of those with pancreatitis and is more sensitive early on. Lipase is more sensitive if symptoms have been present for more than 24 hours. Both amylase and lipase levels may be normal in a patient with CT-proved pancreatitis.

B. Ultrasonography or CT of the pancreas is definitive.

C. Radiography may reveal a "sentinel loop," a localized ileus in the midepigastric region. Pleural effusions may also be present.

IV. LABORATORY STUDIES

CBC, electrolytes, liver enzymes, calcium, magnesium, PT/PTT.

1. May have hemoconcentration secondary to third spacing of fluid.
2. May have hypocalcemia caused by "soap" formation (saponification of triglycerides and calcium).
3. Frequently have hypomagnesemia.
4. White blood cell count usually elevated.
5. Liver enzymes may be elevated from biliary obstruction.

V. PROGNOSIS

Based on Ranson's criteria, the presence of three or four signs on admission is associated with a mortality of 15% to 20%. If 7 or more signs are present, mortality approaches 100%.

A. On admission.

1. Age >55 years.
2. WBC count >16,000.
3. Blood glucose >200 mg/dl.
4. LDH >350 IU/L.
5. AST >250 IU/L.

B. At 48 hours.

1. Fall in HCT >10%.
2. Rise in BUN >5 mg/dl.
3. Serum calcium <8 mg/dl.
4. Arterial Po_2 <60 mm Hg.

5. Base deficit >4 mEq/L.
6. Estimated fluid third spacing of >6 liters.

VI. ACUTE MANAGEMENT

Treat underlying cause!

A. **Treat shock.** See Chapter 1 for guidelines. Invasive hemodynamic monitoring may be required. May need up to 8Liters of fluid per day. Antibiotics should only be used for infectious complications and should not be used routinely.

B. **NG tube useful for those with vomiting.** However, NG tubes have not been shown to reduce the duration of hospitalization nor do they decrease pain intensity associated with pancreatitis. Keep NPO.

C. Prevent hypocalcemia and hypomagnesemia.

D. Manage pain with parenteral patient-controlled narcotics (see Chapter 9 for details).

E. Keep stomach pH close to neutral.

F. Octreotide has been shown *not to be useful* in treating pancreatitis.

G. Surgical approach may be needed for trauma, infection, and abscess or pseudocyst formation.

VII. LONG-TERM SEQUELAE

A. **Chronic pancreatitis.** Characterized by chronic and progressive loss of pancreatic parenchyma. Both endocrine (diabetes mellitus) and exocrine (steatorrhea, azotorrhea) insufficiency develop when 80% to 90% of the gland is destroyed. Pancreatic calcification (resulting from intraductal calcium carbonate deposition) may be apparent on plain abdominal radiography. Patients may require therapy with insulin, pancreatic enzyme replacement (Creon), and medium-chain triglycerides.

B. **Pseudocyst formulation.** Result from the formation of granulation tissue within the pancreas. They may be asymptomatic and resolve spontaneously. Treatment (drainage, resection) is indicated if they persist for more than 6 weeks, are enlarging, or are symptomatic.

C. **Pleural fistulas and pancreatic ascites.** These entities result from pancreatic fluid entering the pleural space or abdomen respectively. Treatment includes repeated aspiration, diuretics, carbonic anhydrase inhibitors, octreotide, or surgical correction.

DIFFERENTIAL DIAGNOSIS OF ELEVATED LIVER ENZYMES

1. *Viral agents* including hepatitis (A, B, C, D, E), CMV, Epstein-Barr, and other viruses.
2. *Drugs and chemicals.* Acetaminophen overdose, INH, griseofulvin, anticonvulsants, NSAIDs, etc.; chemicals (carbon tetrachloride etc.), alcohol, etc.

3. *Primary liver diseases.* Sclerosing cholangitis, primary biliary cirrhosis (positive antimitochondrial antibody).
4. *Metabolic diseases* such as Gilbert's disease (mild elevation in unconjugated bilirubin, especially with dehydration), Wilson's disease (decreased ceruloplasmin), hemochromatosis (see Chapter 5), alpha$_1$-antitrypsinase deficiency.
5. *Mechanical difficulties.* Ductal obstruction secondary to common duct stone or carcinoma (especially pancreatic, hepatoma, metastatic).
6. *Cholestasis* from central venous nutrition, pregnancy, or ceftriaxone therapy.
7. *Infiltrative processes.* Fatty liver (especially in those with diabetes, hypothyroidism, obesity; can see on ultrasonogram), liver abscess (including amebic or echinococcal; diagnosis by ultrasonogram or CT; may have eosinophilia), AIDS-related lymphoma.
8. *Trauma secondary to CHF.*

HEPATITIS

I. CLINICALLY

Fever, nausea, anorexia, vague RUQ abdominal pain, jaundice. Smokers may find tobacco tastes bad. There is a pronounced elevation of liver enzymes.

II. ETIOLOGIC AGENTS (Table 4-2)

A. Hepatitis A.

1. 50% to 75% of adults in the U.S. are positive for antibodies to hepatitis A. Hepatitis A is a picornavirus and often produces subclinical disease. Transmission can be parenteral but usually occurs by means of contaminated food and water in areas of the world where sanitation is poor.
2. Diagnosis is based on elevated IgM (acute disease) or elevated IgG (prior disease) antibodies to hepatitis A.
3. Prophylaxis is IgG (gamma globulin) 0.02 ml/kg IM for close contacts. Immunization can be achieved with an inactivated hepatitis A vaccine (Havrix) and should be given IM at least 4 weeks before anticipated exposure, with a second dose 6 months to 1 year later.

B. Hepatitis B. For children 2 to 18 years of age, give 3 doses with repeat doses at 1 month and at 6 to 12 months.

1. Especially frequent in drug abusers, male homosexuals, and chronic dialysis patients. 5% to 10% of U.S. adults have had the disease.
2. 10% develop chronic carrier state and constitute an infectious pool.
3. ***Diagnosis.***
   a. Hepatitis B surface antigen (HBsAg) is found in acute illness and becomes positive 1 to 7 weeks before clinical disease. It remains positive 1 to 6 weeks after clinical disease and in chronic carrier states. Blood containing HBsAg is considered potentially infectious.

TABLE 4-2
Comparisons of Type A, Type B, and Type C Hepatitis

Feature	Hepatitis A	Hepatitis B	Hepatitis C
Incubation	15 to 45 days (mean 30)	30 to 180 days (mean 60 to 90)	15 to 160 days (mean 50)
Onset	Acute	Often insidious	Insidious
Age preference	Children, young adults	Any age	Any age but more common in adults
Transmission route			
Fecal-oral	+++	−	Unknown
Other nonpercutaneous	+/−	++	++
Percutaneous	+/−	+++	+++
Severity	Mild	Often severe	Variable
Prognosis	Generally good	Worse with age, debility	Moderate
Progression to chronicity	None	Occasional (5% to 10%)	Occasional (10% to 50%)
Prophylaxis	Immunoglobulin or hepatitis A vaccine	Standard IG (not documented) HBIG, hepatitis B vaccine	?
Carrier	None	0.1% to 30%	Exists but prevalence unknown

b. Hepatitis B antibody (Anti-HBs) is an antibody against the surface antigen of hepatitis B and appears weeks to months after clinical illness. The presence of this antibody confers immunity and indicates prior disease or vaccination.
c. Anticore antibody (Anti HBc) appears during the acute phase of the illness and can be used to diagnose acute disease. IgM appears acutely and IgG chronically. The latter may be protective against reinfection.
d. Hepatitis B e antigen (HBeAg) is a mark of infectivity both acutely and chronically.
e. Those who are hepatitis B carriers or have chronic active hepatitis will be HBsAg positive.

4. ***Prophylaxis.*** Hepatitis B vaccine at time 0, 1 and 6 months given in the deltoid muscle. An acute exposure by needle stick should be treated with hepatitis B immune globulin

and vaccination. See Chapter 10 for pediatric immunization schedule.

C. Hepatitis C.

1. Accounts for 20% to 40% of acute hepatitis in the U.S. Most patients with hepatitis C have a history of intravenous drug abuse. Hepatitis C also causes 90% of post-transfusional hepatitis. Epidemiologic evidence suggests that it can be transmitted sexually with risk of transmission increasing with duration of a relationship. The virus has an extremely high mutation rate and is thus not easily neutralized by antibody responses.
2. Acute infection is usually asymptomatic. 20% of patients develop jaundice. 75% of those infected develop chronic disease with chronically elevated ALT (2- to 8-fold normal). 20% of patients eventually develop cirrhosis. This can take several years to decades to occur. The degree of ALT elevation does not correlate with the severity of disease. The severity of disease can be evaluated only with a liver biopsy. Hepatitis C infection is a risk factor for the development of hepatocellular carcinoma.
3. Serologic tests that probe for antibodies produced in response to several viral antigens are now available for the diagnosis of hepatitis C. These tests are now highly sensitive and specific. HCV RNA may be more directly detected with polymerase chain reaction technology.
4. Alpha-interferons can be useful in treating chronic hepatitis C but should be administered under the care of a gastroenterologist. The usual dose is 3 million units 3 times per week for 6 months. There is a 40% to 50% response rate, and multiple courses may be necessary to achieve normalization of ALT. There is no other therapy currently available to patients who do not respond to interferon alfa-2b. There may be multiple side effects of therapy, including myelosuppression, fatigue, myalgias, fever, and hair loss.

D. Hepatitis D.

1. Requires coinfection with hepatitis B.
2. Diagnosis made with hepatitis D viral antibody.
3. Clinical course is identical to that of hepatitis B, since it requires coinfection to be active.

E. Chemical agents that can cause hepatitis include acetaminophen toxicity, carbon tetrachloride, alcohol, isoniazid, oral contraceptives, and halothane.

III. MANAGEMENT

Management is supportive and includes nutritional support but limitation of protein intake. Discontinue hepatotoxic drugs, prescribe prophylaxis for contacts. Those with hepatitis A should be prescribed enteric precautions, whereas those with hepatitis B and C should be prescribed blood and body fluid precautions.

ALCOHOLIC LIVER DISEASE

- **A.** Cause is chronic alcohol ingestion.
- **B.** See chronic liver disease below for symptoms and signs.
- **C.** Clinically resembles hepatitis and progresses to cirrhosis.
- **D.** Must abstain from alcohol.
- **E.** See chronic liver disease below for manifestations and treatment.

LIVER FAILURE AND CHRONIC LIVER DISEASE

I. CIRRHOSIS

Cirrhosis is a diffuse process consisting of islands of regenerated liver surrounded by dense fibrosis that occurs after a protracted insult (such as alcohol, chronic active hepatitis).

II. SYMPTOMS OF CIRRHOSIS

Weight loss, malnutrition, fatigue, easy bruising (caused by reduced levels of factors II, VII, IX, and X), jaundice, encephalopathy, pruritus, edema, and ascites. The patient may also have GI bleeding from esophageal varices (caused by portal hypertension) or coma. Look for fetor hepaticus, asterixis, and hyperreflexia. *GI bleeding is a common cause of encephalopathy and coma in liver failure patients because of the large gastrointestinal protein load.*

III. LABORATORY EVALUATION

Laboratory evaluation may show normal liver enzymes in end-stage disease because of the small amount of residual hepatic tissue. These patients will usually have low serum levels of total protein and albumin. Anemia and thrombocytopenia may also be present. Blood ammonia levels may be elevated, but these correlate poorly with clinical manifestations of coma. *Electrolyte abnormalities include hyponatremia, hypokalemia, and water overload (see also sections on these topics). There may also be concomitant acidosis or alkalosis.*

IV. TREATMENT

Consists in removal of the offending agent (such as alcohol).

A. Acute treatment (for coma or encephalopathy).

1. Clean bowels with enemas.
2. Neomycin 4 to 6 g PO QD in divided doses to reduce bacterial toxins. May be given via NG tube.
3. Lactulose 30 to 45 g PO TID to produce two or three loose stools per day.
4. Limit total protein intake to 20 to 40 g/day.
5. Vitamin K 5 to 10 mg/day for 2 or 3 days may help coagulation.

6. Potassium supplements may be used for hypokalemia.
7. Potassium-sparing diuretics such as spironolactone 100 to 300 mg/day divided into 2 or 3 doses will reduce ascites without decreasing potassium. Hydrochlorothiazide or furosemide may be added to this regimen if needed (see section on ascites below).

B. Chronic treatment. Chronic treatment includes the prevention of coma or encephalopathy with the measures outlined above as well as chronic management of electrolyte disorders.

1. Watch for spontaneous peritonitis, which can occur with ascites (see section on ascites below).
2. Acetaminophen toxicity is common in this population with doses that are generally considered nontoxic.

ASCITES

A. Ascites is a pathologic accumulation of serous fluid within the abdomen. It may be caused by decompensated liver disease (alcohol- and virus-related cirrhosis), heart failure, abdominal carcinomatosis, tuberculosis, and pancreatic disease. Cirrhosis is the cause for the most number of cases of ascites.

B. Diagnostic paracentesis can confirm the diagnosis of portal hypertension or rule out the possibility of infection. The following tests should be performed on ascites fluid: cell count, cytology, culture (in blood culture bottles), Gram stain, total protein, glucose, lactate dehydrogenase, amylase, and, if warranted, mycobacterial smear and culture. Samples with >250 neutrophils per milliliter are assumed to be infected, and broad-spectrum antibiotic therapy should be initiated. Patients with a total protein concentration <1.0 g/dl are at high risk for spontaneous bacterial peritonitis. There is good evidence that Bactrim (1 DS tablet daily 5 days a week) is effective in preventing spontaneous bacterial peritonitis and decreasing mortality. Norfloxacin has been used as well, but its use is discouraged because of the rapid development of resistant organisms.

C. Therapeutic paracentesis with the removal of 5 or moreLiters is indicated if the patient presents with early satiety or shortness of breath. After the procedure, give 40 g of albumin IV to prevent hyponatremia and renal failure.

D. The serum-ascites albumin gradient is equal to $[\text{albumin}]_{\text{serum}} - [\text{albumin}]_{\text{ascites}}$. If the gradient exceeds 1.1 g/dl, the patient has portal hypertension.

E. Treatment consists in restricting sodium intake and the promotion of natriuresis with oral diuretics. Combinations of furosemide and spironolactone have been shown to be optimal for promoting sodium excretion and sparing potassium. Doses should be titrated to a maximum of 400 mg/day and 160 mg/day of spironolactone and furosemide respectively. Serial determinations of urinary sodium excretion may help to guide dosing. Other therapies include portal shunting and liver transplantation. *Overaggressive diuresis is associated with hepatorenal syndrome* (a relatively acute, progressive renal failure in the patient with advanced liver disease secondary to decreased renal perfusion) *and is discouraged. Large-volume paracentesis is preferable.*

CROHN'S DISEASE (REGIONAL ENTERITIS, GRANULOMATOUS COLITIS)

A. Definition. A transmural inflammatory process potentially involving any portion of the GI tract.

B. Involvement. Most commonly involves the ileum but frequently also involves the colon, anus (perianal fistulas and abscesses), and mouth (oral ulcerations).

C. Clinical presentation. Diarrhea (rarely guaiac positive), abdominal pain especially in the right lower quadrant, fever, fatigue, and bowel obstruction. Fistulous tract and abscess formation is not uncommon.

D. May have anemia, elevated sedimentation rate. ANCA may be positive.

E. Diagnosis. By endoscopy and biopsy or x-ray contrast studies showing typical areas of stricture with regions of normal bowel. *Contrast studies should not be done in patients who present with fulminant disease because of the possibility of inducing a toxic megacolon.*

F. Complications.

1. Toxic megacolon (more common with ulcerative colitis).
2. Dehydration and malnutrition from diarrhea and malabsorption. Fat-soluble vitamins and vitamin B_{12} tend to be particularly affected.
3. Bowel perforation and abscess formation.
4. Chronic fistula formation.
5. Bowel cancer (five time the rate of age-matched controls).
6. Renal disease including urolithiasis (not found with ulcerative colitis).

G. Extraintestinal manifestations include joint disease, erythema nodosum, pyoderma gangrenosum, episcleritis or keratoconjunctivitis, and sclerosing cholangitis.

H. Differential diagnosis. See section on diarrhea on p. 155.

I. Treatment.

1. ***Acute treatment.***
   a. Steroids. Start prednisone 40 to 60 mg PO QD or its IV equivalent. In severe or fulminant case most patients will respond to 7 to 10 days of IV steroid therapy. When bowel function is restored and the patient is tolerating a diet, IV steroids may be discontinued and the patient switched to oral prednisone or prednisolone therapy with rapid tapering down and discontinuation. In an

effort to decrease the severity of steroid side effects, new steroid preparations that minimize systemic effects have been developed. Budesonide (a steroid with high receptor affinity and high first-pass hepatic metabolism) is particularly promising and is available as both an enema and an oral controlled-release preparation that target the ileum and colon. Corticosteroid enemas can be used in patients with isolated rectal or left colic disease.

b. Metronidazole has been shown to be useful in doses of 10 to 30 mg/kg/day divided into 3 or 4 doses when perianal disease develops.
c. Intravenous cyclosporin A (4 mg/kg/day IV for 6 days followed by 8 mg/kg/day orally for 3 to 6 months) or surgery should be considered for patients with severe disease who are refractory to steroid therapy.
d. Total parenteral nutrition may be needed during the acute phase of disease.
e. Tincture of opium and other antidiarrheal agents may be useful during therapy. These should be avoided, however, if the possibility of toxic megacolon is present.

2. ***Long-term management.***
   a. Steroids should be tapered and discontinued as quickly as possible because of their significant side effects. Many will require long-term steroids, however.
   b. Long-term metronidazole use has been associated with a reversible peripheral neuropathy but can be used to keep steroid doses at the lowest possible levels.
   c. Azathioprine and 6-mercaptopurine have been used when steroids fail and facilitate steroid tapering, but these drugs have significant side effects, including bone marrow suppression and pancreatitis (3% to 15%).
   d. Aminosalicylates such as sulfasalazine and mesalamine are frequently used to treat mild to moderate Crohn's disease and to maintain remission. Sulfasalazine 3 to 4 g PO QD divided Q8h may be used to help induce a remission but is seldom effective on its own. Sulfasalazine decreases folate absorption and patients receiving sulfasalazine should receive folate supplementation.
   e. Olsalazine (250 to 500 mg PO QID) or mesalamine (Asacol 200 to 400 mg PO TID; Pentasa 1 g PO QID) provide the active moiety (5-ASA) without the sulfapyridine, which causes most of the side effects. Olsalazine may cause diarrhea in some patients.
   f. Antidiarrheal agents including loperamide or atropine sulfate–diphenoxylate HCl can be helpful.
   g. Hyperbaric oxygen therapy may be considered for patients with poorly healing fistulas.

ULCERATIVE COLITIS

A. Defined as inflammation limited to the mucosal surface and submucosa (as opposed to Crohn's disease, which is transmural).

B. Involvement is limited to the colon and rectosigmoid area in a continuous pattern without skip areas.

C. Clinical presentation is manifested by diarrhea (frequently bloody), passage of blood and mucus per rectum, abdominal pain, fever, tenesmus, and toxic megacolon.

D. Diagnosis is by endoscopy and biopsy or contrast studies showing superficial ulcerations. Carcinoembryonic antigen is elevated in chronic cases and is not suggestive of the development of a carcinoma. Bowel ANCA may be positive. Eosinophilia is also common (15% to 30%). As with Crohn's disease, contrast studies are contraindicated in those with acute disease, since barium may induce a toxic megacolon.

E. Complications include those listed above for Crohn's disease. Additionally the development of a toxic megacolon or anemia from hemorrhage is more common with ulcerative colitis as is the development of malignancy.

F. Extracolonic manifestations are the same as those found in Crohn's disease except for renal disease, which is exclusively found in those with Crohn's disease.

G. Treatment.

1. ***Acute management.***
   a. Asymptomatic treatment with antidiarrheal agents (see section on diarrhea, p. 155). These should be avoided if there is any evidence of toxic megacolon.
   b. If disease is moderate or mild, hydrocortisone enemas (100 mg BID) may be helpful. Mesalamine enemas, 4 g in 100 ml QHS, have been shown to be efficacious. Mesalamine suppositories (1 g QHS) may be used for isolated rectal disease. Oral mesalamine, olsalazine, sulfasalazine, and prednisone can be used in doses similar to those noted above for Crohn's disease.
   c. For more severe disease (systemic signs and symptoms, severe abdominal pain) parenteral steroids should be administered. In patients who have not had prior therapy with corticosteroids, ACTH 75 to 120 units/day IV by continuous drip may be more effective. Either treatment for severe disease should be continued for 7 to 10 days and then tapered as disease allows.
   d. Cyclosporin A 4 mg/kg/day IV added to steroids will frequently induce remission when steroids alone fail.
2. Long-term management includes the treatments noted for Crohn's disease. Oral forms of 5-ASA (olsalazine, mesalamine, sulfasalazine) are effective for treating mild to moderate ulcerative colitis and in maintaining its remission.

3. Surgical management for uncontrolled hemorrhage, toxic colitis, and perforation. Total proctocolectomy is curative.

LACTOSE INTOLERANCE

I. DEFINITION

Lactose intolerance is caused by a jejunal deficiency of lactase, a disaccharidase responsible for hydrolyzing lactose into glucose and galactose. Lactose is unabsorbable and increases the osmotic gradient within the small intestine. This produces a net flow of water and electrolytes into the small intestine. Bacteria within the colon ferment lactose into a variety of gases (hydrogen, carbon dioxide, and methane).

II. SYMPTOMS

A. Because of the increased volume of bowel gas and water, as well as the decreased intestinal transit time produced by the increased small intestinal water and solute load, patients may develop abdominal pain and bloating, distension, borborygmi, diarrhea, and flatulence.

B. People who are "lactose intolerant" by their own report rarely have symptoms if they limit themselves to about 240 ml of milk per day.

III. TYPES

Intestinal lactase activity varies by age and ethnic origin.

A. Primary. Adult lactase deficiency. Inherited as an autosomal recessive trait. Onset most common in adolescence and early adulthood. Symptom severity is dependent on intestinal lactase activity and the size of the lactose load.

B. Secondary. Temporary lactase deficiency produced during acute infectious gastroenteritis or mucosal damage from NSAIDs or other medications. Chronic small intestinal disorders (celiac sprue, cystic fibrosis, Whipple's disease, regional enteritis, HIV-induced enteropathy) may also cause a lactase deficiency because of brush border mucosal damage.

C. Congenital (alactasia). This condition is extremely rare and results in the complete absence of lactase expression because of a genetic defect.

IV. EVALUATION

A. Lactose tolerance test. Withdraw lactose from the diet for 1 to 2 weeks and see if symptoms resolve.

B. Breath hydrogen test.

C. Small-bowel biopsy.

D. Stool pH of less than 5.3 is diagnostic of carbohydrate intolerance.

V. MANAGEMENT

A. **Dietary measures.** Study ingredient labels on foods and avoid products that contain milk, lactose, and dry milk solids. Use lactose-reduced milks.

B. Lactase supplements (Lactaid, Lactrase, Dairy Ease) may be taken 30 minutes before the consumption of a lactose-containing product. Two capsules provide enough lactase to hydrolyze the lactose in an 8 oz glass of whole milk.

C. The consumption of yogurt containing live bacterial cultures can result in the release of bioactive bacterial lactase into the gut.

CLOSTRIDIUM DIFFICILE INFECTION

A. *Clostridium difficile* is a gram-positive anaerobic bacterium most often responsible for antibiotic-associated diarrhea.

B. The infection clinically ranges from asymptomatic carrier states to severe pseudomenbranous colitis.

C. **Clinical manifestations.** *Any of these manifestations may be absent, and pseudomembranous colitis should be considered in any patient with otherwise unexplainable diarrhea.*

1. Profuse watery diarrhea that may be foul smelling.
2. Abdominal pain, cramping, and tenderness.
3. Stools may be guaiac positive and occasionally grossly bloody.
4. Fever.
5. White blood cell count 12,000 to 20,000.
6. In severe cases toxic megacolon, colonic perforation, and peritonitis may develop. Other complications include electrolyte abnormalities, hypovolemic shock, anasarca caused by hypoalbuminemia, sepsis, and hemorrhage.

D. Although classically associated with clindamycin use, *C. difficile* colitis can be caused by almost any antibiotic. Symptoms may develop within a few days or even 6 to 10 weeks after antibiotic therapy is completed.

E. Toxin detection by latex agglutination, immunobinding assay, or ELISA make the diagnosis. Since *C. difficile* may be a normal bowel organism (especially in children), simply culturing the organism does not mean that diarrhea is caused by *C. difficile.*

F. Those patients with mild symptoms will usually resolve infection spontaneously once the causative antibiotic is withdrawn. More severe cases warrant therapy with oral antibiotic therapy. Both vancomycin (500 mg PO QID) and metronidazole (250 mg PO QID) for 10 days are effective therapies. Patients with relapse may be treated with another course of the aforementioned antibiotics.

GIARDIASIS

A. General. Disease varies from asymptomatic colonization (15%) to explosive diarrhea (25% to 50%) with weight loss and malabsorption. Approximately 50% of those ingesting *Giardia* will not become colonized or develop diarrhea. Generally transmitted through water especially from wells on farms, streams, or lakes. Has also occurred from public water systems (especially Eastern Europe), but this is uncommon in the United States.

B. Clinically. Fever (initially), nausea, abdominal cramping, diarrhea, increased flatus but may be asymptomatic, and any of the above may be absent.

C. Diagnosis. Stools for O & P, duodenal biopsy. These have been replaced by assay for *Giardia* antigen in the stool.

D. Treatment. Metronidazole 250 (standard) to 750 mg (for treatment failures) PO TID for 5 to 10 days. The 250 mg dose has about an 85% cure rate.

BIBLIOGRAPHY

Agarwal N et al: Evaluating tests for acute pancreatitis, *Am J Gastroenterol* 85:356-366, 1990.

Aurisicchio LN, Pitchumoni CS: Lactose intolerance: recognizing the link between diet and discomfort, *Postgrad Med* 95:113-120, 1994.

Berkow R et al: *The Merck manual,* ed 16, Rahway, N.J., 1992, Merck Research Laboratories.

Besson I et al: Schlerotherapy with or without octreotide for acute variceal bleeding, *N Engl J Med* 333:555-559, 1995.

Camilleri M, Prather CM: The irritable bowel syndrome: mechanisms and a practical approach to management, *Ann Intern Med* 116:1001-1008, 1992.

Camilleri M et al: Clinical management of intractable constipation, *Ann Intern Med* 121:520-528, 1994.

Caputo GM et al: *Clostridium difficile* infection: a common clinical problem for the general internist, *J Gen Intern Med* 9:528-533, 1994.

Dale DC, Federman DD, editors: *Scientific American Medicine,* New York, 1996, Scientific American, Inc.

Donatelle EP: Constipation: pathophysiology and treatment, *Am Fam Physician* 42:5, 1990.

Donowitz M et al: Evaluation of patients with chronic diarrhea, *N Engl J Med* 332:725-729, 1995.

Dupeyron C et al: Rapid emergence of quinolone resistance in cirrhotic patients treated with norfloxacin to prevent spontaneous bacterial peritonitis, *Antimicrob Agents Chemother* 38(2):340-344, 1994.

DuPont HL, Ericsson CD: Prevention and treatment of traveler's diarrhea, *N Engl J Med* 328:1821-1827, 1993.

Eastwood GL, Avunduk C: *Manual of gastroenterology,* Boston, 1988, Little, Brown & Co.

Ericsson CD et al: Treatment of traveler's diarrhea with sulfamethoxazole and trimethoprim and loperamide, *JAMA* 263:257-261, 1990.

Graham DY et al: Duodenal and gastric ulcer prevention with Misoprostol in arthritis patients taking NSAIDS, *Ann Intern Med* 119:257-262, 1993.

Graham DY et al: Effect of treatment of *Helicobacter pylori* infection on the long-term recurrence of gastric or duodenal ulcer, *Ann Intern Med* 116:705-708, 1992.

Graham DY et al: Effect of triple therapy (antibiotics plus bismuth) on duodenal ulcer healing: a randomized controlled trial, *Ann Intern Med* 115:266-269, 1991.
Gumaste V et al: Serum lipase: a better test to diagnose acute alcoholic pancreatitis, *Am J Med* 92(3):239, 1992.
Hanauer SB: Inflammatory bowel disease, *N Engl J Med* 334:841-848, 1996.
Hastings G, Weber J: Inflammatory bowel disease: Part I. Clinical features and diagnosis, *Am Fam Physician* 47(93):598, 1993.
Hastings G, Weber J: Inflammatory bowel disease: Part II. Medical and surgical management, *Am Fam Physician* 47(4):811, 1993.
Hertervig E et al: Anti-neutrophil cytoplasmic antibodies in chronic inflammatory bowel disease: prevalence and diagnostic role, *Scand J Gastroenterol* 30(7):693-698, 1995.
Imperiale TF et al: A meta-analysis of somatostatin versus vasopressin in the management of acute esophageal variceal hemorrhage, *Gastroenterology* 109:1289-1294, 1995.
John DJB et al: Evaluation of new occult blood tests for detection of colorectal neoplasia, *Gastroenterology* 104(6):1661, 1993.
Kuipers EJ el al: Long-term sequelae of *Helicobacter pylori* gastritis, *Lancet* 345:1525-1528, 1995.
Lankisch PG et al: Undetected fatal acute pancreatitis: Why is the disease so frequently overlooked? *Am J Gastroenterol* 86(3): 322, 1991.
Lichtiger S et al: Cyclosporine in severe ulcerative colitis refractory to steroid therapy, *N Engl J Med* 330:1841-1845, 1994.
Manabe YC: *Clostridium difficile* colitis: an efficient clinical approach to diagnosis, *Ann Intern Med* 123(11):835, 1995.
Mandell GL et al, editors: *Principles and practice of infectious disease,* ed 4, New York 1995, Churchill Livingston.
Marshall JB: Polyps in the colon, *Postgrad Med* 92:6, 1992.
McCarthy DM: NSAID-induced gastrointestinal damage: a critical review of prophylaxis and therapy, *J Clin Gastroenterol* 12:S13-S20, 1990.
McEvoy GK et al: *AHFS drug information,* Bethesda, Md., 1993, American Society of Hospital Pharmacists.
Miller-Catchpole R: Transjugular intrahepatic portosystemic shunt (TIPS): diagnostic and therapeutic technology assessment (DATTA), *JAMA* 273:1824-1830, 1995.
Murphy GS et al: Ciprofloxacin and loperamide in the treatment of bacillary dysentery, *Ann Intern Med* 118:582-586, 1993.
NIH Consensus Development Panel on *Helicobacter pylori* in Peptic Ulcer Disease: *Helicobacter pylori* in peptic ulcer disease, *JAMA* 272:65-69, 1994.
O'Brien B et al: Cost-effectiveness of *Helicobacter pylori* eradication for the long-term management of duodenal ulcer in Canada, *Arch Intern Med* 155:1958-1964, 1995.
Owens DM et al: The irritable bowel syndrome: long-term prognosis and the physician patient interaction, *Ann Intern Med* 122:107-112, 1995.
Pezzilli R et al: Serum lipase assay: a test of choice in acute pancreatitis, *Panminerva Med* 34(1)30, 1992.
Pope CE Acid-reflux disorders, *N Engl J Med* 331:656-660, 1994.
Raskin JB et al: Misoprostol dosage in the prevention of nonsteroidal anti-inflammatory drug-induced gastric and duodenal ulcers: a comparison of three regimens, *Ann Intern Med* 123:344-350, 1995.
Rigas B, Spiro HM: *Clinical gastroenterology,* ed 4, New York, 1995, McGraw-Hill.
Rössle M et al: The transjugular intrahepatic portosystemic stent-shunt procedure for variceal bleeding, *N Engl J Med* 330:165-171, 1994.
Rubenstein E, Federman DD, editors: *Scientific American Medicine,* New York, 1996, Scientific American, Inc.
Runyon BA: Care of patients with ascites, *N Engl J Med* 330:337-342, 1994.
Rutgeerts P et al: A comparison of budesonide with prednisolone for active Crohn's disease, *N Engl J Med* 331:842-845, 1994.

Sacher DB et al: *Pocket guide to gastroenterology,* Baltimore, 1991, Williams & Wilkins.

Sanford SP: *Guide to antimicrobial therapy,* Dallas, 1996, Antimicrobial Therapy, Inc.

Singh N et al: Trimethoprim-sulfamethoxazole for the prevention of spontaneous bacterial peritonitis in cirrhosis: a randomized trial, *Ann Intern Med* 122(8)595-598, 1995.

Soffer EE et al: Misoprostol is effective treatment for patients with severe chronic constipation, *Dig Dis Sci* 39(5):929, 1994.

Stahl TJ: Office management of common anorectal problems, *Postgrad Med* 92:2, 1992.

Steer ML et al: Chronic pancreatitis, *N Engl J Med* 332:1482-1490, 1995.

Steinberg W, Tenner S: Acute pancreatitis, *N Engl J Med* 330:1198-1210, 1994.

Suarez FL et al: A comparison of symptoms after the consumption of milk or lactose hydrolyzed milk by people with self-reported severe lactose intolerance, *N Engl J Med* 333(1):1, 1996.

The Mesalamine Study Group: An oral preparation of mesalamine as long-term maintenance therapy for ulcerative colitis: a randomized, placebo-controlled trial, *Ann Intern Med* 124:204-211, 1996.

Taha AS et al: Famotidine for the prevention of gastric and duodenal ulcers caused by nonsteroidal antiinflammatory drugs, *N Engl J Med* 334(22):1435, 1996.

Thomas GA et al: Transdermal nicotine as maintenance therapy for ulcerative colitis, *N Engl J Med* 332(15):988-992, 1995.

Tintinalli JE: *Emergency medicine: a comprehensive study guide,* New York, 1996, Health Professions Div., McGraw-Hill.

Trier JS: Celiac sprue. In Sleisenger MH, Fordtran JS, editors: *Gastrointestinal disease,* vol 2, Philadelphia, 1993, Saunders.

Truszkowski JA, Summers RW: Colorectal neoplasms, *Postgrad Med* 98:97-110, 1995.

Tytgat GNJ: *Helicobacter pylori* infection and duodenal ulcer disease, *J Intern Med* 231(3):199-203, 1992.

Villaneueva C et al: Nadolol plus isosorbide mononitrate compared with sclerotherapy for the prevention of variceal rebleeding, *N Engl J Med* 334(25):1624-1629, 1996.

Walsh JH, Peterson WL: The treatment of *Helicobacter pylori* infection in the management of peptic ulcer disease, *N Engl J Med* 333:984-991, 1995.

5

Hematologic, Electrolyte, and Metabolic Disorders

JAMES SCHLICHTMANN AND MARK A. GRABER

BLEEDING DISORDERS

I. PRESENTATION

Can often determine type of bleeding disorder by history and physical.

A. Is there a family history of bleeding after minor surgical procedures, dental procedures, childbirth, or other trauma?

B. Is this an isolated event or has the patient had other bleeding episodes?

C. Is the patient receiving medications that can cause a bleeding problem? Many drugs can contribute to a bleeding problem and included semisynthetic penicillins, cephalosporins, dipyridamole, thiazides, alcohol, quinidine, chlorpromazine, sulfonamides, INH, rifampin, methyldopa, phenytoin, barbiturates, warfarin, heparin, thrombolytic agents, NSAIDs and ASA, diuretics, allopurinol, TMP/SMX, among many others.

D. Look for physical signs and symptoms of diseases related to capillary bleeding and fragility. Examples include Cushing syndrome and Marfan's syndrome. Consider also "senile purpura," petechiae secondary to coughing, sneezing, Valsalva maneuver, blood pressure measurement, vasculitis ("palpable purpura"), scurvy (vitamin C deficiency), or exogenous steroids.

E. Telangiectasias are suggestive of Osler-Weber-Rendu syndrome.

II. DIFFERENTIATION OF PLATELET VERSUS COAGULATION DEFECT

Bleeding can be attributable to either platelet problems or coagulation defects.

A. Platelet defects. Generally have immediate onset of bleeding after trauma. Bleeding is predominantly in skin, mucous membranes, nose, GI and urinary tracts. Bleeding may be observed as petechiae (<3 mm) or ecchymoses (>3 mm). Must differentiate from vasculitic "palpable purpura."

B. Coagulation system defects. "Deep" bleeding (in the joint spaces, muscles' and retroperitoneal spaces) is common. Observed on exam as hematomas and hemarthroses.

III. PHYSICAL EXAM

A. Assess volume status and correct shock if present (see hypovolemic shock, p. 48).

B. Look for hepatosplenomegaly (evidence of platelet destruction, extramedullary hematopoiesis).

C. Do rectal exam for evidence of GI bleeding and examine oropharynx for evidence of bleeding.

IV. TESTS OF COAGULATION

A. PT (INR) to assess extrinsic system. Elevated in DIC, warfarin use, liver failure, myelofibrosis, vitamin K deficiency, fat malabsorption, circulating anticoagulants, factor deficiencies (vitamin K dependent), etc.

B. PTT to assess intrinsic system. Elevated in factor deficiencies (such as hemophilia), circulating anticoagulants as in lupus (mix patient's serum with equal amount of normal serum, if it corrects PTT elevation not caused by circulating anticoagulant, which will prevent coagulation even with adequate clotting factors present), heparin use, other drugs such as antipsychotics. PTT is the best screening test for coagulation defects and is elevated in 90% of those with coagulopathy. May have increased thrombotic events depending on cause.

C. Platelet count and bleeding time. If <100,000/mm^3, expect a mild prolongation of bleeding time. <50,000 results in easy bruising and <20,000 is associated with an increased incidence of spontaneous bleeding. If bleeding time is lengthened and there is normal platelet count, consider qualitative platelet defect. Can also perform tests of platelet aggregation.

D. Fibrin degradation products (or fibrin split products). Provides a measure of fibrin activation. Elevated in DIC but may also be elevated in other states such as trauma and inflammatory diseases.

E. Fibrin D-dimer. A byproduct of clot breakdown, D-dimer is a more sensitive measurement to prove intravascular coagulation (and therefore fibrinolysis) is present. Will be present in most individuals so sensitive but not specific.

F. Can also assay for specific factors.

V. DIFFERENTIAL DIAGNOSIS OF ABNORMAL BLEEDING

A. Bleeding caused by qualitative platelet disorders.

1. ***Von Willebrand's disease.***

a. Most common hereditary coagulation disorder. Autosomal dominant. Abnormal synthesis of von Willebrand's factor (vWf) causing decreased platelet adhesion and decreased serum levels of factor VIII:C (vWf is carrier for factor VIII:C). Type I is absent vWf; type II is abnormal, nonfunctional vWf.
b. **Treatment** involves administering factor VIII:C to achieve 30% to 50% activity (*Humate-P or Koate-HS contains some von Willebrand factor; others factor VIII:C concentrates do not!* See hemophilia below for calculations). Another alternative is cryoprecipitate (1000 to 1250 units of factor VIII:C, generally about 10 bags). However, this carries the risk of virus transmission. A single infusion is enough to control mild bleeding. If bleeding persists, repeat the infusion every 12 hours. Desmopressin also useful for Type I von Willebrand's (see hemophilia below for dose). If neither of these modalities works, consider platelet transfusion.

2. ***Defective aggregation.*** Rare
3. ***Defective activation or secretion.***
   a. Ingestion of aspirin or NSAIDs.
   b. High-dose penicillin.
   c. Storage pool defects. Vary rare. The platelet's are activated but secrete "inactive" granules, that is, gray platelet syndrome and dense granule deficiency syndrome.
   d. Can treat these with platelet transfusion.

B. Bleeding caused by quantitative platelet disorders.

1. ***Thrombocytosis.*** Occurs in myeloproliferative disease (including polycythemia vera, myeloid metaplasia with myelofibrosis, essential thrombocytosis). In these states platelets are often poorly functioning with abnormal aggregation leading to a bleeding disorder. The platelets in those with a reactive thrombocytosis (such as cancer, inflammation) function well. Treatment of bleeding is by platelet transfusion to bring the pool of *normal* platelets to >50,000/ml (generally about 6 platelet packs).
2. ***Thrombocytopenia.*** Causes include decreased production, increased splenic sequestration, or increased platelet destruction. Consider also HELLP syndrome and preeclampsia in pregnant females.
   a. Decreased production can be caused by:
      (1) Marrow aplasia. Infiltration secondary to malignancy or fibrosis. Also from vitamin deficiency. Diagnose by bone marrow biopsy.
      (2) Multiple drugs including ethanol, estrogens, thiazides, and cytotoxic drugs (cytosine arabinoside, daunorubicin, cyclophosphamide, busulfan, methotrexate, 6-mercaptopurine, etc.).

(3) Infectious causes including sepsis, AIDS, EBV, ehrlichiosis, Colorado tick fever, Rocky Mountain spotted fever, babesiosis, malaria, etc.

b. Increased sequestration in spleen secondary to portal HTN (that is, secondary to cirrhosis), myeloproliferative disease.

c. Increased platelet destruction caused by:

(1) Immunologic destruction. After bacterial or viral infections, drugs (sulfonamides, quinidine, INH, sedative or hypnotics, chlorpromazine, digoxin, methyldopa, heparin), idiopathic thrombocytopenic purpura (ITP).

(2) Nonimmunologic destruction. Vasculitis, DIC, thrombotic thrombocytopenic purpura (TTP), hemolytic uremic syndrome (HUS), and prosthetic heart valves.

d. **Idiopathic thrombocytopenic purpura** (ITP). Antibodies form against platelets.

(1) **Frequently preceded by** URI or other viral infection. More frequent in women, those with HIV, those with mononucleosis (EBV), Graves' disease, hyperthyroidism.

(2) **Presents as** petechiae; women may have increased uterine bleeding, other bleeding such as CNS, gums.

(3) **Diagnosis.** By bone marrow showing increase in megakaryocytes. Also may have antiplatelet antibodies (90% sensitive but only 25% specific). Many clinicians will not order this and make the diagnosis by marrow alone.

(4) **Treatment.**

- May choose to follow and not treat if no bleeding.
- In children 70% recover in 4 to 6 weeks.
- Platelet transfusions are not helpful, and infused platelets will be destroyed along with the patient's platelets. May want to use to try to stop acute bleeding, though.
- If bleeding or platelet count <20,000, treat with prednisone 1 to 2 mg/kg/day or methylprednisolone 1 g/day for 3 days. May take 2 to 3 weeks to see response.
- Intravenous IgG concentrates transiently increase platelet count (1 g/kg IV for 2 days). Rh_0(D) immune globulin (WinRho-SD) has recently been released and is indicated as IV therapy for ITP in nonsplenectomized patients who are *Rh positive.* The dose is 250 IU/kg given either at one time or as split doses and must be reduced for those with anemia. *See package information for details.*

- Splenectomy for patients who are bleeding and are not responding to other measures and bleeding.
- Other options include danazol, vincristine/vinblastine, cyclophosphamide, and azathioprine.

e. **Disseminated intravascular coagulation** (DIC).

(1) Occurs as a result of:
- Complications of obstetrics including abruptio placentae, saline abortion, retained products of conception, amniotic fluid embolism, eclampsia.
- Infection especially gram negative with endotoxin release.
- Malignancy especially adenocarcinoma of pancreas and prostate, acute leukemia.
- Rarely head trauma, prostatic surgery, venomous snake bites, etc.

(2) Clinically.
- Subacute. Thromboembolic events including DVT, heart valve thrombosis, stroke, extremity infarction, etc.
- Acute. Serious bleeding complications with depletion of clotting factors.

(3) Diagnosis. Elevated PT/INR or elevated PTT, thrombocytopenia, reduced level of fibrinogen, elevated D-dimer, and elevated fibrin degradation products (fibrin split products). Will also have evidence of microangiopathic hemolysis including schistocytes, helmet cells, etc.

(4) **Treatment.**
- Correct the problems that led to DIC in the first place.
- If no complications of DIC (no bleeding or thrombosis), no need to institute replacement therapy.
- For bleeding complications, can infuse platelets to replace platelets, cryoprecipitate or fresh frozen plasma to replace clotting factors. Maintain fibrinogen level at 100 to 150 mg/dl and other factors above 50% activity if possible.
- If have thrombotic complications, use heparin 500 units/hour (about 5 to 10 U/kg/hour) after a 500 to 1000 U bolus *(note these are lower doses than with usual heparin use)* but only if able to correct underlying process. This should be followed in 2 to 3 hours by fresh frozen plasma. Consider increasing heparin to 750 to 1000 U/hour after administering fresh frozen plasma.

- Aminocaproic acid and tranexamic acid (prevent fibrinolysis), though used in the past, have fallen out of favor because may increase thrombotic complications.

C. Bleeding caused by defects of the intrinsic pathway.

1. ***Products available for factor replacement.***
   a. **Fresh frozen plasma.** Contains all the coagulation factors in nearly normal concentrations. This is useful for patients with liver disease who have multiple factor deficiencies and require infrequent therapy. Contains about 200 to 250 units of each factor (about 1 unit of factor VIII per milliliter).
   b. **Cryoprecipitate.** Contains factor VIII, vWf, and fibrinogen. This is treatment of choice for von Willebrand's disease if virus-free factor VIII not available. Contains about 100 U of factor VIII per bag.
   c. **Factor VIII concentrate.** A lyophilized powder prepared from multiple donors that contains a high concentration of factor VIII and a variable amount of vWf *(Humate-P or Koate-HS have adequate amounts).* Most preparations have some risk of transmission of hepatitis and HIV. Virus-free preparations are available (that is, Monoclate-P and Hemofil-M) though they are much more expensive.
   d. **Genetically engineered factor VIII** available. Carries no risk of disease transmission.
   e. **Prothrombin complex concentration.** Contains 500 to 1000 IU of prothrombin factor X and factor IX.
2. ***Hemophilia A.*** *Deficiency of factor VIII,* X-linked recessive. Diagnose by factor VIII assay. PT and thrombin clot time are normal. PTT generally elevated but may be normal if >30% activity (mild disease).
   a. **Treatment of factor VIII deficiency.**
      (1) *Minor cuts and abrasions,* superficial ecchymosis, and nontraumatic hematuria may require no therapy. *CNS trauma requires prophylactic therapy.*
      (2) *Uncomplicated hemarthrosis,* noncritical hematomas, and traumatic hematuria are treated with factor VIII to achieve a factor VIII level of 25% to 50% for at least 72 hours.
      (3) *Life-threatening hemorrhage* and hematomas in critical locations require factor VIII to achieve a factor VIII level of >50% for 2 weeks.
      (4) *If mild hemophilia* (baseline factor VIII activity of 5% to 10%), Desmopressin 0.3 mg/kg in 50 ml NS IV over 15 to 30 minutes will transiently increase factor VIII and von Willibrand's factor enough for minor surgery. Levels will return to baseline value

with a half-life of 8 to 10 hours. Epsilon-aminocaproic acid 75 mg/kg PO 6 hours (4 g Q6h in adults) should be used to prevent fibrinolysis. An alternative is tranexamic acid 25 mg/kg TID (1.5 g PO TID in adults).

(5) *To calculate factor VIII dose needed:* 1 U/ml = 100% activity; 0.5 U/ml = 50% activity; etc. Units of factor VIII needed = Wt in kg × 44 × (Required activity in U/ml − Patient's current activity in U/ml). For example if a 25 kg patient has 10% activity and you want to raise it to 50% activity for an uncomplicated hemarthrosis: Units of factor VIII needed = 25 kg × 44 × (0.5 U/ml − 0.1 U/ml) = 440 U. To raise it from 0% activity to 100% activity: Units of factor VIII needed = 25 kg × 44 × (1 U/ml − 0 U/ml) = 1100 units.

(6) Consider use ϵ-aminocaproic acid or tranexamic after factor infused (see above for dose).

3. ***Hemophilia B.*** Deficiency of factor IX (Christmas disease), X-linked recessive. Diagnose by factor IX assay.
   - **Treatment of factor IX deficiency.**
     (1) Minimal bleeding can be treated with FFP.
     (2) Major hemorrhage is treated with prothrombin complex concentrate or FFP.
4. ***Factor XI deficiency.*** Autosomal recessive disease occurring primarily in Ashkenazi Jews.
   - Treatment generally not required because bleeding tends to be minor.

D. Bleeding caused by defects of the extrinsic and common pathway.

1. ***Hepatocellular insufficiency.*** Have decreased production of vitamin K–dependent factors II, VII, IX, X.
2. ***Vitamin K deficiency from:***
   a. Cholestasis and other GI disease causing impaired absorption of lipid-soluble vitamin K.
   b. Poor dietary intake of vitamin K.
   c. Broad-spectrum antibiotics. Gut bacteria produce vitamin K. Loss of these bacteria from antibiotics can lead to vitamin K deficiency.
3. ***Coumarin anticoagulants.***
4. ***Treatment.***
   a. **Vitamin K deficiency.**
      (1) For serious hemorrhage, infuse FFP 15 ml/kg IV and then 5 to 8 ml/kg IV Q8-12h.
      (2) Mild vitamin K deficiencies can be treated with 10 to 15 mg IM or IV QD for 1 to 3 days. The administration of vitamin K may make it difficult to achieve anticoagulation with warfarin again for several days.

b. **Liver disease.**
   (1) Fresh frozen plasma.
   (2) Vitamin K 10 to 15 mg IV or SQ for 1 to 3 days.
c. **Warfarin overdose.**
   (1) Treat like vitamin K deficiency. However, if use vitamin K, will not be able to anticoagulate well with warfarin for at least several days.
   (2) Do not treat the INR. If the patient is not bleeding, watchful waiting is adequate.

E. Bleeding caused by vascular defects.

1. ***Paraproteinemias.*** Cryoglobulinemia, macroglobulinemia, myeloma.
2. ***Thrombotic thrombocytopenic purpura.*** (TTP and hemolytic uremic syndrome may be variants of the same disease.)
   a. Presents with thrombocytopenia, microangiopathic hemolytic anemia (schistocytes, helmet cells on smear), with elevated LDH, fever, renal failure, mental status changes, focal neurologic deficits.
   b. Generally occurs in those 10 to 40 years of age with peak about 25 years. May occur in postpartum period.
   c. Diagnose by biopsy of vessels, clinical presentation.
   d. Mortality 60% to 80%, and most adults die within 10 days of disease onset.
   e. Forty percent 10-year recurrence rate if survive initial insult.
   f. Therapy includes exchange transfusion or intensive plasmapheresis along with infusion of fresh frozen plasma (45 ml/kg or so), aspirin (325 mg Q6h) and dipyridamole (75 to 100 mg Q6h) to inhibit platelet aggregation. High-dose steroids (prednisone 200 mg/day) have also been used.
3. ***Hemolytic uremic syndrome.***
   a. Usually in infants, children, or pregnant or postpartum women.
   b. Presents with thrombocytopenia, fever, microangiopathic hemolytic anemia, hypertension, acute renal failure with anuria.
   c. Etiology.
      (1) In some cases, indicated by a diarrheal illness caused by *Escherichia coli* O157:H7 which produces Shiga toxin (also known as verocytotoxin). Has been found in pond water, apple cider and uncooked or undercooked hamburger. Day care is also a risk.
      (2) Some cases are related to use of cytotoxic drugs (especially chemotherapeutic agents) drugs or cancer.
   d. 5% mortality in children, 60% to 80% in adults.
   e. Treatment is high-dose steroids (that is, prednisone 200 mg/day), plasmapheresis.

4. ***Henoch-Schönlein purpura.*** A generally self-limited IgA vasculitis.
   a. May follow URI or streptococcal infection.
   b. Presents with purpura, arthralgias, colicky abdominal pain, and hematuria (from nephritis).
   c. Aspirin and corticosteroids have been used for joint pain and GI symptoms respectively. Corticosteroids do not change the course of the associated renal disease.
5. ***Miscellaneous.*** Causes of vascular defects include SLE, rheumatoid arthritis, Sjögren syndrome, amyloidosis.

F. Bleeding caused by heparin. Treatment is protamine sulfate, which forms an inactive complex with heparin. 1 mg of protamine zinc will neutralize about 90 to 115 U of heparin depending on derivation of heparin. Calculate dose and administer over 10 minutes. Do not exceed 50 mg. Heparin half-life is 30 to 180 minutes; so dose of protamine needed will decrease rapidly with time. *Administer slowly to prevent hypotension. Protamine is an anticoagulant when not complexed with heparin. Therefore follow dosing guidelines carefully.*

ANEMIA

I. OVERVIEW

A. Definition.

1. Normal hematocrit (HCT) = 36% to 48%, hemoglobin (Hb) = 12 to 16 g/dl. Anemia is defined as a low HCT and Hb.
2. Changes in intravascular volume can be reflected in the hematocrit. Fluid overload leads to hemodilution and a lower HCT, whereas volume contraction can yield a spuriously elevated HCT even in the face of anemia.

B. Signs and symptoms of anemia.

1. ***Symptoms.*** Dyspnea on exertion, palpitations, angina pectoris, light-headedness, syncope, anorexia, tinnitus.
2. ***Signs.*** Pallor of mucous membranes and skin, mild tachycardia, peripheral edema, systolic ejection murmurs from increased flow though not sensitive or specific.

C. History. Obtain history including presence of jaundice or gallstones (hemolysis), history of blood loss, alcohol abuse, diarrhea, other chronic disease, drugs. etc.

D. Laboratory evaluation.

1. All anemic patients should have the following labs:
   a. Differential CBC.
   b. Platelet count.
   c. Mean corpuscular volume (MCV). In hemolysis, elevated MCV reflects reticulocytosis.
   d. Serum ferritin (estimate of Fe stores).
   e. Reticulocyte count.
      • The reticulocyte count is expressed as a percentage of total cells counted and must be corrected to a total

number of reticulocytes per microliter. This is done by multiplying the red blood cell count by the percentage of reticulocytes. Normal is 50 to 100,000 reticulocytes per microliter.

- Reticulocyte counts that are normal or low (in the face of anemia) are suggestive of the inability of the bone marrow to respond to anemia (marrow failure).
- Reticulocyte counts that are increased are indicative of acute blood loss or hemolysis with a marrow that is able to respond.
- If reticulocyte count is low or normal reflecting the inability of the marrow to respond to anemia ("marrow failure"), the MCV is helpful in diagnosing anemia. The MCV is either normocytic at 80 to 100 femtoliters, microcytic <80 fl, or macrocytic >100 fl.
- Consider serum haptoglobin, serum free hemoglobin to evaluate for hemolysis.

II. MICROCYTOSIS AND UNRESPONSIVE MARROW

Low or normal reticulocyte count and anemia.

A. Iron deficiency anemia generally has microcytic MCV but may occasionally be normocytic.

1. ***Causes.*** Increased iron requirements (during infancy, adolescence, pregnancy, etc.), inadequate iron intake, decreased iron absorption (gastrectomy, achlorhydria, chronic diarrhea), blood loss from menses or GI tract.
2. ***Exam.*** Skin and conjunctivae may show pallor; nails may be dry and brittle with ridges; cardiovascular exam may reveal tachycardia and flow murmur. Stomatitis or glossitis may be present. However, physical signs and symptoms are not sensitive enough to rule in or out the diagnosis of anemia.
3. ***Lab tests.***
   a. CBC will show microcytic, hypochromic cells.
   b. Low serum ferritin (overall best test for outpatients). Serum ferritin elevated by fever, cancer, other inflammatory processes and is therefore a poor predictor of iron deficiency anemia in hospitalized patients.
   c. Increased TIBC with transferrin saturation <15%.
   d. Low serum iron.
   e. Bone marrow biopsy specimen will show decreased iron stores.
   f. Must differentiate from the thalassemias and anemia of chronic disease.
4. ***Other work-up.*** All adults with iron deficiency anemia should be evaluated for upper and lower GI bleeding. If a source is found in the upper GI tract, there is little chance of there being a second lower GI source. However, use clinical judgment when deciding whether to work up both upper and lower GI.

5. ***Treatment.*** Ferrous sulfate 325 mg PO TID. Enteric-coated and timed-release products are poorly absorbed. Better absorbed if administered between meals on an empty stomach, but less GI upset if taken with meals. Vitamin C will increase absorption. Calcium and magnesium may impair Fe absorption. Iron may impair absorption of thyroxin. Treat for 6 months to replace body stores. Iron is very toxic and should be kept away from children.
6. If marrow does not respond to iron, consider another superimposed cause of anemia such as inflammation, vitamin B_{12} or folate deficiency, continued bleeding, etc.

B. Anemia of chronic disease. Microcytic in 30% of cases. See IIIB later in this section for details.

C. Thalassemias.

1. Hemoglobin made up of paired alpha and beta chains. Thalassemia caused by a defect in the synthesis of either alpha or beta chains. Normally have 4 genes to produce alpha chains but only 2 to produce beta chains.
2. ***Alpha-thalassemia.*** Caused by decreased synthesis of alpha subchain of Hb. Since normally have 4 copies, generally a mild disease.
   a. **Silent carrier state.** One of the four genes is deleted. No hematologic abnormalities.
   b. **Alpha-thalassemia trait.** Two of four genes are deleted. RBCs are microcytic, hypochromic. No significant anemia. Hemoglobin shows a decrease in Hb A_2.
   c. **Beta-thalassemia minor.** Caused by decreased synthesis of beta chains. One of two genes not present (heterozygous).
      (1) **Presentation.** Symptoms of anemia, splenomegaly, icterus. Cells are microcytic. Examination of peripheral smear shows target cells, cigar-shaped cells, and basophilic stippling.
      (2) **Diagnosis.** Hb electrophoresis shows increased Hb A_2, usually >4% and possibly an increase of hemoglobin F. May occur with a normal Hb A, however.
      (3) **Treatment.** None. Genetic counseling is necessary.
3. ***Beta-thalassemia major (Cooley's anemia).***
   a. Both genes for beta-chain synthesis defective or missing.
   b. **Presentation.** Manifestations begin at approximately 4 to 6 months of life. Usually present with severe anemia (HCT less than 20%). There is pronounced wasting, jaundice, slow growth and development, and delayed onset of secondary sex features. The patient will have skeletal abnormalities secondary to bone marrow expansion.
   c. **Diagnosis.** Hb electrophoresis shows large amounts of Hb F, variable amounts of Hb A, and increased Hb A_2. Nucleated RBCs.

d. **Treatment.** Transfusion, splenectomy, deferoxamine, folic acid supplementation. Watch for development of hemochromatosis.
e. **Prognosis.** Many die before puberty secondary to hemochromatosis.

D. Sideroblastic anemia.

1. ***Causes.*** Anemia and ineffective erythropoiesis.
   a. **Hereditary.** Likely X-linked recessive.
   b. **Acquired.** Drugs and toxins (alcohol, lead, INH, chloramphenicol), neoplasia and inflammation (rheumatoid arthritis, carcinoma, lymphoma, leukemia), malnutrition (folate deficiency), idiopathic. May also represent a myelodysplastic syndrome with deletion of either chromosome 5 or chromosome 7.
2. ***Lab tests.*** CBC may show normochromic or hypochromic cells; anisocytosis and poikilocytosis are pronounced. Sideroblasts may or may not be present. Iron studies will show increased serum iron, increased ferritin, increased transferrin saturation, decreased TIBC. LDH may be elevated. If appropriate, determine if there is chromosomal abnormality.
3. ***Clinically.*** May have anemia or hemochromatosis.
4. ***Treatment.***
   a. Withdraw offending agent, especially alcohol.
   b. Pyridoxine 200 mg QD × 2 to 3 months with or without folate. May work.
   c. Androgens may be of benefit.

III. NORMOCYTOSIS AND UNRESPONSIVE MARROW

Low or normal reticulocyte count and anemia.

A. Iron deficiency. Generally there is microcytosis but may be normal (see above).

B. Anemia of chronic disease.

1. ***Causes.*** Chronic infections (subacute bacterial endocarditis, osteomyelitis, AIDS), chronic inflammatory disorders (RA, SLE, sarcoidosis, renal failure), neoplasms, hypothyroidism, liver disease, alcoholism, CHF, diabetes though some authors do not include diseases associated with liver, kidney, and endocrine systems in this classification.
2. ***Multifactorial causes.*** Decreased RBC life-span, unresponsive bone marrow, inability to mobilize iron stores.
3. ***Lab tests.*** Hemoglobin generally between 9 and 11 mg/dl. Cells may be normocytic or microcytic. Serum ferritin usually increased but may be normal. TIBC and serum iron will be decreased.
4. ***Treatment.*** Treat underlying disease. Transfuse only as needed for symptoms. Erythropoietin may be used as well. Start with 100 to 150 U/kg SQ 3 × per week and increase to 300 U/kg SQ 3 × per week if no response in 3 weeks. If

no response by 12 weeks, the patient isn't going to respond, and erythropoietin should be discontinued. Reduce dose when HCT reaches 36% and hold dose if HCT = 40.

C. Primary marrow disorders.

1. Include congenital aplastic anemia, acquired aplastic anemia, and marrow depression from drugs and toxins (antineoplastic agents, immunosuppressive drugs, ionizing radiation, benzene, chloramphenicol, antithyroid agents, oral hypoglycemics, TMP/SMX, etc.), infections including hepatitis, mononucleosis, graft versus host disease, lupus, HIV.
2. ***Clinical manifestations.*** Weakness and fatigue from anemia, bleeding from thrombocytopenia, infection from leukopenia.
3. ***Aplastic anemia.***
   a. In aplastic anemia, course may be mild or severe though predicting the course based on marrow cellularity etc. is imprecise. 70% mortality by 1 year with "severe" disease.
   b. **Diagnosis.** CBC may show pancytopenia with normochromic-normocytic anemia. Reticulocyte count will be very low. Serum iron will be elevated with normal TIBC. Bone marrow will be hypocellular.
   c. **Therapy.** Requires hematology consultation.

IV. MACROCYTOSIS WITH UNRESPONSIVE MARROW

Low or normal reticulocyte count and anemia.

A. Causes.

1. *Vitamin B_{12} deficiency* (malabsorption from pernicious anemia, gastrectomy, Crohn's disease, celiac sprue). Strict vegetarians are at high risk but not a problem in Ovo-Lacto vegetarians. In the elderly, achlorhydria and lack of intrinsic factor may decrease vitamin B_{12} absorption.
2. *Folic acid deficiency* (usually caused by poor intake in alcoholics, indigent; or increased demand in pregnancy).
3. *Drugs* (including methotrexate, trimethoprim, pentamidine, AZT, hydroxyurea, alkylating agents, chloramphenicol).
4. *Alcohol* also causes macrocytosis independent of nutritional effects.
5. *Arsenic.*
6. *Endocrine including hypothyroidism.*

B. Clinical presentation.

1. ***Vitamin B_{12} deficiency.***
   a. *Symptoms of anemia.* Gastrointestinal symptoms (glossitis, taste bud atrophy, anorexia, weight loss, diarrhea). Neurologic symptoms including numbness, paresthesias, weakness, ataxia, sphincter dysfunction, positive Babinski sign (toe upgoing).
   b. *Signs* include those of anemia (pallor, tachycardia, etc.) and neurologic signs of hyperreflexia or hyporeflexia,

positive Romberg sign, impaired positional and vibratory sensation, depressed mentation, hallucinations, and personality changes. Neurologic disease may occur with normal hematocrit.

c. Some would suggest periodic screening of those >55 years of age, since can have symptoms of deficiency before have hematologic changes. If use 258 pmol/L as cutoff, 40.5% may be deficient.

2. ***Folate deficiency.*** Signs and symptoms are the same as in vitamin B_{12} deficiency, except that the patient is more likely to be malnourished. Neurologic abnormalities are generally absent as is glossitis.

C. Diagnosis. Elevated MCV, low reticulocyte count. *However, many have normal indices because of coexistent thalassemia or iron deficiency, etc.* Low vitamin B_{12} or RBC folate levels respectively *(check both vitamin B_{12} and folate!).* Serum folate level varies with meals and is an unreliable indicator of base state. Thrombocytopenia (50%) and leukopenia are late findings. Smear shows anisocytosis, poikilocytosis, basophilic stippling, hypersegmentation of neutrophils. Once the diagnosis of vitamin B_{12} deficiency is made, a Schilling test can identify the pathophysiologic characteristics.

D. Therapy.

1. ***Vitamin B_{12} deficiency.*** IM cyanocobalamin 1000 μg per week for 6 weeks and then 1000 μg IM every month for life.
2. ***Folate deficiency.*** One milligram of folic acid PO QD is sufficient.
3. Blood transfusions are usually not required.
4. Empiric therapy before a diagnosis is established can be dangerous. A patient deficient in vitamin B_{12} may have a hematologic response to folic acid but an exacerbation of neurologic symptoms.
5. Esophageal, stomach, and colorectal tumors have a higher incidence in those with pernicious anemia. They also have a higher rate of hypothyroidism; so screen these patients.

V. ANEMIA WITH INCREASED RED BLOOD CELL PRODUCTION

A. Usually acute anemias primarily associated with blood loss or hemolysis. May be caused by prolonged running or marching as well as microangiopathic changes as with HUS/TTP or artificial valves.

B. Hemolytic Anemia.

1. ***Presentation.*** Patients usually present with classic signs of anemia. See section IB for symptoms. Hemolytic crisis, which is rare, presents with fever, chills, tachycardia, tachypnea, backache, hemoglobinuria. Can progress to renal failure from hemoglobinuria. In addition to the causes below, consider malaria, ehrlichiosis, etc.

2. ***Lab tests.***
   a. Often normochromic-normocytic but may be macrocytic.
   b. Generally have an elevated indirect bilirubin with normal direct bilirubin.
   c. Haptoglobin is decreased; serum LDH is increased; hemosiderinuria and hemoglobinuria may be present.
   d. Serum free hemoglobin may be increased.
   e. Coombs' tests. Direct Coombs' test measures antibody that is attached to RBCs (antibody directly on RBC). Indirect Coombs' tests for circulating anti-RBC antibodies in serum. Example: In Rh disease, mother has positive indirect Coombs (circulating anti-D antibody). Rh-positive child has positive direct Coombs because mother's antibodies are coating cells (tested after birth).
3. ***Hemolytic anemia secondary to acquired hemolytic disorders.***
   a. **Warm-antibody induced hemolytic anemia.** Antibodies most active at temperature of 37° C. About 70% of those with antibody-related hemolytic disease have warm antibodies.
      (1) May be primary (60%) or secondary (40%) to underlying disease affecting the immune system (such as CLL, non-Hodgkins lymphoma, SLE, myeloma, HIV, ulcerative colitis). Commonly occurs with drugs (penicillin, alpha-methyldopa, INH, sulfonamides).
      (2) Usually have positive direct Coombs' test, generally an IgG antibody.
      (3) Often severe with Hb of 7.0 or less; can be fatal.
      (4) May have enlarged spleen, liver, jaundice.
      (5) No therapy required if disease is mild. With significant hemolysis, prednisone at dose of 1 to 1.5 mg/kg/day, transfusions, splenectomy (50% to 75% response; may relapse), and cytotoxic agents (cyclophosphamide 50 to 150 mg/day or azathioprine 50 to 200 mg/day) have been used with some success as have androgens. Hematology consultation is recommended.
   b. **Cold-antibody induced hemolytic anemia.** Represent about 15% of those with antibody-related hemolysis. Generally get agglutination of cells followed by hemolysis.
      (1) These IgM antibodies agglutinate RBCs at temperature <37° C (most reactive <30° C). Seen with *Mycoplasma pneumoniae*, infectious mononucleosis, and lymphoid neoplasms.
      (2) May note cold-related symptoms such as acrocyanosis, which gets better on warming.

(3) Maintain patient in warm environment. Chlorambucil is the most common agent used. If related to infectious process, generally resolve spontaneously in weeks.

c. **Trauma in the circulation.**

(1) Abnormalities of the vessel wall: seen in malignant hypertension, eclampsia, TTP, valve prostheses, and microvascular thrombi.

(2) Diagnosis. Fragmented and nucleated RBCs. See appropriate book section on underlying disease.

(3) **Therapy.** Directed toward underlying illness.

d. **Red blood cell defects.** Hereditary spherocytosis, hereditary elliptocytosis, hereditary stomatocytosis can cause a hemolytic anemia.

e. Paroxysmal nocturnal hemoglobinuria.

SICKLE CELL ANEMIA

A. Incidence. 0.3% of African Americans are homozygotes (have sickle cell disease); 13% of African Americans are heterozygotes (carriers)

B. Genetics. Autosomal recessive. Have abnormal hemoglobin S, leading to sickling of RBCs

C. Clinically.

1. Have anemia (see IA and IB for clinical symptoms).
2. ***Sickle crisis*** (sickling of cells causing vaso-occlusive disease with bone, lung, renal infarctions) often precipitated by exposure to cold and, *importantly, infection!* Most common sites of pain are lumbar spine, abdomen, femur, knees, and sternum, ribs, shoulder and elbows. May be associated with abdominal distension or ileus. May have fever, pulmonary infarctions (see acute chest syndrome below). May be difficult to differentiate sickle cell acute abdominal pain from a surgical acute abdomen.
3. ***Fever.*** From infections especially pneumonia and especially in children. If temperature >38° C (101° F), start broad-spectrum antibiotics while searching for a cause of infection.
   - Are de facto splenectomized secondary to repeated infarction. Need to treat fever aggressively because encapsulated organisms such as pneumococci and *Haemophilus influenzae* cause high mortality.
4. Have increased bilirubin secondary to increased RBC destruction.
5. Cholelithiasis is common (75%).
6. ***Acute chest syndrome.***

   a. Characterized by "pleuritic" chest pain, fever, hypoxia, cough, dyspnea, rales and rhonchi (any combination). Occurs in 30%.

b. Is a major source of mortality in those with sickle cell disease (15% of deaths in adults).
c. May have delayed development of infiltrates on CXR. Must differentiate from pneumonia.

7. Acute splenic sequestration syndrome, which causes a hemoglobin drop from 3 to 6 g/dl.

D. Microscopic examination of blood smear shows typical sickle-shaped RBCs.

E. Treatment.

1. ***Acute treatment of sickle crisis.***
   a. Pain control (such as IV morphine), hydration, transfusion for evidence of cardiopulmonary failure or a Hb <5 mg/dl. Admission as required to treat infection, maintain hydration, or for parenteral analgesics.
   b. If fever >38° C (101° F), start antibiotics (by ceftriaxone) while looking for source of infection.
2. ***Chronic treatment.***
   a. Infection prophylaxis including pneumococcal and *H. influenzae* vaccine during childhood. Start prophylactic antibiotics (penicillin or ceftriaxone) for fever starting at 4 months. This has been shown to reduce mortality.
   b. Hydroxyurea has been shown to increase fetal hemoglobin and decrease frequency of sickle cell crises.
   c. Bone marrow transplantation has been used with success in some cases.

GLUCOSE-6-PHOSPHATE DEHYDROGENASE (G6PD) DEFICIENCY

A. Incidence. X-linked disorder that is expressed in 10% of African-American men and fewer African-American women. Also occurs in people of Mediterranean ancestry.

B. Clinically. Get variable degree of hemolysis in RBCs after exposure to substances that cause oxidative stress including:

1. ***Drugs.*** Sulfonamides, nitrofurantoin, salicylates, vitamin C, quinine, and quinidine.
2. ***Foods.*** Fava beans.
3. ***Infections.*** Fever, viral illnesses, bacterial infections.
4. ***DKA and renal failure.***

C. Diagnosis. Check G6PD levels *when reticulocyte count is normal.* If checked after acute hemolysis, those cells surviving in the circulation and the young reticulocytes may have a normal G6PD level.

D. Treatment.

1. Since only old RBCs are vulnerable, generally <25% of the RBC mass is affected.
2. May develop renal failure secondary to hemolysis.
3. Maintain hydration and withdraw offending agents.

IRON-STORAGE DISEASES

I. HEREDITARY HEMOCHROMATOSIS

A. General. Inherited disorder that results from excessive iron absorption from food. Generally presents in those 40 to 60 years of age. Men more commonly symptomatic than women (not from menstrual loss of iron, probably secondary to X-linked gene that suppressed enhanced iron absorption).

B. Clinically. May have evidence of liver failure (cirrhosis), pancreatic failure (diabetes, specifically "bronze diabetes"), joint symptoms, congestive heart failure, hypothyroidism, impotence (secondary to hypogonadism), CNS symptoms, nonspecific right upper quadrant abdominal pain.

C. Alcohol intake may exacerbate the disease and hasten the onset of symptoms.

D. Diagnosis. Elevated serum iron, elevated transferrin saturation (>50%), elevated serum ferritin (>700 ng/dl).

E. Treatment. Based on phlebotomy. Remove 500 ml of blood every week until HCT stabilized at 35 to 40, Hb about 12 g/dl). Avoid iron-fortified foods; consider drinking tea, yes tea, with meals because it reduces iron absorption.

II. TRANSFUSION-RELATED HEMOCHROMATOSIS

A. General. Related to iron overload from transfusions especially in those with sickle cell disease, aplastic anemia, thalassemia.

B. Diagnosis. Blood testing as in idiopathic hemochromatosis.

C. Treatment. Deferoxamine, 1 to 4 g/day IV or SQ. Hematology consultation is suggested.

TRANSFUSION MEDICINE: AVAILABLE PRODUCTS AND TRANSFUSION REACTIONS

I. BLOOD PRODUCTS AND INDICATIONS

May need to use diuretics (such as furosemide, dose determined by underlying function) to maintain hemodynamic stability in those with CHF, etc.

A. Packed red blood cells. Used to reverse hemodynamically significant anemia in patients without compatibility problems. Expect the Hb to increase by 1 g/dl/unit in the patient without active bleeding. Rate of transfusion dependent on clinical setting (faster with acute blood loss, over 3 to 4 hours with CHF).

B. Leukocyte-poor RBCs. Used in those with a history of 2 or more febrile reactions to packed RBCs and in those requiring a large number of transfusions to prevent immunization against donor WBCs.

C. Washed RBCs. Used in those with a history of anaphylactic or allergic reactions to transfusions (such as those with IgA deficiency).

D. Irradiated RBCs. Used in those with immunodefiency to prevent transfusion associated graft versus host disease (>90% mortality, rash, pancytopenia, diarrhea). Examples include those with bone marrow transplants, premature infants. No need to use this in patients with AIDS.

TRANSFUSION REACTIONS

A. Hemolytic reactions.

1. May be acute or delayed.
2. Symptoms include fever, back pain, pain in the extremity that is accepting the transfused blood, DIC, renal failure, chest pain, wheezing, nausea, vomiting.
3. If suspected, immediately discontinue transfusion and return transfused unit to blood bank along with specimen of patient's blood.
4. ***Treatment.*** Fluids and mannitol (0.5 to 2.5 g/kg) to maintain urine output and prevent renal failure. Furosemide also useful. Treat pain with narcotic analgesics, wheezing (with albuterol), etc. as appropriate for those symptoms.

B. Febrile reactions.

1. Complicate about 2% of transfusions.
2. Symptoms include fever within 5 hours of transfusion; may have shaking chills. Must differentiate from sepsis.
3. ***Treatment.*** Stop transfusion; use meperidine in 25 mg IV aliquots to control symptoms such as chills, acetaminophen for fever. Can try to pretreat with acetaminophen and ASA and meperidine to prevent febrile reactions. After 2 febrile transfusion reactions, consider use of leukocyte-poor cells in future transfusions.

C. Allergic reactions.

1. Complicate about 2% of transfusions, especially in those who are IgA deficient. True anaphylaxis is 1 in 20,000.
2. Symptoms include allergic manifestations such as pruritus, urticaria, bronchospasm with wheezing, possibly shock.
3. *See Chapter 1 for treatment of anaphylaxis.*
4. Use washed cells if reacting to plasma protein.

D. Graft versus host disease.

1. ***Rare.*** Clinically have diarrhea, rash, pancytopenia, elevated liver enzymes.
2. Most common in those with lymphoma, bone marrow transplants, hereditary immune deficiencies, premature infants *but not AIDS.*
3. ***Treatment.*** High mortality rate (>90%). Treatment not generally effective; requires consultation with hematology staff. Prevent by using irradiated cell products in those at risk.

E. Transfusion-related pulmonary injury.

1. Pulmonary infiltrates and noncardiogenic CHF (ARDS) related to lung injury.

2. Clinically note fever, chills, cough, hypoxia.
3. ***Treatment.*** Symptomatic and includes respiratory support, including mechanical ventilation if required.

POTASSIUM

I. OVERVIEW

Total body potassium is approximately 50 mEq/kg of body weight. 98% is intracellular; serum decrease of 1 mEq of K^+ corresponds to a 10% to 20% deficit in total body potassium. Serum K^+ concentration is not always a reliable indicator of total body K^+. Distribution affected by:

A. Na^+, K^+-ATPase activity within cell membranes.

B. H^+ concentration in extracellular fluid: acidosis increases serum potassium.

C. An increase in both insulin and epinephrine reduce serum potassium.

D. Elevated aldosterone decreases serum potassium (increases serum sodium).

E. Cell-membrane permeability (an increase in permeability, increases serum K). Total body K^+ is largely controlled by the kidney with 90% of ingested K^+ excreted in the urine, 10% of the daily K^+ load is excreted in the GI tract (in uremic patients this may increase to 33%). Normally there is no significant K^+ loss through the skin. However, with profuse sweating the K^+ loss through the skin may approach 24% of the daily K^+ load. 5 to 15 mEq of K^+ are lost daily in the urine even with no K^+ intake.

II. HYPOKALEMIA

Serum K^+ level below the lab's normal level.

A. Etiology.

1. *GI losses* of K^+ seen in vomiting, NG suction, diarrhea, malabsorption syndrome, laxative or enema abuse. Villous adenomas may excrete K^+ and are associated with a large amount of mucus in the stools. GI losses distal to the stomach result in a low urine K^+ concentration and metabolic acidosis secondary to high bicarbonate losses. GI losses from the stomach result in a high urine K^+ concentration (usually >40 mEq/L) and metabolic alkalosis secondary to high hydrochloride loss.
2. ***Diuretics.*** Thiazides, furosemide, ethacrynic acid, and bumetanide. Maximal decrease in serum K^+ concentration is usually seen after 7 days of treatment. Degree of K^+ depletion dependent on Na^+ ingestion with severe salt restriction (<2 g/day) or excessive Na^+ intake (10 g/day) resulting in increased K^+ loss. More likely to be significant K^+ loss if patient has edema (edematous states associated with elevated aldosterone level, which stimulates K^+ excretion). Serum K^+ concentration should be measured before

initiation of a diuretic and 1 week after initiation of increase in dose of the diuretic.

3. ***Other causes of hypokalemia.***
   a. Insufficient dietary K^+ is an unusual cause, seen occasionally in alcoholics or cachectic patients.
   b. Excessive renal losses. Hypokalemia occurs with a urine K^+ concentration >20 mEq/L. *Causes*: hyperaldosteronism, Bartter's syndrome, glucocorticoid excess, magnesium deficiency, osmotic diuresis, renal tubular acidosis, diuretics, and many antibiotics (carbenicillin, aminoglycosides).
   c. Maldistribution of K^+. Alkalosis, increases in insulin, glucose, and adrenergic excess (MI, inhaled beta-agonists) cause a shift of K^+ from the ECF into the cells without depletion of total body K^+.
   d. Hyperaldosteronism. May have hypertension, edema when severe. To evaluate, stop all antihypertensives if possible and liberalize diet (must have normal Na intake), get baseline serum aldosterone value and then give fludrocortisone 0.2 mg PO TID for 3 days. Recheck serum aldosterone, which should be <3 ng/dl. Other protocols are used as well, such as spironolactone challenge.

B. Presentation. Weakness (especially of proximal muscles), perhaps areflexia, orthostatic hypotension, decreased GI motility resulting in ileus. Hyperpolarization of the myocardium occurs with hypokalemia and may cause ventricular ectopy, reentry phenomena, and conduction abnormalities. The ECG frequently shows flattened T waves, U waves, and ST-segment depression. Hypokalemia also causes increased sensitivity of cardiac cells to digitalis preparations and may result in toxicity at therapeutic plasma levels of digitalis.

C. Treatment.

1. It is difficult or impossible to correct a potassium deficit in the face of hypomagnesemia, a frequent occurrence with potassium-wasting diuretics. A magnesium level should be checked if there is any difficulty increasing the serum potassium, and magnesium should be replaced if the serum level is low. Since serum magnesium levels do not reflect total body stores, empiric use of magnesium is indicated if despite a normal serum magnesium it is still difficult to increase the serum potassium (see section on hypomagnesemia, p. 224).
2. ***Oral therapy.*** K^+ supplementation (20 mEq KCl) should be given at start of diuretic therapy if indicated. Recheck K^+ concentration 2 to 4 weeks after starting supplementation. Check periodically thereafter. In hypokalemic-hypochloremic metabolic alkalosis, a chloride supplement

should be given as well (KCl). Consider potassium-sparing diuretics in patients with hypokalemia caused by renal losses, but do not use in those with renal insufficiency, with potassium supplements, or with ACE inhibitors except under very close control (that is, hospitalization with daily potassium measurements).

3. *IV therapy* should be used for severe hypokalemia and in patients unable to tolerate oral supplementation. If serum K^+ concentrations >2.4 mEq/L and no ECG changes, K^+ can be given at a rate up to 10 to 20 mEq/hr with maximum daily administration of 200 mEq. Rapid treatment required if K^+ concentration <2 mEq/L with ECG changes (up to 40 mEq/hr on monitor, through peripheral line, diluted). Serum K^+ concentrations should be measured every 4 to 6 hours with the patient under continuous ECG monitoring until ECG changes resolve. Use nondextrose solution to prevent insulin release.

III. HYPERKALEMIA

A. Definition. Serum K^+ above laboratory normal (generally 5.5 mEq/L).

B. Causes.

1. ***Inadequate renal excretion.*** Acute or chronic renal failure, potassium-sparing diuretics, ACE inhibitors.
2. *Potassium load* from massive cell death caused by crush injuries, major surgery, burns, acute arterial emboli, hemolysis, GI bleeding, or rhabdomyolysis. Exogenous sources such as ingestion of potassium supplements and salt substitutes, blood transfusions, IV potassium administration and high dose penicillin therapy must also be considered. Also consider water softeners as a potential source of exogenous potassium.
3. ***Intracellular to extracellular shift.*** Acidosis, digitalis, overdose, insulin deficiency, or rapid increase of blood osmolality.
4. ***Adrenal insufficiency*** (Addison's disease).
5. ***Pseudohyperkalemia.*** Secondary to hemolysis of blood sample or prolonged tourniquet time.
6. ***Hypoaldosteronism.***

C. Presentation. Most important effect is a change in cardiac excitability. ECG shows sequential changes with a rising serum potassium level. Initially, tall peaked T waves are seen (K^+ >6.5 mEq/dl). This is followed by prolonged PR intervals, diminished P-wave amplitude, widened QRS complexes (K^+ = 7 to 8 mEq/L). Eventually the QT interval prolongs and leads to a sine-wave pattern. Ventricular fibrillation and asystole are likely with K^+ >10 mEq/L. Other findings include paresthesias, weakness, areflexia, and ascending paralysis.

D. Treatment. Continuous ECG monitoring is warranted if ECG changes are present or if serum potassium >7 mEq/L.

1. *Calcium gluconate* may be administered IV as 10 ml of a 10% solution over 10 minutes to stabilize myocardium and cardiac conduction system. This can be repeated twice at 5-minute intervals if no response. *Administration of calcium may cause digitalis toxicity in patients receiving digitalis therapy and should not be used in the face of digitalis toxicity.*
2. *Sodium bicarbonate* alkalinizes the blood causing a shift of potassium from the extracelluar fluid to the intracellular space. This is given as 40 to 150 mEq of $NaHCO_3$ IV over 30 minutes or as an IV bolus in an emergency; may worsen CHF because of sodium load. The effect is temporary but will work even when serum pH is normal.
3. *Insulin* causes a shift of potassium from the extracellular fluid into cells. 5 to 10 units of regular insulin should be administered with 1 ampule of 50% glucose IV over 5 minutes. A response may not be seen for 50 to 60 minutes, and the effect usually lasts for several hours.
4. *Cation-exchange resins* such as sodium polystyrene sulfonate (Kayexalate and others) remove potassium from the body by binding potassium in the GI tract in exchange for another cation (sodium in the case of sodium polystyrene sulfonate and most other drugs in this class). These drugs may be given orally or rectally. The initial oral dose is 15 to 30 g of sodium polystyrene sulfonate mixed with 50 to 100 ml of 70% sorbitol to counteract its constipating effect. The dose may be repeated every 3 to 4 hours to a total of 4 or 5 per day if needed. A retention enema is given as 50 g of sodium polystyrene sulfonate mixed with 200 ml of 20% sorbitol or $D_{20}W$ and may be repeated every 1 to 2 hours initially and then every 6 hours or as necessary. These agents cause a significant sodium load.
5. *Dialysis* may be required in severe, refractory cases of hyperkalemia.
6. *Aerosolized beta$_2$-agonists.* Will drive K^+ intracellularly and are particularly useful in renal failure. Can use constant nebulization of albuterol.
7. *Potassium restriction* is indicated in the late stages of renal failure (GRF <15 ml/min).
8. *Adrenal insufficiency* is treated acutely with hydrocortisone succinate. See p. 244 for a discussion of adrenal insufficiency.

SODIUM

I. HYPONATREMIA

Defined as a serum sodium below normal (generally 135 mEq/L).

A. Four possible states. Initial assessment is to measure serum osmolality and classify as hyposmotic (<280 mOsm), hyperosmotic (>285 mOsm) or isosmotic (280 to 285 mOsm). Then assess the patient's volume status based on clinical exam and lab data such as urine specific gravity and BUN/Cr. Hyposmotic states are then classified as euvolemic, hypervolemic, or hypovolemic.

1. Artifactual or spurious.
2. Dilutional. Hypervolemic with expansion of total body water.
3. Hypovolemic. Sodium depletion in excess of water depletion.
4. Euvolemic. Sodium and water depletion in equal amounts.

B. Artifactual or spurious. Lab reporting error secondary to:

1. ***Hyperglycemia.*** Correct sodium (each increase of blood glucose of 100 mg/dl decreases serum sodium by 1.7 mEq/L).
2. ***Hyperlipidemia.*** Measured serum osmolality will be normal and greater than the calculated osmolality (Osm = [2 × Na] + [Glucose/18]+[BUN/2.8]).

C. Dilutional or hypervolemic.

1. ***Caused by defect in water excretion.***
   a. *Sodium-retaining (edematous) states.*
      (1) CHF.
      (2) Renal failure and nephrotic syndrome.
      (3) Cirrhosis and ascites.
      (4) Diagnosis.
         (a) Clinical situation and underlying disease are key to cause.
         (b) Urine sodium concentration usually very low (<10 mEq/L). However, with acute and chronic renal failure, may have urine Na and Cl concentrations >20 mEq/L.
         (c) Urine osmolality elevated (only valid in absence of diuretics).
         (d) Generally will manifest edema from underlying cause.
   b. *Excessive water intake without sodium retention in the presence of:*
      (1) Renal failure.
      (2) Hypothyroidism.
      (3) Addison's disease.
      (4) Nonosmotically driven ADH secretion (SIDH) such as that seen with stress, postoperatively, drugs including MAO inhibitors, desmopressin, paregoric, oral hypoglycemic agents, opioids, barbiturates, vincristine, clofibrate, carbamazepine, NSAIDs. Postoperative hyponatremia is more common and more severe in menstruating females.
2. ***Diagnosis of dilutional or hypervolemic hyponatremia.***
   a. To diagnose most causes of hypervolemic or dilutional hyponatremia (renal failure, hypothyroidism, and

Addison's disease), see the section appropriate to the individual illness.

b. *SIADH.*

(1) *Clinically.* May be caused by lung and other cancers, pulmonary (pneumonia, TB, contusion) and CNS disorders including Guillain-Barré and subarachnoid hemorrhage, acute intermittent porphyria, multiple drugs including those noted above. Isovolemic or hypervolemic without edema. May find inciting factor. Have normal GFR.

(2) *Diagnosis.* Have inappropriately hypertonic urine with respect to serum sodium (urine osmolality should be <130 mOsm/kg if hyponatremic [kidneys should be conserving sodium and getting rid of free water]); in SIADH, urine osmoles are >130 mOsm/kg).

(3) *Treatment for SIADH.* Fluid restriction to 1 liter per day. If this is unacceptable to patient, demeclocycline 3.25 to 3.75 mg/kg Q6h to antagonize the effect of ADH on the kidney may help. Doses up to 1200 mg/day (400 mg Q6h) have been used. Use with caution in those with liver disease (because may cause renal failure), CHF, or renal failure.

D. Hypovolemic hyponatremia.

1. ***Causes.*** Combined water and sodium loss.
   a. GI loss such as vomiting, NG suction, diarrhea.
   b. Third-space losses as with burns, surgery.
   c. Excessive sweating.
   d. Renal and adrenal disease including uncontrolled diabetes mellitus, hypoaldosteronism, Addison's disease, recovery phase of renal disease.
2. ***Diagnosis.***
   a. If renal function intact, the urine osmolality is high and the urine Na usually less than 10 to 15 mEq/L. The fractional excretion of sodium (FE_{Na}) is <1%. (See p. 246 for calculations.)
   b. If renal or adrenal disease is present, the urine Na usually >20 mEq/L and is not helpful. (See section on renal failure, p. 506.)
   c. In the presence of metabolic alkalosis: urine Na may be high with a low urine chloride <10 mEq/L.

E. Euvolemic hyponatremia.

Causes. SIADH; see above for diagnosis and treatment. May also be caused by water intoxication but usually requires intake of >10 L/day, hypothyroidism, stress, adrenal insufficiency with a urine Na >20 mEq/L. Fluid restriction will be diagnostic (see diabetes insipidus for protocol, p. 219).

F. Clinical presentation of hyponatremia.

Depends on severity and time course of onset.

1. Rapidly developing hyponatremia is more symptomatic.
2. If plasma Na drops 10 mEq/L over several hours, patients may have nausea, vomiting, headache, muscle cramps.
3. If plasma Na drops 10 mEq/L in an hour, may have severe headache, lethargy, seizures, disorientation, and coma.
   a. Mortality 50% if Na concentration falls to <113 mEq/L rapidly.
   b. Any geriatric patient presenting with a change in mental status should have serum electrolytes to check for hyponatremia.
4. May have signs of the underlying illness (such as CHF, Addison's disease). If secondary to fluid loss, may have signs of shock including hypotension and tachycardia.

G. Treatment of hyponatremia.

1. Treat underlying condition (CHF, Addison's disease, hypothyroidism, SIADH). See specific section on treatment of underlying disease.
2. Stop any contributing drugs.
3. Correct a long-standing hyponatremia slowly and a rapidly developing hyponatremia more aggressively. Do not overcorrect hyponatremia. May precipitate central pontine myelinolysis.
   a. Do not raise serum Na more than 12 mEq/L in 24 hours in asymptomatic patients. If patient symptomatic, can increase by 1 to 1.5 mEq/L/hour until symptoms resolve.
   b. To calculate the amount of Na needed to raise the serum Na to 125 mEq/L:

$$\text{Amount of Na (mEq)} = 125\ \text{mEq/L} - \text{Actual serum Na (mEq/L)} \times \text{TBW (in liters)}$$

$$\text{TBW} = 0.6 \times \text{Body weight in kg}$$

   c. May replace Na with 3% or 5% NaCl solution (provide 0.51 mEq/ml and 0.86 mEq/ml respectively).
   d. In those with ECF volume expansion, the use of diuretics may be necessary.

II. HYPERNATREMIA

Defined as a serum sodium above normal (generally 135 to 140 mEq/L).

A. Causes.

1. Occurs if hypotonic fluid losses are not adequately replaced.
   a. If fluid losses are extrarenal (GI losses, perspiration, or hyperventilation), the urine osmolality will be greater than that of the serum, and urinary Na^+ will be <20 mEq/L.
   b. A urine osmolality less than or equal to that of the serum implies renal fluid losses (diuretic therapy, osmotic diuresis, diabetes insipidus, acute tubular

necrosis, postobstructive uropathy, hypokalemic nephropathy, or hypercalcemic nephropathy).

2. Hypernatremia may occur with hyperalimentation or other hypertonic fluid administration.

B. Signs and symptoms. Muscle irritability, confusion, ataxia, tremulousness, seizures, and coma secondary to the hypernatremia. Additional manifestations usually occur secondary to the underlying abnormality and volume status (tachycardia and orthostatic hypotension with volume depletion; edema with fluid excess).

C. Treatment.

1. Hypernatremia with volume depletion should be treated by administration of isotonic saline until hemodynamic stability is achieved. Can then correct the remaining water deficit with D_5W or hypotonic saline.
2. Hypernatremia with volume excess is treated with diuresis or, if necessary, with dialysis. D_5W is then administered to replace the water deficit.
3. Body water deficit is estimated by:
   a. Deficit = Desired TBW (liters) − Current TBW.
   b. Desired TBW = (Measured serum Na) × (Current TBW/Normal serum Na).
   c. Current TBW = 0.6 × Current body weight (kg).
4. One half the calculated water deficit should be given in the first 24 hours, and the remaining deficit is corrected over 1 or 2 days to avoid cerebral edema secondary to abrupt change in serum sodium concentration.
5. *Diabetes insipidus* (may also have normal sodium if no access to free water): Caused by either renal resistance to ADH or decreased secretion of ADH (including granulomatous disease, CNS trauma or hypoxia, tumor, drugs (especially lithium carbonate), etc. May have polyuria and polydipsia.
   a. **Diagnosis.** An initial urine osmolality of <300 mOsm/kg indicates possibility of diabetes insipidus (though occasionally will have urine osmolality of 300 to 500 mOsm/kg). Patients with hypernatremia *should* have a maximally concentrated urine (800 to 1200 mOsm/kg). Next step is water deprivation *under direct observation because of risk of hypovolemia* for 6 to 12 hours. Check urine and serum osmolality. If concentrate urine to normal with fluid deprivation (>800 mOsm/kg), problem not diabetes insipidus (consider water intoxication, etc.). If not able to concentrate urine, probably diabetes insipidus. Confirm by administration of 10 to 20 microunits of DDAVP by nasal spray *or* 5 U SQ. If concentrate urine by 50%, have diagnosis. If not able to concentrate, consider nephrogenic diabetes insipidus or other diagnosis causing hypernatremia.

b. **Treatment.** DDAVP 10 to 25 μg intranasally BID to reduce polydipsia or polyuria.

CALCIUM

I. HYPERCALCEMIA

An elevated serum calcium of over 10.5 mg/dL after correction for serum albumin. Corrected calcium = Serum calcium + (0.8 × [Normal serum albumin − Patient's albumin]).

A. History. "Bones, stones, abdominal groans."

1. If mild, may be asymptomatic. Frequently found on routine screening labs.
2. *Moderate elevations.* Constipation, anorexia, nausea, vomiting, abdominal pain, ileus.
3. *More severe elevations* (>12 mg/dl). Emotional lability, confusion, delirium, psychosis, stupor, coma. Weaknesses and seizures. Nephrolithiasis or urolithiasis common. May have associated renal failure, QT shortening.
4. No symptom complex is sensitive enough to be diagnostic.

B. Etiology and pathophysiology. Either overabsorption of calcium as with milk-alkali syndrome; too little calcium excretion as with thiazide use; excess mobilization of bone as with hyperparathyroidism, metastatic cancer.

C. Differential diagnosis. See specific topic for additional information.

1. ***Spurious.*** High calcium meal before blood draw, long tourniquet application time; 53% will be found to be normocalcemic when calcium level is repeated.
2. ***Hyperparathyroidism.*** Generally have high calcium, low phosphate, elevated serum parathyroid hormone.
3. ***Malignancy.*** Breast cancer (50% of cases from malignancy), lung cancer, multiple myeloma, renal cancer, colon cancer, prostate cancer, ovarian cancer, others.
4. Together, hyperparathyroidism and malignancy account for 80% to 90% of cases of hypercalcemia in adults.
5. ***Drugs.*** Lithium carbonate, vitamin D, vitamin A, thiazide diuretics; milk-alkali syndrome.
6. ***Hyperthyroidism or hypothyroidism.*** Will have low TSH, elevated free T_4 (hyperthyroidism), high TSH (hypothyroidism).
7. ***Immobilization and bedrest.***
8. ***Addison's disease.*** Should have weakness, fatigue, weight loss, hypotension and may have hyperpigmentation, low sodium and high potassium levels.
9. ***Cushing's disease.*** Should have physical stigmas such as truncal obesity, striae, moon facies.
10. ***Multiple endocrine neoplasia.*** *MEN type I:* tumors of parathyroid, pituitary, pancreas, and possibly Zollinger-Ellison syndrome; *MEN type II:* medullary thyroid carcinoma, hyperparathyroidism, pheochromocytoma.

11. ***Paget's disease of the bone.*** Usually asymptomatic but may have gradual onset of aching bone pain, deformity, hearing loss, pain from entrapment neuropathy secondary to abnormal bone formation. Will have radiographic abnormality, increased serum alkaline phosphatase, increased urine excretion of total peptide hydroxyproline.

D. Work-up.

1. History and physical exam including drug and vitamin history.
2. Repeat calcium to rule out artifact. Get fasting A.M. calcium, electrolytes, BUN, creatinine, and alkaline phosphatase; look for evidence of renal failure, adrenal failure, bone disease. TSH to rule out hyperthyroidism or hypothyroidism. If repeat calcium is elevated and no other abnormality noted, continue work-up.
3. Check parathyroid hormone level preferably using a two-site, double antibody, immunoradiometric assay (immunoassay for intact parathyroid hormone). Obtain a simultaneous calcium. If parathyroid hormone is high, the diagnosis is hyperparathyroidism. Consider surgical referral for parathyroidectomy. If parathyroid hormone normal or low, it is suggestive of malignancy: continue work-up.
4. Search for malignancy including breast exam, mammogram, chest radiograph, stool guaiac, PSA value, abdominal CT, bone scan, bone radiographs, etc. as dictated by patient history and physical. Serum and urine protein electrophoresis looking for myeloma if indicated (urine dip stick will not pick up Bence Jones proteins).
5. If this work-up negative and have uveitis or erythema nodosum and have bilateral hilar adenopathy on CXR, can assume sarcoid. Serum ACE levels unreliable (see sarcoid section, p. 150).
6. If work-up is negative and patient asymptomatic, repeat calcium value, work-up, in 6 months.
7. If work-up remains negative and high calcium maintained, consider neck exploration for parathyroid adenoma.

E. Laboratory results.

1. High chloride and low phosphate levels are suggestive of hyperparathyroidism.
2. Anemia, high sedimentation rate, abnormal serum globulins, low albumin level, proteinuria, suggestive of malignancy.
3. Elevated parathyroid hormone defines hyperparathyroidism.
4. Elevated BUN and creatinine suggestive of renal failure.
5. Elevated alkaline phosphatase suggestive of a bone process such as Paget's disease of the bone or metastatic breast or prostate cancer.

F. Treatment for hypercalcemia. Address underlying disorder (see under specific diagnosis)

1. ***Acute treatment.***

a. If patient severely symptomatic or if serum Ca >15 mg/dl, need to reduce serum Ca rapidly.
b. *Promote diuresis* and replace intravascular volume with normal saline. If renal function intact, give 1 to 2 liters of normal saline and furosemide 80 to 100 mg IV Q2-12h for the first 24 hours. Adjust furosemide and saline rates to prevent fluid overload *and* intravascular depletion. Replace urine losses with normal saline and KCl to prevent hypokalemia. Avoid thiazide diuretics, which can cause calcium retention.
c. If renal function compromised, try acute hemodialysis.
d. *Calcitonin* 4 to 8 units SQ Q6-12h. Not very potent but rapid acting; will lower serum calcium by 1 to 3 mg/dl. Use 1 or 2 doses as emergency therapy while waiting for other modalities to work. Short acting. Side effects include abdominal cramping, nausea, flushing, allergic reaction (to salmon calcitonin). Calcitonin nasal spray is now available for maintenance.
e. *Bisphosphonates* (inhibit osteoclastic activity), helpful in hyperparathyroidism, malignancy.
   (1) *Pamidronate* 60 to 90 mg IV over 4 to 24 hours. More potent than etidronate; achieves control in 70% to 100% of cases. Effective within 2 days and reaches nadir at 7 days. Side effects are mild and include a transient increase in temperature (<2° C), transient leukopenia, and a small decrease in serum phosphate. Generally preferred over etidronate and plicamycin.
   (2) *Disodium etidronate* 7.5 mg/kg IV daily over 4 hours for 3 to 7 days. May cause increase in serum creatinine and phosphate. Long-term administration may lead to osteomalacia. Calcium will drop within 2 days and reach nadir at 7 days. Achieves control in 60% to 100%.
f. *Plicamycin (mithramycin)* 25 μg/kg IV in 500 ml of D_5W over 3 to 6 hours is useful. May repeat several times at 24- to 48-hour intervals. Especially useful in hypercalcemia from malignancy. Side effects include nausea, local irritation, and cellulitis if extravasation occurs, hepatic toxicity, nephrotoxicity, thrombocytopenia. Contraindicated in hepatic or renal dysfunction, thrombocytopenia, other coagulopathy. Works in 12 hours with peak at 72 hours. Use becoming less common as bisphosphonates become more common. Is less well tolerated and less effective than pamidronate.
g. *Steroids.* Prednisone 60 mg/day PO, or hydrocortisone succinate 200 to 300 mg IV. Helpful for hypercalcemia from vitamin-D intoxication, myeloma, and breast carcinoma.

h. A very risky approach is to administer 1 liter of disodium phosphate and monopotassium phosphate (0.5 to 1 g can be given over 24 hours). This can cause soft-tissue calcification, renal failure, and death. This approach should be tried only if all other measures fail, hypercalcemia is life threatening, and you are unable to arrange for hemodialysis. A nephrology or endocrinology consultation is suggested before you use this modality.

2. ***Chronic treatment.***
   a. Oral calcium binders including phosphates (1 to 3 g of elemental phosphorus per day). Do not use in those with renal failure.
   b. Oral etidronate 1200 to 1600 mg/day. May cause osteomalacia.
   c. Pamidronate. May be repeated in initial dose (see above) weekly if needed. Does not cause osteomalacia.

II. HYPOCALCEMIA

Defined as serum Ca <8.8 mg/dl (usually <7 mg/dl when symptoms present). Must correct for serum albumin. Corrected calcium = Measured serum calcium + (0.8 × [Normal serum albumin − Patient's albumin]).

A. Causes.

1. Hypoparathyroidism.
2. Spurious.
3. Vitamin D deficiency or resistance.
4. Renal tubular acidosis, renal failure.
5. Magnesium depletion.
6. Acute pancreatitis.
7. Septic shock.
8. Drugs: cisplatin, pentamadine, foscarnet, ketoconazole.

B. Clinical symptoms.

1. Primarily neurologic.
2. If develops slowly, get confusion, encephalopathy, depression, psychosis. May also note tetany, convulsions, laryngospasm, carpopedal spasm, muscle aches.
3. *Look for Chvostek's sign.* Contraction of facial muscles elicited by light tapping of facial nerve.
4. *Trousseau's sign.* Carpopedal spasms elicited by application of tourniquet for 3 minutes to extremity. Avoid in those with vascular disease or coagulopathy.

C. Treatment.

1. If tetany present, can administer 10 ml of 10% calcium gluconate over 15 to 30 minutes.
2. Lasts only a few hours and may require repeat infusions (60 ml of Ca gluconate in 500 ml of D_5W at 0.5 to 2 mg/kg/hour. Measure calcium every couple of hours.
3. May cause arrhythmias in those taking digitalis.

4. Must correct hypomagnesemia if present (see below and hypokalemia, p. 211, for discussion).
5. Administer oral calcium 1 to 7 g/day divided with meals.
6. If secondary to renal failure:
   a. Need to add phosphate binders (aluminum hydroxide gel).
   b. Dietary restriction of phosphate.
   c. Vitamin D may be hazardous in renal failure.
7. If secondary to vitamin D deficiency, give vitamin D replacement, such as Rocaltrol (calcitriol), Calderol, etc.
8. If vitamin D resistant, treat with inorganic phosphate 1 to 3.5 g/day and calcitriol 0.25 to 1 µg/day.

MAGNESIUM

I. HYPERMAGNESEMIA

Serum magnesium >2.5 mg/dl. Fifty-percent of body stores is in bone; the remainder mostly in the muscle. Less than 1% in ECF with 20% to 30% protein bound, and the remainder as free cation. Most absorbed in small bowel, excreted by kidneys.

A. Causes.

1. Renal failure in patients administered magnesium-containing products (laxatives and antacids).
2. Administration IV (as in preeclampsia).

B. Clinically. Get impairment of neuromuscular transmission. Presents as muscle weakness, respiratory depression, absence of deep tendon reflexes, widened QRS and prolonged PR interval, hypotension, heart block, asystole.

C. Treatment.

1. IV administration of 10 to 20 ml of 10% calcium gluconate IV over 10 minutes or 10% $CaCl_2$ 5 to 10 mg/kg IV to temporize. Without severe renal dysfunction 20 ml of 10% calcium gluconate in a liter of 0.9 NS can be given at 100 to 200 ml/hour.
2. Administration of furosemide or ethacrynic acid may enhance excretion.
3. Hemodialysis is effective.

II. HYPOMAGNESEMIA

Serum magnesium <1.9 mg/dl. However, serum levels do not reflect total body stores, and a patient (especially in CHF, using a diuretic, etc.) may be total body depleted with normal serum levels of magnesium.

A. Causes.

1. Relatively common in stress situations as in myocardial infarction, shock.
2. Alcoholism and nutritional deficiency (chronic TPN).
3. Loss from diarrhea, diuretics *(diuretics major cause of hypomagnesemia in those with CHF)*, osmotic diuresis (diabetes).

4. ***Renal.*** Hyperaldosteronism and hypoparathyroidism. Hypercalcemia causes increased renal Mg^{++} excretion.
5. Amphotericin B and cyclosporin A.

B. Clinically. Anorexia, lethargy, vomiting, tetany, arrhythmias, seizures, prolonged PR and QT intervals.

C. Treatment.

1. In emergency, can give 2 to 4 g of magnesium sulfate in 50 ml of D_5W over 5 to 15 minutes. Can repeat to a total of 10 g over the next 6 hours. Continue replacement for 3 to 7 days with 48 mEq/L/24 hours.
2. If less severe situation, replace 0.03 to 0.06 g/kg/day in 4 to 6 doses until serum magnesium normal.
3. Continue oral replacement therapy as long as precipita-ting factor is present (such as oral Mag-Ox one PO QD BID).

GLUCOSE

I. HYPOGLYCEMIA

A. Definition. Plasma glucose <50 mg/dl. May be asymptomatic.

B. Categories.

1. ***Postprandial hypoglycemia.***
   a. **Clinically.**
      (1) Generally have symptoms of adrenergic stimulation including diaphoresis, anxiety, irritability, palpitations, tremor, and hunger.
      (2) Occurs 2 to 4 hours postprandially.
      (3) Occurs suddenly and generally subsides in 15 to 20 minutes.
      (4) Caused by stimulation of epinephrine release.
   b. **Etiology.** Often idiopathic but may be caused by early diabetes, alcohol intake, status post gastrectomy, renal failure, drugs such as salicylates, beta-blockers, pentamidine, ACE inhibitors.
2. ***Fasting hypoglycemia.***
   a. **Clinically.**
      (1) Generally have symptoms of neuroglycopenia including headache, mental dullness, and fatigue. If hypoglycemia is more severe, may progress to confusion, visual blurring, loss of consciousness and seizures.
      (2) Occurs with fasting greater than 4 hours.
   b. **Etiology.**
      (1) Excess insulin including insulinoma, self-administered insulin or oral hypoglycemic agents.
      (2) Alcohol abuse and liver disease (decreased gluconeogenesis).
      (3) Pituitary or adrenal insufficiency.

3. ***Iatrogenic or exogenous.*** May occur in diabetic patients with changes in dosage of medications or level of physical activity.

C. Evaluation of hypoglycemia.

1. ***Postprandial hypoglycemia.***
   a. 5-hour glucose tolerance test (GTT). Give 75 g glucose load and measure serum glucose every 30 minutes for 5 hours. 25% of asymptomatic individuals will have hypoglycemic symptoms and a blood glucose <50 mg/dl when challenged this way. Many have blood glucose <50 mg/dl but remain asymptomatic.
   b. If cause of postprandial hypoglycemia is:
      (1) *Early diabetes.* Normal or elevated fasting glucose; glucose is greatest during first 2 hours, an indication of diabetes, but may have low plasma level at glucose hours 3 to 4.
      (2) *Status post gastrectomy.* Rapid elevation of glucose by 1 hour; rapid decline with trough at 2 to 3 hours.
      (3) *Idiopathic hypoglycemia.* Normal plasma glucose hours 1 to 2, low glucose hour 3, return to baseline value by hour 5.
      (4) Idiopathic postprandial syndrome. Have postprandial adrenergic symptoms with normal GTT.
2. ***Fasting hypoglycemia.***
   a. For screening, measure plasma glucose after overnight fast.
      (1) If overnight value normal (>50 mg/dl), can try 72-hour fast (observed).
      (2) Some premenopausal women will normally have serum glucose <50 mg/dl after a 72-hour fast.
   b. If cause for fasting hypoglycemia is:
      (1) Insulinoma. Will have hunger, weight gain, hypoglycemic symptoms. Consultation with an endocrinologist important.
      (2) Surreptitious insulin or oral hypoglycemic administration.
         - Usually a diabetic or person with medical background.
         - Needle marks usually evident (with insulin).
         - Can measure for oral hypoglycemic agents in the blood.
         - Measure insulin C-peptide; will be low if exogenous insulin being administered to patient.
         - The presence of anti-insulin antibodies supports the diagnosis of exogenous insulin being given.
      (3) Alcohol abuse. Should have other stigmas of alcohol abuse.

(4) Liver disease.
- Have elevated liver enzymes; other signs liver failure.
- Any patient with cirrhosis and hypoglycemia should be evaluated for a hepatoma.

(5) Pituitary or adrenal insufficiency. See below for evaluation.

D. Treatment of hypoglycemia.

1. ***Acute management.***
   a. Oral carbohydrates if possible.
   b. IV D_{50} at 1 ampule or more. No predictable response of blood glucose to D_{50}.
   c. If no IV access, glucagon 1 mg IM (may cause nausea, vomiting, aspiration).
   d. Monitor blood glucose Q15-30 min.
   e. Those with hypoglycemia secondary to oral agents should be admitted for observation.
2. ***Long-term management.***
   a. Adjust drug dosages; give diabetic training where applicable.
   b. Institute an ADA diet with high proportion of complex carbohydrates.
   c. Propantheline 7.5 to 15 mg PO ½ hour before meals may delay gastric emptying in postgastrectomy patient avoiding rapid peaks in serum glucose. This is not an approved use.

II. DIABETES MELLITUS

A. Overview.

1. ***Definition.*** Diabetes mellitus (DM) is hyperglycemia secondary to decreased insulin production or peripheral tissue resistance to insulin.
2. ***Classification.***
   a. Insulin-dependent DM (IDDM, or type I DM) usually occurs in childhood or early adulthood and results in ketoacidosis when patients are without insulin therapy. This accounts for 10% of cases of DM.
   b. Non–insulin dependent DM (NIDDM, or type II DM) usually occurs in people >40 years of age, and 60% of the patients are obese. These patients are not ketosis prone but may develop it under conditions of stress.
   c. Gestational onset DM (GODM) occurs when diabetes onset is during pregnancy and resolves with delivery. These patients are at a higher risk for developing DM at a later date. See Chapter 8 for details on GODM diagnosis and management.
   d. Secondary DM can be caused by steroid therapy, Cushing's syndrome, pancreatectomy, pancreatic

insufficiency secondary to pancreatitis, or endocrine disorders.

3. The long-term complications of diabetes are now considered to be related to the level of diabetic control achieved as shown in the Diabetes Control and Complications Trial. The conclusion of the study was that intensive therapy delays the onset and slows the progression of diabetic retinopathy, nephropathy, and neuropathy in patients with IDDM. Although it seems reasonable that these same conclusions would apply to NIDDM, these studies are currently lacking in the literature.

B. Etiology.

1. ***Type I DM (or insulin-dependent DM, or IDDM).*** This is caused by beta islet cell failure of multifactorial causes such as genetic predisposition, viral and autoimmune attacks on the beta islet cells.
2. ***Type II DM (or non–insulin dependent DM, or NIDDM).*** This occurs with intact beta islet cell function but peripheral tissue resistance to insulin. There may be some decrease in insulin production or a hyperinsulin state.

C. Evaluation.

1. ***Symptoms.*** Presentations may include polyuria, polydipsia, polyphagia associated with weight loss, blurred vision, recurrent candidal vaginitis, soft-tissue infections, or dehydration. Many cases will be asymptomatic and picked up on routine screening.
2. Normal 2-hour postprandial blood glucose varies depending on patient's age. Also, consider reversible factors before establishing the diagnosis of DM.
3. The diagnosis of diabetes mellitus is made if:
   a. Random plasma glucose of >200 mg/dl.
   b. Fasting plasma glucose of >140 mg/dl on more than one occasion, or if the oral glucose tolerance test (OGTT) is abnormal.
   c. Elevated HbA_{1c}.
4. The GTT must be done when the daily carbohydrate intake is >150 g, physical activity is unrestricted, and the patient is not under stress.
5. The patient must fast for 10 to 16 hours before the ingestion of a 75 g glucose load. Plasma glucose is measured initially and at half-hour intervals until 2 hours after glucose administration. The test is normal if the fasting plasma glucose is <115 mg/dl, the 2-hour plasma glucose is <140 mg/dl, and no value is >200 mg/dl. The diagnosis of DM can be made if the 2-hour sample and at least one other sample is >200 mg/dl. The patient is said to have impaired glucose tolerance if the plasma glucose values are above normal but not diagnostic for DM. Of these patients, 1% to 5% per year will develop DM.

6. The hemoglobin A_{1c}, which is a reflection of blood glucose over the past several months, is elevated.
7. It is usually possible to differentiate between type I and type II DM based on clinical situation. On occasion, however, this may be difficult. The diagnosis can be clarified by the use of the C-peptide, a product of the cleavage of pro-insulin to insulin. This will be present in those with type II DM and low or absent in those with type I DM. If the C-peptide is borderline, checking it after a glucose load may help. In those with type II DM, it will increase significantly after glucose load; this response will be absent in those with type I DM.

D. Treatment.

1. ***Goal of therapy.*** Eliminate symptoms and prevent the complications of diabetes. After the initial diagnosis of DM, there often occurs a "honeymoon" period during which small amounts of hypoglycemic agent or insulin is needed. Frequently, diabetes first presents during a situation of metabolic stress (such as infection or pregnancy). With the return to baseline metabolic demands, the pancreatic reserve may be adequate to maintain a normal or near-normal blood glucose.
2. ***Patient education.*** Crucial to proper management of DM. Patients must understand diet planning, home glucose-monitoring techniques, proper foot care, symptoms and treatment of hypoglycemia.
3. ***Diet therapy.*** Patients should receive instruction from a registered dietitian. Alcohol ingestion should be limited. Diet should include a 60% to 65% carbohydrates, 25% to 35% fat, and 10% to 20% protein.
   a. *Type I DM.* A fairly rigid dietary pattern must be followed to avoid wide fluctuations in plasma glucose. There can be some flexibility if intensive conventional therapy is used. If a meal must be delayed, the patient should ingest 10 g of carbohydrate per half hour. Caloric needs may be estimated at 40 kcal/kg/day for an adult with average activity. Modest excercise requires 10 g of extra carbohydrate per hour, whereas vigorous excercise requires 20 to 30 g/hour.
   b. *Type II DM.* In the obese patient, diabetes is usually reversible with weight loss. If the patient is not obese, the same rigid type I DM diet applies. If patients are receiving oral drug or insulin therapy, their appetite may be stimulated causing weight gain. This is not the case with the use of metformin.
4. ***Pharmacologic therapy.*** Type I DM patients must be started on insulin at the time of diagnosis. However, type II DM patients may need insulin, oral hypoglycemics, or

metformin if control of hyperglycemia is not achieved by diet alone. The hemoglobin A_{1c} level may be helpful in deciding the need for drug therapy in relatively mild hyperglycemia.

a. *Insulin.* Beef, pork, and recombinant human insulin (Humulin) are available. Humulin is generally preferable and tends to be less immunogenic than beef or pork insulin and therefore there is less insulin resistance secondary to anti-insulin antibodies. Although there was some thought that those using Humulin are less likely to manifest and therefore recognize symptoms of hypoglycemia, this has proved not to be the case.
   (1) Preparations.
      (a) Short-acting insulin (regular or Semilente): onset (SQ) 15 to 30 minutes; peaks 2 to 4 hours; duration 6 to 8 hours.
      (b) Intermediate-acting insulin (NPH or Lente): onset 1 to 3 hours; peak action 6 to 12 hours; duration 18 to 26 hours.
      (c) Long-acting insulin (Ultralente PZI): onset 4 to 8 hours; peak action 14 to 24 hours; duration 28 to 36 hours.
   (2) *In type I DM,* glucose control is initially obtained with a sliding scale of regular insulin. Measure serum glucose every 6 hours and give SQ regular insulin to cover sugars. Once the glucose is stabilized with Q6h injections, a split-dosing regimen is introduced with ⅔ of the total insulin requirement given as an A.M. dose and ⅓ given as a P.M. dose. This should be given as NPH insulin. If the intermediate-acting agent doesn't give adequate control of daytime blood glucose, a short-acting agent should be added. The two types of insulin can be given in the same syringe unless they are regular and protamine zinc insulin (PZI).
      (a) Intensive insulin therapy involves either an insulin pump, which administers continuous SQ insulin infusion with mealtime boluses, or multiple daily insulin injections with frequent blood glucose determinations. Another option is the use of a long-acting insulin (such as Ultralente) to provide a base of insulin delivery augmented by regular insulin at mealtimes.
      (b) While adjusting insulin regimen, measure preprandial blood glucose 4 times daily (including bedtime).
      (c) *Only regular insulin can be given IV.*

(3) *In type II DM,* insulin is usually added to an oral agent when glycemic control is suboptimal at maximal doses of oral medications. An intermediate-acting agent is used starting with a low dose and increasing as needed for glycemic control (such as 5 to 10 units of NPH increasing as needed). Adding NPH at bedtime is generally more efficacious than using it during the day. If using only insulin, start with an A.M. injection. The dose can be increased by 5 units every 3 to 7 days until adequate control is achieved. If fasting hyperglycemia is a problem, intermediate-acting insulin can be given twice daily as a split dose.

b. *Oral hypoglycemic agents.*

(1) *Mechanism of action.* These agents stimulate insulin secretion and reduce insulin resistance of tissues. *These drugs are indicated in the management of NIDDM only.*

(2) *Sulfonylureas.* Glyburide 2.5 to 20 mg or glipizide 5 to 40 mg are good choices for an oral hypoglycemic. There is little evidence that glipizide doses of greater than 20 mg/day are helpful and may actually result in decreased beta-cell function. Both can be dosed once a day. However, glyburide is more likely to result in glycemic control when used once a day than glipizide is. Glyburide should be used in a twice-daily dosing if 20 mg/day total is required. Glipizide should be divided into twice-daily dosing if more than 15 mg is needed for glycemic control.

(a) *Contraindications* include IDDM, severe renal or hepatic disease, pregnancy, lactation. They should not be used in children.

(b) *Complications* of sulfonylureas.
- Hypoglycemia, which may occur and may be severe and prolonged.
- A disulfiram-like effect may be seen when taken with alcohol with symptoms of flushing, headache, tachycardia, nausea, and vomiting.
- Severe hyponatremia and fluid retention may result from the use of chlorpropamide in the elderly (drug-induced SIADH).

(c) Drug interactions.
- Propranolol and clonidine mask the signs and symptoms of hypoglycemia.
- Thiazide diuretics, chlorthalidone, furosemide, ethacrynic acid, and phenytoin may have antagonistic effects on sulfonylureas.

- Hypoglycemic effects of the sulfonylureas may be potentiated by ACE inhibitors, salicylates, sulfonamides, phenylbutazone, methyldopa, clofibrate, warfarin, monoamine oxidase inhibitors, and chloramphenicol.

(3) *Metformin.* A new antihyperglycemic biguanide drug for NIDDM that is used alone or with sulfonylureas to enhance their effect. Metformin reduces blood glucose levels by improving hepatic and peripheral tissue sensitivity to insulin without affecting the secretion of insulin. Hypoglycemia and increased body weight, which are seen with sulfonylureas and insulin, are not a problem with metformin. Metformin also appears to improve plasma lipid and fibrinolytic profiles associated with NIDDM. Initial dosage is 500 mg PO QD until initial nausea and anorexia are tolerated and then advanced to 500 mg BID and then increased 500 mg/day weekly to maximum dose of 2500 mg if needed to control sugars. Use with or after food may lessen the GI side effects. The main risk of metformin is the rare induction of lactic acidosis. This risk is minimized if the use of metformin is avoided in patients with renal disease (decreased creatinine clearance), or patients with CHF or pulmonary disease.

(4) *Acarbose,* an oral agent that reduces the absorption of carbohydrates, is an alternative method of treating type II (NIDDM) diabetes. Start with 50 mg PO TID with meals and increase weekly to 300 mg PO TID. Main side effects include asymptomatic elevation of liver enzymes, flatulence, and diarrhea. Acarbose is generally added to treatment with another agent such as a sulfonylurea.

(5) *Troglitazone (Rezulin).* Troglitazone is a new class of oral hypoglycemic agent that increases the body's sensitivity to endogenous insulin. It is used for type II diabetes and may reduce or eliminate the need for insulin in some type II diabetics.

c. *Symptoms of hypoglycemia* may develop with the use of insulin or oral hypoglycemics. Symptoms include shakiness, tachycardia, weakness, sweating, and nightmares. If not treated with glucose, manifestations may progress to stupor and coma.

d. ***Somogyi phenomenon.*** This refers to hyperglycemia secondary to a period of drug-induced hypoglycemia with metabolic compensation (increased gluconeogenesis and sympathetic outflow). If controlling high blood glucose becomes a problem (especially A.M. glucose), consider checking for hypoglycemia in the time leading up to high readings.

E. Complications of DM.

1. The DCCT study found that intensive glycemic control delayed the onset and progression of diabetic retinopathy, nephropathy, and neuropathy. Current recommendations are to treat patients with IDDM with closely monitored regimens to maintain blood glucose levels as close to their normal state as possible, with recognition that the number of hypoglycemic episodes may increase. Patient education and compliance are crucial.
2. ***Diabetic nephropathy.*** Diabetic nephropathy is the most common cause of end-stage renal disease in the United States. There is clear evidence to indicate that the use of ACE inhibitors (captopril and others) in those diabetics with microalbuminuria can delay the development of renal failure; this is true even in the absence of hypertension. Accordingly, all diabetics over 12 years of age should be screened for microalbuminuria at least yearly and should start using an ACE inhibitor when microalbuminuria develops. Dipsticks are not considered sensitive enough for screening.
3. ***Atherosclerosis*** of the coronary and peripheral arteries is three times more common in diabetics and increases with time.
   a. *Coronary artery disease.* The leading cause of death in DM patients is myocardial infarction. 30% of myocardial infarctions in diabetic patients are "silent" (that is, painless). Therefore the possibility of a MI must be considered whenever a diabetic patient presents with CHF, dyspnea, diabetic ketoacidosis, or other secondary event.
   b. *Peripheral vascular disease.* This disease results in ischemia with ulceration, polymicrobial infection, and gangrene of the lower extremities.
4. ***Diabetic neuropathy.***
   a. *Peripheral sensory neuropathy* is the most common type and results in hypesthesia (diminution of all sensation) first in distal lower and later distal upper extremities. Hypesthesia may be preceded by hyperesthesia and dysesthesias, especially burning sensations.
   b. *Peripheral motor neuropathy* may occur particularly involving the interosseous muscles of the feet and hands.
   c. *Mononeuropathies* can occur in any superficial nerve with sudden onset of intense pain in the distribution of the affected nerve. The pain is usually worse at

night. Muscle weakness and atrophy may occur, usually with complete recovery with a few months. The cranial nerves may be involved; pupillary function is usually spared with third nerve palsy. Pain management may require potent analgesics. Tricyclic antidepressants are helpful for peripheral neuropathy pain. Other agents that have been used include carbamazepine and capsaicin cream.

d. *Autonomic neuropathy* may be manifested by hyperhydrosis of the upper body with anhydrosis of the lower body or by generalized anhydrosis. Other symptoms may include resting tachycardia, impotence, neurogenic bladder, diarrhea, and urinary or fecal incontinence. Orthostatic hypotension may be treated with fludrocortisone, 0.1 to 0.3 mg/day or with NaCl 1 to 4 g PO QID; care must be taken to avoid recumbent hypertension and cardiac failure if these measures are adopted.

e. *Diabetic amyopathy* is a rare complication of DM with proximal muscle weakness and pain, most commonly involving the pelvic girdle. Onset may be rapid, and the patient may have a low-grade fever and an elevated ESR. Prognosis for improvement is good over months.

5. ***Neuropathic arthropathy (Charcot's joint).*** Degenerative changes of the joints of the feet and ankles that occasionally progresses to complete joint destruction. This is frequently a painless process secondary to recurrent trauma, which may have gone unnoticed by the patient.
6. ***Gastroparesis diabeticorum (gastric atony).*** May be asymptomatic or manifested by nausea and vomiting. Gastric emptying time may be unpredictable, making diabetic control difficult in an insulin-dependent patient. Metoclopramide 10 mg ½ hour AC and HS may be effective treatment. Erythromycin and cisapride have also been used to promote gastric emptying.
7. ***Diabetic foot problems.*** Diabetic foot problems caused by sensory neuropathies, arthropathies, and peripheral vascular disease make care of diabetic foot important. Feet should be inspected daily for ulcerations, and shoes must be properly fitted. Foot ulcers commonly become infected, and osteomyelitis may also develop. Straphylococci and streptococci are the most common pathogens, but gram-negative and anaerobic bacteria may also be involved. For early infection, can use cefotaxime. If patient is septic, consider imipenem, ticarcillin-clavulanate, or clindamycin and fluoroquinolones. Aggressive therapy with dressing changes and débridement is essential. Surgical revascularization should be considered if indicated. Amputation of the foot is occasionally necessary.

TABLE 5-1
Summary of Diabetic Follow-up

Follow-up	IDDM	NIDDM
Eye exam by ophthalmologist	5 years after diagnosis and then every year	At time of diagnosis and every year thereafter
HbA_{1c}	Every 3 months	Every 3 months
Blood pressure	Every visit	Every visit
Foot check	Every visit	Every visit
Urine microalbumin	Every 6 months to 1 year after 12 years of age	Every 6 months to 1 year

8. ***Diabetic retinopathy.*** Leading cause of blindness. Typical lesions include microaneurysms, punctate retinal hemorrhages, hard exudates, soft exudates ("cotton wool" spots), microvascular anomalies, and macular edema. With proliferative retinopathy, new vessels and fibrous tissue grow along the posterior surface of the vitreous; this may lead to contraction of the vitreous, causing traction on the vessels and on the retina, resulting in vitreous hemorrhages and retinal detachment. Diabetes should be evaluated annually by an ophthalmologist.
9. ***Summary of diabetic follow-up*** (Table 5-1).

III. DIABETIC KETOACIDOSIS

A. Overview. When severe insulin deficiency occurs, a starvation-like state develops with breakdown of free fatty acids and increasing blood levels of acetoacetic acid, beta-hydroxybutyric acid, and acetone, resulting in acidosis. This occurs predominantly in type I DM but can occur in anyone who requires insulin to control glucose.

B. Causes. DKA frequently results from intercurrent infection, poor compliance with insulin, or dehydration.

C. Evaluation.

1. ***Symptoms.*** Mental status changes, rapid respirations, acetone ("fruity") odor of breath, nausea and vomiting, dehydration, and a history of diabetes (unless first presentation). Frequently complain of abdominal pain.
2. ***Hyperglycemia can be diagnosed*** with rapid blood glucose determination, and ketosis can be determined with bedside reagents. These and the symptoms are adequate for initiation of treatment.
3. Additional laboratory evaluation should include true glucose, serum ketones, electrolytes, BUN, creatinine, serum osmolarity, and arterial blood gases. CXR, urine and C&S, blood cultures should also be done.

a. Generally hypokalemic and hypomagnesemic.
b. Acidosis will give a spuriously elevated potassium.

D. Treatment.

1. ***Acute management (adults).***
   a. *Supportive therapy.* Airway maintenance, supplemental oxygen as needed, and treatment of shock.
   b. *Fluid.* Initially 1 liter of normal saline should be given over a half hour if no cardiac compromise is present. The rate should then be decreased to 1 liter/hour if patient is clinically stable. This will result in a decrease in blood glucose and restoration of adequate renal perfusion. If cardiac compromise is present, central venous pressure monitoring is indicated to guide fluid resuscitation.
   c. *Potassium replacement* in acidotic adults (Table 5-2). Monitor potassium; use judgment. This is only a guide.
   d. *Insulin* (0.1 unit/kg IV) 5 to 10 units of regular insulin IV bolus in adults should be given with the initial fluid resuscitation. This should be followed by an insulin infusion of 3 to 10 units/hour (or more if needed), adjusted according to subsequent glucose and electrolyte determinations.
      - Ideal rate of fall in serum glucose is not greater than 100 mg/dl/hour. If the glucose fails to fall by at least 10%, insulin infusion should be increased each hour until response occurs. When blood glucose reaches a range of 250 to 300 mg/dl, glucose should be added to IV fluids so that infusing solution includes 10% glucose ($D_{10}W$). Insulin infusion should be adjusted if needed to maintain glucose level *but should not be stopped. It is preferable to give $D_{10}W$ with the infusion than it is to stop the insulin!*
   e. *Bicarbonate.* Bicarbonate is controversial but may be indicated for coma, arterial pH of less than 7.0, or severe hyperkalemia. May be administered with one of

TABLE 5-2
Potassium Replacement in Acidotic Adults

If Serum K^+ (mEq/dl)	mEq/hr KCl in NS
<3	40
3-4	30
4-5	20
5-6	10
>6	0

the initial liters of fluid by mixing of 2 ampules of bicarbonate (88 mEq) in a liter of 0.45% saline, which is substituted for one of the liters of normal saline. *Bicarbonate may induce hypokalemia and does not seem to change outcomes.*

f. Monitor serum glucose and potassium as well as urine output hourly. If bicarbonate therapy was administered, arterial blood gases should also be followed. Otherwise monitor DKA by following plasma bicarbonate levels.

g. *Phosphate.* Supplementation may be required if patient is not able to initiate oral intake within first few hours. Potassium phosphate (4 mEq of K^+ per 93 mg of phosphorus) may be added to maintenance fluids if necessary. Should not exceed total dose of 20 mEq K^+, and great caution required with renal insufficiency.

h. *Magnesium.* Should replace. Can give magnesium sulfate 2.5 g in 50 ml of NS over first hour.

i. Maintenance fluids should consist of 0.45% saline with additives as indicated; 150 to 200 ml/hour adjusted according to urine output.

j. Evaluate for potential precipitating factors, including infection, pregnancy, MI, inappropriate use of insulin.

k. *Diet.* Oral intake may resume when mental status and nausea and vomiting allow. Initial diet should consist of fluids, and full diet not resumed until ketoacidosis corrected.

2. ***For children.***

a. Assume 10% to 15% deficit (100 to 150 ml/kg). Want to replace 50% in first 8 hours.

(1) For first hour give 20 ml/kg boluses of normal saline until patient out of shock.

(2) Hours 2 to 8. Give enough normal saline to replace 50% total deficit taking into account percentage already replaced in first hour. Change to D_5W 0.5 NS when serum glucose <250 mg/dl.

(3) Hours 9 to 24. Use 0.3 to 0.5 NS to replace remaining deficit (50% of baseline deficit) plus maintenance fluids (see Chapter 10 on fluid management, p. 466 to 471).

b. *In most children* a bolus of regular insulin 0.1 unit/kg followed by 0.1 unit/kg/hour is a good starting point.

IV. HYPERGLYCEMIC-HYPEROSMOLAR NONKETOTIC SYNDROME

A. Overview. Severe hyperglycemia leads to mental status changes and dehydration with absence of serum ketones; occurs primarily in type II diabetics.

B. Causes. Hyperglycemic-hyperosmolar nonketonic syndrome occurs because of osmotic diuresis from severe hyperglycemia with elevation of plasma osmolarity, dehydration, and hypernatremia.

C. Evaluation.

1. ***Symptoms.*** Mental status changes, obtundation or coma, dehydration or shock.
2. ***Laboratory studies.*** Serum glucose, ketones, osmolarity, electrolytes, BUN, creatinine, and arterial blood gases. ECG should also be obtained. Treatment should not be delayed pending the results of these studies.

D. Treatment.

1. ***Acute management.***
   a. Supportive measures to provide adequate airway and ventilation and treatment of shock.
   b. *Fluid.* Initial therapy should be with normal saline at 1 liter/hour until intravascular volume is restored. If hypernatremia is present, this may be switched to 0.45% saline. Caution must be exercised in the setting of renal impairment, CHF, possible MI.
   c. *Insulin.* Treatment is initiated with 5 to 10 units of regular IV bolus for serum glucose greater than 600 mg/dl and begin insulin drip as above under DKA.
2. ***Long-term management.***
   a. Monitor glucose and electrolytes initially every hour. Urine output should be monitored continuously. ABGs should be followed if bicarbonate is given. Serum osmolarity should be checked every 2 to 3 hours initially to aid in fluid therapy.
   b. *Fluid.* After intravascular volume is restored, therapy should be guided by electrolyte determinations. Generally 0.45% saline will be appropriate. If significant hypernatremia is present, the initial resuscitation with 0.45% saline should be followed by 0.2% saline or D_5W. Fluid should be administered at 150 ml/hour, adjusted according to vitals and urine output.
   c. *Electrolytes.* Potassium depletion may occur, and supplementation should be provided if levels approach low normal; 10 mEq/hour of KCl initially, adjusted accordingly.
   d. *Insulin.* After initial bolus, constant infusion should be started at 5 to 10 units of regular insulin per hour. Gradual decline in blood glucose (around 75 mg/dl/hour) is the desired goal. Glucose should be added to the maintenance fluids when blood glucose drops to the 200 to 300 mg/dl range.
   e. Patient should be evaluated for possible precipitating causes, including infection, MI, stroke.

HYPERTHYROIDISM

I. OVERVIEW DEFINITION

Hyperthyroidism is a disease caused by high levels of circulating thyroid hormone.

II. ETIOLOGY

Common causes of hyperthyroidism include:

A. **Graves' disease.** Most common cause of hyperthyroidism in the *third and fourth decades.* Causes diffuse symmetrically enlarged thyroid gland with normal to slightly soft consistency. The classic infiltrative ophthalmopathy may occur with or without overt hyperthyroidism.

B. **Toxic multinodular goiter.** Results in an irregular, asymmetric, nodular thyroid gland. It usually develops insidiously in the *sixth or seventh decade* in a patient who has had a nontoxic nodular goiter for years. A thyroid scan may be useful in establishing the diagnosis.

C. **Solitary hyperfunctioning adenomas.** Usually occur during the *fourth and fifth decades.* The thyroid gland contains a smooth, well-defined, soft to firm nodule that shows intense radioactive uptake on scan with absence of uptake in the rest of the gland. Most patients with solitary adenomas do not become thyrotoxic. When they do, they are usually less toxic than those with Graves' disease, and they don't develop ophthalmopathy or pretibial myxedema.

D. **Autoimmune thyroiditis.** Normal-sized or enlarged nontender thyroid gland. Thyroid antibodies, when present, are high in titer. ^{131}I uptake is suppressed or zero. This disorder improves spontaneously but frequently recurs. Autoimmune thyroiditis, painless thyroiditis, lymphocytic thyroiditis, and Hashimoto's thyroiditis are probably all the same disorder.

E. **Excess exogenous thyroid.** May occur because of dosage errors or occasionally in individuals taking large doses of thyroid hormones to lose weight or increase their energy. The thyroid gland is normal or small in size, and ^{131}I uptake is suppressed.

F. **Subacute thyroiditis and viral thyroiditis.** Tender, diffusely enlarged thyroid gland with a normal or elevated T_4, a depressed ^{131}I uptake, and an elevated ESR. Probably of viral origin and may present as a sore throat.

G. **Rare causes.** Radiation thyroiditis, thyroid carcinoma, excessive TSH stimulation, excessive iodine intake, struma ovarii, and trophoblastic disease.

III. EVALUATION

A. **Symptoms.** Patients may present with nervousness, heat intolerance, palpitations, tachycardia, weight loss, weakness, dyspnea on exertion, emotional lability, poor concentration, itching and burning of eyes, fullness in the throat, diarrhea, and dysmenorrhea or amenorrhea. Diarrhea is a bad sign and can herald the onset of thyroid storm. Frequently geriatric patients may show withdrawal or depression (apathetic hyperthyroidism).

B. Laboratory evaluation of hyperthyroidism.

1. ***Ultrasensitive TSH.*** Best method for diagnosing hyperthyroidism. Will be decreased in response to increased circulating thyroid hormone in 98%.
2. ***Free T_4.*** A measure of the active thyroid hormone, unaffected by changes in the thyroxine-binding globulin (TBG), will be elevated in most cases of hyperthyroidism.
3. ***Total T_4.*** Measurement affected by increases in TBG. Therefore, elevated total T_4 is not sensitive or specific. Will be elevated in states that increase the TBG including pregnancy, estrogen therapy and oral contraceptives, infectious hepatitis, cirrhosis, breast carcinoma, hypothyroidism, acute intermittent porphyria.
4. ***Free T_4 index.*** Corrects the total T_4 for the serum TBG to allow one to estimate the free T_4.
5. ***Free T_3/T_3 RIA.*** About 5% of hyperthyroid individuals will have a normal T_4 level but an elevated T_3 level, indicating an isolated T_3 hyperthyroidism. If the patient is clinically hyperthyroid but the free T_4 is normal, checking a T_3 RIA is prudent.
6. ***Antithyroid antibodies (antimicrosomal antibody and antifollicular cell antibody, antithyroglobulin antibody).*** Elevated especially in autoimmune thyroiditis (such as Hashimoto's thyroiditis). May be slightly elevated in other thyroid diseases.

IV. TREATMENT

A. Graves' disease.

1. *Propylthiouracil* 100 to 150 mg every 8 hours, or *methimazole* 15 to 60 mg divided BID or TID every 12 hours depending on severity of illness. Clinical improvement may be seen in 1 to 2 weeks, and the patient becomes euthyroid 2 to 3 months after beginning therapy. After the euthyroid state is reached, the medication dose should be decreased by a third every few months if the patient remains euthyroid. A free T_4 level should be checked after 1 month of therapy and then every 2 to 3 months. These drugs are usually continued for 6 months to 1 year. Low-dose thyroxine may be needed during therapy. A significant number of patients will experience permanent remission of hyperthyroidism after discontinuing these medications. Side effects include rashes, agranulocytosis, thrombocytopenia, anemia, hepatitis, arthritis, fever. A white blood cell count and liver enzymes should be obtained before drug therapy is started

and rechecked after 1 month and 3 months of treatment; after that recheck labs only if new symptoms arise. These drugs cause no permanent thyroid damage.

2. *Inorganic iodine* rapidly controls hyperthyroidism by inhibiting hormone synthesis and release from the gland. One drop of saturated potassium iodide solution in juice is taken daily. This should not be used as the sole form of therapy. It may be used alone for 7 to 10 days before surgery to decrease the vascularity of the thyroid gland. It should not be used for at least 3 days after ^{131}I therapy but thereafter may be used alone until the ^{131}I becomes effective.
3. *Propranolol,* 80 to 200 mg/day in divided doses Q6h, will reduce symptoms of tachycardia, palpitations, heat intolerance, and nervousness but will not normalize the metabolic rate. It should not be used alone except in the case of transient hyperthyroidism secondary to autoimmune thyroiditis.
4. *Iodine 131,* 5 to 15 mCi, renders most patients euthyroid within 3 to 6 months. Therefore treatment should be preceded and followed by antithyroid therapy. Most will eventually become hypothyroid. Pregnancy is an absolute contraindication to ^{131}I therapy.
5. ***Surgery.*** Usually reserved for those who are unable to take antithyroid drugs.
6. ***Ophthalmopathy.*** Symptomatic treatment only. Artificial tears or methyl cellulose drops for the discomfort, patching or prisms for diplopia, diuretics and raising the head of the bed for circumorbital edema.

B. *Toxic multinodular goiter* is treated with ^{131}I or surgery. Antithyroid drugs will not induce permanent remission and should be used only as interim therapy. Large multinodular goiters do not respond well to ^{131}I. Hypothyroidism is rare after ^{131}I therapy because normal thyroid tissue is suppressed and so does not in this condition take up the ^{131}I.

C. *Solitary hyperfunctioning adenomas* are treated with ^{131}I or surgery with antithyroid drugs used only as interim therapy when needed. Hypothyroidism is rare after therapy.

D. *Autoimmune thyroiditis* is transient and does not require definitive treatment except in those patients with recurrent hyperthyroidism. Propranolol may be used alone if symptoms are mild. Antithyroid drugs may be needed for a short time in some patients.

E. *Subacute thyroiditis and viral thyroiditis* generally self-limited but should be treated with aspirin 650 mg QID. In more severe cases, prednisone may be used at 40 mg PO QD, tapering to 10 mg each day over 2 weeks, and then continued for 1 month after patient becomes asymptomatic. Resolution of symptoms usually occurs in 1 to 6 months, and relapse is common. Hypothyroidism may occur but is rare.

THYROID STORM

I. OVERVIEW

A severe life-threatening form of hyperthyroidism.

II. CAUSE

Increasing stress such as trauma or illness may cause this in a previously mildly hyperthyroid patient.

III. CLINICALLY

Have signs and symptoms consistent with thyrotoxicosis (tachycardia, heat intolerance, weight loss) as well as fever, confusion, agitation, weakness, diarrhea, and shock.

IV. TREATMENT

A. When suspected, treatment should be instituted immediately. If defervescence of fever doesn't occur within several hours, concurrent infection should be suspected. Other signs of hyperthyroidism may require several days of therapy before improvement is seen.

B. Treatment is propranolol 20 to 40 mg Q4h to control tachycardia, tremor, etc. (can give 0.5 to 1.0 mg IV Q5 min to keep pulse about 100). Give propylthiouracil 250 mg PO or per NG Q6h (alternative is methimazole 20 to 40 mg PO or per NG Q6-8h) and SSKI 30 gtt PO *1 hour after giving PTU to avoid iodine being used for additional thyroid hormone synthesis. Continue with 5 to 10 gtt QID.* Alternative is 0.5 g of sodium iodide in 1 liter of NS over 12 hours. Fluid and electrolytes should be replaced and fever controlled with acetaminophen and a cooling blanket.

C. Avoid aspirin because may increase T_3 and T_4 by reducing protein binding.

D. Give steroids equivalent to about 300 mg of hydrocortisone per day (100 mg IV Q6h). Dexamethasone has some theoretical advantage because prevents conversion of T_4 to T_3 peripherally. (This would be about 11.25 mg of dexamethasone divided TID.)

HYPOTHYROIDISM

I. OVERVIEW

A. Definition. Primary hypothyroidism refers to a thyroid hormone deficiency as a result of thyroid gland disease. Secondary hypothyroidism results from TSH deficiency. Tertiary hypothyroidism results from thyrotropin releasing hormone (TRH) deficiency.

B. Prevalence. Present in 1% to 6% of population.

II. ETIOLOGY

A. Without thyroid enlargement. Commonly caused by ^{131}I therapy, thyroidectomy for hyperthyroidism. The second most common cause is idiopathic hypothyroidism. Developmental defects and TSH or TRH deficiency are less common causes.

B. **With thyroid enlargement.** Most commonly caused by Hashimoto's thyroiditis. Drugs, iodine deficiency, and inherited defects in thyroid hormone snythesis are rare causes.

III. EVALUATION

A. **Signs and symptoms.** Fatigue, weakness, slow movement, cold intolerance, constipation, hair loss, menorrhagia, carpal tunnel syndrome, dry skin, edema of the face and extremities, memory impairment, hearing loss, hoarseness, and occasionally bradycardia and hypothermia. Sparse eyebrows with loss of the lateral half is a nonspecific sign. Pericardial effusion and ascites occasionally occur. A delay in the relaxation phase of the deep tendon reflexes, especially at the ankles, is a specific finding. May have myalgias and arthralgias. Psychosis may develop with long-standing hypothyroidism and may be precipitated by thyroid hormone replacement. Infants may present with hypotonia, umbilical hernia, delayed mental and physical development, and other signs and symptoms typical of adult patients. Mental retardation may result if hypothyroidism goes untreated in the first few years of life.

B. **Laboratory findings.** A low free T_4 (see hyperthyroidism, p. 239, for discussion of thyroid tests). A low TSH value indicates secondary or tertiary hypothyroidism, whereas a high TSH value is diagnostic of primary thyroid failure. The ^{131}I uptake is not helpful. Other laboratory abnormalities may include high AST, low sodium, low blood glucose, elevated CPK, elevated cholesterol and triglycerides, mild anemia, elevated prolactin levels secondary to high TRH levels, and flat or inverted T waves with minor ST-segment depression and low amplitude on ECG.

IV. TREATMENT

Treatment is by levothyroxine with the average daily dose being 0.1 to 0.15 mg every day. Patients over 40 years of age or those with heart disease should be started on 1/4 to 1/3 (0.025 mg) of this dose with increases every 2 to 4 weeks until a maintenance dose is reached. The goal is to normalize the TSH, and the serum TSH usually returns to normal within a few months after a maintenance dose is reached. Elective surgery should be avoided in hypothyroid patients because respiratory depression commonly occurs. Increased sensitivity to narcotics and hypnotics is also common in the hypothyroid patient.

MYXEDEMA COMA

I. OVERVIEW

Myxedema coma occurs with severe chronic hypothyroidism and is life threatening.

II. ETIOLOGY

The coma is precipitated in chronically hypothyroid patients by exposure to cold, infection, hypoglycemia, respiratory depressants, allergic reactions, or other metabolic stress.

III. TREATMENT

A. 500 µg of thyroxine (T_4) IV followed by oral thyroxine 0.1 mg QD. May substitute 40 µg of T_3 IV for the IV T_4 if available.

B. Hyponatremia and hypoglycemia frequently occur and should be treated appropriately.

C. Hypothermia or heat loss should be avoided.

THYROID ENLARGEMENT

I. GOITER

A goiter is a simple enlargement of the thyroid gland. It is more common in females with the highest incidence in the second through sixth decades of life.

A. Diffuse goiters are caused by iodine deficiency or excess, congenital defects in thyroid hormone synthesis, and drugs (such as lithium carbonate).

B. Most are asymptomatic. Unusual to have pain and rare to have hoarseness and tracheal obstruction. Thyroid function tests should be performed on all patients with goiter because it can be associated with hypothyroidism, euthyroidism, or hyperthyroidism.

II. MULTINODULAR GOITER

Multinodular enlargement of the thyroid gland.

A. Cause unknown.

B. Clinical presentation.

1. ***Symptoms.*** Thyromegaly, occasionally with rapid enlargement and tenderness secondary to hemorrhage into a cyst. Rarely, tracheal compression may occur, causing coughing or choking. Some patients may complain of a lump in the throat.
2. ***Physical exam.*** Many nodules of varying sizes are usually palpable. Occasionally it may be difficult to distinguish from the typically lobulated, irregular Hashimoto's gland.
3. ***Thyroid function tests.*** Performed to rule out toxicity. A thyroid scan is useful only if the diagnosis of multinodular goiter is in doubt based on physical exam. A scan will show a patchy radioisotope distribution. Malignancy is rare but should be considered if the gland is enlarging rapidly or hoarseness develops.

C. Treatment. Exogenous thyroid hormone suppression of TSH to prevent further growth of the gland. The gland usually will not shrink significantly with therapy, but it is worth a try. Levothyroxine is begun as per hypothyroidism, and TSH should be monitored. Oversupression of the TSH can cause bone demineralization. Occasionally hyperthyroidism may develop in a patient with multinodular goiter. Levothyroxine suppression should not be given to patients with angina or other known heart disease unless the patient is hypothyroid. If thyroid enlargement persists despite adequate TSH suppression, a needle biopsy or subtotal thyroidectomy should be considered.

III. SOLITARY NODULES

Usually benign. Suspect malignancy in a patient with a history of radiation exposure, rapid enlargement, hoarseness or obstruction, and a solid nodule that is cold on scan.

A. Diagnosis. History and a thyroid scan should be done on every patient with a solitary nodule. Hot nodules that take up the radioisotope are generally benign.

B. Treatment.

1. High-risk lesions should be surgically removed.
2. Low-risk lesions may be aspirated for cytologic examination if the pathologist is experienced.
3. Thyroid hormone has been used in an attempt to shrink the isolated thyroid nodule. However, this is generally ineffective.

IV. SUBACUTE THYROIDITIS

Presents with diffuse enlargement of the thyroid gland and may be associated with hyper-, hypo-, or euthyroidism. See section on hyperthyroidism for the discussion of this entity, p. 238.

V. EUTHYROID SICK SYNDROME

Have decreased T_3, increased reverse T_3, decreased T_4, normal TSH. Patients are euthyroid but suffering from chronic disease.

ADRENAL DISEASE

I. HYPOADRENALISM (Addison's disease)

A. Etiology. Most idiopathic (autoimmune), others from adrenal destruction (neoplasm, TB, amyloidosis, inflammatory necrosis), iatrogenic (discontinuation steroids, ketoconazole, other drugs). Primary Addison's: from adrenal destruction. Secondary Addison's: from pituitary destruction. Those with pituitary Addison's are more tolerant to metabolic stress because mineralocorticoids are intact.

B. Clinically.

1. Weakness, fatigue, orthostatic hypotension.
2. Hyperpigmentation, freckling (not with central hypoadrenalism; requires elevated ACTH to stimulate melanocytes).
3. Nausea, weight loss, dehydration, hypotension, small heart size.
4. Decreased cold tolerance, hypometabolism.

C. Diagnosis.

1. Serum Na <130 mEq/L, K >5 mEq/L, elevated BUN and creatinine. May be hypoglycemic. Electrolyte abnormalities may be found only in Addison's secondary to adrenal destruction. Requires loss of aldosterone to give abnormal electrolytes.
2. Low fasting A.M. cortisol.
3. ***Cosyntropin stimulation test.*** Get baseline level.
   a. Give cosyntropin 0.25 mg IV before 9:00 A.M.
   b. Cortisol should increase from baseline value of 5 to 25 μg/dl and be doubled by 60 to 90 minutes. Any level of >20 μg/dl is considered normal responsiveness. If still suspect hypoadrenalism, do metyrapone test.
4. ***Metyrapone test.*** Get baseline serum cortisol value.
   a. Administer 3 g of metyrapone orally at midnight.
   b. Measure cortisol and deoxycortisol at 8:00 A.M. the next day. If the pituitary-adrenal axis is intact, the plasma cortisol level should be less than 5 mg/dl and the 11-deoxycortisol level grater than 10 mg/dl.
   c. Measure serum ACTH. Will be elevated if primary adrenal failure; will be normal or low if primary pituitary failure.

D. Treatment.

1. ***Emergency.*** Institute therapy immediately!
   a. *Administer hydrocortisone succinate* 100 mg IV push and another 100 mg in NS over the next 2 hours and a total of 300 mg hydrocortisone succinate IV over the first 24 hours.
   b. Administer NS IV to correct hypotension and shock.
2. ***Long-term therapy.***
   a. Hydrocortisone succinate 150 mg IV over the second 24 hours.
   b. Hydrocortisone succinate 75 mg IV over the third 24 hours.
   c. Maintenance doses are hydrocortisone 30 mg PO QD plus fludrocortisone acetate 0.1 mg PO QD.

II. HYPERADRENALISM (CUSHING'S DISEASE)

A. Cause. Administration of exogenous steroids, ACTH secretion by pituitary or extrapituitary source (such as small cell carcinoma of lung).

B. Clinically. "Moon" facies, plethora, truncal obesity with wasted extremities, atrophic skin with senile purpura, abdominal striae, poor wound healing, hypertension, glucose intolerance, psychiatric symptoms.

C. Diagnosis.

1. Elevated A.M. fasting cortisol and lack of diurnal variation.
2. Check 24-hour free cortisol (usually >150 μg/24 hours in Cushing's). 17-OHS not helpful because can be falsely positive in obesity.

3. ***Dexamethasone test.***
   a. Administer dexamethasone 1 mg PO at midnight. Measure serum cortisol at 7:00 A.M. the next day. Should be <5 μg/dl.
   b. If this is equivocal, can give dexamethasone 0.5 mg PO Q6h for 2 days. Will not have decrease of urinary free cortisol.
   c. Can also administer dexamethasone IV 1 mg/hour for 7 hours by constant infusion. At the end of this time, a normal person should have reduced plasma cortisol by at least 7 mg/dl over baseline value.
4. Further diagnosis and therapy should be done under the guidance of an endocrinologist.

ELECTROLYTE FORMULAS

I. HYPERGLYCEMIA EFFECT ON SERUM Na^+

Correct serum Na^+ = Measured sodium + 1.6 × ([Measured serum glucose − 100]/100)
for serum glucose over 100 mg/dl

II. HYPERLIPIDEMIA OR HYPERPROTEINEMIA EFFECT ON Na^+

Correct serum Na^+ = Measured sodium × (93 ÷ % of serum water)
% serum H_2O = 99 − 1.03(Lipids in g/L) − 0.73(Protein in g/dl)

III. FRACTIONAL EXCRETION OF Na^+ (FE_{Na})

% FE_{Na} = (Urine Na/Serum Na)/(Urine Cr/Serum Cr) × 100

IV. SERUM Na^+ REQUIREMENT IN HYPONATREMIA

Desired Na^+ mEq/L = (Desired serum Na − Measured Na) × TBW
TBW (total body water in liters) = 0.6 × Body weight in kg

V. BODY WATER DEFICIT IN HYPERNATREMIA

Deficit = Desired TBW − Current TBW
Desired TBW = Measured Na × (Current TBW/normal serum Na)
Current TBW = 0.6 × Current body weight in kg
or Deficit = 0.6 (Current weight in kg) × ([Serum Na/140] − 1)

VI. CREATININE CLEARANCE

Creatinine clearance = (140 − Age)(Wt in kg)/(72 × Serum Cr in mg/dl)
Normal male = 125 ml/min
Normal female = 105 ml/min

METABOLIC FORMULAS

1. *Serum osmolarity* = 2(Na + K) + BUN/2.8 + Glucose/18
   a. Normal value 280 to 296 mOsm/kg of water
   b. A difference between the measured and calculated

osmolarity (osmolar gap) can indicate a circulating osmotically active substance such as ethanol, methanol, or ethylene glycol (antifreeze).

2. *Anion gap* = Na − (Cl + Bicarbonate)
   Normal is up to 15. Greater than this in presence of acidosis indicates an anion gap acidosis (see next section on acid-base disorders).

ACID-BASE DISORDERS

I. METABOLIC ACIDOSIS

A. Definition. pH <7.4 and implies a loss of bicarbonate or accumulation of fixed acids. Divided into two groups based on the calculated anion gap (see calculation above) described. Compensatory response is hyperventilation with drop in P_{CO_2}.

B. Normal anion-gap acidosis.

1. ***GI bicarbonate*** (HCO_3^-) losses, including causes relating to diarrhea, ileostomy, and colostomy.
2. Renal tubular acidosis (RTA).
   a. **Distal (type I) RTA.** Will be hypokalemic with urine pH >5.3. Caused by distal nephron acidification defect. Causes include familial and idiopathic hypercalciuria, Sjögren's syndrome, rheumatoid arthritis, primary hyperparathyroidism, multiple myeloma, and severe dehydration. Also lithium, amphotericin B, and toluene. Occasionally seen is a *hyper*kalemic form with SLE, obstructive uropathy, or sickle cell uropathy. Treat with bicarbonate repletion at 1 to 2 mEq/kg/day with any acute K^+ deficit corrected and maintenance oral K^+ if needed.
   b. **Proximal (type II) RTA.** Caused by a defect in the ability of proximal tubules to recover bicarbonate. Acutely the urine pH is usually >5.5, but it decreases with falling serum bicarbonate levels, resulting in increased proximal reabsorption of bicarbonate; final result is pH 5.5. Causes include autoimmune diseases (as in type I RTA), multiple myeloma, heavy metals, acetazolamide, and outdated tetracycline. Treatment is to identify the primary cause and treat it. Bicarbonate at 5 to 15 mEq/kg/day may be required and can result in severe hypokalemia. Consider use of thiazide diuretics to cause ECF volume contraction to promote HCO_3^- reabsorption proximally.
   c. **Type IV RTA.** Generally caused by moderate renal insufficiency with renal resistance to aldosterone (as in diabetes). Similar presentation to hyporeninemic hypoaldosteronism. K^+ may be normal but generally is increased. Bicarbonate will typically be >15 mEq/L. Urine pH, done under mineral oil at time of collec-

tion, is usually <5.5. Treat with K^+ restriction and consider use of loop diuretics such as furosemide (Lasix and others). Bicarbonate may be needed (see above for dosing). Florinef (fludrocortisone) at 0.1 to 0.2 mg PO QD may be useful if primary adrenal insufficiency is the cause.

3. ***Interstitial renal disease.*** Same as type IV RTA; serum K^+ is increased.
4. ***Ureterosigmoid loop.***
5. Ingestion of acetazolamide, ammonium chloride, cholestyramine, calcium chloride or magnesium chloride.
6. Small bowel drainage or fistula, biliary drainage or fistula, or pancreatic drainage or fistulas.
7. Calculating the urine ion gap (Urine Na + Urine K− Urine Cl) may help to determine if acidosis is renal related. A negative gap implies normal renal NH^{4+} excretion and a nonrenal cause for the acidosis. A positive gap denotes the opposite. CAVEAT: Only valid in absence of diuretics. Also, if volume depleted secondary to GI losses, may be a false-positive urine ion gap.

C. Increased anion-gap acidosis.

1. Methanol.
2. Uremia or renal failure.
3. Lactic acidosis.
4. Ethanol or ethylene glycol (antifreeze).
5. Paraldehyde.
6. Alcoholic ketoacidosis or diabetic ketoacidosis.
7. Others. Salicylates, cyanide (may be caused by nitroprusside). Can measure for these substances directly, but the first step is to determine the osmolal gap as noted previously. Treatment depends on the underlying condition.

II. METABOLIC ALKALOSIS

A. Definition.

Serum pH >7.40. Implies a loss of acid or gain of bicarbonate. ECF volume contraction, hypokalemia, and increased mineralocorticoids or glucocorticoids all impair the normal kidney's ability to excrete excess HCO_3^- and may result in a metabolic alkalosis. Additionally, excess exogenous bicarbonate should be in the differential. Metabolic alkalosis is separated into the two categories of chloride-responsive and non–chloride responsive. The urinary Cl^- level is measured to help differentiate the causes of metabolic alkalosis. ECF contraction is usually rapid and because of overzealous diuretic use is commonly termed "contraction alkalosis."

B. Clinical findings.

Carpal-pedal spasms, tetany, neuromuscular irritability, hypotension, hypoventilation, impaired cognition, cardiac arrhythmias, and decreased levels of ionized Ca^{++}.

C. Diagnosis.

Elevated serum HCO_3^- levels and alkalotic serum pH. There may be a compensatory respiratory acidosis with a decrease in the respiratory rate. The urine may be alkaline or paradoxically acidic, especially in the presence of K^+ wasting (hyperaldosteronism and diuretic use).

D. Treatment.

1. ***Chloride-responsive alkalosis.*** This alkalosis is the more commonly seen form with urine Cl^- <10 mEq/L. Usually secondary to contraction alkalosis caused by GI HCl losses (emesis, NG suctioning), or diuretic use. Occasionally seen with villous adenomas or cystic fibrosis. Treat underlying cause and correct concurrent hypokalemia (for IV KCl see section on hypokalemia, p. 211). Chloride may be administered as NaCl tablets or as 0.9 NS if volume depleted. Use caution in those with CHF and those who are fluid overloaded. Consider acetazolamide if renal function is intact. Some physicians also recommend use of H_2-blockers to decrease gastric HCl losses.
2. ***Non–chloride responsive alkalosis.*** Seen in primary hyperaldosteronism, Cushing's syndrome, and renal artery stenosis. Occasionally seen in patients who consume excessive amounts of licorice, or secondary to severe hypokalemia (<2.0 mEq/L) or Bartter's syndrome. The primary treatment is to determine the underlying cause and to correct it. See hypokalemia, p. 211, for treatment of low levels of potassium.
3. Other rare causes include massive citrated blood transfusions, hypercalcemia of malignancy, sarcoidosis, vitamin D toxicity, and high-dose penicillin-carbenicillin. Also consider milk-alkali syndrome.
4. If the metabolic alkalosis is severe (pH >7.55) with systemic effects, consider HCl acid therapy, which is typically done in an ICU setting.

BIBLIOGRAPHY

Allen LH et al: Vitamin B_{12} deficiency in elderly individuals: diagnosis and requirements, *Am J Clin Nutr* 60(1):12, 1994.

Bennett PH et al: Screening and management of microalbuminuria in patients with diabetes mellitus, *Am J Kidney Dis* 125(1):107, 1995.

Berkow R et al, editors: *The Merck manual of diagnosis and therapy,* ed 16, Rahway, N. J., 1992, The Merck Co.

Bilezikian JP: Management of acute hypercalcemia, *N Engl J Med* 326(8):1196, 1992.

Butkiewicz EK et al: Insulin therapy for diabetic ketoacidosis: bolus injection versus continuous insulin infusion, *Diabetes Care* 18(8):1187, 1995.

Colagiuri S, Miller JJ, Petocz P: Double-blind crossover comparison of human and porcine insulins in patients reporting lack of hypoglycaemia awareness, *Lancet* 339:1432-1435, 1992.

Coniff RF et al: Reduction of glycosylated hemoglobin and postprandial hyperglycemia by acarbose in patients with NIDDM: a placebo-controlled dose-comparison study, *Diabetes Care* 18(6):817, 1995.

Coniff RF et al: A double-blind placebo-controlled trial evaluating the safety and efficacy of acarbose for the treatment of patients with insulin-requiring type II diabetes, *Diabetes Care* 18(7):928, 1995.

Dale DC, Federman DD, editors: *Scientific American Medicine,* New York, 1996, Scientific American, Inc.

Diabetes Control and Complications Trial Research Group: The effect of intensive treatment of diabetes on the development and progression of long-term complications of diabetes mellitus, *N Engl J Med* 329(14):977, 1993.

Dorup I et al: Oral magnesium supplementation restores the concentrations of magnesium, potassium and sodium-potassium pumps in skeletal muscle of patients receiving diuretic treatment, *J Intern Med* 233(2):117, 1993.

Ewald GA, McKenzie CR, editors: *Manual of medical therapeutics: Department of Medicine, Washington University School of Medicine,* ed 28, Boston, 1995, Little, Brown & Co.

Glover JJ et al: Conservative treatment of overanticoagulated patients, *Chest* 108(4):987, 1995.

Goni MH et al: Hypercalcemia of cancer: an update [review], *Anticancer Res* 13(4):1155-1160, 1993.

Goodman LS, Gilman AG, et al editors: *The pharmacological basis of therapeutics,* ed 8, New York, 1990, Pergamon Press.

Gordon SR et al: The role of endoscopy in the evaluation of iron deficiency anemia in patients over the age of 50, *Am J Gastroenterol* 89(11):1963, 1994.

Greenspan FS, editor: *Basic and clinical endocrinology,* East Norwalk, Conn., 1991, Appleton & Lange.

Guthrie JA et al: Is it worth doing barium enemas on patients with unexplained iron deficiency anemia? *Clin Radiol* 49(6):375, 1994.

Hassell KL et al: Acute multiorgan failure syndrome: a potentially catastrophic complication of severe sickle cell pain episodes, *Am J Med* 96(2):155, 1994.

Hord JD et al: Long-term granulocyte-macrophage colony-stimulating factor and immunosuppression in the treatment of acquired severe aplastic anemia, *Pediatr Hematol Oncol* 17(2):140-144, 1995.

Horowitz E et al: Etidronate for hypercalcemia of maligancy and osteoporosis [review], *Am Fam Physician* 43(6):2155-2159, 1991.

Isselbacher KJ et al, editors: *Harrison's principles of internal medicine,* ed 13, New York, 1994, McGraw-Hill.

Kellihan MJ: Pamidronate [review], *Ann Pharmacol* 26(10):1262-1269, 1992.

Kilo C et al: Glyburide versus glipizide in the treatment of patients with non-insulin-dependent diabetes mellitus, *Clin Ther* 14(6):801, 1992.

Kinirons MT: Newer agents for the treatment of malignant hypercalcemia [review], *Am J Med Sci* 305(6):403-406, 1993.

Meyers AR, editor: *National Medical Series for Independent Study: Medicine,* ed 3, Philadelphia, 1997, Williams & Wilkins.

Nardone DA et al: Usefulness of physical examination in detecting the presence or absence of anemia, *Arch Intern Med* 150(1):201, 1990.

Orland MJ, Saltman RJ, editors: *Manual of medical therapeutics,* ed 25, Boston, 1986, Little, Brown & Co.

Panzer, RJ et al, editors: *Diagnostic strategies for common medical problems,* Philadelphia, 1991, American College Of Physicians.

Pollack CV et al: Usefulness of empiric chest radiography and urinalysis testing in adults with acute sickle cell pain crisis, *Ann Emerg Med* 20(11):1210, 1991.

Rakel RE, Conn HF, editors: *Textbook of family practice,* ed 3, Philadelphia, 1995, Saunders.

Rockey DC et al: Evaluation of the gastrointestinal tract in patients with iron deficiency anemia, *N Engl J Med* 329(23):1691, 1993.

Sanford JP: *Guide to antimicrobial therapy, 1995,* Dallas, 1995, Anti-Microbial Therapy, Inc.

Schrier RW: *Renal and electrolyte disorders,* ed 4, Boston, 1992, Little, Brown & Co.

Serjeant GR et al: The painful crisis of homozygous sickle cell disease: clinical features, *Br J Hematol* 87(3):586, 1994.

Shank ML et al: Bedtime insulin/daytime glipizide: effective therapy for sulfonylurea failures in NIDDM, *Diabetes* 44(2):165, 1995.

Shumak KH, Rock GA, Nair RC: Late relapses in patients successfully treated for thrombotic thrombocytopenic purpura. Canadian Apheresis Group, *Ann Intern Med* 122(8):569-572, 1995.

Stenman S et al: What is the benefit of increasing the sulfonylurea dose? *Ann Intern Med* 118(3):169, 1993.

Tintinalli JE et al: *Emergency medicine: a comprehensive study guide,* New York, 1996, McGraw-Hill.

Van Agtmael MA et al: Acute chest syndrome in adult Afro-Caribbean patients with sickle cell disease, *Arch Intern Med* 154(5):557, 1994.

Viberti G et al: Effect of captopril on progression to clinical proteinuria in patients with insulin-dependent diabetes mellitus and microalbuminuria, *JAMA* 271(4):275, 1994.

Wallach J: *Interpretation of diagnostic tests: a synopsis of laboratory medicine,* ed 5, Boston, 1992, Little, Brown & Co.

Wilimas JA et al: A randomized study of outpatient treatment with ceftriaxone for selected febrile children with sickle cell disease, *N Engl J Med* 329(7):472, 1993.

Wilson et al, editors: *Harrison's principles of internal medicine,* ed 13, New York, 1994, McGraw-Hill.

Wyngaarden JB et al, editors: *Cecil textbook of medicine,* ed 19, Philadelphia, 1996, Saunders.

Yao Y et al: Prevalance of vitamin B_{12} deficiency among geriatric outpatients, *J Fam Pract* 35(5): 524, 1992.

6

Rheumatology

HAJIME TOYOSHIMA, PETER P. TOTH, AND MARK A. GRABER

RHEUMATOID ARTHRITIS

I. OVERVIEW

Chronic systemic inflammatory disease principally involving joints but also with extra-articular manifestations. Rheumatoid arthritis (RA) affects 0.03% to 1.5% of the population, with females affected 2 to 3 times more often than males. Life-span is decreased on average by 7.5 years for men and 3.5 years for women.

II. DIAGNOSIS

A. To make a diagnosis of RA, symptoms must have been present for at least 6 weeks. Four of seven criteria of the American Rheumatism Association (ARA) must be satisfied. Criteria include:

1. Morning stiffness in and around joints, lasting more than 1 hour.
2. Arthritis of 3 or more joint areas involved simultaneously.
3. Arthritis of at least 1 area in a wrist, MCP, or PIP joint.
4. Symmetric arthritis involving the same joint areas.
5. Rheumatoid nodules.
6. Positive serum rheumatoid factor.
7. Radiographic changes typical of RA on hand and wrist radiographs, including erosions, or unequivocal bony decalcification in or adjacent to the involved joints.

B. Be aware that a positive rheumatoid factor is only one criterion and a positive rheumatoid factor need not be present for a diagnosis of rheumatoid arthritis to be made. Also should not have evidence of other disease that may account for symptoms such as polyarteritis nodosa or lupus.

C. Most patients have an insidious onset; however a third of patients experience rapid onset in days or weeks. The disease may be rapidly progressive causing joint destruction and other sequelae (see below) or may progress slowly; many have a fluctuating course of exacerbations and remissions.

III. CLINICAL FEATURES

A. Articular movement.

1. Synovium (synovial membrane) is the site of onset of inflammation, with proliferation of synovia ("pannus") and inflammatory destruction of soft tissue resulting in laxity of ligaments and tendons. Joint destruction occurs with erosion of juxta-articular bone around the margins of pannus and invasion of subchondral tissue by pannus. Can see cysts, loss of cartilage, and bony erosion. Thickened pannus may be palpated around joints with joint effusion present.
2. The most common sites of joint lesions are metacarpophalangeal (MCP) and proximal interphalangeal (PIP) joints and wrists. Distribution is symmetric, and small joints are predominantly involved.
3. ***Manifestations in specific joints.***
   a. *Cervical spine.* Frequently affected (40%). This may lead to atlantoaxial subluxation or, less commonly, subluxation at lower levels. Symptoms are those of a radiculopathy, including pain radiating up into the occiput, paresthesia, sudden deterioration in hand function, sensory loss, abnormal gait, and urinary retention or incontinence.
   b. *Joint involvement.*
      (1) Hand involved >85% of patients. May notice fusiform swelling of fingers and MCP joints, ulnar deviation of fingers, palmar subluxation of proximal area of phalanges. Distal interphalangeal (DIP) joints are most often spared. Ulnar deviation at MCP joints often is associated with radial deviation at wrist. Swan-neck and boutonnière deformities are also common.
      (2) Hip involved in 50% of cases.
      (3) Knee involved in 80% of patients.
      (4) Foot and ankle involved in 80% of cases.
      (5) Metatarsophalangeal (MTP), talonavicular, and ankle joints are affected in descending order of frequency.
   c. *Constitutional features.* Fatigue, weight loss, muscle pain, excessive sweating, or low-grade fever are common. Most patients with active disease complain of morning stiffness for more than 1 hour.

B. Extra-articular complications.

1. ***Rheumatoid nodules.*** Characteristic of RA and seen in up to 25% to 50% of patients especially those with more severe disease. They occur in the lungs, heart, kidney, and dura mater, in addition to the extensor surface of the forearm, olecranon, Achilles tendons, and ischial area. Usually asymptomatic.
2. ***Rheumatoid vasculitis.*** Usually occurs in patients with severe deforming arthritis and a high titer of rheumatoid factor. Vasculitic lesions include rheumatoid nodules, small

nail fold infarcts, and palpable purpura. May also be manifest by mononeuritis multiplex, organ ischemia, CNS infarctions, MI.

3. ***Sjögren's syndrome.*** Keratoconjunctivitis sicca is the most common eye complication and results in dry eyes with slight redness and normal vision.
4. ***Episcleritis and scleritis.*** Eye irritation and pain. May cause vision loss.
5. ***Pleuropericarditis or obstructive pulmonary disease including pulmonary nodules.*** Diffuse interstitial fibrosis with pneumonitis is common. COPD is more common than in the general public. However, pleural disease is usually asymptomatic; can see subpleural nodules, and exudative pleural effusions.
6. ***Cardiac.*** Symptomatic cardiac disease is not common. Most common type is acute pericarditis, usually in seropositive individuals (unrelated to duration of arthritis). Rheumatoid nodules can involve valves and myocardium and may have MI secondary to vasculitis.
7. ***Neurologic.*** May have entrapment neuropathy secondary to tissue swelling (as in carpal tunnel). Mononeuritis multiplex may occur and is related to ischemic neuropathy from vasculitis.
8. ***Miscellaneous.*** RA is a common cause of carpal tunnel syndrome.

C. Laboratory findings.

1. May have anemia of chronic disease (normochromic or hypochromic, normocytic), thrombocytosis reflecting inflammation, elevated ESR, elevated C-reactive protein, elevated ferritin as acute-phase reactant, low serum iron, low total iron binding capacity, elevated serum globulin.
2. ***Presence of rheumatoid factor.*** Occurs in 90% of patients but is neither specific nor sensitive for the diagnosis of RA. Rheumatoid factor is an immunoglobulin directed against IgG. Generally higher titers in those with more generalized disease and destructive arthritis. Extremely high titers are associated with the presence of rheumatoid nodules.
3. ***Synovial fluid white blood cell count.*** 5000 to 20,000 per mm^3 with 50% to 70% neutrophils; cultures should be negative.
4. ***Felty's syndrome.*** Combination of (generally severe) seropositive RA, splenomegaly, and leukopenia (WBC <3500/µl). It is associated with serious infections, vasculitis (leg ulcers, mononeuritis), anemia, thrombocytopenia, and lymphadenopathy.

D. Radiographic findings. Characteristic changes in RA include periarticular osteoporosis, symmetric narrowing of the joint space, and marginal bone erosions.

IV. TREATMENT

A. Education. The basic treatment program consists in patient education, balancing rest, exercise (often with physical and occupational therapy), and medication. More than 95% of seropositive patients respond to therapy, and 70% of patients have partial or complete remissions.

B. Aspirin and NSAID. Provide symptomatic relief but do nothing to suppress the rate of cartilage erosion or to alter the course of the disease. Doses should be increased to the recommended maximum over 1 to 2 weeks; a medication should not be abandoned until the patient has been on a maximal dose for at least 2 weeks, since medications may take this much time to reach maximal efficacy. If after 2 weeks of receiving a maximal dose the results are disappointing, an alternative NSAID should be tried. Zero-order release aspirin products such as ZORpin and Easprin may make aspirin products easier to take. Naproxen 500 mg PO BID or ibuprofen 600 mg PO TID are some of the least expensive NSAIDs. Use of misoprostol with NSAIDs reduces incidence of severe side effects (see section on ulcers, p. 169).

C. Steroids. Glucocorticoids have anti-inflammatory and immunosuppressive effects and reduce joint erosion. They are used especially for life-threatening manifestations such as vasculitis. Low-dose corticosteroids (<10 mg of prednisone QD or its equivalent) are sometimes useful for patients who are unable to work or care for themselves, but steroid doses should be kept to a minimum because of osteopenia and other side effects such as skin thinning, increased susceptibility to infection, ecchymoses, and cushingoid appearance. Intra-articular steroids may be helpful. Combinations of steroids with other slow-acting antirheumatic drugs may be beneficial.

D. SAARDs (slow-acting antirheumatic drugs). Believed to modify the fundamental pathologic process. Although no consensus exists as to which SAARDs should be used in what order, treatment must be individualized, and the initial use of less toxic medications such as minocycline, hydroxycholoroquine, and sulfasalazine are preferred. Oral gold sodium thiosulfate tends to be less toxic than other medications but is less effective. Injectable gold sodium thiomalate is more toxic and no more effective than hydroxychloroquine and sulfasalazine are. Because of the spontaneous waxing and warning of RA, these drugs should be used for 6 months or so before one decides on efficacy. Disease-modifying drugs should be considered for use early in the course of RA.

1. ***Antibiotics.*** Minocycline 100 mg PO BID has been shown to be effective for mild to moderate RA in a double-blind placebo-controlled trial.
2. ***Antimalarials.*** Hydroxychloroquine 400 to 600 mg PO daily for 4 to 6 weeks and then 200 to 400 mg daily.

Baseline ophthalmologic examination with subsequent examinations every 6 months can allow one to detect early eye changes. May have ciliary muscle dysfunction or corneal opacities. Having the patient view an Ansler grid daily will give an early warning of visual changes. As safe as NSAIDs.

3. ***Sulfasalazine.*** (Not approved by FDA for RA.) 500 mg PO QD and then increasing doses to a maximum of 3000 mg daily. Back down to 500 mg QID for maintenance. Contraindications include sulfonamide allergy. Side effects include bone marrow toxicity, hepatitis, reversible oligospermia, yellow discoloration of urine and of soft contact lenses, nausea, headache, and abdominal discomfort. Monitoring CBCs and liver enzymes is recommended.
4. ***Penicillamine.*** Start with 125 to 250 mg PO QD 1 hour before or 2 hours after eating and then increase the dose by 125 to 250 mg/day every 1 to 2 months to a maximum of 750 to 1000 mg daily. Metallic taste and nausea are common early problems but resolve with continued use. Skin rashes, bone marrow toxicity, and proteinuria may occur. Autoimmune syndromes, including myasthenia gravis, polymyositis, pemphigus, and Goodpasture's syndrome have been reported as a result of penicillamine. A monthly urinalysis and CBC count are recommended, and penicillamine should not be used in those with renal disease.
5. ***Gold salts.***
   a. *Parenteral gold salts.* Gold sodium thiomalate and aurothioglucose. *Intramuscular:* single dose of 10 mg, followed by 25 mg 1 week later to test for sensitivity. Maintenance therapy is 25 to 50 mg weekly. If there is no improvement with a cumulative dose of 1 or 2 g or if toxicity develops, therapy should be discontinued.
   b. *Auranofin.* 3 to 6 mg PO QD. Diarrhea is a common side effect. Monthly urinalysis and CBC counts should be performed.
   c. *Side effects.*
      (1) *Common.* Pruritic skin rash, mouth ulcers, transient leukopenia, eosinophilia, diarrhea (oral). Treatment can sometimes be temporarily halted and then restarted at lower doses, and side effects may not recur, but you need to let the rash clear because it can lead to an exfoliative dermatitis.
      (2) *Transient proteinuria.* 3% to 10% of patients. Usually require only cessation of treatment until the urine clears.
      (3) *Less common.* Thrombocytopenia, pancytopenia, agranulocytosis, and aplastic anemia. Usually responds to stopping drug. Gold-chelating agent (dimercaprol) can be used if response is not fast enough.

6. ***Methotrexate.*** 7.5 to 15 mg PO weekly. *Contraindications:* concomitant therapy with sulfonamide containing antibiotics or HIV seropositivity. Alcohol consumption, gross obesity, and diabetes are aggravating factors to hepatic toxicity. May have nausea, vomiting, abdominal cramps. Serious side effects are bone marrow toxicity, alveolitis, and hepatic fibrosis. Monthly CBCs and liver enzyme studies every 2 to 3 months are recommended. Persistent elevation of liver enzymes or significant hypoalbuminemia may indicate the need for a liver biopsy. Should be administered with folic acid, at least 5 mg/week, which decreases side effects but not efficacy.
7. ***Azathioprine.*** 50 to 100 mg PO QD (1.0 to 1.5 mg/kg/day, which may be increased by 0.5 mg/kg/day weekly to 2.0 to 2.5 mg/kg/day after 3 months). Nausea is the main limiting factor. Monthly CBC and quarterly liver function tests are recommended. The concomitant use of allopurinol increases toxicity and should be avoided. Dosage should be reduced if renal impairment is present.

OSTEOARTHRITIS

I. OVERVIEW

Osteoarthritis (OA) is the most common joint disease. OA is a condition of snyovial joints characterized by focal cartilage loss and an accompanying reparative bone response. Typical radiographic features are joint space narrowing and the presence of osteophytes and sclerosis. OA is strongly related to age. It is uncommon under 45 years of age, but at 65 at least half the people have radiographic evidence of OA.

II. TYPES

A. Primary OA. Primary OA is a wear-and-tear phenomenon. OA generally spares the shoulders and MCP joints.

B. Secondary OA. May involve joints that are generally not involved with primary OA including MCP joints, shoulder, or isolated large joints. It may be related to chondrocalcinosis or another secondary cause (below).

1. ***Traumatic arthritis*** secondary to slipped capital femoral epiphysis, congenital hip dislocation, destruction secondary to septic joint, hemophilia, or other injury.
2. ***Paget's disease.*** A defect in older individuals of bone resorption and redeposition. Radiograph shows typical scalloped pattern of bone deposition. May have elevated alkaline phosphatase, elevated urine hydroxyproline. Alendronate may be used for treatment.
3. ***Alkaptonuria with ochronosis.*** Rare disorder of tyrosine metabolism.
4. ***Hemochromatosis.*** 50% of cases show chronic progressive arthritis, affecting predominantly MCP and wrist joints

as well as large joints, including shoulders, hips, and knees. Treatment is symptomatic, but refer to Chapter 5.

5. ***Wilson's disease.*** 50% of adults with Wilson's disease have arthropathy, characterized by mild OA of the wrists, MCP joints, knees, and spine.
6. ***Neuroarthropathy (Charcot's joint).*** Severe destructive arthropathy caused by impaired joint sensation. Diabetes mellitus, tabes dorsalis, and syringomyelia are common causes. The foot is involved most commonly.

III. CLINICAL FEATURES

A. Pain after joint use progressing to pain with minimal movement and at rest and at night. As opposed to RA, there is generally no early morning stiffness or gelling.

B. Patients often have pain on passive movement with crepitus and joint enlargement.

C. May develop genu valgus or varus deformity at knee if there is a disproportionate loss of cartilage on one side.

D. Pseudolaxity of collateral ligaments develops with degeneration of cartilage.

IV. RADIOGRAPHIC FEATURES

Characteristic progressive changes include joint-space narrowing, subchondral osteosclerosis, marginal osteophyte formation, and subchondral cysts. Spondylolisthesis (subluxation of one vertebra on another with lateral spondylosis) may occur.

V. LABORATORY

None.

VI. TREATMENT

A. Goal of treatment. Relieve pain, preserve joint motion and function, and prevent further injury and wear of cartilage.

B. Biomechanical factors. Weight loss, use of canes or crutches, correction of postural abnormalities, and proper shoe support are helpful corrective measures.

C. Pain control.

1. *Analgesics,* such as acetaminophen 1g PO QID as needed, are important. OA is not an inflammatory disorder, and acetaminophen is equal or superior to NSAIDs in efficacy without NSAID side effects.
2. *NSAIDs* are helpful in those who have failed acetaminophen. However, they have many side effects and may hasten joint destruction. When an NSAID is being chosen, patient side effects and cost should be considerations, since, in all likelihood, they will be used long term. Two weeks at maximal dose is needed before one decides that a particular drug is a therapeutic failure. Naprosyn 500 mg PO BID or ibuprofen 600 mg PO QID are relatively inexpensive and well tolerated.

3. ***Corticosteroids.*** Oral or parenteral corticosteroid therapy is not indicated. Intra-articular injection of steroid may be helpful in acute flares.
4. ***Surgery.*** Joint arthroplasty may relieve pain, stabilize joints, and improve function. Total joint arthroplasty is successful for the knee and hip.

CRYSTAL-INDUCED SYNOVITIS

I. PRIMARY GOUTY ARTHRITIS

A. Overview. An illness secondary to a chronic increase in the serum uric acid. Deposition of uric acid crystals occur throughout the body and results in:

1. Multiple acute episodes.
2. Chronic, low-grade inflammation of joints.
3. Accumulation of articular, osseous, soft tissue, and cartilaginous crystalline deposits (tophi).
4. Renal injury (gouty nephropathy).
5. Uric acid kidney stones.

B. Acute gouty arthritis.

1. ***Clinical features.*** Onset is usually acute with (generally) nocturnal onset of monoarticular pain; rarely more than one joint can be acutely involved. Involved joints are red, swollen, warm, and exquisitely tender. Fever and leukocytosis may occur. The big toe (first MTP) joint is the classic site of gout (also called podagra). Other sites, such as foot, knee, hand, or shoulder, may also be involved. Acute attack lasts 3 to 10 days without treatment. It may be difficult to differentiate from a septic joint, and so joint aspiration for synovial fluid examination is critical, especially with the first attack.
2. ***Precipitating events.*** Trauma, surgery, major medical illness (myocardial infarction, cerebrovascular accident, pulmonary embolus), fasting, alcohol use, and infection. Overindulgence in food and emotional stress may also trigger attacks.
3. ***Differential diagnosis.*** Septic arthritis, other arthritis including pseudogout, RA.
4. ***Diagnosis.*** Definite diagnosis can be made by demonstration of the presence of monosodium urate (MSU) crystals within synovial leukocytes or in material derived from tophi under polarizing microscopy.
   a. Recommendation is to demonstrate crystals in joint aspirate.
      (1) Synovial fluid typically reveals 2000 to 100,000 cells/mm^3, predominantly PMNs.
      (2) Urate crystals are rod or needle shaped and negatively birefringent.
      (3) Crystals may be recovered from joints during asymptomatic periods.

   (4) Examined fluid should be sent for Gram stain and culture to rule out infection.
- b. *Serum uric acid levels are generally not helpful in acute attacks and may be normal.* However, when levels are chronically greater than 10 mg/dl, the chance of an acute attack is >90%.

5. ***Treatment.*** Do not administer allopurinol or probenecid until acute attack completely subsides; these may prolong the attack. Although colchicine has classically been used for acute attacks of gout, NSAIDs have replaced it as initial therapy. Steroids are another option for acute treatment.
   - a. **NSAIDs.** There is no advantage to using ketorolac in an acute flare of gout. It is equal to indomethacin in time of onset and control of symptoms.
     - (1) **Indomethacin (Indocin).** 50 to 75 mg PO and then 50 mg Q6h, tapering to 50 mg Q8h and to 25 mg Q6h and maintained until symptoms have completely resolved.
     - (2) **Ketorolac (Toradol).** 30 to 60 mg IM, followed by 15 to 30 mg Q6-8h to maximum of 120 mg a day.
     - (3) **Ibuprofen**. 800 mg PO Q8h.
   - b. **Corticosteroids.** Methylprednisolone 125 mg IV or IM followed by prednisone 40 to 60 mg a day PO with colchicine 0.5 mg PO once or twice a day until symptoms resolve. Taper rapidly.
   - c. **Colchicine.**
     - (1) Colchicine should be reversed for cases in which the diagnosis of gout is not confirmed and a response may have diagnostic value and for cases in which NSAIDs steroids are contraindicated or have failed.
     - (2) Administer 1 mg PO initially, followed by 0.5 mg Q2h up to 6 times on first day. On second day, give 0.5 mg Q6h and then twice a day until side effects occur. Side effects include abdominal cramps, diarrhea, nausea, and vomiting. If diarrhea develops, the drug is discontinued.
     - (3) Given *intravenously* 1 to 2 mg in 10 ml of saline in 0.5 mg doses repeated once or twice every 6 hours. Total cumulative IV dose of colchicine should not exceed 4 mg for a course of therapy. Venous extravasation and venous sclerosis may occur. Courses of IV therapy should not be repeated for several days to several weeks because of risk of toxic accumulation. *IV Colchicine should not be given to patients who are already receiving maintenance therapy with colchicine.*
     - (4) The dose should be reduced in older patients and in patients with renal or hepatic disease.

6. ***Intercritical period.*** The goal is to prevent recurrent attack of acute gout. Oral colchicine 0.5 to 1.5 mg QD

is the most effective dosing. Side effects are uncommon at this dose, and it may be discontinued after the serum urate level becomes normal and stable for 2 to 3 months. A low dose of NSAIDs (indomethacin 25 mg PO BID) is effective, but the incidence of side effects is higher than that of colchicine.

C. Chronic gout.

1. ***Clinical features.*** Chronic changes are the result of persistent hyperuricemia and recurrent acute attacks of gout. Tophi develop mainly in the helix of the ear. Other locations include the ulnar aspects of the forearm, olecranon, and prepatellar bursae, Achilles tendons, and hands. Extra-articular locations for tophus formation included myocardium, pericardium, aortic valves, and extradural spinal regions.
2. ***Clinical picture.*** May mimic rheumatoid arthritis though generally less symmetric.
3. ***Characteristic radiographic appearance.*** Bony erosion with an overhanging margin of the involved joint.
4. ***Treatment of hyperuricemia.*** Treatment depends on cause: increased uric acid (about 10%) production versus decreased excretion (about 90%). Asymptomatic hyperuricemia should not be treated. Treatment should be undertaken only after the second attack of gout or in the presence of a history of uric acid stones. The goal is to reduce serum uric acid level below its saturation point in extracellular fluid (6.4 mg/dl).
   a. There are two classes of drugs to reduce uric acid: *uricosurics,* such as probenecid, which increases excretion, and *xanthine oxidase inhibitors,* such as allopurinol, which reduce production. Before deciding on therapy, obtain a 24-hour urine specimen for uric acid. This will help determine if the patient is an overproducer of uric acid or an underexcreter. If excretion is >800 mg/day, patient is an overproducer of uric acid and will require allopurinol to prevent production. Those with decreased excretion can be treated with either class of drug.
   b. Drugs that increase excretion.
      (1) **Probenecid.** Blocks tubular reabsorption of filtered uric acid. Initial dose is 250 mg PO BID and gradually increased by 500 mg every 4 weeks, until daily maximum dose of 2000 mg is achieved. The goal is to decrease serum uric acid levels to between 5 and 6 mg/dl. It is recommended for patients under 60 years of age and those with normal renal function, uric acid excretion of less than a range of 800 to 1000 mg/day, and no history of kidney stones. Advise the patient to increase fluid intake and consider alkalinization of the urine to a pH of 6.5 or more with sodium bicarbonate, 2 to 6 g/day, or acetazolamide (Diamox) 250

mg/day PO. Aspirin blocks probenecid's effect. Continue colchicine for prophylaxis as above.

(2) **Sulfinpyrazone** (Anturane) 50 to 100 mg PO BID may be given. Its dose may be gradually increased by 100 mg every week until the maximal dose of 800 mg/day is attained. This is especially useful for those patients who must take aspirin.

c. Drug that decreases production. *Allopurinol (Zyloprim):* starting dose is 100 mg PO QD. Usual dose is 200 to 300 mg/day, and maximum is 800 mg/day. Indications include a history of kidney stones, presence of tophi, renal insufficiency (GFR <60 ml/min), inability to lower the serum urate level below 7 mg/dl with other agents, urinary urate excretion >800 to 1000 mg/day, allergy to uricosurics, and hyperuricemia caused by hypoxanthine-guanine phosphoribosyltransferase deficiency. Side effects are rare but can be serious. These include drug fever, rash (including Stevens-Johnson syndrome), bone marrow depression, vasculitis, and hepatitis.

II. CALCIUM PYROPHOSPHATE DEPOSITION DISEASE

A. Overview. A degenerative joint disease characterized by the accumulation of calcium pyrophosphate crystals in articular cartilage and periarticular tissues. May be idiopathic or associated with a variety of metabolic diseases.

1. ***Pseudogout.*** An acute inflammatory attack that involves one or more joints that can last for several days. Attacks can be very similar to gout, though usually not so severe. The knees are involved in about half of patients, but any joint can be affected. Patients may have less severe attacks between acute flares. Crystal deposition can occur in tendons, ligaments, and synovia as well as in cartilage. Surgery or illness can predispose to attacks.
2. ***Pseudo-osteoarthritis.*** Chronic calcium pyrophosphate disease may appear similar to osteoarthritis (termed "pseudo-osteoarthritis") with progressive degeneration of multiple joints. Knees are most commonly affected, followed by wrists, MCP joints, hips, shoulders, and elbows. May have symmetric involvement.
3. ***Pseudorheumatoid arthritis.*** In 5%, calcium pyrophosphate disease presents with symptoms similar to rheumatoid arthritis including morning stiffness, fatigue, synovial membrane thickening, and elevated ESR. About 10% of patients with CPPD have a positive rheumatoid factor.
4. ***Diagnosis.***

a. *Laboratory.* Joint should be tapped and will note crystals composed of calcium pyrophosphate dihydrate (CPPD). Crystals are rod shaped, often intracellular, and positively birefringent, or blue when parallel to the axis of a polarizing microscope compensator. Evaluation should include serum calcium, magnesium, phosphorus, alkaline phosphatase, ferritin, serum iron and iron-binding capacity, glucose, T_4, TSH, and uric acid.

b. *Radiographic findings.* Typical findings are punctate and linear densities in articular hyaline or fibrocartilaginous tissues. Characteristic sites include articular cartilage of knee, acetabular labrum, symphysis pubis, articular disk of wrist, and anulus fibrosus of intervertebral disks. Radiologic screen for CPPD disease should include AP view of both knees, AP view of pelvis including hips and symphysis pubis, and a PA view of both hands.

B. Treatment of pseudogout by NSAIDs.

1. ***Effective.*** No one drug is superior. May be used in similar fashion as that in acute episodes of gouty arthritis.
2. ***Colchicine.*** See gout above for dosing.
   a. Particularly effective when given intravenously.
   b. Oral form is less predictable than when used with gout but has been proved to reduce the number and duration of attacks (with 1.2 mg daily).
   c. Corticosteroid injections are often combined with aspiration for large joints.

SPONDYLOARTHROPATHIES

Characterized by involvement of spine and entheses (insertions of tendons and ligaments). Associated with HLA-B27.

I. ANKYLOSING SPONDYLITIS

A. Clinical features. A disease primarily affecting the sacroiliac joints with varying involvement of the spine and less so the appendicular skeleton.

1. ***Clinically.*** Onset is usually insidious, generally between 10 and 40 years of age. Patients generally present with back pain that is worse after rest and improves with exercise. Patients may notice morning back stiffness that improves during the day; the pain may be so severe at night that it keeps the patient awake or prompts the patient to get up and become mobile to reduce the symptoms. By definition, the back is always involved. However, peripheral joints are involved in up to 25% of cases. Proximal, large joints, such as hips, knees, shoulders, and ankles, are preferentially affected. Involvement is usually asymmetric but not always. May have mild systemic manifestations such as fever, malaise, or anorexia.
2. Associated with HLA-B27 in >90% of cases. The diagnosis is made according to clinical and radiologic criteria. Offspring of those with the disease have a 10% to 20% risk of having disease.

3. ***Enthesopathy.*** Involvement of the sites of insertion of ligaments and tendons (entheses) is manifested clinically as Achilles tendinitis, plantar fasciitis, and costochondritis.
4. ***Extra-articular manifestions.*** May include uveitis (25%), cardiac involvement in 10%, especially aortic insufficiency, cardiomegaly, conduction defects, as well as cavitating fibrosis of the lung, heart block, and amyloidosis.
5. ***Late complications*** secondary to bone involvement. Can include (a) cord compression caused by spinal fractures and (b) cauda equina syndrome (neurogenic bladder, fecal incontinence, leg pain).

B. Diagnosis.

1. ***Physical examination.***
   a. *Flexion test.* Mark two points on the back: at the lumbosacral junction and 10 cm above with patient standing erect. Have the patient bend forward and measure the distance between the two points. Normally, flexible spine should show an increase of >5 cm. Less than 5 cm is suggestive of decreased spinal mobility.
   b. *Chest expansion.* Normally, chest circumference increases by 5 cm with full inspiration. This will be decreased in those with ankylosing spondylitis.
2. ***Radiographic findings.*** Sacroiliitis with sclerosis and fusion of the sacroiliac joints. May have an asymmetric erosive arthropathy. Spine involvement may be manifested by squaring of superior and inferior margins of vertebral body, syndesmophytes, and "bamboo spine."
3. ***Lab tests.*** Immunofluorescence will show IgM deposition in the superficial vessels of the skin. HLA-B27 present not only in 95% of whites with ankylosing spondylitis but also 6% to 8% of normal population. HLA-B27 should not be obtained as a screening measure; diagnosis is made on clinical and radiographic findings.

C. Treatment.

1. ***NSAIDs.*** Indomethacin is the drug of choice, with a starting dose of 25 mg PO TID. This may be increased to 50 mg TID. Side effects include nausea, gastric discomfort and diarrhea, headache, vertigo, and depression common in elderly. Other NSAIDs, such as naproxen and sulindac are also effective.
2. ***Aspirin.*** For unknown reasons generally not effective.
3. ***Sulfasalazine*** 2 to 3 g PO QD. May be helpful, especially for peripheral joint disease.
4. ***Education*** about good posture. Exercise to promote extension of the back. Stop smoking. Avoiding pillows at night and encouraging sleep in the prone position are important.
5. ***Physical therapy exercises*** (especially swimming) and attention to posture is critical. Range-of-motion exercises,

especially of the back, are important to maintain flexibility.

6. ***Genetic counseling should be recommended.***

II. REITER'S SYNDROME

A. Clinical features.

1. ***Reiter's syndrome.*** Seronegative arthropathy that preferentially involves the lower extremities. It may present as insidious joint pain or acutely with fever and swollen, hot joints. The onset may temporally be related to urethritis, diarrhea, or other infection with organisms such as *Yersinia, Salmonella, Shigella, Campylobacter,* or *Chlamydia.* The triad of arthritis, conjunctivitis, and urethritis should be suggestive of a diagnosis of Reiter's syndrome.
2. ***Other associated findings.*** Skin disorders (balanitis, oral ulcerations, or keratoderma blennorrhagicum), conjunctivitis, and urethritis. In chronic disease, heart block or aortic regurgitation may occur. As noted above, diarrhea may precede the development of Reiter's syndrome. There is an association of Reiter's disease with HIV infection, and arthritis may be present before symptoms or signs related to the HIV infection appear.
3. ***Lab tests.*** Findings may include an elevated ESR and anemia of chronic disease; 80% of patients are HLA-B27 positive. Stool cultures as well as urethral cultures should be done. Offer HIV testing in the appropriate population.

B. Treatment.

1. ***NSAIDs.*** Indomethacin 25 mg PO QID (can be increased to 50 mg PO QID).
2. ***Antibiotics.*** Treatment of the underlying bacterial infection may hasten resolution. A 3-month course of tetracycline has been shown to hasten resolution of symptoms in those with disease related to *Chlamydia* organisms.
3. ***Immunosuppressive drugs,*** such as methotrexate or azathioprine, may be effective.

III. ARTHRITIS ASSOCIATED WITH INFLAMMATORY BOWEL DISEASE (ENTEROPATHIC ARTHRITIS)

There are two types of arthritis associated with ulcerative colitis and Crohn's disease: a nondestructive oligoarthritis of peripheral joints and ankylosing spondylitis.

IV. PSORIATIC ARTHRITIS

A. Clinical features. Occurs in up to 7% of patients with psoriasis and is strongly associated with the presence of nail pitting. Most patients (95%) have involvement of multiple small joints of the hands and feet. Others have solely spine involvement or, more commonly, a combination of spine involvement and peripheral joint involvement.

B. Treatment. Basic management utilizes NSAIDs, exercise, physical therapy, and education; control of psoriasis is important. Other possible therapies include methotrexate, antimalarials, and sulfasalazine.

SEPTIC ARTHRITIS

I. OVERVIEW

A. Any infectious agent can cause arthritis, but bacterial arthritis is the most rapidly destructive form. The major responsible organisms are *Neisseria gonorrhoeae* or *Neisseria* species and *Staphylococcus aureus. Streptococcus* species including pneumococcal infections are much less common. Brucellosis is rarely found as joint pathogen in those who work with cattle.

B. Source of infection.

1. ***Hematogenous spread.*** Secondary to a puncture wound, skin infection, or an adjacent osteomyelitis. Rarely, septic arthritis may be secondary to intra-articular injection or joint aspiration (incidence ranges from 1 in 500 to 1 in 5000).
2. ***IV drug use.*** May cause infections in unusual joints such as the sternoclavicular or sacroiliac joints. Infections in IV drug users are frequently secondary to unusual organisms such as *Pseudomonas, Serratia,* and methicillin-resistant staphylococci.
3. ***Underlying illness.*** Steroid use, RA, and the presence of joint prosthesis also predispose to the development of septic arthritis. Those with underlying illness such as lupus, RA, renal failure, and diabetes may have gram-negative organisms.

II. GONOCOCCAL ARTHRITIS

A. Clinical features. May have an acute arthritis involving one or more joints, usually the knees, ankles, or wrists, with the knee being the most commonly involved. Two thirds of patients have a dermatitis with multiple, usually asymptomatic lesions that progress from macular to papular and finally vesicular, or pustular. Any new acute inflammatory monarthritis in a sexually active person should be considered related to gonococcal infection until proved otherwise. Fever may be present, and genitourinary symptoms occur in 25%. Physical exam reveals an acute arthritis, synovitis, or tenosynovitis, or all three.

B. Laboratory features.

1. The synovial fluid white blood cell count averages over 60,000/ml, but low WBC counts have been reported. Gram stain may be positive, but only 25% of synovial fluid cultures are positive.
2. Blood cultures should be done as cultures of the throat, joint, anorectum, blood, and genitourinary tract should be.

III. NONGONOCOCCAL ARTHRITIS

A. Clinical features. The acute onset of arthritis with a hot, swollen joint or joints. Generally one or two joints are involved. The knee is most commonly affected in adults, whereas the hip and knee are the most commonly involved joints in children. Fever is common but may be of low grade; chills are less common.

B. Diagnosis.

1. ***Obtaining synovial fluid sample is critical.*** The definitive test is joint aspiration with fluid sent for Gram staining (positive in 75% for gram-positive cocci), culture, synovial fluid leukocyte count, and differential (greater than 50,000 cells/ml in 70% of patients, with over 80% neutrophils), and decreased synovial fluid glucose.
2. ***Blood cultures should be done.*** Positive in 50% of patients with nongonococcal arthritis.
3. ***An elevated white blood cell count*** with a left shift and an elevated ESR often occur but are nonspecific.
4. ***Radiographic examination.*** Plain films obtained for baseline view and to look for osteomyelitis. Usually no initial changes are visible except effusions and perhaps juxta-articular osteopenia. The changes of osteomyelitis take 10 to 20 days to appear on plain films. Radionuclide imaging, gallium scanning, and computerized tomography can be helpful, particularly with suspected hip or axial joint infections. *Ultrasonography may be used to establish the presence of effusion in the hip joint and aid with aspiration.*
5. ***Surgical exploration.*** May be necessary to obtain fluid from joints such as the sternoclavicular or sacroiliac.

IV. TREATMENT

A. Antibiotic therapy.

1. ***Gonococcal arthritis.*** Ceftriaxone 1 g IV QD for at least 3 days, followed by cefuroxime axetil 500 mg PO BID. For penicillin-allergic patients, an alternative is spectinomycin 2 g IM Q12h.
2. ***Nongonococcal arthritis.***
   a. *In adults.* Make the initial choice based on Gram-stain results and clinical likelihood. Essentially all antibiotics reach high levels of activity within an inflamed joint after oral or parenteral administration. Consider a penicillinase-resistant penicillin (such as methicillin or nafcillin) or vancomycin plus an aminoglycoside or aztreonam. Imipenem has been proposed for single-agent therapy.
   b. *Neonates.* (Methicillin, nafcillin, or vancomycin) plus a third-generation cephalosporin.
   c. *Infants and young children.* (Methicillin, nafcillin, or vancomycin) plus cefuroxime.
   d. *Prosthetic joint infections.* Vancomycin plus aztreonam.

B. Drainage.

1. ***Needle drainage.*** As good as open drainage in most situations but is not adequate for hip infections, especially in children. Aspirate with a large-bore needle daily while effusions accumulate rapidly. Can irrigate with sterile saline.
2. ***Open drainage.*** Method of choice for hip infections.
3. ***Arthroscopy.*** Early arthroscopy has been reported to be helpful with bacterial arthritis of the knee.

C. Immobilize the joint in the functional position during the acute phase of infection, with early mobilization and muscle-strengthening exercises.

D. Reassess therapy if:

1. Synovial fluid cultures are not negative within 72 hours, or
2. Synovial fluid leukocyte count is not greatly lower after 7 days.

E. Prognosis.

1. Up to 10% mortality.
2. Only 60% recover completely; many are left with a joint problem especially if symptomatic for >7 days before therapy. *Staphylococcus aureus* and gram-negative bacilli tend to be more destructive. *Neisseria gonorrhoeae* and pneumococcus are rarely destructive.
3. Sterile synovitis may develop after treatment but is usually self-limited and responds to NSAIDs.

FIBROMYALGIA

I. CLINICAL FEATURES

A. Characterized by diffuse aches, stiffness, and fatigue, coupled with multiple, symmetric tender spots in specific areas (Fig. 6-1). Over 75% of patients are women, and the peak incidence is between 20 to 60 years of age. There is often discordance between symptoms and objective findings. The cause may actually be sleep disturbance.

B. Pain is often aggravated by stress, cold, and activity. Patients often complain of subjective swelling of hands and feet as well as paresthesia and dysesthesia of hands and feet.

C. Fatigability is often extreme, occurring after minimal exertion.

D. Sleep disturbance. Patients complain of nonrestorative sleep, waking unrefreshed. May have depression and irritability and be weepy.

E. Headache is common as are diffuse abdominal pain and alternating diarrhea or constipation.

II. DIAGNOSIS

Fibromyalgia is a diagnosis of exclusion. CBC, ESR, thyroid functions, rheumatoid factor, electrolytes, creatinine, calcium, and phosphorus are usually all normal.

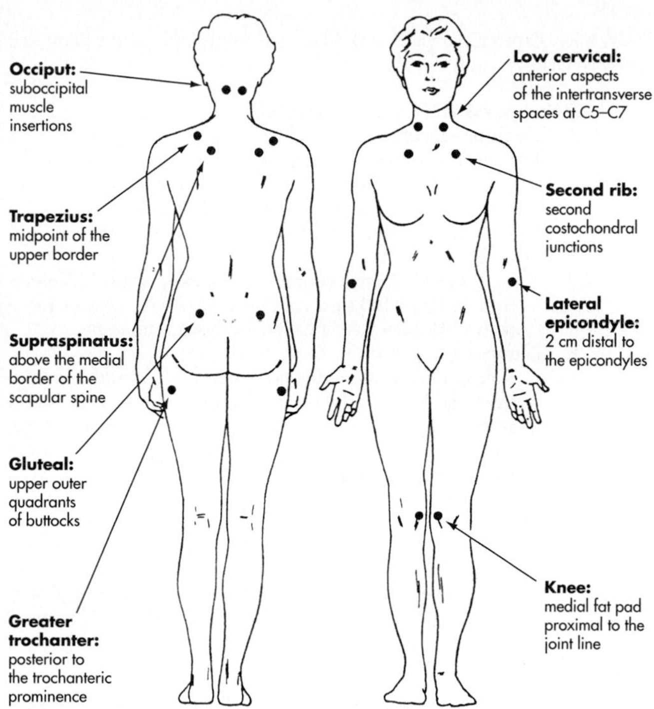

FIG. 6-1 Location of specific tender points in fibromyalgia. (From Schumacher HR Jr, Klippel JH, Koopman WJ, editors: *Primer on the rheumatic diseases,* ed 10, Atlanta, 1993, Arthritis Foundation.)

III. TREATMENT

A. There is no specific treatment but treatment is aimed at controlling symptoms and restoring adequate sleep.

B. Treatment includes reassurance, education, graded aerobic exercise, and increased flexibility. Patients may be assured that fibromyalgia is a self-limited illness that resolves with time.

C. Low-dose amitriptyline (Elavil), 10 to 75 mg PO QHS, or other TCA may be helpful for sleep and is the drug of choice for treatment. Benzodiazepines should be avoided. NSAIDs are useful for achiness.

POLYMYALGIA RHEUMATICA AND GIANT CELL ARTERITIS

Polymyalgia rheumatica (PMR) and giant cell arteritis form a spectrum of disease and affect patients of >50 years of age; up to 15% of patients with

PMR have giant cell arteritis and 40% of patients with active giant cell arteritis have symptoms of PMR.

I. POLYMYALGIA RHEUMATICA

A. Clinical features.

1. Pain and stiffness in the neck, shoulder, and pelvic girdle. Symptoms are bilateral and symmetric and more prolonged in the morning. May have diffuse aching.
2. Systemic features such as low-grade fever, fatigue, and weight loss.
3. ESR and C-reactive protein are elevated with ESR elevation of 50 to 100 mm common. However, 15% of those with PMR may have a normal sedimentation rate.

B. Diagnosis.

1. Rule out other causes such as claudication, hypothyroidism, myositis. In PMR thyroid functions are normal, CPK and aldolase are not elevated, ANA should be "normal" for age, and rheumatoid factor will be negative. Patients may have normocytic, normochromic anemia.
2. Giant cell arteritis should be excluded.

C. Treatment

Prednisone. Initial dose of 10 to 20 mg PO QD for 1 month and then reduce by 2.5 mg every 2 to 4 weeks until the dose is 10 mg. The maintenance dose is about 10 mg PO QD and may be decreased to a range of 5 to 7.5 mg PO QD after 6 months. Most patients require treatment for 3 to 4 years, but withdrawal after 2 years is worth attempting.

II. GIANT CELL ARTERITIS (TEMPORAL ARTERITIS)

A. Clinical features. Predominantly affects persons >50 years of age with early symptoms of headache, fever, fatigue, and perhaps upper-limb girdle pain. May have associated ocular symptoms including partial visual loss and field cuts, diplopia, ptosis, and blindness. Tongue or jaw claudication may occur.

B. Laboratory abnormalities. Greatly elevated ESR, but 10% may have normal ESR, moderate normochromic anemia, and thrombocytosis.

C. Diagnosis. Temporal artery biopsy is most useful within 24 hours of starting treatment; however, steroids have little effect on the sensitivity of the biopsy, and treatment should not be delayed. A positive result helps to prevent later doubt about the diagnosis. Sensitivity of a biopsy is determined by length of artery taken and thinness of sections on microscopy.

D. Treatment. Prednisone: initial dose of 20 to 40 mg PO QD for 8 weeks. Patients with ocular symptoms may need up to 80 mg PO QD. Reduce the dose by 5 mg every 3 to 4 weeks until it is 10 mg QD and then taper slowly. The maintenance dose is about 3 mg PO QD.

RAYNAUD'S PHENOMENON

I. OVERVIEW

A. Episodic, biphasic or triphasic color change: white (ischemia), then often blue (stasis), then red (reactive hyperemia), of fingers or toes in response to cold or emotion.

B. More than 90% of patients with Raynaud's phenomenon are female.

II. TYPES

A. Raynaud's disease (primary Raynaud's phenomenon). The cause is unknown, and the symptoms are usually stable.

B. Secondary Raynaud's phenomenon. Predisposing factors include atherosclerosis, arteritis, cancer, collagen vascular disease, thoracic outlet syndrome, embolic occlusions, occupational disease (working outdoors, using vibrating tools), and certain drugs (β-adrenergic blockers, nicotine, ergotamine).

III. DIAGNOSIS

Diagnosis is made on clinical grounds.

IV. TREATMENT

A. Treat the underlying condition.

B. Simple conservative measures include dressing warmly, avoiding exposure to cold, and cessation of cigarette smoking.

C. Medications may be helpful.

1. Nifedipine extended release (such as Adalat CC) 30 mg PO daily.
2. Captopril 6.25 mg PO daily; may increase to 25 mg daily.

SYSTEMIC LUPUS ERYTHEMATOSUS

I. OVERVIEW

Systemic lupus erythematosus (SLE) is a systemic illness characterized by chronic inflammation; clinical manifestations are protean. It most commonly has its onset between 15 and 40 years of age and has an 8:1 female-to-male ratio. Genetic, environmental, and hormonal factors play a role in its etiology. The prevalence is 2.9 to 4 per 100,000; SLE is more common in blacks and some Asian populations.

II. DIAGNOSIS

Diagnosis of SLE requires the presence of four of 11 criteria below. Keep in mind that a positive ANA is neither required for a diagnosis of lupus nor sufficient in itself to make a diagnosis of lupus.

1. Malar rash
2. Discoid rash
3. Photosensitivity
4. Oral ulcers
5. Arthritis
6. Serositis (pleuritis or pericarditis)
7. Renal disorder (proteinuria >0.5 g/day or cellular casts)

8. Neurologic disorder (seizures or psychosis)
9. Hematologic disorder (hemolytic anemia, leukopenia, lymphopenia, or thrombocytopenia)
10. Immunologic disorder (positive LE cell, anti–double stranded DNA antigen, anti-Smith antigen, or false results of VDRL test) and
11. Positive results of fluorescent antinuclear antibody

III. CLINICAL FEATURES

A. Symmetric arthritis and arthralgias that are nondeforming and nonerosive. Can be confused with RA early in course. May have deformity secondary to contractures. Tenosynovitis occurs in up to 10%, sometimes in absence of arthropathy.

B. Mucocutaneous manifestations.

1. ***Acute cutaneous lupus.*** Characteristic butterfly malar rash, often accompanied by a more widespread morbilliform eruption. Will flare with exacerbation of systemic disease or from sun exposure.
2. ***Discoid lupus.*** Erythematous plaques with scale, mostly on scalp, face, or neck and occasionally on chest and arms. May be pigmented early with later central depigmentation and atrophy. Alopecia and scarring are common. Many with discoid lupus have no other systemic involvement.
3. ***Subacute cutaneous lupus.*** Skin lesions are symmetric, superficial, nonscarring, often annular, occurring on shoulders, upper arms, chest, back, and neck. Over half will have diffuse nonscarring alopecia, and 20% will have discoid lesions. Photosensitivity is prominent, but the incidence of nephritis is low.
4. ***Mucosal manifestations.*** Include recurrent oral and vaginal ulcers.

C. Cardiac involvement.

1. ***Pericarditis.*** May occur in up to 30% and may be asymptomatic. Often accompanied by pleural effusions. Rarely complicated by tamponade or restrictive pericarditis.
2. ***Myocarditis.*** May occur in up to 25%, often associated with pericarditis. Suggested by tachycardia, ST-T wave changes, and cardiomegaly. CPK-MB elevation may occur and can result in CHF or arrhythmias.
3. ***Endocarditis.*** First described by Libman and Sachs. Typically asymptomatic without murmur or hemodynamic dysfunction. Mitral and aortic are the most commonly involved valves, and damage can be severe. Emboli are relatively rare.
4. ***Myocardial infarction.*** Usually considered secondary to accelerated atherosclerosis from long-term steroid use.

D. Renal involvement. Affects 50% of patients, with the glomerulus the most commonly affected site. Any pathologic form of glomerulonephritis can occur, with variable dysfunction and prognosis. Clinical presentations include hematuria, proteinuria, hypertension, and uremia. Only 0.5% go on to end-stage renal disease. However, lupus nephritis is a poor prognostic marker, producing a survival rate of 85% at 5 years and 65% at 10 years.

E. **Pulmonary.** Lung or pleura involved in 40% to 50%, with pleuritis or pleural effusion most common. Myopathy may affect the diaphragm.

F. **Central nervous system.** Frequently involved with highly varied presentation; depression is common. Headaches, strokes, TIAs, and memory loss or encephalopathy may occur. Seizures, chorea, and frank psychosis also occur.

G. **Gastrointestinal.** Less commonly involved. Serositis, oral ulcerations, and esophageal dysmotility may occur. Liver involvement not uncommon, but jaundice is rare.

H. **Raynaud's phenomenon.** Present in about half of patients at presentation.

I. **Other symptoms.**
   1. ***Vascular.*** Terminal arterioles may be involved in vasculitis.
   2. ***Reticuloendothelial.*** Lymphadenopathy is common.

IV. LABORATORY FINDINGS

A. **Presence of ANA.** This result is found in 95% of those with SLE. Most common pattern is homogeneous and diffuse (pattern resulting in "LE cell"). Anti–double stranded DNA and anti-Smith antigens are found only in SLE, whereas other antibodies such as anti–single stranded DNA may also be present in other illnesses. Other antibodies such as anti-Ro, and anti-La may also be present.

B. **Hematologic abnormalities.** A normochromic, normocytic anemia is seen in up to 40% of patients. Evidence of hemolytic anemia may be present, including elevated serum haptoglobin (see Chapter 5). Thrombocytopenia is found in up to 25% of patients. The ESR may be elevated but does not correlate with disease activity.

C. **Lupus anticoagulant.** Characterized by circulating anticoagulant with an elevated PTT or with circulating antiphospholipid (50% of those with lupus)/anticardiolipin antibodies (see below). Associated with venous or arterial thrombosis (see below).

D. Patients with SLE may have a false-positive VDRL test. However, FTA will be negative.

E. Hypocomplementemia (CH50, C3, C4) may be present and correlates with disease activity.

V. TREATMENT

Generally a rheumatologist should participate in setting out a course of treatment though these patients can be followed by a primary care physician. Treatment should be individualized according to the activity of the disease and organs involved.

A. **Preventive care.**
   1. ***Regular monitoring.*** Patients should be seen every 3 to 6 months even if they are doing well.

2. ***Energy conservation.*** Fatigue is a common complaint.
3. ***Photoprotection.*** Sunscreen and avoidance of excess sun.
4. ***Infection control.*** Pneumococcal vaccine and yearly influenza vaccine. Consider antibiotic prophylaxis for procedures.
5. ***Contraception.*** Avoid pregnancy at time of increased disease activity or while using immunosuppressive therapy.

B. Medication.

1. ***NSAIDs.*** Useful for symptomatic relief of joint pain and the pain associated with pleurisy and pericarditis. Are also useful for treatment of systemic symptoms such as fever and fatigue. May combine with a low-dose steroid to minimize side effects of both. Watch for adverse renal effects especially in those who already have lupus nephritis.
2. ***Antimalarial drugs (chloroquine, hydroxychloroquine).*** Hydroxychloroquine is the most commonly used. Effective for cutaneous, musculoskeletal, and mild systemic symptoms. Mechanism of action is unknown. Begin 400 mg PO daily for 4 weeks and then taper to maintenance dose. Relapse is frequent with discontinuation of drug, but control can be maintained at a low dose. Ocular toxicity, including corneal deposits (which are not necessarily a contraindication to continued use) and retinopathy, may occur. Having patient view an Ansler grid every day may give an early indication of eye disease.
3. ***Steroids.*** Topical preparations are effective for cutaneous manifestations. Low-dose oral prednisone can be used for minor disease activity. Dose should be once daily in A.M. to reduce effect on pituitary-adrenal axis and high dose limited to 4 to 6 weeks if possible. Maintenance should be the lowest possible dose, using alternate-day therapy if possible. NSAIDs are used to try to lower steroid dose or for symptomatic treatment on the off day of alternate-day therapy. Prednisone at 1 mg/kg/day may be used for severe flares of joint symptoms, CNS symptoms, and nephritis. IV therapy with methylprednisolone may be needed in particularly severe disease.
4. ***Immunosuppressive drugs (azathioprine, cyclophosphamide).*** For severe flare and renal or CNS involvement. These are generally reserved for patients who failed conventional therapy.

DRUG-INDUCED LUPUS

I. CLINICAL FEATURES

A drug-induced lupus-like syndrome characterized by arthralgias, myalgias, fever, and serositis (pleurisy and pericarditis). CNS and renal disease are rare.

II. LABORATORY TESTS

Lab tests reveal cytopenias, ANA, LE. Anti-dsDNA is typically *not* present. Antihistone antibodies are present in >90% of cases but not specific for drug-induced lupus.

III. CAUSATIVE AGENTS

Hydralazine and procainamide have been strongly implicated in drug-induced lupus. 50% of those using procainamide will develop a positive ANA result; of these half will be symptomatic. Other drugs include phenytoin, primidone, isoniazid, chlorpromazine, penicillamine, practolol, propylthiouracil, methylthiouracil, and methyldopa.

IV. TREATMENT

Symptoms usually resolve when the offending drug is withdrawn. Antinuclear antibodies may persist for months.

LUPUS WITHOUT ANTINUCLEAR ANTIBODIES

1. High incidence of photosensitive cutaneous involvement (subacute cutaneous lupus).
2. Arthritis and Raynaud's phenomena common.
3. Low frequency of renal and CNS involvement.
4. Many have latex rheumatoid factor.
5. Survival better than with lupus with ANA.

ANTIPHOSPHOLIPID SYNDROME

I. GENERAL

Antiphospholipid syndrome (APS) is a disorder characterized by recurrent venous or arterial thrombosis, recurrent fetal loss, and thrombocytopenia associated with the presence of lupus anticoagulant or anticardiolipin antibody, or both. The female-to-male ratio is 2:1. May occur as a manifestation of lupus or may occur as an isolated, discrete syndrome. Anticardiolipin and antiphospholipid are essentially interchangeable terms. Depending on the assay used to detect them, they cross-react. Several subtypes that do not cross-react have been identified but are currently of little clinical significance.

II. CLINICAL FEATURES

A. Pregnancy loss. Obstetric complications include recurrent fetal loss, often but not always in the late second or third trimester, severe preeclampsia, premature delivery, chorea gravidarum, and intrauterine growth retardation. They may also have "postpartum syndrome," which is manifested by pleuropericarditis and fever.

B. Thrombosis. All venous and arterial systems can be involved. The most common site for venous thrombosis is in the lower extremities. Patients may have recurrent DVT or PE. The most common arterial complication is embolic cerebrovascular accidents and transient ischemic attacks.

C. **Other features described.** Endocardial valvular vegetations, livedo reticularis, migraine headache, thrombocytopenia, and Coombs'-positive hemolytic anemia.

III. DIAGNOSIS

A. **Criteria for the presence of lupus anticoagulant (LA).** Prolonged partial thromboplastin time (PTT) not corrected by addition of normal plasma but corrected by freeze-thawed platelets or phospholipids.

B. Anticardiolipin antibody (aCL) as measured by ELISA.

C. Clinical diagnosis of APS can be made if the patient has experienced unexplained thromboembolism, thrombocytopenia, or recurrent fetal loss in conjunction with persistently elevated titers of aCL or LA.

IV. MANAGEMENT

A. For thrombotic events chronic anticoagulation with warfarin and antiplatelet drugs (such as ASA) may be used. Heparin may need to be substituted for warfarin during pregnancy.

B. Steroids and immunosuppressive drugs have been used for acute flares.

C. There is no evidence that prophylactic therapy is helpful in patients who have been and are asymptomatic.

SYSTEMIC SCLEROSIS AND SCLERODERMA

I. GENERAL

Scleroderma is characterized by fibrosis of the skin and visceral organs.

II. CLINICAL FEATURES

A. **Skin.** Bilateral symmetric swelling of the fingers and hands is often an early manifestation. Edema is replaced by induration in a few weeks to several months, resulting in thick, hard skin. Skin thickness spreads rapidly and within months may affect the forearms, upper arms, face, and finally the trunk.

B. **Raynaud's phenomenon.** Occurs in almost all patients.

C. **Joints.** Nondeforming symmetric polyarthritis similar to rheumatoid arthritis.

D. **Lung.** Diffuse interstitial fibrosis occurs in 70% of patients.

E. **Heart.** Cardiac abnormalities, such as conduction defects and supraventricular arrhythmias, are seen in up to 70%.

F. **Gastrointestinal.** Esophageal dysfunction is the most frequent gastrointestinal abnormality but may have malabsorption, etc.

G. **Kidney.** Renal involvement frequently results in fulminant hypertension, renal failure, and death.

III. TREATMENT

No curative therapy available. Penicillamine 750 mg PO QD may decrease skin thickness, delay internal organ involvement, and prolong life expectancy. Other treatments are directed against symptoms including Raynaud's phenomenon, hypertension, gastroesophageal reflux (see Chapter 4), and digital sympathectomy for a critically ischemic finger.

ORTHOPEDICS

LOW BACK PAIN

I. OVERVIEW

Low back pain is the second most common cause of lost work time. Most cases (90%) resolve within 6 weeks; 5% of cases of low back pain become chronic in nature.

II. ETIOLOGY

A. **Mechanical causes.** Account for up to 98% of cases of back pain.

1. ***Disk injury.*** Herniation of the nucleus pulposus usually occurs posteriorly. May impinge upon nerve roots, particularly at the L4-L5-S1 levels. Typically pain increases with coughing, sneezing, or trunk flexion and includes radicular symptoms and signs.
2. ***Degenerative changes in facet joints.*** Result in nerve root impingement at the foramina. Sudden attacks lasting for a few days with symptom-free intervals. Typically pain is worse with trunk extension.
3. ***Spondylosis.*** Degenerative changes in vertebral bodies and disks that may result in nerve root impingement.
4. ***Spondylolisthesis.*** Slippage of the anterior portion of the superior vertebral body on the inferior vertebral body. 80% occur at L5-S1.
5. ***Spondylolysis.*** A defect in the pars interarticularis. More common in younger patients especially those who exercise vigorously.
6. ***Vertebral body fracture.*** After trauma or spontaneous "wedge" fractures in elderly with osteoporosis or those using steroids.
7. ***Spinal canal stenosis.*** Irritation during activity results in pain in one or both extremities while walking (similar pain to claudication). Relieved with rest. Tends to be worse with back extension, better with flexion.
8. ***Myofascial or soft-tissue injury or disorder.*** May have history of trauma, heavy work, or unusual activity.
9. ***Arachnoiditis and postoperative scarring.***
10. ***Children.*** *Under 10 years old:* diskitis (see Chapter 10), tumor, AV malformations, osteomyelitis. *Over 10 years old:* spondylolisthesis, herniated disks, Scheuermann's disease, overuse syndrome, tumor, spondylolysis.

B. Systemic disorders.

1. ***Malignancy***
   a. *Primary tumors.* Multiple myeloma most common.
   b. *Metastatic disease.* 85% are from the breast, prostate, lung, kidney, and thyroid and cause lytic lesions, except for the prostate and treated thyroid carcinomas, which are sclerotic. About 30% bone loss required before lytic changes will be visible on radiographs.
2. ***Miscellaneous.*** Osseous, disk, or epidural infection, spondyloarthropathy (p. 263), metabolic bone disease, including osteoporosis, vascular disorders such as atherosclerosis or vasculitis.

C. Neurologic causes.

1. Myelopathy from intrinsic or extrinsic processes
2. Lumbosacral plexopathy, especially for diabetes
3. Neuropathy, including inflammatory demyelinating type
4. Mononeuropathy, including causalgia
5. Myopathy, including myositis and metabolic causes

D. Referred pain. Including GI disorders such as pancreatitis and perforated ulcer; GU disorders including nephrolithiasis, prostatitis, and pyelonephritis; gynecologic disorders, including ectopic pregnancy and pelvic tumors; abdominal aortic aneurysm, or hip disorder.

III. WORK-UP

A. Physical examination.

1. ***Standing.*** Examine for obvious defects. Palpate for tenderness or muscle spasm. Test the mobility of the lumbar spine with flexion, extension, and lateral flexion. Observe the patient's gait and have the patient walk on his toes (foot plantar flexion test S1) and up on his heels (foot dorsiflexion test L5).
2. ***With the patient sitting.*** *Sitting straight-leg raising (SLR) test:* passive extension of the knee. A positive test is radicular pain at less than 60 degrees. "Crossover" pain with radicular symptoms in the leg *not* lifted is fairly specific for disk disease.
3. ***Reflexes.*** Patellar reflex tests the L4 root; Achilles tendon reflex tests the S1 root (L5-S1 disk). *Babinski sign:* if present, indicates disorder above the lumbar region such as cord tumor or CVA.
4. ***Sensation.*** *L4:* medial border of the feet; *L5*: triangular area at the base of middle toes on the dorsum of the feet; *S1:* lateral margin of the feet and distal portion of the calf.
5. ***Sensation.*** Check hip abduction (L5 motor), perianal sensation (S3-5: also controls anal and urethral sphincter tone), hip extension (L5 motor). *Saddle anesthesia, decreased anal sphincter tone, and crossover leg pain are signs of a central disk herniation, which is considered a surgical emergency. Must be suspected if there is a history of new bowel or bladder incontinence.*

B. Laboratory and imaging studies.

1. Lumbar spine films are not necessary in most patients. Plain films should be obtained if symptoms last more than 6 weeks, there is suspicion or history of malignancy, or the patient is using steroids, is over 50 years of age, has a history of trauma, or has neurologic deficits. There is no need to obtain radiographic evaluation for history consistent with muscle strain.
2. Patients suspected of having infectious or neoplastic causes of low back pain should have an imaging study such as a bone scan, CT, or MRI.
3. If severe symptoms persist for several weeks despite conservative therapy and disk herniation or another surgically correctable disorder is suspected, then CT or MRI imaging may be useful. Generally, since will not want to intervene surgically unless pain is present for at least 6 weeks, no need for these imaging studies unless there is some indication other than pain (that is, neurologic symptoms such as loss of bowel and bladder function). MRI and CT have replaced myelography except in rare circumstances.
4. ***Electromyogram and nerve conduction velocity.*** Can be used to evaluate suspected nerve root involvement.
5. ***Blood tests.*** Differential CBC with ESR, and biochemical screening (calcium phosphate, alkaline phosphatase) should be performed when a systemic cause for back pain is suspected.
6. ***Immunoelectrophoresis of serum and urine samples.*** Allows diagnosis of most cases of myeloma.

IV. TREATMENT

A. Acute back pain (no longer than 6 weeks).

1. There is no difference in outcome when patients with acute back pain are treated by a family physician, a chiropractor, or an orthopedic surgeon. Therapy by a family physician is the most cost effective.
2. Regardless of the method of treatment, 40% better within 1 week, 60% to 85% in 3 weeks, and 90% in 2 months. Negative prognostic factors include more than 3 episodes of back pain, gradual onset of symptoms, and prolonged absence from work.
3. ***Bed rest.*** Should be kept to a minimum, and early mobilization encouraged. If symptoms recur or considerable pain develops in relation to a specific activity or level of activity, the patient should temporarily limit activity for several days but should *not* cease all activity.
4. ***Analgesia.*** NSAIDs most commonly used. Provide pain relief and decrease inflammation. Acetaminophen provides analgesia but has no anti-inflammatory properties. May be used with or instead of NSAIDs. Narcotics should be used for short term only for severe pain. Muscle relaxants such as cyclobenzaprine 10 mg PO TID or QID

work mostly by sedating patients and preventing activity. However, they probably have little effect on muscle spasm.

5. ***Physical therapy.*** Although classically several modes have been used to hasten resolution of back pain, most physical therapy modes have no effect when rigorously tested. Traction, local application of heat, cold, and ultrasound, and corsets have been shown to have no effect. Transcutaneous nerve stimulation may provide short-term symptomatic relief but have no proved long-term benefit.
6. ***Epidural steroid injections.*** May speed recovery from radicular pain.
7. ***Rehabilitation exercises.*** Trunk extensors, abdominal muscles, aerobic conditioning. Main benefit is that they promote early mobilization, which is critical in treating acute back pain. The specific exercise doesn't matter as much as the mobilization.

B. Chronic back pain. Once back pain has been established for more than 1 year, the prognosis is poor. Mild analgesia should be used, avoidance of chronic or repeated reliance on narcotics for pain control is a key management priority. If depression is encountered, it should be treated.

C. Indications for admission and referral. Cauda equina syndrome (urinary retention, sphincter incontinence, saddle anesthesia), severe neurologic deficits (footdrop, gastrocnemius-soleus or quadriceps weakness), progressive neurologic deficit, or multiple nerve root involvement.

SHOULDER PAIN

After knee pain, shoulder pain is the second most common type of orthopedic pain in patients seen by family physicians. Most shoulder problems are attributable to overuse and trauma. The shoulder is composed of one articulation, the scapulothoracic, and three true joints: the sternoclavicular, acromioclavicular, and glenohumeral.

I. ROTATOR CUFF SYNDROME

The rotator cuff muscles are the supraspinatus, infraspinatus, teres minor, and subscapularis, which envelop the scapula.

A. Stage I rotator cuff syndrome.

1. This occurs in persons 25 years of age or younger.
2. This is a rotator cuff tendinitis caused by forceful or repetitive motion.
3. Pain is noted over the anterior aspect of the shoulder and is maximal when the arm is raised from 60 to 120 degrees of elevation.
4. Treatment consists in avoiding aggravating positions and activities, applying ice packs, and taking analgesics.

B. Stage II rotator cuff syndrome.

1. This usually occurs in patients 25 to 40 years of age with multiple previous episodes.

2. In addition to inflammation of the rotator cuff, some permanent fibrosis, thickening, or scarring is present.
3. Calcific deposits may be noted within the rotator cuff on radiographs.
4. Initial treatment is the same as that of stage I. If unsuccessful, the subacromial bursa can be injected with corticosteroids. If symptoms persist, referral to an orthopedist should be considered for surgery.

C. Stage III rotator cuff syndrome.

1. This is a complete tear of the supraspinatus tendon and usually occurs after 40 years of age.
2. The patient may relate feeling a sudden pop in the shoulder and then suffering severe pain. The patient notes increasing weakness when trying to abduct and externally rotate his or her arm.
3. The diagnosis is confirmed by magnetic resonance imaging or a shoulder arthrogram.
4. Treatment is usually surgical repair depending on whether there is significant loss of function. More likely to repair in young patients than in the elderly, for example. Many elderly patients have progressive rotator cuff loss over years as a result of the aging process.

II. ADHESIVE CAPSULITIS (FROZEN SHOULDER)

A. Clinical features.

1. This chronically stiff and painful shoulder begins without any significant injury.
2. The cause is prolonged immobilization from either protracted use of a sling or disuse because of pain in the arm.
3. Shoulder motion is limited in one or more directions, with pain occurrring at the limits of motion. The physical examination is otherwise relatively unremarkable.
4. Treatment involves extended, aggressive physical therapy and NSAIDs.

III. TENDINITIS AND BURSITIS

The supraspinatus and long end of the biceps are especially susceptible.

A. Clinical features. The primary symptom is a painful, aching shoulder of rather nondescript type. With supraspinatus tendinitis, the pain is aggravated when the shoulder is abducted and externally rotated against resistance. With bicipital tendinitis, pain is aggravated when the patient flexes forward against resistance.

B. Treatment.

1. Most of the conditions about the shoulder can be relieved by injection of 1% bupivacaine into the subacromial bursa or tendon region and application of ice.
2. Overuse syndrome in the shoulder should be treated with NSAIDs and rest for 5 to 7 days.

IV. ACROMIOCLAVICULAR INJURIES

Usually result from a direct blow or fall on the tip of the shoulder.

A. Grade I (sprain). Partial tear of the joint capsule without joint deformity and minimal ligamentous disruption and instability. AC joint films (with and without weights) are normal. Treatment includes ice, pain medication, a sling for comfort, and early mobilization.

B. Grade II (subluxation). Complete tear of the acromioclavicular ligaments.

- The AC joint is locally tender and painful with motion. The distal end of the clavicle may protrude slightly upward. Stress radiograph of the AC joint with the patient holding a 10-pound weight in both hands reveals widening of the joint. Treatment is symptomatic in the same manner as the grade I injury but usually requires a longer period of immobilization (2 to 4 weeks).

C. Grade III (dislocation). Complete tear of the acromioclavicular and coracoclavicular ligaments with pain on any attempt at abduction. There is an obvious "step-off" on physical examination. Radiographs show superior displacement of the clavicle and complete dislocation of the joint with weights. Conservative treatment with a sling is appropriate, provided that the patient understands that permanent deformity may result. Patients usually return to normal function. Surgical treatment is important if symptomatic treatment fails or if it will interfere with the patient's life (as in an athlete or person who does heavy work).

V. GLENOHUMERAL DISLOCATIONS

A. Clinical features. 95% are anterior, most commonly subcoracoid and then subglenoid. The usual mechanism is forced abduction and external rotation. Patients complain of severe pain and usually hold the arm in tightly against their body. The shoulder appears flattened laterally and prominent anteriorly. The acromion process is prominent, and so the shoulder appears to be "squared off." The examiner must check associated injuries, including proximal humeral fractures, avulsion of the rotator cuff, and injuries to the adjacent neurovascular structures. Axillary nerve injury is most common and is associated with decreased active contraction of the deltoid muscle.

B. Radiographs taken in two planes (AP and lateral scapula or axillary views) will confirm the dislocation and should be done to rule out fracture if mechanism suggestive.

C. Treatment. The dislocation should be reduced as soon as possible. Adequate analgesia and relaxation can be obtained by a 20 ml intra-articular injection of 1% lidocaine. This is superior to 10 mg of IV morphine and 2 mg of midazolam. Narcotics and muscle relaxants (such as morphine and diazepam) can be used as adjuncts.

1. ***External rotation method (Hennipen technique).*** The patient is placed supine, with the arm abducted and the elbow flexed to 90 degrees. The examiner holds the elbow in position and guides the forearm of the patient outward, externally rotating the shoulder. No pressure is applied to the forearm to force external rotation. If necessary, the arm can be abducted while in external rotation. Reduction usually occurs silently, unnoticed by the patient. This method has the lowest rate of complications.
2. ***Modified Stimson reduction.***
    a. Analgesia or relaxation as noted above.
    b. Patient placed prone on a table with the injured shoulder hanging free.
    c. Weight (up to 10 pounds) is suspended from the wrist, and the patient is left for 5 to 15 minutes.
    d. Further manipulation often required consisting of gentle internal and external rotation with downward traction.

D. Postreduction care. Postreduction radiographs are obtained to ensure good relocation. The patient's arm is immobilized in a sling-and-swathe dressing for 6 weeks. Early orthopedic follow-up care is recommended. Recurrent dislocation or subluxation is common and may require surgical repair.

PROBLEMS OF THE ELBOW, WRIST, AND HAND

I. ELBOW

A. Lateral epicondylitis (tennis elbow). Very common and occurs as an inflammatory process at the extensor origin of the lateral epicondyle. May be secondary to overuse or repetitive use. Pain at the lateral epicondyle, with referred pain to the extensor surface of the forearm is typical. The pain is exacerbated by resisted extension of the wrist or fingers. Treatment includes avoiding exacerbating activities, NSAIDs, and placing a constrictive band on the elbow (commercial "tennis elbow" bands are available). Occasionally immobilization of the wrist in a volar splint is required. Local steroid injection and orthopedic referral may be advised in recalcitrant cases.

B. Medial epicondylitis. This results from repeated flexion activities of the wrist and fingers. Pain is at the medial epicondyle and exacerbated by resistant flexion of the fingers. Treatment is the same as that of lateral epicondylitis.

C. Radial head subluxation (nursemaid's elbow).

1. The ***mechanism*** is a sudden pull on the extended pronated elbow of a child (for example, when one picks up a child by the forearm or swings the child), usually under 4 years of age. The child holds his arm in pronation and usually refuses to move it with pain on supination and palpation of the radial head.
2. ***Although radiographic findings*** are usually normal, one must be sure to rule out undisplaced supracondylar fracture.

3. ***Treatment*** is firm supination of the forearm, flexing the elbow gently to 90 degrees with pressure over the radial head. Reduction is achieved with a palpable click over the radial head, and the pain is immediately relieved. The patient should resume full activity within several minutes of reduction.

D. Little Leaguer's elbow. Results from overuse of an adolescent's pitching elbow. Will feel pain over the medial aspect over the medial humeral condyle. The most effective management is prevention. If loose bodies develop in the elbow, they need to be removed surgically.

E. Olecranon bursitis. May be secondary to trauma (such as laying on carpet with elbows propped up while watching TV). May be septic or sterile. With septic type, generally have fever, warmth over the olecranon bursa; may have local skin disruption indicating an area from which infection could have spread.

1. ***Cause.*** For septic bursitis, majority are *Staphylococcus aureus*. May also be secondary to sterile inflammation from gout or pseudogout.
2. ***Diagnosis.*** Tap bursa under sterile conditions and send fluid to lab for Gram stain, culture, cell count, crystals. If septic type, should look similar to fluid from septic joint (above).
3. ***Treatment.*** If no predisposing factors (DM, steroid use, immunosuppression from malignancy, etc.) may choose to treat as outpatient with an agent to cover *Staphylococcus* (dicloxacillin, amoxicillin/clavulanate [Augmentin]). If patient is toxic, admit for IV antibiotics. Warm soaks or hot packs will aid resolution. For either infectious or noninfectious bursitis, needle drainage, repeated if needed, will aid in resolution. Such drainage is critical for infectious bursitis. Occasionally, an olecranon bursa must be opened surgically.

II. WRIST AND HAND

A. Ganglion cyst. The most commonly noted nodule in the hand. Typical locations include the dorsal aspect of the wrist, radial volar aspect of the wrist, dorsal aspect of the hand, and palmar aspect of the fingers near the MCP joints. If the cyst is small, aspiration of the cyst contents may be performed with a 22-gauge needle and injection of a steroid. However, multiple aspirations may be required for resolution. If the cyst is painful or large or if there is a question of cause, orthopedic referral for surgical removal should be considered.

B. Carpal tunnel syndrome.

1. ***Clinical features.*** The symptoms are a result of median nerve dysfunction because of increased pressure within the carpal tunnel. The causes include overuse, ganglion cyst, synovial proliferation, pregnancy, rheumatoid arthritis,

and hypothyroidism. Typical symptoms are pain, paresthesia, numbness, or a pins-and-needles sensation in the median nerve distribution of the hand, usually in the thumb, index and middle fingers, and radial aspect of the ring finger. Nocturnal paresthesia is characteristic.

2. ***Exam.*** Tinnel's sign, which is a painful sensation of the fingers induced by percussion of the median nerve at the level of the palmar wrist, may be positive, but specificity only 54% and sensitivity 50%. Phalen's sign, keeping both wrists in a palmar-flexed position may reproduce symptoms. Sensitivity varies from 10% to 88% depending on study; it has an 80% specificity.
3. ***Treatment.*** The patient without thenar atrophy can be treated with conservative therapy, which includes a resting splint with the wrist in neutral position and NSAIDs. Although cock-up splints have been the classic form of immobilization, they have been shown to be inferior to a simple, neutral splint. Steroid injections of the carpal tunnel may be effective. If EMG shows impaired conduction of the median nerve at the wrist, or the carpal tunnel symptoms do not improve in 6 weeks, or if there is evidence of thenar muscle weakness or atrophy, surgical referral is indicated.

C. Mallet finger.

1. Injury resulting from forced flexion of distal tip of a finger. Result is a stretching or rupture of the tendon of the extensor digitorum profundus or avulsion of part of the distal phalanx with tendon attached.
2. ***Exam*** reveals swelling, tenderness, DIP joint held in flexion with patient unable to extend it.
3. ***Treatment.***
   a. Splint finger in extension across DIP joint leaving PIP joint free to allow continued function. Splint for several weeks (6 to 12); longer times for injuries with delayed diagnosis.
   b. Operative repair is necessary for the minority of cases that don't respond to splinting.

KNEE PAIN

The majority of knee injuries in adults are of a ligamentous nature. In children, however, a bloody effusion after injury frequently indicates bony injury.

I. LIGAMENTOUS INJURIES

A. Collateral ligament injury.

1. Typically caused by direct trauma to the contralateral side of the knee, or excessive indirect force to the knee in a varus or valgus manner.
2. Pain and a sensation of tearing may have been noted by the patient at the time of injury. In case of medial collateral ligament injury, there may be tenderness along the distal femur extending to the joint line. Medial

collateral ligament injuries may be associated with meniscus tears.

3. Valgus and varus tests provide assessment of the collateral ligaments. With the knee in 30 degrees of flexion, the collateral ligaments can be isolated.
4. Grade I sprains are caused by microtears of the ligament and correspond to less than 5 mm of increased joint opening and no instability. Grade II sprains are a partial macrotear of the ligament with the presence of instability and significant increased joint opening with a point. A grade III sprain is a complete tear of the ligament with no end point distinguishable on examination.
5. ***Treatment*** of isolated grade I and II injuries involves conservative measures, such as ice application for 15 to 20 minutes TID and elevation for the first 24 to 72 hours, rest with an immobilizer for 7 to 14 days, and NSAID therapy. The patient should be placed on crutches with weight bearing as tolerated. Prompt initiation of physical therapy should be included in initial treatment. Grade III injuries can be treated nonoperatively, but an orthopedic referral is recommended to assess the need for surgical intervention.

B. Anterior cruciate ligament injury.

1. There is a history of a twisting injury accompanied by a pop or tearing feeling and a subsequent effusion. A hemarthrosis is found in 75% of cases. Frequently associated with a medial collateral ligament injury.
2. The Lachman and pivot shift tests are useful. The Lachman test is performed with the knee at 30 degrees in a supine position and involves anterior displacement of the tibia on the femur. The pivot shift test involves flexion of the knee while the lower leg is internally rotated and a valgus stress is applied, resulting in subluxation of the tibia. The tibia can be relocated abruptly when the knee is extended.
3. Treatment should be supervised by an orthopedist. Treatment of acute injuries depends on the severity. Patients without associated meniscal, collateral ligament, or posterior cruciate ligament injury should be treated by immobilization of the knee for comfort and crutches. Patients with associated ligament injury or meniscal injury should be referred immediately to an orthopedist because surgery may be necessary.

C. Posterior cruciate ligament injury.

1. Most injuries are the result of direct trauma to the proximal tibia when the flexed knee is decelerated rapidly, as in a dashboard injury.
2. The posterior drawer and tibial sag tests are used. In the posterior drawer test, the knee is flexed 90 degrees and pos-

terior displacement of the tibia on the femur is attempted. In the tibial sag test, the knee is flexed to 90 degrees; in case of posterior cruciate ligament rupture, the tibia is displaced posteriorly on the femur.

3. Isolated tears should be managed conservatively. If radiographs, particularly the lateral view, reveal displaced bony avulsions, posterior cruciate ligament injury may require surgical fixation.

II. MENISCAL TEARS

A. Clinical features.

1. Medial meniscal injuries are one of the most common causes of knee joint pain. The medial meniscus is much more susceptible to tears than the lateral meniscus is. More than one third of meniscal injuries are associated with an anterior cruciate ligament tear and possibly medial collateral ligament injuries.
2. Patients complain of pain at the time of injury, which persists and interferes with weight-bearing activity. The most consistent physical finding is tenderness to palpation along the joint line. Patients often complain of the knee "locking," which may be attributable to pain or a physical inability to extend the knee because the torn meniscus prevents extension.
3. Several clinical tests help determine if meniscal injury is present. In the McMurray's test, the knee is fully flexed, with the leg externally rotated when one is testing for medial meniscal tears and internally rotated when testing for lateral meniscal tears. While maintaining rotation, extend the knee with a firm controlled movement. A painful click signifies a positive test. The Apley's test is performed with the patient in a prone position. The knee is flexed to 90 degrees, and an axial load is placed on the heel of the foot while the lower leg is rotated internally and externally. If pain results, the test is positive.

B. Diagnosis. If there are any diagnostic doubts, patients should be referred for evaluation by magnetic resonance imaging or arthroscopy.

C. Treatment. The knee should be immobilized if there is pain with motion. Crutches, quadriceps exercises, NSAIDs, or analgesics can be used. If the knee remains locked or if symptoms of pain, giving way (a sense that the knee is going to collapse), and swelling persist, orthopedic referral should be made for surgical intervention.

III. PATELLOFEMORAL PAIN SYNDROME

A. Clinical features. Most common anterior knee problem seen by the family physician. The problem is anterior knee pain, which is worse with sitting in a tight space with the knee flexed, or on descending stairs or slopes. Patients may complain of some snapping, popping, or crepitus about the patella.

B. Radiographs of the knee are usually negative. However, lateral displacement of the patella on sunrise films may be present.

C. Treatment. NSAIDs, ice application, and appropriate exercises including those that strengthen the medial quadriceps and stretch the hamstrings are useful (such as straight leg raising with the ankle and hip externally rotated.

IV. PATELLAR DISLOCATIONS

A. Clinical features. Patients complain of the knee giving way or popping out. The patella may remain dislocated when patient is seen, but many spontaneously reduce. An effusion (hemarthrosis) may be present. The medial retinaculum is tender. *Apprehension test:* displace the patella laterally; patients feel as though the patella is going to dislocate and will be very apprehensive. Between occurrences the patella is observed to have considerable lateral mobility, particularly during active extension. The patellar ligament may be noted to angulate laterally from the axis of the quadriceps muscle.

B. Reduction. Encourage the patient to relax the quadriceps and push the patella medially back into place. If unable to get the patella over the lateral femoral condyle, push the patella anteriorly while passively flexing the knee (the patella usually reduces by 30 degrees of flexion). If the effusion is tense, aspiration may reduce discomfort.

C. Postreduction care. Many believe that adequate immobilization is obtained with the use of a knee immobilizer for 6 weeks. Some believe that a full-leg cylinder cast is required. Have patients fully weight bearing as well as performing quadriceps isometric exercises while immobilized. After immobilization, patients are placed on partial weight bearing while quadriceps strengthening is initiated. Rehabilitation needs to include the vastus medialis, which operates only in the last 15 degrees of extension. Resume full weight bearing when flexion to 30 degrees is painless. An elastic knee support may add some patellar stability during strenuous activity.

D. Dislocation more than three times may require surgical treatment.

PROBLEMS OF THE FOOT AND ANKLE

I. ANKLE SPRAIN

A. Clinical features. Sprains usually result from an inversion force; an eversion injury may result in a fracture. The most common ligament injured is the anterior talofibular ligament. A history of popping or a painful snap with ankle injury may be indicative of a significant ligament injury.

B. Radiography. The Ottawa ankle rules (Fig. 6-2) have been developed and validated to determine who needs a radiograph. Using these rules, an occasional fracture will be missed. However, these are generally of no clinical significance (as with an avulsion injury). They apply only to an individual older than 17 years of age.

C. Treatment. In most ankle sprains, treatment includes external support such as the application of an air splint, ice application for 20 minutes every 4 hours, and elevation above the heart. NSAIDs or acetaminophen with or without hydrocodone or codeine can be used for pain control. The patient should be allowed partial weight bearing with crutches or a cane. Early mobilization and weight bearing hasten resolution. Patients with recurrent problems of instability or an acute grade III problem should be referred to an orthopedist for evaluation and the possibility of reconstructive surgery. However, recent data have called the need for reconstructive surgery into doubt.

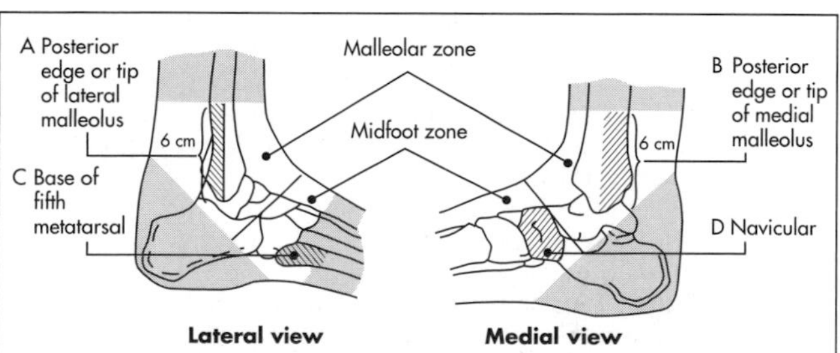

An ankle radiographic series is required only if there is any pain in the malleolar zone and any of these findings is present:
(1) bone tenderness at A
(2) bone tenderness at B
(3) inability to bear weight both immediately and in the ED

A foot radiographic series is required only if there is any pain in midfoot zone and any of these findings is present:
(1) bone tenderness at C
(2) bone tenderness at D
(3) inability to bear weight both immediately and in the ED

FIG. 6-2 Ottawa ankle rules. (From Stiell IG, Greenberg GH, McKnight RD, Wells GA: *Ann Emerg Med* 27(1):103-104, 1996.)

FRACTURES

I. TYPES

- **A. Closed fracture.** Fracture that does not communicate with the outside.
- **B. Open fracture:** Fracture that communicates with the external environment.
- **C. Comminuted fracture.** Consisting of three or more fragments.
- **D. Avulsion fracture.** Fragment of bone pulled from its normal position by a muscular contraction or resistance of a ligament.
- **E. Greenstick fracture.** Incomplete angulated fracture of a long bone, particularly in children.
- **F. Torus fracture.** Compression of the bone without cortical disruption. Seen especially in the forearms of children.

II. EPIPHYSEAL PLATE FRACTURES

Described using the Salter and Harris classification (Fig. 6-3).

A. Salter I (approximately 6%).

1. Separation of the epiphysis from the metaphysis without evidence of a metaphyseal fragment.
2. Usually the result of a shearing force, can be associated with birth injury.
3. Most common in infants and young children.
4. High index of suspicion is necessary because spontaneous reduction can occur.
5. Prognosis is excellent because epiphyseal blood supply is usually intact and growing cells of epiphyseal plate are undisturbed.

B. Salter II (approximately 75%).

1. Fracture extends transversely through the epiphyseal plate and then out through the metaphysis on the side opposite the fracture initiation resulting in a triangular metaphyseal fragment.
2. Most frequent in children over 10 years of age.
3. Usually treated with closed reduction.
4. Prognosis is excellent because the blood supply is almost always intact.

C. Salter III (8%).

1. Intra-articular fracture that extends from the joint surface across the epiphysis to the epiphyseal plate and out to the periphery.
2. Commonly involves the lower tibial epiphysis.
3. Caused by an intra-articular shearing force.
4. Often requires open reduction.
5. Prognosis is good if the blood supply is intact and reduction is maintained.

D. Salter IV (10%).

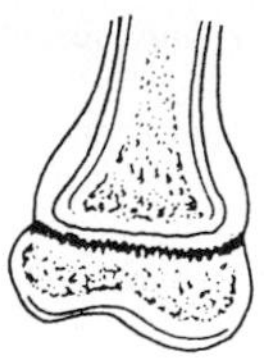

Type 1
Pure epiphyseal separation

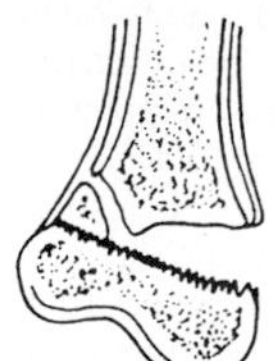

Type 2
Partial epiphyseal separation with fracture of diaphysis

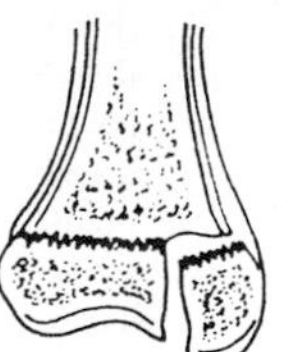

Type 3
Partial epiphyseal separation with fracture of epiphysis

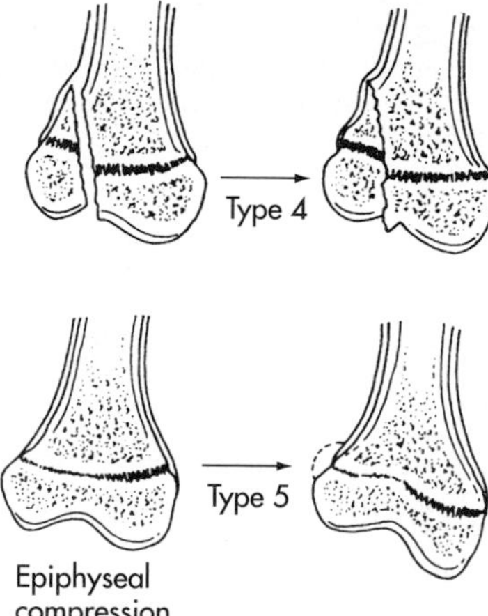

FIG. 6-3 Salter-Harris classification of epiphyseal fractures.

1. Intra-articular fracture consisting of a vertical fracture through the epiphysis that crosses the epiphyseal plate and leaves through a portion of the metaphysis.
2. Frequently involves lateral condyle of humerus.
3. Treated with anatomic reduction and internal fixation.
4. Prognosis is poor unless reduction is maintained.

E. Salter V (1%).

1. Results from a crush injury through the epiphysis to a portion of the epiphyseal plate.
2. Usually occurs in a joint that has only one plane of movement.
3. Most commonly seen in the knee and ankle.

4. Initial radiographs tend to be normal and so must suspect this fracture from the mechanism of injury.
5. Results are poor with premature cessation of growth.
6. Nontraumatic events causing a Salter V type of injury are metaphyseal osteomyelitis and epiphyseal aseptic necrosis.
7. Salter V can occur in conjunction with Salter I, II, and III fractures and not be recognized until growth arrest occurs.
8. Treat with 3 weeks of no weight bearing.

III. REPAIR

A good rule of thumb is that most bones join in 6 to 8 weeks; lower limb bones may take longer; fractures in children may take less time.

IV. COMPLICATIONS

A. **Immediate complications,** within the first few hours, include hemorrhage, damage to arteries, and damage to surrounding soft tissues.

B. **Early complications,** within the first few weeks, include wound infection, fat embolism, shock lung, chest infection, DIC, and exacerbation of general illness. May also have compartment syndrome from casting (see p. 44).

C. **Late complications,** months and years later, include deformity, osteoarthritis of adjacent or distant joints, aseptic necrosis, traumatic chondromalacia, and reflex sympathetic dystrophy.

V. MANAGEMENT OF SOME SPECIFIC FRACTURES

A. **Fracture of radial head.** Usually caused by a fall onto an outstretched hand. Patients are reluctant to pronate the hand or to flex the elbow beyond 90 degrees. The only roentgenographic evidence may be an anterior or posterior fat pad sign. The posterior fat pad is more specific but less sensitive. Management of nondisplaced fractures includes a sling and posterior elbow splint for 1 to 2 weeks with range-of-motion exercises after 1 week. Continue in sling for another week and do follow-up radiograph to document that no displacement has occurred with mobilization. Displacement of the head should be referred to an orthopedist for operative repair.

B. **Radial fractures.**

1. In children, the most common injury is the torus (buckle) fracture, which occurs with a fall onto an outstretched hand. Radiographic findings may show only a slight cortical disruption on the lateral film. Treatment is a short arm cast for 3 weeks.
2. In adults, the most common radial fracture is the Colles' fracture, which is extra-articular and occurs 2.5 to 3 cm proximal to the articular surface of the distal radius. This fracture occurs with the hand dorsiflexed; the distal

fracture segment is angulated dorsally and causes a "silver-fork" deformity. Reduction by traction and manipulation can be performed. After reducing the fracture, a plaster short-arm cast is applied for 5 to 8 weeks. If nondisplaced, casting for 6 weeks without reduction is indicated.

C. Metacarpal fractures. A boxer's fracture is a fracture of the distal neck of the fifth metacarpal and is generally the result of punching something with a closed fist (generally a wall or refrigerator). Tenderness is localized to the injured metacarpal bone. Radiographs reveal a fracture of the involved metacarpal or subluxation at the carpometacarpal joint. Nondisplaced fractures of the base of the metacarpals are treated with immobilization in a short arm cast. Displaced fractures are reduced by traction with local pressure over the prominent proximal end of the distal metacarpal fracture. A follow-up radiograph is necessary within 7 days. If any instability is noted after reduction or the fracture is comminuted, the patient should be referred to an orthopedist for open reduction and internal fixation.

D. Fracture of a finger.

1. ***Distal tip fractures*** are usually crush injuries to the tip of the finger. Protective splinting of the tip for several weeks is usually satisfactory.
2. ***Middle and proximal phalangeal fractures*** should be examined for evidence of angulation (by roentgenography) or rotation (by clinical examination), which require reduction. Nondisplaced extra-articular fractures can be managed by 1 to 2 weeks of immobilization followed by dynamic splinting with buddy taping to the adjacent finger. Large intra-articular or displaced fractures are usually unstable and require orthopedic referral.
3. ***Small (<25%) avulsion fractures of the middle phalangeal base*** occur with a hyperextension injury. These injuries are managed by 2 to 3 weeks of immobilization with up to 15 degrees of flexion at the PIP joint, followed by buddy taping for 3 to 6 weeks.

BURSITIS OF THE HIP

Bursitis of the hip largely involves the trochanteric bursa. Patients present with a history of pain with walking, running, or climbing, They may also complain of pain when lying on the affected side. There is a tenderness over the greater trochanter. NSAIDs and corticosteroid injection (triamcinolone 20 to 40 mg infiltrated around area with bupivacaine 0.5% 5 ml) are very effective.

MEDICAL CLEARANCE FOR SPORTS PARTICIPATION

There are several clinical entities that require modification or exclusion from sports. See Table 6-1 for recommendations.

TABLE 6-1
Recommendations for Participation in Competitive Sports

	Contact/ collision	Limited contact/impact	Noncontact*		
			S	MS	NS
Atlantoaxial instability	No	No	Yes	Yes	Yes
^ Swimming: no butterfly, breaststroke, or diving starts					
Acute illness	•	•	•	•	•
• Needs individual assessment, such as contagiousness to others, risk of worsening illness					
Cardiovascular					
Carditis	No	No	No	No	No
Hypertension					
Mild	Yes	Yes	Yes	Yes	Yes
Moderate	•	•	•	•	•
Severe	•	•	•	•	•
Congenital heart disease	■	■	■	■	■
Eyes					
Absence or loss of function of one eye	•	•	•	•	•
Detached retina	■	■	■	■	■
• Availability of American Society for Testing and Materials (ASTM)–approved eye guards may allow a competitor to participate in most sports, but this must be judged on an individual basis					

■ Consult an ophthalmologist					
Inguinal hernia	Yes	Yes	Yes	Yes	Yes
Kidney: absence of one	No	Yes	Yes	Yes	Yes
Liver: enlarged	No	No	Yes	Yes	Yes
Musculoskeletal disorders	•	•	•	•	•
• Needs individual assessment					
Neurologic					
History of serious head or spine trauma, repeated concussion, or craniotomy	•	•	Yes	Yes	Yes
Convulsive disorder					
Well controlled	Yes	Yes	Yes	Yes	Yes
Poorly controlled	No	No	Yes	Yes	Yes
• Needs individual assessment					
No swimming or weight lifting					
No archery or riflery					
Ovary: absence of one	Yes	Yes	Yes	Yes	Yes
Respiratory					
Pulmonary insufficiency	•	•	•	•	•
Asthma	Yes	Yes	Yes	Yes	Yes
• May be allowed to compete if oxygenation remains satisfactory during a graded stress test					

(Footnote symbols on p. 296)

Continued.

TABLE 6-1
Recommendations for Participation in Competitive Sports—cont'd

	Contact/ collision	Limited contact/impact	Noncontact*		
			S	MS	NS
Sickle cell trait	Yes	Yes	Yes	Yes	Yes
Skin: boils, herpes, impetigo, scabies	•	•	Yes	Yes	Yes
• No gymnastics with mats, martial arts, wrestling, or contact sports until not contagious					
Spleen: enlarged	No	No	No	Yes	Yes
Testicle: absent or undescended	Yes	Yes	Yes	Yes	Yes

Adapted from American Academy of Pediatrics: *Sports medicine: health care for young athletes*, Elk Grove Village, Ill., 1991, American Academy of Pediatrics.

**S*, Strenuous; *MS,* moderately strenuous; *NS,* nonstrenuous.

^ Certain sports may require a protective cup.

• Needs individual assessment.

■ Patients with mild forms can be allowed a full range of activities; patients with moderate or severe forms or those who are postoperative need evaluation by a cardiologist before athletic participation.

BIBLIOGRAPHY

Brooks PM: Clinical management of rheumatoid arthritis, *Lancet* 341:286-290, 1993.

Burke DT et al: Tinel's sign and Phalen's test in carpal tunnel syndrome, *Orthopedics* 15(11):1297, 1992.

Carey TS et al: The outcomes and costs of care for acute low back pain among patients seen by primary care practitioners, chiropractors, and orthopedic surgeons, *N Engl J Med* 333(14):913, 1995.

Cash JM, Klippel JH: Second-line drug therapy for rheumatoid arthritis, *N Engl J Med* 330:1368-1375, 1994.

Dalakas MC: Polymyositis, dermatomyositis, and inclusion-body myositis, *N Engl J Med* 325:1487-1498, 1991.

Dale DC, Federman DD, editors: *Scientific American medicine,* New York, 1996, Scientific American, Inc.

Deyo RA et al: Lumbar spine films in primary care: current use and effects of selective ordering criteria, *J Gen Intern Med* 1(1):20, 1986.

Dieppe P et al: A two year, placebo-controlled trial of nonsteroidal antiinflammatory therapy in osteoarthritis of the knee joint, *Br J Rheumatol* 32(7):595, 1993.

Doherty M: ABCs of rheumatology: fibromyalgia syndrome, *Br Med J* 310:386-389, 1995.

Donovan PJ, Paulos LE: Common injuries of the shoulder: diagnosis and treatment, *West J Med* 163:351-359, 1995.

Escalante A: Ankylosing spondylitis, *Postgrad Med* 94:153-166, 1993.

Furst DE: Are there differences among nonsteroidal antiinflammatory drugs? *Arthritis Rheum* 37:1-9, 1994.

Gam AN et al: Ultrasound therapy in musculoskeletal disorders: a meta-analysis, *Pain* 63(1):85, 1995.

Glockner SM: Shoulder pain: a diagnostic dilemma, *Am Fam Physician* 51:1677-1687, 1995.

Goroll AH et al, editors: *Primary care medicine,* ed 3, Philadelphia, 1995, Lippincott.

Hughes, GR: The antiphospholipid syndrome: ten years on, *Lancet* 342:341-344, 1993.

Indahl A et al: Good prognosis for low back pain when left untampered: a randomized clinical trial, *Spine* 20(4):473, 1995.

Isenberg DA, Black C: ABC of rheumatology: Raynaud's phenomenon, scleroderma, and overlap syndrome, *Br Med J* 310:795-798, 1995.

Jones A, Doherty M: ABC of rheumatology: osteoarthritis, *Br Med J* 310:457-460, 1995.

Keat A: ABC of rheumatology: spondyloarthropathies, *Br Med J* 310:1321-1324, 1995.

Kirchner JT: Reiter's syndrome, *Postgrad Med* 97:111-122, 1995.

Kuschner SH et al: Splinting for carpal tunnel syndrome: in search of the optimal angle, *Arch Phys Med Rehabil* 75(11):1241, 1994.

Kuschner SH et al: Tinel's sign and Phalen's test in carpal tunnel syndrome, *Orthopedics* 15:1297, 1992.

Malmivaara A et al: The treatment of acute low back pain: bed rest, exercise, or ordinary activity? *N Eng J Med* 332:351-355, 1995.

Matelic TM et al: Acute hemarthrosis of the knee in children, *Am J Sports Med* 23(6):668, 1995.

Mills JA: Systemic lupus erythematosus, *N Engl J Med* 330:1871-1879, 1994.

Morgan SL et al: Supplementation with folic acid during methotrexate therapy for rheumatoid arthritis: a double-blind, placebo-controlled trial, *Ann Intern Med* 121(11):833-841, 1994.

Munk B et al: Long-term outcome after ruptured lateral ankle ligaments: a prospective study of three different treatments in 79 patients with 11-year follow-up, *Acta Ortho P Scand* 66(5):452, 1995.

Ohi JA: Treatment of ganglia by aspiration alone, *J Hand Surg* 17b:660, 1992.

Pinals RS: Polyarthritis and fever, *N Engl J Med* 330:769-774, 1994.

Pope MH et al: A prospective randomized three-week trial of spinal manipulation, transcutaneous muscle stimulation, massage and corset in the treatment of subacute low back pain, *Spine* 19(22):2571, 1994.

Pountain G, Hazelman B: ABC of rheumatology: polymyalgia rheumatica and giant cell arteritis, *Br Med J* 310:1057-1059, 1995.

Prakash UBS, editor: *Mayo Internal Medicine Board Review 1996-97,* Rochester, Minn., 1996, Mayo Foundation for Medical Education and Research.

Rakel RE, editor: *Textbook of family practice,* ed 5, Philadelphia, 1995, Saunders.

Reese RE, Betts RF: A practical approach to infectious disease, Boston, 1996, Little, Brown & Co.

Riggs BL, Melton LJ III: The prevention and treatment of osteoporosis, *N Engl J Med* 327:620-627, 1992.

Schumacher HR Jr et al, editors: *Primer on the rheumatic diseases,* ed 10, Atlanta, Ga., 1993, Arthritis Foundation.

Shrestha M et al: Randomized double-blind comparison of the analgesic efficacy of intramuscular ketorolac and oral indomethacin in the treatment of acute gouty arthritis, *Ann Emerg Med* 26(6):682, 1995.

Smith BW, Green GA: Acute knee injuries: Part I: History and physical examination, *Am Fam Physician* 51:615-621, 1995.

Smith BW, Green GA: Acute knee injuries: Part II: Diagnosis and management, *Am Fam Physician* 51:799-806, 1995.

Snaith ML: ABC of rheumatology: gout, hyperuricemia, and crystal arthritis, *Br Med J* 310:521-524, 1995.

Steinberg GG et al, editors: *Ramamurti's orthopedics in primary care,* ed 2, Baltimore, 1992, Williams & Wilkins.

Stiell IG et al: Implementation of the Ottawa ankle rules, *JAMA* 271:827-832, 1994.

Stiell IG et al: Prospective validation of a decision rule for the use of radiography in acute knee injuries, *JAMA* 275:611-615, 1996.

Tan N et al: Acute gouty arthritis, *Postgrad Med* 94:73-87, 1993.

Taylor RB, editor: *Family medicine: principles and practice,* ed 4, New York, 1994, Springer-Verlag.

Tilley BC et al: For the Mira Trial Group: minocycline in rheumatoid arthritis: a 48-week, double-blind, placebo-controlled trial, *Ann Intern Med* 122:81-89, 1995.

Vawter RL, Antoneli MAS: Rational treatment of gout, *Postgrad Med* 91:115-127, 1992.

Wheeler AH: Diagnosis and management of low back pain and sciatica, *Am Fam Physician* 52:1333-1341, 1995.

Williams HJ et al: Comparison of naproxen and acetaminophen in a two-year study of treatment of osteoarthritis of the knee, *Arthritis Rheum* 36(9):1196, 1993.

7

Gynecology

PETER P. TOTH AND A. JOTHIVIJAYARANI

GENERAL GYNECOLOGY

I. GYNECOLOGIC HISTORY

See Chapter 8.

CONTRACEPTIVES (Table 7-1)

I. COMBINED PILL

A. **Mechanism of action.** Ovarian ovulation suppression through inhibition of the hypothalamic-pituitary-ovarian axis and alteration of the cervical mucus, retarding sperm entry and discouraging implantation into an unfavorable endometrium.

B. **Risks and adverse effects.** Thromboembolism, thrombosis-induced myocardial infarction, gallstone formation, breast cancer (particularly if age <25 and treatment >8 years), hypertension, and cervical cancer.

C. **Side effects.** Nausea, breast tenderness, weight gain, loss of libido, leg cramping, headache, bloating, and acne.

D. **Absolute contraindications.** Pregnancy, history of thromboembolic disease, ischemic heart disease, severe hypertension, history of breast cancer, estrogen-dependent neoplasms, cerebral ischemia (transient cerebral ischemia, focal or severe migraine), hepatic dysfunction, porphyria.

E. **Relative contraindications.** Smoking, diabetes, hyperlipidemia, active gallbladder disease, sickle cell anemia, active mononucleosis, major surgery within 1 month, long leg cast, >40 years with cardiovascular risk factors, abnormal vaginal bleeding of unknown cause.

F. **Noncontraceptive benefits of oral contraceptives.** More regular and predictable menses, reduced prevalence and severity of dysmenorrhea, reduction in days and amount of menstrual flow, increased iron stores in woman with menorrhagia, restoration of regular menses in anovulatory women; protection from benign breast disease, PID, ectopic

TABLE 7-1
Methods of Contraception

Method	Mechanism of action	Failure rate (%)*		Some adverse effects
		Low	High	
No method		85	85	
Spermicide alone	Inactivation of sperm	21.6	25.6	Irritation can occur
Sponge with spermicide	Mechanical barrier to sperm; inactivation of sperm	16	51.9	Increased risk of vaginal infection
Withdrawal		14.7	27.8	
Periodic abstinence	Avoidance of coitus during presumed fertile days	13.8	19.2	
Diaphragm or cervical cap with spermicide	Mechanical barrier to sperm; inactivation of sperm	12	38.9	Increased risk of urinary or vaginal infection
Condom	Mechanical barrier to sperm	9.8	18.5	Allergic reactions
Oral contraceptives				
Combined	Suppression of ovulation, changes in cervical mucus and endometrium			Estrogen-related risk of thromboembolism, stroke, myocardial infarction in smokers, hypertension

Progestin only	Changes in cervical mucus and endometrium, possibly suppression of ovulation			Irregular, unpredictable bleeding in some
Intrauterine device Progsterone T Copper-T 380A	Inhibition of sperm migration, fertilization, or ovum transport	2.5	4.5	Pelvic inflammatory disease, uterine perforation, increase in menstrual blood loss of copper
Medroxyprogesterone acetate (Depo-Provera)	Changes in cervical mucus and endometrium, suppression of ovulation	<1	<1	Menstrual irregularities, headache, weight gain
Levonorgestrel subdermal implants (Norplant)	Same as medroxyprogesterone acetate	<1	<1	Menstrual irregularities, headache, weight gain

From Abramowicz M, editor: *Medical Letter* 34:885, 1992.

*Percentage of accidental pregnancy during first year of use. *Low* and *high* refer to rates among women in the USA more and less likely than average to use the method correctly and consistently.

pregnancy, epithelial ovarian cancer, endometrial carcinoma, and increased bone mineral density.

II. PROGESTIN-ONLY PILL

Because of their reduced potential to cause clotting abnormalities, they are used in women with risk factors for cardiovascular disease, such as smokers, women >35 years, and diabetics. They also have little effect on lactation.

III. MANAGING THE PATIENT TAKING THE PILL

A. **Starting regimens.** Day 1 after menses in most menstruating women, fourth week in the nonlactating postpartum woman, the day after an induced or spontaneous abortion, 2 weeks after full mobilization after major or leg surgery. Some will start on the Sunday after last menses for convenience. Exclude pregnancy and supplement with alternative contraception during the first month.

B. **Missed pill.** If a pill is missed, it should be taken as soon as possible, and the next dose should be taken as usual. Alternative contraception should be used for 7 days.

IV. NEWER PROGESTINS

Three new 19-nortestosterone gonane progestogens, with low androgenicity and minimal metabolic effects and good cycle control, have been introduced. They are desogestrel, norgestimate, and gestodene. However, these are more expensive, and there is evidence that the risk of thromboembolic disease is increased with desogestrel and gestodene (Orthocept and Desogen).

V. INTRAUTERINE DEVICES

A. Progestasert releases progesterone, leading to less menstrual blood loss and less dysmenorrhea. Replace annually.

B. ParaGard copper-T 380A can be left in place 8 years.

C. **Contraindications.** Mucopurulent cervicitis, history of PID or ectopic pregnancy. Risk of ectopic pregnancy lower than in women using no contraceptives but higher than in those using oral contraceptives.

VI. SPERMICIDES containing nonoxynol-9 destroy sperm cell walls and provide some protection against STDs but may increase the risk of HIV transmission.

VII. BARRIER DEVICES (condoms, diaphragms, caps, sponges, and new female condoms) decrease the risk of STDs when used properly.

VIII. PERIODIC ABSTINENCE during presumed fertile times requires long periods of abstinence. Highest failure rates occur in women with irregular menstrual cycles.

IX. MEDROXYPROGESTERONE ACETATE (Depo-Provera) 150 mg IM every 3 months is FDA approved. Most women are amenorrheic after 1 year with some irregular bleeding during that year. Long-term safety unclear. Possible increased risk of breast cancer and osteoporosis.

X. PROGESTIN IMPLANTS (Norplant) involves subcutaneous insertion of six Silastic capsules containing levonorgestrel for slow release providing contraception for 5 years. Removal possible at any time, though can be difficult if capsules embedded in fibrotic tissue. Long-term safety unclear.

A. **Absolute contraindications.** Pregnancy, history of thromboembolic disease or breast cancer, estrogen-dependent neoplasms, CVA or coronary artery disease, liver tumor, impaired liver function.

B. **Relative contraindications.** Can include hypertension, smoking, severe headaches, diabetes, hyperlipidemia, active gallbladder disease, sickle cell anemia, active mononucleosis, major surgery within 1 month.

C. **Fertility.** Usually returns 2 months after removal.

XI. POSTCOITAL CONTRACEPTION

Morning-after pill: Four tablets of Ovral, an OCP containing 50 μg of ethinyl estradiol, begun within 72 hours of intercourse can usually prevent pregnancy by causing shedding of the endometrium and preventing implantation of the fertilized ovum. Mifepristone (RU 486) 600 mg within 72 hours is more effective with fewer side effects but is not yet available in the United States.

COMMON GYNECOLOGIC INFECTIONS

I. VULVOVAGINITIS

Vulvovaginitis is the most common outpatient gynecologic complaint. Organisms commonly responsible are *Gardnerella, Candida,* and *Trichomonas.* Diabetes mellitus, pregnancy, multiple sexual partners, high-dose estrogen oral contraceptives, corticosteroid therapy, use of intrauterine devices, and tight-fitting undergarments may predispose to the development of vulvovaginitis as well as other gynecologic infections. Consider HIV in women with recurrent episodes of candidiasis. See Table 7-2 for differential characteristics.

A. Clinical manifestations of vaginitis.

1. ***Candidal vaginitis.*** Nonmalodorous, thick, white, cottage cheese–like discharge that adheres to vaginal walls. Presence of hyphal forms or budding yeast cells on wet-mount microscopic evaluation. However, microscopy lacks sensitivity; so may want to treat those with typical symptoms (pruritis) and in absence of watery discharge.

TABLE 7-2
Characteristics of Vaginitis

Organism	Discharge	Wet prep	Symptoms
Candida	White, thick	Pseudohyphae (lack sensitivity)	Pruritus
Trichomonas	Thin, green/yellow copious	Motile trichomonads	Copious discharge, pruritus
Nonspecific or bacteria	Scant, gray, pH >4.5	Clue cells, positive whiff test	Discharge with fishy odor

2. ***Bacterial vaginosis.*** Thin, dark or dull gray, homogeneous malodorous discharge that adheres to the vaginal walls. Elevated pH (>4.5). Positive whiff or amine test. Presence of clue cells on saline wet mount. Polymicrobial (*Gardnerella vaginalis, Mycoplasma hominis, Mobiluncus, Bacteroides,* etc.).
3. ***Trichomonas vaginalis.*** Copious, yellow gray or green, homogeneous or frothy, malodorous discharge. Elevated pH (>4.5). Presence of mobile, flagellated organisms and leukocytes on wet mount. Vulvovaginal irritation, dysuria.

B. Evaluation. History, exam, microscopic exam of secretions with saline and KOH (wet prep), vaginal pH with nitrazine.

C. Treatment.

1. ***Candida.*** The following vaginal suppositories can be used at bedtime for 3 days: clotrimazole 200 mg (100 mg × 2), miconazole 200 mg, or terconazole 80 mg. Cream formulations also effective when used at bedtime for 7 days: clotrimazole 1% 5 g, miconazole 2% 5 g, or terconazole 0.4% 5 g. A single oral dose of fluconazole 150 PO or itraconazole 200 mg PO QD for 3 days are also effective.
2. ***Bacterial vaginosis.*** *Oral:* metronidazole 500 mg PO BID for 7 days or 2 g PO as single dose; clindamycin 300 mg PO BID for 7 days. *Vaginal:* metronidazole 0.75% gel 5 g BID for 5 days or clindamycin 2% cream QHS for 1 week.
3. ***Trichomoniasis.*** Metronidazole 500 mg PO BID for 7 days or 2 g PO as single dose.

II. CERVICAL INFECTIONS

A. Range of symptoms. Asymptomatic, mucopurulent cervicitis; may have associated urethritis or infection of Bartholin's gland.

B. Collecting specimens. Collect specimen for gonococcus culture first, since this organism will be found in the mucus. Endocervical cells are needed for *Chlamydia,* which is an intracellular organism. These should be taken from the endocervix. See Chapter 11 for treatment details.

III. SYPHILIS

Incidence increasing in U.S. See Chapter 11 for details on diagnosis and treatment.

IV. PELVIC INFLAMMATORY DISEASE

PID includes a wide variety of infections, such as puerperal and postoperative infections, septic abortions, and salpingitis. Term used interchangeably with acute salpingitis. This is a sexually transmitted ascending infection of the upper genital tract.

A. **Pathogenesis.** Ascending infection from cervix to fallopian tubes with initial mucosal damage often by *Neisseria gonorrhoeae* with secondary infection by other organisms including *Chlamydia, Mycoplasma, Ureaplasma,* gram-negative enterics, and anaerobes. Often polymicrobial.
B. **Predisposing factors.** Multiple sexual partners, nonbarrier contraceptive use (especially IUD), transvaginal instrumentation of cervix and uterus, recent menstrual period, history of PID, douching.
C. **Diagnosis.**
   1. ***Differential diagnosis.*** Appendicitis, ectopic pregnancy, septic abortion, pyelonephritis, inflammatory bowel disease, endometriosis, hemorrhagic corpus luteum, ovarian cyst, adnexal torsion.
   2. Obtain UA, CBC, pregnancy test, ESR, Gram stain of cervical discharge, and appropriate cultures: endocervix, rectum, urethra, blood, and peritoneal fluid as indicated.
   3. ***Criteria for diagnosis.***
      All 3 of the following:
      a. Lower abdominal pain and tenderness with or without rebound
      b. Cervical motion tenderness
      c. Adnexal tenderness

      Plus one or more of the following (secondary criteria):
      a. Temperature >38.0° C
      b. WBC >10,500/mm^3
      c. Culdocentesis with WBCs and bacteria
      d. Mass on bimanual exam or ultrasonography
      e. Elevated ESR
      f. Endocervical Gram stain with gram-negative intracellular diplococci or positive rapid assay for *Chlamydia*
D. **Treatment.** *Because of the risk of infertility, treat presumptively while awaiting cultures even if they do not meet secondary criteria.*
   1. ***Outpatient therapy.***
      a. Ceftriaxone 250 mg IM or cefoxitin 2 g IM plus probenecid 1 g PO. Ofloxacin 400 mg PO or ciprofloxacin 500 ng PO are acceptable alternatives.
      b. Either of above followed by doxycycline 100 mg PO BID × 14 days. *Single-dose azithromycin is not adequate therapy for* Chlamydia *in the setting of PID!*

2. ***Inpatient therapy.***
   a. Cefoxitin 2 g IV Q6h plus doxycycline 100 mg IV Q12h or cefotetan 2 g IV Q12h plus doxycycline 100 mg IV Q12h until improvement. Either followed by doxycycline 100 mg PO BID to complete 14 days.
   b. Alternative preferred in IUD-related infection, suspected abscess, or procedure-related infection: clindamycin 900 mg IV Q8h plus gentamicin loading dose 2 mg/kg IV followed by gentamicin 1.5 mg/kg Q8h until improvement. Then doxycycline 100 mg PO BID or clindamycin 450 mg PO QID to complete 14 days. Gentamicin dose needs to be adjusted in the presence of renal insufficiency.
3. ***Criteria for hospital admission.***
   a. Uncertain diagnosis
   b. Suspected pelvic abscess
   c. Concurrent pregnancy
   d. Severity of illness precludes outpatient therapy
   e. Inability to comply with outpatient treatment including necessary follow-up exam after 48 to 72 hours of therapy
   f. Failure of outpatient therapy

E. Complications. Infection rarely remains confined to fallopian tubes, and peritonitis is common. Increased risk of ectopic pregnancy, infertility, rupture of a tubo-ovarian abscess. adnexal torsion, bowel obstruction secondary to adhesions, and septicemia.

BARTHOLIN GLANDS

1. The Bartholin's glands are pea-sized organs situated at the 5 and 7 o'clock positions of the vaginal introitus. When normal they are nonpalpable.
2. A Bartholin gland may become enlarged from cystic dilatation, abscess, or adenocarcinoma (generally in women >40 years).
3. ***Symptoms and treatment.***
   a. Cystic dilatation of the Bartholin's duct can result from trauma or inflammation. These cysts are usually asymptomatic, and in women under 40 years of age they generally do not require treatment.
   b. A Bartholin's gland abscess is accompanied by dyspareunia, vulvar pain, pain during walking, erythema, edema, and possibly cellulitis of the surrounding tissue. The abscess tends to recur after simple incision and drainage. The therapies of choice are to marsupialize the duct or to insert a Word catheter for 4 to 6 weeks. Antibiotics are not prescribed unless the abscess is accompanied by cellulitis. The gland should be excised if the abscess reforms on multiple occasions. The gland should also be removed for histologic evaluation if it is enlarged in a woman >40 years because of its potential for being an adenocarcinoma.

PELVIC PAIN

I. DIAGNOSTIC APPROACH TO PELVIC PAIN

A. History.

1. Pain onset, location, duration, description, intensity, relationship to menses.
   a. Sudden onset is suggestive of torsion, *Mittelschmerz,* urolithiasis, ruptured corpus luteum cyst, ruptured ectopic pregnancy.
   b. More gradual onset is suggestive of appendicitis, PID, abscess, etc.
2. Menstrual history changes, LMP, spotting, birth control, sexual activity, signs of pregnancy (nausea, breast tenderness, urinary frequency).
3. Systems-specific questions with above differential diagnosis in mind (GU, GI, GYN systems). Evidence of hypovolemia.

B. Physical exam.

1. ***Abdomen.*** Peritoneal signs, masses, tenderness, bowel sounds, rectal exam with occult blood testing, flank tenderness.
2. ***Pelvic.*** Complete vulvar and vaginal exam, cervix (dilatation, tissue at os, lesions, motion tenderness), uterine size and tenderness, and adnexa (masses, tenderness, unilateral or bilateral).

C. Diagnostic aids.

1. ***Blood.*** CBC with differential, ESR (which is elevated with infection or inflammation); Hb and HCT may be decreased with hemorrhage. Repeat testing over time can be informative.
2. ***Cultures.*** Blood, cervix, urine, as indicated.
3. ***Urinalysis.*** Helpful to differentiate GU disorders. May be negative if complete obstruction is present.
4. ***Stool guaiac.*** Points toward GI tract if positive.
5. ***Pregnancy test.*** Must know sensitivity of the test you are using. Urine pregnancy test may miss very early ectopics. Serum RIA is very sensitive and picks up virtually all pregnancies.
6. ***Culdocentesis.*** Positive with any intraperitoneal bleeding (such as ectopic pregnancy, bleeding corpus luteum cyst, ruptured liver adenoma, ruptured spleen, peptic ulcer). The absence of fluid is nondiagnostic and does not help in differentiating the cause of pain.
7. ***Ultrasound.*** Useful to distinguish intrauterine from extrauterine pregnancy, also helpful in diagnosing appendicitis, luteal cysts, PID, spontaneous abortion. Be sure to check blood flow to both ovaries to rule out ovarian torsion.
8. Abdominal films may show ureteral stone, bowel obstruction.
9. Radiologic studies such as barium enema, IVP, CT scan.
10. Laparoscopy when indicated.

II. MANAGEMENT

A. Assess vital signs; stabilize hemodynamically if necessary.

B. If there is evidence of peritoneal irritation (surgical abdomen), intraperitoneal bleeding with signs or symptoms of pregnancy, positive pregnancy test, consult gynecologist. If suspect hemorrhage (unstable vital signs), do not order more time-consuming tests (such as ultrasonography) before surgical consultation.

III. DIFFERENTIAL DIAGNOSIS OF PELVIC PAIN

Appendicitis, pyelonephritis, ectopic pregnancy, diverticulitis, ureteral stone, spontaneous abortion, inflammatory bowel, cystitis, pelvic inflammatory disease, irritable bowel, bleeding corpus luteum cyst, bowel obstruction, adnexal torsion, inguinal hernia, Mittelschmerz, endometriosis, among other causes.

ENDOMETRIAL ABNORMALITIES

I. ENDOMETRITIS

A. Can cause abnormal bleeding and uterine tenderness.

B. Diagnosis. Made by endometrial biopsy specimen that reveals plasma cells or etiologic microbes.

C. Types. Puerperal (see Chapter 8), chlamydial or gonococcal, with or without concomitant salpingitis, secondary to curettage or other instrumentation, IUD-induced endometritis, tuberculous.

D. Therapy.

1. Submit endometrial and cervical specimens for *Chlamydia* and gonorrhea cultures. Treat patient for these organisms as detailed above.
2. If caused by an IUD, remove. Treat for *Actinomyces israelii* with ampicillin or tetracycline. Patient at risk for tubo-ovarian abscess.
3. Chronic endometritis is treated with doxycycline 100 mg PO BID for 14 to 21 days.

II. ENDOMETRIAL ADENOCARCINOMA

A. Endometrial carcinoma. The most frequent malignancy of the female pelvis in the United States. The presence of AGCUS cells on a Pap smear, abnormal bleeding in a perimenopausal female (prolonged or heavy bleeding, or intermenstrual bleeding), or postmenopausal bleeding may all herald the development of an endometrial adenocarcinoma. The probability that postmenopausal bleeding is caused by an endometrial carcinoma increases as a given patient's age increases.

B. Risk factors. Chronic anovulation (as in polycystic ovarian syndrome), obesity (increased conversion of androstenedione to estrone by adipose tissue aromatase), unopposed exogenous estrogen use, diabetes mellitus, nulliparity, late menopause, and hypertension.

C. Diagnosis. Diagnose with endometrial biopsy or dilatation and curettage. If histologic evaluation reveals simple or complex hyperplasia, risk of malignancy is low. However, if the biopsy specimen shows atypical hyperplasia or evidence of adenocarcinoma, the patient should be referred for total abdominal hysterectomy and bilateral salpingo-oophorectomy with staging biopsies as indicated.

D. Women receiving hormone replacement therapy who have regular withdrawal bleeding in response to exogenous progestins do not require scheduled monitoring with endometrial biopsy.

ENDOMETRIOSIS

I. OVERVIEW

A. Definition. Endometriosis is the presence of functioning endometrial tissue outside its normal location, most frequently confined to the ovaries, uterosacral ligaments, cul-de-sac, and occasionally uterovesical peritoneum.

B. Pathogenesis. Three major theories.

1. Retrograde transport and implantation.
2. Retrograde transport with metaplastic transformation of adjacent peritoneum.
3. Lymphatic or hematogenous dissemination.

II. EVALUATION

A. History.

1. The most common symptoms associated with pelvic endometriosis are dysmenorrhea (66%), dyspareunia (33%), infertility (70%), and pelvic pain. May have progressively more heavy menses with irregular menses.
2. Less common symptoms include dyschezia (painful defecation), premenstrual spotting, dysfunctional uterine bleeding, infertility, and dysuria.
3. One third of women have no symptoms.

B. Physical examination.

1. Fifty percent of women have a normal clinical examination.
2. Findings may include a fixed, tender, retroverted uterus; tender nodules along the uterosacral ligaments (with obliteration of the cul-de-sac); nodules on the back of the uterus and cervix; bilateral fixed adnexal masses.

C. Diagnostic aid: laparoscopy. Since clinical diagnosis may be wrong 30% to 40% of the time, it is necessary to confirm the diagnosis of endometriosis by laparoscopy before intensive treatment is begun. Laparoscopy will help assess the extent and stage of the disease as well as tubal patency.

III. MANAGEMENT

A. Mild disease.

1. Endometriosis with peritoneal cul-de-sac involvement is often not progressive, particularly when the ovaries are not involved.
2. Treatment options.
   a. Observation.
   b. Mild analgesics.
   c. Cyclic birth control pills (estrogen and progesterone) to create anovulatory cycles.

B. Treatment options in moderate disease.

1. ***"Pseudomenopause."*** Danazol treatment for 6 months. This treatment suppresses gonadotropins and causes endometrial tissue to slough. 10% of women get side effects comparable to menopause.
2. ***"Pseudopregnancy."*** Estrogen and progesterone in 2 to 10 times the dose in birth control pills. Treat for 6 months to a year. This treatment has antigonadotrophic effects as well as a direct effect on endometrial tissue. All patients have severe side effects.
3. Conservative surgery to selectively remove extrauterine endometrial tissue. May use hormones 6 weeks before and 3 to 6 months after surgery.
4. Pseudomenopause and conservative surgery have a better success rate for subsequent pregnancy than pseudopregnancy has.

C. Severe disease.

1. Treatment options are as above in III B.
2. ***Radical surgery.*** Hysterectomy with removal of ovaries if they are involved.
3. Lupron (GnRH analog) is very effective in treating endometriosis, but discussion of this therapy is beyond the scope of this book.

OVARIAN MASSES

I. OVERVIEW

A. The uterine adnexae include the ovaries, fallopian tubes, and uterine ligaments.

B. Normal structures.

1. Ovaries usually 3 to 5 cm in length but influenced by hormones.
2. Fallopian tubes normally cannot be felt.
3. Ninety percent of adnexal masses involve the fallopian tube or ovary.

II. EVALUATION

A. History.

1. Family history on both sides of family is critical because of the familial relationship of some ovarian neoplasms.
2. Ovarian neoplasms are often clinically silent, except for nonspecific "pressure" symptoms including urinary frequency, constipation, and pelvic heaviness.
3. Very large tumors may cause increased abdominal girth and may be confused with pregnancy.
4. Pain may result from stretching of the ovarian capsule, torsion, rupture, or intracystic hemorrhage.
5. Functional cysts may cause menstrual abnormalities.
6. Multiparity, late menarche, early menopause, and the use of oral contraceptive pills have all been shown to be protective against ovarian surface epithelial cell tumors.

B. Physical exam.

1. Benign tumors are characteristically unilateral, cystic, and mobile and do not cause ascites.
2. Malignancies are usually solid, fixed, and nodular and may cause ascites.

C. Diagnostic evaluation. Generally ultrasonography is first line. Other tests as indicated by diagnosis.

III. TREATMENT OF OVARIAN MASSES

A. Women of childbearing age with clinically benign ovarian cysts under 6 cm in diameter may be observed monthly. *If an ovarian "mass" persists, is greater than 6 cm, or increases in size during an observation period of 2 months, proceed with ultrasound evaluation and consider surgical excision.* If the cyst persists but decreases in size, it may be observed through another cycle.

B. Premenstrual (germ cell tumors) and postmenopausal (surface epithelial or stromal tumors) females are at high risk for malignancy. A palpable ovary in a postmenopausal female is abnormal, and one should proceed to full evaluation without a period of observation. Early diagnosis is essential and usually necessitates surgical excision.

C. Cysts greater than 10 cm in diameter are more likely to be malignant and require immediate evaluation and probable excision.

D. Solid ovarian tumors (by ultrasonography) are almost always malignant and demand immediate and aggressive evaluation and treatment. An exception to this is the rare luteoma of pregnancy.

PEDIATRIC GYNECOLOGY

Gynecology of infancy and childhood is often neglected, primarily because problems are uncommon before the onset of puberty; however, when such problems arise, they must be appropriately evaluated. If child abuse is suspected, document the exam carefully and report to the appropriate authorities. Consultation with a specialist in pediatric gynecology may be helpful in cases with legal ramifications.

I. COMMON DISORDERS OF INFANCY AND CHILDHOOD

A. Vulvovaginitis. Most common complaint.

1. ***Symptoms.*** Soreness, pruritus, discharge, burning.
2. ***Exam.*** Microscopic exam of vaginal secretions, UA, and possible cultures. Recurrent or refractory infections of foul-smelling, bloody discharge require vaginoscopy to exclude foreign body or tumor.
3. ***Causes.***
   a. Nonspecific polymicrobial infection secondary to poor hygiene or foreign body.
   b. Primary infections *(Candida, Gardnerella, Trichomonas,* gonorrhea, syphilis, herpes, etc.).
   c. Pinworms.
   d. Neoplasms rare.
4. ***Treatment.***
   a. Remove foreign body with warm saline irrigation or bayonet forceps. Obtain cultures and treat concurrent infection.
   b. Treat specific infections. *Candidiasis:* see section on common gynecologic infections, p. 303. *Gardnerella and Trichomonas vulvovaginitis:* metronidazole 35 to 50 mg/kg/day up to 750 mg divided TID for 7 days. *Gonorrhea:* probenecid 25 mg/kg PO plus amoxicillin 50 mg/kg or procaine penicillin G 100,000 U/kg IM or spectinomycin 40 mg/kg IM. *UTI:* amoxicillin 20 to 40 mg/kg/day divided TID × 10 days if sensitive. *Scabies and pediculosis pubis:* see Chapter 13.
   c. Sitz baths.
   d. Educate about perineal hygiene.

B. Pinworms *(Enterobias vermicularis).*

1. May cause vulvovaginitis; rectal itching common; frequently have vaginal pain.
2. See Chapter 10 for diagnosis and treatment.

C. Diaper dermatitis (primary contact irritant dermatitis).

1. Caused by irritants in urine, producing red, papulovesicular, shiny rash sparing skin folds; may fissure.
2. Treat with frequent changes allowing skin to dry fully and good hygiene and protection with zinc oxide or white petroleum jelly. Treat secondary infections caused by *Streptococcus, Staphylococcus,* or *Candida* organisms.

D. Labial adhesions.

1. Related to low estrogen levels, poor hygiene and vulvar irritation. Usually asymptomatic. Symptomatic when interfering with urination leading to dysuria and recurrent vulvar and vaginal infections.

2. Treat with topical estrogen cream BID for 7 to 10 days, which will lyse adhesions. Use surgical intervention only as a last resort.

E. Neonatal vaginal bleeding. May occur at 3 to 5 days, representing withdrawal of placental estrogens. No treatment except reassurance of parents.

F. Urethral prolapse.

1. Prolapse of estrogen-dependent distal urethral mucosa forming painful, friable mass at vaginal orifice. Catheter passed through center enters bladder.
2. Treat initially with topical estrogens and antibiotic creams. If urinary retention is present or lesion is large and necrotic, surgical excision may be required.

II. RARE BUT SERIOUS DISORDERS OF INFANCY AND CHILDHOOD

A. Sarcoma botryoides (embryonal carcinoma of vagina).

1. Presents as bloody vaginal discharge most commonly in very young girls (<3 years) with polypoid growth, which may look like a cluster of grapes.
2. Survival rare but improving with use of combination chemotherapy and radical surgery.

B. Ovarian tumors.

1. Symptoms include pain, mass, pressure; may cause vaginal bleeding or the precocious development of secondary sex characteristics if hormonally active.
2. Requires complete evaluation by experienced gynecologist.

ABNORMAL VAGINAL BLEEDING AND AMENORRHEA

I. TERMINOLOGY

A. Menorrhagia. Heavy or prolonged bleeding.

B. Metrorrhagia. Intermenstrual bleeding, spotting, or breakthrough bleeding.

C. Polymenorrhea. Menstrual interval <21 days.

D. Oligomenorrhea. Menstrual interval >35 days.

E. Amenorrhea. Absence of menstrual bleeding.

II. CAUSES OF VAGINAL BLEEDING

A. Dysfunctional uterine bleeding. Usually associated with anovulatory cycles and irregular sloughing of estrogen-stimulated endometrium. Represents abnormal hormonal regulation with tonic hormone levels rather than cyclical fluctuating gonadotropins and sex hormones. Common causes include puberty, climacteric, anorexia nervosa, polycystic ovarian disease, and obesity.

B. Benign organic lesions. Chronic cervicitis, cervical polyps, endometrial polyps, leiomyomas, chronic endometritis including low-grade form associated with IUD use.

C. **Malignant lesions.** Vaginal, uterine, cervical carcinomas; estrogen-producing ovarian neoplasms.
D. **Coagulopathies.** Most common is von Willebrand's disease. Also consider leukemias, thrombocytopenias.
E. **Pregnancy-related bleeding.** Ectopic pregnancy, threatened abortion, molar pregnancy, abruptio placentae, placenta previa.
F. **Miscellaneous.** Viral illnesses, hypothyroidism, liver disease, oral contraceptive breakthrough bleeding, ovulatory bleeding.

III. EVALUATION

A. **History.** Menstrual history, drug history, pregnancy, bleeding tendencies, contraceptive use (OCPs or IUD).
B. **Physical exam.** Pelvic noting hirsutism, virilization, vaginal or cervical lesions, uterine size and shape, adnexal masses. Obtain Pap smear and consider endometrial biopsy.
C. **Initial lab tests.** CBC with platelets, PT, PTT, pregnancy test, and T_4/TSH. Consider FSH/LH and androgens as indicated.

IV. TREATMENT OF IRREGULAR BLEEDING

A. **Adolescent or young women with anovulatory bleeding.**
   1. After exclusion of organic disease and pregnancy, treat with any combined progestin-estrogen OCP pack taking 1 pill QID until gone (7 days). Expect cessation of flow in 12 to 24 hours. Heavy withdrawal flow with cramping will start 2 to 4 days after regimen completed. On day 5 of withdrawal flow, begin daily low-dose combination OCP for at least 3 months and longer if continued contraception is indicated. If contraception not needed, may use cyclic medroxyprogesterone acetate 10 mg QD × 10 days each month for 3 months. Reconsider need for therapy in 1 year.
   2. Profuse bleeding (Hb <10, orthostatic hypotension) may require IV conjugated estrogens 25 mg Q4h (maximum 3 doses) followed by medroxyprogesterone acetate 10 mg PO QD × 7 to 10 days to initiate withdrawal bleeding. On day 5 of withdrawal bleeding begin low-dose OCP as above.
   3. Special situations requiring estrogen alone include those patients with atrophic endometrium. Patients fitting this category include those with prolonged bleeding, biopsy with scant tissue, breakthrough bleeding from progestin-only pills, Norplant or Depo-Provera. Therapy includes conjugated oral estrogen 1.25 mg QD × 7 to 10 days followed by medroxyprogesterone acetate.

B. **Reproductive mature female.** As above except repeated episodes of irregular bleeding should be treated with D&C and hysteroscopy to evaluate for organic lesions (polyps, submucosal fibroids). Hysterectomy may be considered for recurrent bleeding if reproductive potential is no longer an issue.

C. Postmenopausal bleeding. Always requires complete evaluation for carcinoma, including endometrial biopsy, possible D&C. Treat benign lesions if identified. Refer for definitive treatment of malignant lesions.

V. AMENORRHEA IN REPRODUCTIVE-AGED MATURE FEMALE

Pregnancy must be considered and ruled out by pregnancy test in all reproductive-aged women with amenorrhea.

A. History. Menstrual pattern, obstetric history, weight loss or gain, drug use (phenothiazines), headaches or visual disturbances, hirsutism, exercise.

B. Causes. May include pregnancy, hyperthyroidism, early or physiologic menopause, hypothyroidism, prolactinoma, etc.

C. Exam. Pelvic, noting hirsutism, galactorrhea.

D. If pregnancy test negative. Initial evaluation should include a serum prolactin, TSH, and a progesterone challenge with medroxyprogesterone acetate 10 mg QD × 5 days. Withdrawal bleeding within 7 days indicates ovaries are secreting estrogen.

E. Diagnosis and further evaluation dependent on above results.

1. ***Galactorrhea and hyperprolactinemia.*** Most common lesion is microadenoma of pituitary, but rule out other endocrine causes (hypothyroidism). May have headaches or visual symptoms. High-resolution CT of the sella turcica or MRI are the imaging studies of choice. Refer appropriately if abnormal or, if normal, follow prolactin Q6 months and CT or MRI Q1-2 years. Can treat with bromocriptine to suppress prolactin and shrink adenomas.
2. ***No galactorrhea and positive progestin challenge.*** Expected withdrawal bleed occurs; normal prolactin.
   a. Treat underlying cause if identified, considering polycystic ovarian disease (in PCOD have elevated LH, normal or low FSH, possibly mildly elevated androgens, maybe obesity, hirsutism, acne) and ovarian or adrenal tumors if hirsute.
   b. Combined OCPs can be used. An alternative is the use monthly or every other month of medroxyprogesterone acetate 10 mg QD × 10 days to prevent endometrial hyperplasia.
   c. If fertility desired, clomiphene citrate can be used in PCOD, 50 mg PO QD × 5 days, with ovulation expected 5 to 10 days after last dose.
3. ***No galactorrhea and a negative progestin challenge.*** *No withdrawal bleeding, a normal prolactin level.*
   a. Draw FSH; consider Asherman's syndrome (uterine synechiae) if history of D&C. FSH >40 mIU/ml indicates gonadal failure including menopause. FSH <40 mIU/ml is suggestive of severe hypothalamic dysfunction.

b. Treat hypoestrogenism to maintain bone density and prevent genital atrophy with combined OCPs or one of several hormone replacement regimens (see menopause below).
c. If fertility desired, refer for combined clomiphene and human menopausal gonadotropin therapy.

DYSMENORRHEA

I. CHARACTERISTICS AND ETIOLOGY

A. **Primary.** Menstrual pain with normal pelvic organs. Usual onset before 20 years of age. Pain begins within a day of onset of flow, lasting 24 to 72 hours. Increased prostaglandin activity from hormonal and psychologic factors causes increased uterine contractility.

B. **Secondary.** Menstrual pain with a pelvic pathologic condition on exam or at laparoscopy. Usual onset after 20 years of age, progressive with age, and less characteristically timed with menses. Causes include endometriosis, leiomyomas, endometrial cancer, IUD use, polyps, PID, cervical stenosis, ovarian cysts, imperforate hymen, uterine synechiae.

II. EVALUATION

A. **History.** Past menstrual history, family history, review of systems, level of debility, and psychologic overlay.

B. **Exam.** Pelvic, rectovaginal exam for uterosacral nodules.

C. **Lab tests.** Not usually necessary. If indicated by H&P, consider Pap smear, cultures, wet mount, endometrial biopsy, ultrasonography, laparoscopy.

III. TREATMENT

A. **Primary.**

1. Reassurance.
2. NSAIDs (ibuprofen 400 to 800 mg PO TID; naproxen 500 mg PO BID. Mefenamic acid 500 mg initially and then 250 mg PO TID may be especially effective.): Start 3 days before expected menses and continue through days of flow that patient has pain. Reassess need for medications in 1 year.
3. Consider combined OCPs if above inadequate. Reassess in 1 year.
4. If above unsuccessful, consider organic disorder (possible laparoscopy).

B. **Secondary.**

1. Laparoscopy often indicated.
2. Treat underlying cause.

PREMENSTRUAL SYNDROME

Constellation of physical, emotional, or behavioral symptoms occurring during the second half of the menstrual cycle (luteal phase, 7 to 10 days before menses), with resolution of symptoms soon after flow begins. There must be a symptom-free interval during the first half (follicular phase) of the menstrual cycle to make this diagnosis.

I. GENERAL CONSIDERATIONS

A. 90% of women affected minimally, 10% severely.

B. Affects primarily those in late 20s to early 30s without racial, socioeconomic, or other demographic predilection.

II. CAUSES

A. Hormonal and chemical. Imbalances involving estrogen, progesterone, increased prostaglandins, decreased endorphins, prolactin excess, aldosterone excess with fluid retention, insulin excess with reactive hypoglycemia, vitamin B_6 deficiency, and others.

B. Biopsychosocial. With expectations, beliefs, personality, coping style, sexual experiences, social supports, etc. all playing a role.

III. DIAGNOSIS IS CLINICAL

A. Minimum symptoms and signs. Edema, weight gain, restlessness, irritability, and increased tension. Many other physical and emotional symptoms possible.

B. Symptom calendar. Helpful in diagnosis and response to therapy.

IV. TREATMENT

A. Validation and education. Consider support groups, relaxation.

B. Diet. Limit salt, refined sugar, caffeine, alcohol, fat. Increase complex carbohydrates and fiber. Consider vitamin B_6 50 mg PO TID, keeping in mind risk of peripheral neuropathy.

C. Aerobic exercise. May decrease depressive symptoms.

D. Medications.

1. ***Fluoxetine (Prozac).*** May be titrated to effect from 5 to 20 mg PO QD. Has been shown to be effective in controlling symptom severity in multiple placebo-controlled clinical trials.
2. ***Calcium.*** 1000 mg PO QD or magnesium 400 IU PO QD during the luteal phase have both been shown to be effective in placebo-controlled trials.
3. ***Diuretics.*** Spironolactone 25 mg QID during luteal phase (12 days before menses). Best for those with weight gain, bloating, edema, and breast tenderness.
4. ***Prostaglandin cyclo-oxygenase inhibitors.*** Ibuprofen 400 to 800 mg TID, naproxen 500 mg PO BID, or mefenamic acid 500 mg TID 10 days before period through day 2 of menses. Have been shown to reduce the intensity of both the physical and emotional symptoms.

5. ***Progesterone vaginal or rectal suppository.*** 200 to 400 mg/day during luteal phase.

ABNORMAL PAP SMEARS

I. APPROACH BASED ON PAP SMEAR

ASCUS = atypical squamous cells of undertermined significance. AGCUS = atypical glandular cells of undetermined significance. LSIL = low-grade squamous intraepithelial lesion (same as CIN I, or cervical intraepithelial neoplasia, grade 1).

A. **Normal.** Repeat every year from 18 to 65 years of age. If low risk, may change to every 3 years after 2 consecutive normals. After 65 years may discontinue after 2 consecutive normals.
B. **No endocervical cells present.** Pap test is considered inadequate and should be repeated.
C. **ASCUS secondary to reactive/reparative changes or inflammatory changes.** Look for causative agent on wet mount or cultures and treat. If no agent identified, treat with doxycycline 100 mg BID × 7 days. Repeat Pap test in 3 months. If resolved, repeat Pap in 6 months and then yearly. If abnormal at 3 months, do colposcopy.
D. **ASCUS.** Repeat Pap smear in 3 months and then every 6 months for 2 years reverting to yearly after having 3 consecutive normals. Colposcopy indicated if follow-up smear indicates ASCUS, or patient not able to comply with every 6 month follow-up exam.
E. **LSIL or CIN I:** Proceed to colposcopy.
F. **ASCUS with dysplasia.** Colposcopy indicated.
G. **AGCUS.** Colposcopy with endocervical curettage.
H. **Other indications for colposcopy.** Dysplasia (mild, moderate, severe), squamous cell carcinoma, adenocarcinoma, human papillomavirus infection (cervical or external genitalia), persistent inflammation.

II. METHODS FOR TREATING CERVICAL DYSPLASIA

A. **Ectocervical.**
   1. Cryotherapy.
   2. Laser therapy.
   3. Topical 5-fluorouracil.
   4. Local excision (biopsy forceps) if entire lesion well visualized.
B. **Endocervical.**
   1. Surgical or laser conization.
   2. Loop electrosurgical excision procedure.

MENOPAUSE

Menopause is the physiologic cessation of menstrual function. By definition, diagnosis is made after 6 months of amenorrhea. Hormonal replacement may abolish many of the symptoms and may prevent further health risks including osteoporosis and cardiovascular disease.

I. CLINICAL FEATURES

A. **Average age 51 years.** Symptoms begin in premenopausal years and progress as hormone levels decrease.

B. **Vasomotor symptoms.** Hot flashes, night sweats.

C. **Atrophic symptoms.** Vaginal dryness, pruritus, irritation, and dyspareunia; urinary symptoms of frequency, dysuria, and increased incidence of cystitis.

D. **Emotional symptoms.** Lability, irritability, depression, and insomnia.

E. **Increased risk of coronary artery disease.**

F. **Osteoporosis.** 50% bone loss in first 7 years; resultant fractures (hip, vertebral) major cause of increased morbidity and mortality.

II. MANAGEMENT

A. **Hormone replacement therapy (HRT).**

1. ***Benefits.*** Control of vasomotor, atrophic, and psychologic symptoms. It is cardioprotective, prevents osteoporosis, and may delay or prevent the development of Alzheimer's disease.
2. ***Risks.***
   a. Risk of endometrial hyperplasia or neoplasia doubles if estrogen used alone; however, it progestin added, less risk of cancer compared to non–hormonally treated patients.
   b. Breast cancer: controversial. Most recent data indicate that relative risk of invasive breast cancer is 1.41 in those taking estrogen and progesterone for 5 years or greater. Progesterone does not seem to have any beneficial effect for decreasing the risk of breast cancer.
   c. Other risks include hypertension (reversible) and thromboembolic disease.
   d. Postmenopausal estrogen may reduce incidence of heart disease, but most studies were done without progesterone.
   e. Contraindications include unexplained vaginal bleeding, active liver disease or chronically impaired liver function, carcinoma of the breast, endometrial carcinoma, recent vascular thrombosis, or past history of thromboembolic disease with previous hormone therapy.
   f. Relative contraindications include hypertension, uterine leiomyomas, migraine headaches, familial hyperlipidemia, endometriosis, and gallbladder disease.
3. ***Initial assessment.***
   a. History and physical highlighting breast and pelvic exam.

b. Baseline mammogram.
c. Vaginal smear to cytologist for maturation index (% of superficial, intermediate and parabasal cells). When superficial cells are present, estrogen production is normal.
d. Progestin challenge test (in those with uterus). Give progestin (medroxyprogesterone acetate 10 mg PO QD or norethindrone 2.5 to 5 mg PO QD) for 14 days. No withdrawal bleeding indicates no significant estrogen stimulation. May begin hormone replacement without endometrial biopsy. Withdrawal bleeding in perimenopausal women not receiving hormone replacement may signify inappropriate estrogen stimulation. Proceed to endometrial biopsy to exclude premalignant or malignant lesion before starting hormone replacement therapy (HRT). If estrogen contraindicated or refused, progestin should be given 14 days every month as long as withdrawal bleeding occurs to counteract the risk of endometrial hyperplasia with neoplasia.
e. Serum FSH. If vaginal smear and progestin challenge do not indicate estrogen deficiency, serum FSH >30 should prompt HRT.
f. Endometrial biopsy. Obtain before initiation of HRT if progestin challenge positive. Annual sampling not needed unless bleeding irregular, excessive, or prolonged. Not needed for breakthrough bleeding during first year of continuous combined regimen if initial progestin challenge negative.

4. ***Regimens.***
a. *Continuous unopposed estrogen.* Conjugated equine estrogen (Premarin) (0.625 mg PO QD) for those without a uterus. This may be increased to 1.25 mg PO QD if patient still has menopausal symptoms at 0.625 mg.
b. *Cyclic sequential.* Calendar days 1 to 25 Premarin 0.625 mg or Estrace 1 mg or Estraderm patch 0.05 mg QD plus medroxyprogesterone acetate 10 mg at days 13 to 25. If symptoms reoccur after day 25, continuous estrogen can be used as long as progesterone is given 10 to 14 days each month.
c. *Continuous combined.* Daily natural estrogens as in (b) plus daily medroxyprogesterone acetate 2.5 mg. Irregular bleeding common for 4 to 6 months with 60% to 65% amenorrheic by 6 months.
d. Other regimens less well studied.
e. The Postmenopausal Estrogen/Progestin Interventions Trial has unequivocally demonstrated that (1) estrogen or estrogen-progestin combination therapy

increases serum HDL and decreases serum LDL and fibrinogen levels and (2) the coadministration of a progestin (given either cyclically or continuously) with estrogen protects against endometrial hyperplasia.

OSTEOPOROSIS

1. Refers to postmenopausal bone loss from loss of estrogens. This leads to fractures of the hip and spine. More likely to occur in those who are of short stature, are white, smoke, have a sedentary lifestyle, and have a family history of osteoporosis. Additionally, hyperthyroidism (including iatrogenic) is a risk factor for osteoporosis. Risk decreased by obesity, presence of diabetes mellitus II.
2. **Diagnosis.** Radiograph will show bone loss only after there is 20% to 30% bone loss. Bone densitometry can be used to document bone loss but not recommended as a routine screening test.
3. **Treatment.** Osteoporosis prevention must be started early. Calcium 1000 to 1500 mg QD and vitamin D 400 U/day is useful for all women without contraindications regardless of age. Weight-bearing exercise and hormone replacement therapy can be used (see previous menopause section for details). Alendronate (Fosamax 10 mg PO once a day), a bisphosphonate, has been shown to be effective at preventing and treating osteoporosis. Its simultaneous use with estrogen has not been studied, but many physicians use these drugs together anyway. It must be taken in the morning with 8 oz. of water at least ½ hour before any other foods or fluids are taken. Miacalcin (salmon calcitonin) 1 spray in alternating nostrils each day is also acceptable therapy.
4. Fluoride, though it increases bone density, actually increases hip fracture risk.

INFERTILITY

Involuntary infertility is defined as the inability to conceive during one or more years of unprotected intercourse. It is increasing in incidence. Affects 20% of couples today.

I. GENERAL INFORMATION

A. **Average time to conception.** 3 months.
B. **Contributing factors.** Delay in childbearing, increasing incidence of PID with tubal damage.
C. Acknowledge emotional nature of problem and define infertility as a couple's shared concern.
D. **Common major problems.** Male factors, ovulation disorders, uterine and tubal disease, or a combination of these factors. Less common problems include cervical problems or immune infertility. Since up to 50% of couples have some component of male factor infertility, a semen analysis is a crucial early step in evaluation.

II. DIAGNOSTIC EVALUATION

A. Thorough history and physical examination of both male and female, inquiring about sexual practices and difficulties. Even seemingly innocuous lubricants such as K-Y or petroleum jelly can be spermicidal.

B. Semen analysis. Collected after a 2 or 3-day period of abstinence in glass container. If pyospermia present, search for and treat infections of urethra, epididymis, or prostate. If otherwise abnormal, repeat in 2 weeks. If abnormalities persist, refer to urologist for further evaluation. Other male causes for infertility include testicular disorders, endocrine abnormalities, ductal obstruction, retrograde ejaculation, varicocele, or hypospadias. Treatment is specific to cause.

C. Ovulation assessment.

1. Symptoms of ovulation (such as *Mittelschmerz*, PMS), regularity of menstrual cycle.
2. Basal body temperature charting. Should see 0.5 to 1.0 Fahrenheit degree increase with ovulation. Expect 11 or more days between temperature rise and onset of menses with normal luteal phase.
3. Low serum progesterone level on day 21 of cycle is suggestive of luteal phase defect.
4. Evaluate and treat menstrual abnormalities.
   a. *Amenorrhea.* Rule out premature ovarian failure, confirmed by FSH >40 ng/ml and estradiol <40 picograms/ml in same sample.
   b. *Oligomenorrhea with hirsutism or galactorrhea.* Suspect polycystic ovary disease. Assess for hyperprolactinemia, and, if present, work up to exclude pituitary cause. If idiopathic hyperprolactinemia, treat with bromocriptine 2.5 mg QHS until BBT demonstrates ovulation. Dose can be increased by 2.5 mg every 3 days until prolactin normal with maximum daily dose 15 mg. If no ovulation in 2 months, add clomiphene. Hypothyroidism can be associated with hyperprolactinemia and should be evaluated and treated.
   c. *Luteal phase defect.* Inadequate progesterone secretion by corpus luteum or lack of endometrial responsiveness. Confirm luteal phase defect by endometrial biopsy 1 to 2 days before expected menses. Biopsy will be out of phase >2 days relative to ovulation estimated by BBT. Treat with supplemental vaginal progesterone suppositories 25 mg BID starting 3 days after ovulation. Continue until menses or if pregnancy occurs, continue until week 10 when placental progesterone is sufficient to support pregnancy.

D. Ovulation induction if documented defect found.

1. Clomiphene citrate 50 mg QD for days 5 to 9 after either induced or spontaneous bleeding. Monitor for ovulation

with BBT or ovulation kits that detect LH surge about 12 to 24 hours before ovulation to allow timing of intercourse. During the following cycle the dose can be increased to a range of 100 to 200 mg QD to achieve serum progesterone level on day 21 of >10 ng/ml to counteract any luteal phase defect that might affect implantation. Side effects include ovarian enlargement and hot flashes. 5% to 10% of patients have multiple gestation.

2. If clomiphene alone is not effective, use clomiphene as above plus 10,000 IU HCG 5 to 7 days after clomiphene.
3. Human menopausal gonadotropin (Pergonal) is used for hypothalamic-pituitary insufficiency. Multiple gestations occur at rates higher than those with other ovulation regimens, and close monitoring is required.

E. Tubal functioning related to prior PID, ectopic, abdominopelvic surgery, IUD use.

1. Hysterosalpingogram to assess patency and identify uterine anomalies, fibroids, synechiae.
2. Laparoscopy if no cause found after work-up as outlined above.

F. Cervical factor, postcoital testing, role of sperm antibodies, and cervicitis are controversial.

ECTOPIC PREGNANCY

Ectopic pregnancy is potentially life threatening and, though common, may be difficult to diagnose. It must be suspected in any woman with vaginal bleeding and lower abdominal pain.

I. GENERAL INFORMATION

A. 98% of ectopics are tubal rather than cervical or abdominal.

B. Risk factors: Previous ectopic, current IUD use, prior tubal surgeries, history of PID, prior infertility.

II. EVALUATION

A. Symptoms. Abdominal pain (98%), amenorrhea (65%), vaginal bleeding (80%), with or without symptoms of early pregnancy, nausea, vomiting, syncope, dizziness, referred shoulder pain, tenesmus, low-grade fever.

B. Exam. Check vital signs for orthostatic changes, hemodynamic instability. Pelvic views may be normal early on; only 50% have adnexal mass. Uterus may be enlarged secondary to deciduation or blood. Cervical motion tenderness may be found as well as doughy cul-de-sac secondary to bleeding.

C. Unstable patient. When an acute abdominal emergency or hemorrhagic shock is suspected, immediate culdocentesis will confirm hemoperitoneum (>5 ml of nonclotting blood). When combined with a positive urine pregnancy test, a positive culdocentesis allows one to predict ectopic pregnancy in

>99% cases. Do not waste time getting a serum pregnancy test or an ultrasonogram. Obtain immediate surgical consultation.

D. **Lab tests.** *Pregnancy test.* Sensitivity of assay must be known. Newer urine tests are more sensitive (50 to 200 mIU of HCG/ml). Optimal test is quantitative *beta-HCG,* detecting 15 to 50 mIU of HCG/ml roughly at time of expected menses or 7 days after implantation.

E. **Ultrasonography.** The "discriminatory zone" is the range of serum beta-HCG (6000 to 6500 mIU/ml) above which an intrauterine pregnancy should be detectable by transabdominal ultrasonography in 95% of cases. With the use of transvaginal ultrasonography this is now lowered to about 1500 (though still center dependent) when an intrauterine sac ought to be visible, making ectopic unlikely. Ultrasonographic findings may include the presence of a solid, cystic or complex adnexal mass adjacent to a slightly enlarged uterus, absence of intrauterine sac, and free fluid (blood) in the cul-de-sac. Adnexal mass often not detectable until HCG in 3500 to 6500 mIU/ml range.

F. In stable patient, if unable to exclude ectopic pregnancy by ultrasonography, consider serial measurements of quantitative beta-HCG to distinguish ectopic from early intrauterine. If HCG does not rise by 66% in 48 hours, suspect ectopic. Following serum progesterone levels also can be helpful.

III. TREATMENT

Treatment is surgical though some centers are using methotrexate therapy in patients that have early ectopic pregnancy and no fetal heart motion by ultrasonography.

IV. FERTILITY IMPLICATIONS

On average 30% of patients are infertile after an ectopic pregnancy.

CHRONIC PELVIC PAIN

I. CHARACTERISTICS

Duration of 6 months or longer, incomplete relief by most previous treatments, significantly impaired function at home or at work, signs of depression (early morning awakening, weight loss, anorexia), pain out of proportion to pathologic condition, altered family roles.

II. CAUSES

A. **Causes of noncyclic pelvic pain.** Pelvic inflammatory disease, pelvic adhesions, and uterine displacement. *Musculoskeletal disorders:* poor posture, scoliosis, unilateral standing habits, lumbar lordosis, leg-length discrepancy, abnormal gait. Abdominal wall trigger points, history of low back trauma. *Urinary tract disorders:* urethral syndrome, interstitial cystitis. *Gastrointestinal tract disorders:* irritable bowel syndrome, chronic constipation, and diverticulitis. *Psychogenic and psychologic factors* may also be important as in cases of sexual or physical abuse or if the patient has a history of depression, post–traumatic stress disorder, somatoform disorder, or a panic or anxiety disorder.

B. Predominantly cyclic. *Mittelschmerz*, primary and secondary dysmenorrhea, endometriosis, adenomyosis, cervical stenosis, intrauterine device, leiomyomas, premenstrual syndrome.

III. HISTORY

A. Location of pain.
B. Relationship of the pain to menstruation, sexual activity, bladder and bowel function, and emotional state.
C. Sexual abuse history.
D. Previous abdominopelvic surgical procedures or episodes of PID.
E. Psychologic response to pain and its effect on lifestyle, family, and friends should also be determined.

IV. EVALUATION

A. Physical examination focusing on the abdomen and pelvis. The examiner should probe for abdominal wall trigger points and evaluate for musculoskeletal disorders and tenderness of the bladder, urethra, and other pelvic organs.
B. Psychometric testing (as with Beck Depression Scale) as indicated.
C. Lab tests. UA and urine culture, CBC, stool guaiac, Pap smear, cervical cultures. Endoscopy, colonoscopy, barium enema as indicated.

V. MANAGEMENT

A. Pain.

1. Once a pathologic cause of chronic pelvic pain is ruled out, provide symptomatic relief. Pain relief may be achieved with the scheduled dosing of an NSAID (ibuprofen, naproxen).
2. If a trigger point is identified, it may be injected with 5 to 10 ml of 0.25% bupivacaine and 40 mg of triamcinolone. Trigger-point injections may at first be repeated Q2-4 weeks followed by successively longer intervals until the nidus of pain resolves.
3. Low doses of tricyclic antidepressants (Tofranil, Elavil) taken at bedtime also decrease pain intensity and promote sleep. May exacerbate constipation.
4. Relaxation techniques, stress management, and pain-coping strategies may also be tried.

5. Functional bowel disorders: daily psyllium supplements and increased dietary fiber can reestablish normal bowel motility and relieve the symptoms of irritable bowel syndrome and constipation.

B. Depression. See Chapter 15.

C. Surgical management. Diagnostic laparoscopy, lysis of adhesions, uterine suspension, uterosacral nerve ablation, presacral neurectomy, hysterectomy.

SEXUAL ASSAULT

I. DEFINITION

Sexual assault may be defined as any sexual act performed by one person to another without that person's consent. It may be the result of the use or threat of force, coercion, or the victim's inability to give appropriate consent.

II. HISTORY

It is critical to do this history and examination in a supportive, nonjudgmental environment. Contact with a local rape crisis center that may provide a trained counselor to be at the bedside is helpful. Determine patient's age, description of events (use of force, nature of assault, documentation of physical and emotional condition of the patient), thorough sexual and gynecologic history (menstrual history, birth control regimen, and pregnancy status).

III. PHYSICAL EXAMINATION

A. Obtain informed consent.

B. Collect clothing (if victim has not changed clothes).

C. Body evaluation. Examine for cuts, bruises, and bite marks. Procure photographs or drawings of injured areas. Obtain fingernail scrapings and sample the dried and moist secretions and foreign material on the patient's body. Use a Wood's lamp to detect semen. *Oral cavity:* swab for semen if within 6 hours of the assault; examine for injuries from oral penetration. Culture for gonorrhea. *Genitalia:* hair combing, hair sample, sample vaginal secretions, cultures for GC and other STDs. Examine for gynecologic disease, trauma, and foreign objects. *Rectum:* examine for trauma; culture rectum for gonorrhea.

D. Lab tests. Blood type, RPR, pregnancy test, alcohol/drug screen, UA. Smears of vaginal secretions or a Pap smear should be made to document the presence of sperm. DNA fingerprinting by wet or dry swab. Motile sperm may be present in the vagina for up to 8 hours after intercourse but may be present in the cervical mucus for as long as 2 to 3 days. Nonmotile sperm may be noted in the vagina for up to 24 hours and in the cervix for up to 17 days. If no sperm are noted, evidence of residual acid phosphatase should still be sought, since the attacker may have had a vasectomy.

IV. RAPE-TRAUMA SYNDROME

A. Acute phase. May last for hours to days and is characterized by a distortion or paralysis of the individual's coping mechanism. Generalized body pain, eating and sleeping disturbances, vaginal discharge, itching and rectal pain, depression, anxiety, and mood swings may be present.

B. Delayed or organizational phase. Characterized by flashbacks, nightmares, phobias, and a need for reorganization of thought processes, in addition to gynecologic and menstrual complaints. This phase may occur months or years after the event.

C. Counseling. Should be phase specific.

V. PROPHYLACTIC THERAPY

A single dose of ceftriaxone 250 mg IM plus either doxycycline 100 mg PO BID for 7 days or azithromycin 1 g PO prophylaxes the patient against gonorrhea, chlamydiosis, and syphilis. Spectinomycin could be substituted for ceftriaxone, if required. Erythromycin can be substituted for doxycycline in a pregnant woman. The patient should be instructed to return for repeat serologic tests in 3 to 4 weeks. The patient should be counseled about possible HIV infection. HIV serologic analysis should be obtained at the time of assault and repeated in 6 months. If the patient is at risk for pregnancy, a morning-after regimen should be instituted if desired by patient (see section on contraception, p. 299), and a pregnancy test should be performed during the return visit. If the patient is pregnant, she should be counseled about all available options. Arrange for follow-up medical care and counseling.

VI. CHILD SEXUAL ABUSE

A. Babies, children, handicapped people, and the elderly can be victims of sexual assault. A high index of suspicion is needed for diagnosis.

B. Symptoms. *Behavioral:* anxiety, sleep disturbances, withdrawal, somatic complaints, increased sex play, inappropriate sexual behavior, school problems, acting-out behaviors, self-destructive behaviors, depression, low self-esteem. *Physical:* unexplained vaginal injuries, unexplained vaginal bleeding, bruising, bites, scratches, pregnancy, sexually transmitted disease, recurrent vaginal infections, pain in the anal or genital area, recurrent atypical abdominal pain.

C. Physical findings

1. ***Nonspecific.*** Redness of external genitalia, increased vascular pattern of the vestibule and labia, presence of purulent discharge from the vagina, small skin fissures or lacerations in the area of the posterior fourchette, and agglutination of the labia minora.
2. ***Specific findings.*** Recent or healed lacerations of the hymen and vaginal mucosa, an enlarged hymenal opening

of 1 cm or more, procto-episiotomy, and indentations in the skin indicating teeth marks (bite marks), laboratory confirmation of a venereal disease.

3. ***Definitive findings.*** Any presence of sperm.
4. Colposcopy allows a detailed magnified inspection of the vulva to search for physical signs of abuse that may have escaped detection by unaided examination. However, most findings are visible to the naked eye. *Take pictures and document any findings well.*

BIBLIOGRAPHY

Abbott J: Clinical and microscopic diagnosis of vaginal yeast infection: a prospective analysis, *Ann Emerg Med* 25(5):587-591, 1995.

Blackwell RE: The infertility workup and diagnosis, *J Reprod Med* 34(1;suppl):81-84, 1989.

Brotzman GL et al: The minimally abnormal Pap smear, *Am Fam Physician* 53(4):1154-1162, 1995.

Cervical Cytology, *ACOG Techn Bull*, No 183, 1993 (American College of Obstetricians and Gynecologists, Washington, D.C.).

Colditz GA et al: The use of estrogens and progestins and the risk of breast cancer in postmenopausal women, *N Engl J Med* 332(24):1589, 1995.

D'Amico JF, Gambone JC: Advances in the management of the infertile couple, *Am Fam Physician* 39(5):257-264, 1989.

Gambrell RD: Update on hormone replacement therapy, *Am Fam Physician* 46(5; suppl):87-95, 1992.

Gorol A et al, editors: *Primary care medicine,* ed 2, Philadelphia, 1987, Lippincott.

Gross Z et al: Ectopic pregnancy: nonsurgical, outpatient evaluation and single-dose methotrexate treatment, *J Reprod Med* 40(5):371, 1995.

Herbst AL et al: *Comprehensive gynecology,* St. Louis, 1992, Mosby.

Leach RE, Ory SJ: Management of ectopic pregnancy, *Am Fam Physician* 41(4):1215-1222, 1990.

Lipscomb GH, Ling FW: Chronic pelvic pain, *Office Gynecol* 79:1411-1425, 1995.

Mazur MT, Kurman RJ: *Diagnosis of endometrial biopsies and curettings: a practical approach,* New York, 1995, Springer-Verlag.

McBride WZ: Spontaneous abortion, *Am Fam Physician* 43(1):175-182, 1991.

Menkes DB et al: Fluoxetine treatment of severe premenstrual syndrome, *Br Med J* 305:346, 1992.

Moore TR et al: *Gynecology and obstetrics: a longitudinal approach,* New York, 1993, Churchill Livingstone.

Ory SJ: New options for diagnosis and treatment of ectopic pregnancy, *JAMA* 267(4):534-537, 1992.

Osteoporosis, *ACOG Techn Bull,* No 167, May 1992 (American College of Obstetricians and Gynecologists, Washington, D.C.).

Pelvic organ prolapse, *ACOG Techn Bull* No 214, Oct 1995 (American College of Obstetricians and Gynecologists, Washington, D.C.).

Pernoll ML, editor: *Current obstetric and gynecologic diagnosis and treatment,* Norwalk, Conn., 1991, Appleton & Lange.

Rakel R, editor: *Conn's current therapy,* Philadelphia, 1996, Saunders.

Rivlin ME et al, editors: *Manual of clinical problems in obstetrics and gynecology with annotated key references,* ed 2, Boston, 1986, Little, Brown & Co.

Sanford JP: *Guide to antimicrobial therapy 1996,* Dallas, Texas, 1996, Antimicrobial Therapy, Inc.

Scott JR et al: *Danforth's obstetrics and gynecology,* Philadelphia, 1994, Lippincott.

Sexual assault, *ACOG Techn Bull,* No 172, Sept 1992 (American College of Obstetricians and Gynecologists, Washington, D.C.).

Speroff L et al: *Clinical gynecologic endocrinology and infertility,* Baltimore, 1994, Williams & Wilkins.

The Writing Group for the PEPI Trial: Effects of estrogen or estrogen/progestin regimens on heart disease risk factors in postmenopausal women, *JAMA* 273:199-208, 1995.

The Writing Group of the PEPI Trial: Effects of hormone replacement therapy on endometrial histology in postmenopausal women, *JAMA* 275:370-375, 1996.

Tintinalli JE et al: *Emergency medicine: a comprehensive study guide,* New York, 1995, McGraw-Hill.

Uterine leiomyomata, *ACOG Techn Bull,* No. 192, May 1994 (American College of Obstetricians and Gynecologists, Washington, D.C.).

Wathen PI et al: Abnormal uterine bleeding, *Med Clin North Am* 79:321-341, 1995.

Webb AMC et al: Comparison of Yuzpe regimen, danazol, and mifepristone (RU486) in oral postcoital contraception, *Br Med J* 305(6859):927-931, 1992.

Wells RG: Managing miscarriage, *Postgrad Med* 89(2):207-212, 1991.

Wickes SL: Clinics in office practice, *Prim Care* 15(3):473, 1988.

8

Obstetrics

PETER P. TOTH AND A. JOTHIVIJAYARANI

PRECONCEPTION CARE

Preconception care is intended to prevent congenital anomalies and is offered to all women of childbearing age, since more than 50% of pregnancies are unplanned.

A. **Proved benefits.** Prevention of neural tube defects by folic acid supplementation. Tight glucose control in DM results in lower incidence of congenital abnormalities. Identify and control, when possible, factors leading to previous poor results in pregnancy (such as preterm labor, antiphospholipid antibody syndrome).

B. **Prepregnancy advice.** Proper nutrition, exercise, smoking cessation, abstinence from alcohol and drugs, protection from radiation (x rays) and workplace exposures, information on prescribed and OTC drugs to avoid teratogenicity, infection control (STD protection and treatment, rubella and hepatitis immunity status), and psychosocial counseling for planning a pregnancy.

PRENATAL CARE

I. HISTORY AT INITIAL EVALUATION

A. **Menstrual history.** Cycle length, age of menarche, pain with menses, duration of flow, characteristics of previous two menses, previous methods of contraception. Establish dates carefully based on first day of last menstrual period and uterine size. Obtain ultrasonogram if in doubt.

B. **Medical history.** Underlying problems or illnesses, history of sexually transmitted diseases, medications, family history, and genetic history.

C. **Habits.** Tobacco, alcohol, other recreational drugs, diet, activity. Moderate caffeine intake (100 mg/day or 1 cup of coffee per day) does not appear to increase the risk of spontaneous abortion or IUGR.

D. Obstetric history. Dates of all pregnancies including termination and spontaneous abortions. Outcome and gestational length. Duration of labor, complications. Particular note should be made of previous shoulder dystocia, premature labor, PROM, placenta previa, and postpartum hemorrhage. *Type:* normal spontaneous vaginal delivery (NSVD), forceps, C-section (indication, type of uterine incision). Weight, sex, and Apgar scores of liveborn infants. Neonatal complications. Number of living children.

E. Social history. Occupational hazards, support network, father of child involved, wanted pregnancy, expectations, potential stresses, need of social or financial services.

II. PHYSICAL EXAMINATION

A. General physical exam. Particular attention to height, weight, BP, thyroid gland, dentition, heart, breasts, deep tendon reflexes, signs of underlying heart disease.

B. Pelvic examination.

1. ***External.*** Look for evidence of condylomata acuminata. These lesions may progress during pregnancy, and a small percentage of infants born through involved vaginal tissue will develop laryngeal papillomas. Podophyllin is contraindicated during pregnancy, but cryotherapy, laser, and TCA may be used. Also look for and culture lesions suspicious for herpes simplex.
2. ***Vaginal and cervical.*** Look for evidence of condylomas and herpes. Examine vaginal discharge and evaluate for *Candida*, *Trichomonas,* and bacterial vaginosis (BV); culture cervical discharge for GC and *Chlamydia.* Treat any vaginal infection. It is particularly important to screen for and treat BV, since it is associated with an increased risk of preterm labor, premature rupture of membranes, preterm birth, and histologic chorioamnionitis. Treatment with either metronidazole or erythromycin has been shown to reduce premature births among pregnant women with BV. Rule out cervical anomalies. Pap smear should be obtained if patient has not had one in last 6 months.
3. ***Bimanual.*** Rule out adnexal abnormalities. Determine uterine size: 8 weeks = 2 × normal; 10 weeks = 3 × normal; 12 weeks = 4 × normal; 16 weeks = halfway to umbilicus; 20 weeks = at umbilicus. Thereafter rely on fundal height.
4. ***Urinary tract.*** UA.

III. LABORATORY EVALUATION

A. First visit.

1. ***Routine.*** Pap smear, CBC, UA, and screen for bacteriuria, ABO blood type, Rh type, antibody screen (indirect Coombs'), VDRL test, rubella antibody titer, and hepatitis

B surface antigen. Treat asymptomatic bacteriuria to prevent pyelonephritis during pregnancy. Urine should also be screened for protein and glucose by dipstick at each visit.

2. ***When indicated.*** Cervical culture for GC and *Chlamydia*, Toxoplasmosis antibody test, sickle cell preparation, or hemoglobin electrophoresis in all previously unscreened black women, tuberculin skin testing, HIV antibody testing, and CMV titers.

B. During pregnancy.

1. ***15 to 20 weeks.*** Serum triple-screen (alpha-fetoprotein [AFP], beta-HCG, and estradiol). See below.
2. ***14 to 20 weeks.*** Amniocentesis, when indicated.
3. ***24 to 28 weeks.*** Blood glucose screen after 50 g of oral glucose and urine culture.
4. ***28 to 32 weeks.*** Hematocrit.
5. ***36 weeks.*** Rh antibody screening if indicated. Consider GC, *Chlamydia,* and herpes rescreening in high-risk women. Repeat hematocrit if indicated. Some suggest screening for group B streptococci at 36 to 37 weeks. See protocol below.

IV. EXPECTED WEIGHT GAIN

1. ***First trimester.*** Should gain 2 to 5 lb total.
2. ***After first trimester.*** ¾ to 1 lb per week.
3. ***Average total weight gain.*** 25 ±5 lb.

PRENATAL PATIENT EDUCATION

I. NUTRITION IN PREGNANCY

Periodic dietary recall will identify abnormal nutrition patterns.

A. Caloric requirements.

1. ***Requirements.*** 30 to 35 kcal/kg/day plus 300 kcal/day. Requirements are higher in adolescence and with multiple gestation. Adolescents are at increased risk of giving birth to small-for-gestational-age infants.

B. Calcium.

1. ***Requirements.*** 1200 to 1500 mg of elemental calcium per day.
2. ***Calcium supplement.***
   a. Milk, 8 oz glass: 300 mg of calcium.
   b. Generic calcium carbonate (260 mg Ca[II]/650 mg tablet) (40% elemental Ca[II]).
   c. Calcium gluconate chewable (45 mg Ca[II]/500 mg tablets; 9% elemental calcium).
   d. Tums regular strength (200 mg Ca[II]/500 mg chewable tablet).
   e. May reduce the risk of preeclampsia.

C. Iron.

1. ***Requirements.*** 30 mg of elemental iron per day.

2. ***Additional requirements.*** If the pregnant woman is iron deficient or has a multiple-gestation pregnancy, she should take 60 to 100 mg of elemental iron per day. If her Hg is <10, she requires 200 mg/day.
3. ***Iron Supplements.***
   a. Ferrous sulfate 65 mg of elemental Fe per 324 mg tablet (20% elemental iron).
   b. Ferrous fumarate 106 mg Fe/325 mg tablet (33% elemental iron).
   c. Ferrous gluconate 38 mg Fe/325 mg (11.6% elemental iron).

D. Folic acid.

1. ***Requirements.*** 1 mg/day. All prescription prenatal vitamins contain 1 mg of folate. OTC prenatal vitamins contain >0.8 mg of folic acid.
2. ***Sources.*** Green leafy vegetables, broccoli, mushrooms, liver.
3. *Adequate folate before conception has been shown to reduce the risk of neural tube defects.*

ACTIVITY

A. Occupation. Abstinence from physical work may be recommended if the woman has a history of two previous premature deliveries, an incompetent cervix, or fetal loss secondary to uterine anomalies. No controlled clinical trials have demonstrated efficacy of bed rest for any of these conditions. Women with multiple gestations beyond 28 weeks, premature rupture of membranes, CHF, hemoglobinopathies, Marfan's syndrome, or diabetes with multiple end-organ involvement are also at risk for complications and may benefit from reduced activity. Furthermore bed rest is indicated if there is a suspicion of IUGR, preeclampsia, or preterm labor.

B. Other. There are no routine restrictions on sexual relations, other than comfort and position. Caution should be used if any of the conditions listed above apply.

HABITS AND MISCELLANEOUS

A. Alcohol. Increases the risk of midtrimester abortion, mental retardation, behavior and learning disorders. 10% to 30% risk of fetal alcohol syndrome in offspring of women who drink 3 to 5 drinks per day. Risks with lesser consumption unknown.

B. Tobacco. Increases the risk of low-birth-weight infants, premature labor, spontaneous abortions, stillbirth, and birth defects. Three times greater incidence of upper respiratory infections and otitis media in young children of smoking parents.

C. **Crack cocaine or other illicit drug use.** Associated with perinatal addiction, preterm labor, and cognitive and psychologic difficulties in the infant. Cocaine abuse during pregnancy is associated with a significant increase in the incidence of placental abruption.

D. **Seatbelts.** A seatbelt should be worn such that the belts do not directly cross the gravid uterus.

E. **Medications.** In general, no medications should be used without checking with a physician.

   1. ***FDA classification of medication with regard to adverse fetal effects.*** *Category A,* proved safe for fetus in human studies (such as prenatal vitamins); *category B,* adverse effect not demonstrated in animal studies with no human studies, or adverse effects shown in animal studies have not been reproduced in human studies (as with penicillin); *category C,* no adequate animal or human studies are available, or animal studies show adverse fetal effects with no human data; *category D,* evidence of fetal risk but benefits believed to outweigh the risks (as with carbamazepine); *category X,* drugs with proved fetal risks that outweigh any benefits.
   2. ***Drugs that are used in pregnancy with no known adverse effect at the usual dose (some are class B).*** Antihistamines, various classes of antihypertensives, diuretics, antibiotics, (penicillin, ampicillin, cephalosporins, erythromycin), nonquinine antimalarials, tuberculostatics (INH, PAS, and rifampin), metronidazole (avoid in first trimester if possible, though one study showed no teratogenicity), steroids. Recent additions to the list: aspirin, general anesthetics, oral hypoglycemics. Accidental use of clomiphene, bromocriptine, birth control pills, and vaginal spermicides have shown no adverse effects.

F. **Infections.** Avoid children with viral illnesses, especially if not rubella or CMV immune. Avoid direct contact with cat litter and eating raw meat to minimize contact with *Toxoplasma gondii.*

G. **Potential problems.** Advise patient to contact physician if she experiences vaginal bleeding, leakage of fluid, fever, persistent nausea or vomiting, burning on urination, severe abdominal pain, severe headache or visual disturbance, persistent RUQ pain with peripheral edema, decrease in fetal movement. (Generally after quickening, one should expect 4 or more fetal movements per hour or at least 10 discrete movements in 2 hours.)

Rh SCREENING AND Rh_0(D) IMMUNOGLOBULIN

I. PROTOCOL FOR ROUTINE Rh SCREENING AND ADMINISTRATION OF Rh_0(D) IMMUNOGLOBULIN

A. **Initial visit.** Draw blood for ABO group, Rh type, and antibody screening (indirect Coombs').

B. If patient is Rh negative. Repeat antibody screen at 26 weeks and, if no antibody is detected, give 300 µg of Rh_0(D) immunoglobulin (1 vial = 300 µg) IM. If antibody is detected, see III below.

C. After delivery. Check fetal ABO/Rh type. If infant is Rh positive, mother receives 300 µg of Rh_0(D) immunoglobulin IM within 72 hours of delivery.

D. 1 vial suppresses immunity to approximately 30 ml of whole blood (15 ml of Rh(+) packed RBCs).

II. ADDITIONAL Rh_0(D) IMMUNOGLOBULIN REQUIREMENTS

A. If at anytime during pregnancy a fetal-maternal hemorrhage is suspected, a Kleihauer-Betke (acid elution) test should be performed. If positive, 10 µg of Rh_0(D) immunoglobulin should be administered per milliliter of fetal blood calculated to have entered the maternal circulation. However, the Kleihauer-Betke test is not 100% sensitive, and so if there is trauma and a suggestion of fetal-maternal hemorrhage, presumptive use of Rh_0(D) is indicated.

B. A 50 µg dose of Rh_0(D) immunoglobulin (1 vial microdose = 50 µg) is indicated for an Rh-negative woman after a first trimester terminated or spontaneously aborted pregnancy.

C. A 300 µg dose of Rh_0(D) immunoglobulin is indicated for the Rh-negative woman who undergoes amniocentesis, who undergoes a spontaneous or induced abortion, or who has an ectopic pregnancy.

D. The Kleihauer-Betke test should be performed after delivery if a larger than usual fetal-maternal hemorrhage may have taken place, as with placental abruption. More than the standard 300 µg dose may be required (which protects only up to 15 ml of Rh-positive red blood cells).

III. ISOIMMUNIZATION.

If the patient is Rh negative and the antibody screen is position before Rh_0(D) immunoglobulin administration, obtain an antibody titer and refer to a specialist. These infants are at risk for erythroblastosis fetalis.

PRENATAL DIAGNOSIS OF CONGENITAL DISORDERS

A. Genetic screening. Genetic screening of all pregnant patients using a questionnaire to identify high-risk patients is recommended. Prenatal testing for congenital abnormalities is indicated in:

1. Advanced maternal age (>35 years of age).
2. History of previous pregnancy with chromosomal abnormalities.
3. Parents with chromosomal abnormality.
4. Pregnancies at risk for neural tube defect (NTD), inborn errors of metabolism.

5. Family history of Down syndrome and other chromosomal abnormalities and genetic diseases (such as Duchenne's muscular dystrophy, hemophilia).
6. History of recurrent spontaneous abortions.
7. *Ethnic predisposition:* Ashkenazi Jews and French Canadians for Tay-Sachs disease; African Americans for sickle cell anemia; Mediterranean and Asian descent for alpha-thalassemia; Greek and Italian descent for beta-thalassemia.

B. Methods of diagnosis.

1. Chorionic villus sampling at 10 to 12 weeks (fetal loss rate of 0.5% to 1.5%). No longer associated with increase in limb-reduction defects.
2. Early amniocentesis performed between 12 and 15 weeks with 1% to 2% fetal loss rate.
3. Midtrimester amniocentesis between 15 and 20 weeks with 0.5% to 1% fetal loss rate.
4. Fetal ultrasound examination before the above procedures.
5. Triple screen. Offer to all pregnant women at 15 to 20 weeks (see above).

C. Referral for genetic counseling and perinatal consultation for high risk. The patient's attitude toward termination should not influence the counseling, since foreknowledge of a fetal defect can facilitate psychologic adjustment, and arrangements can be made for management assistance by a perinatologist.

ALPHA-FETOPROTEIN (AFP)

I. OVERVIEW

The measurement of AFP in maternal serum at 15 to 20 weeks of gestation may be used as a screening test to detect fetal NTDs. To evaluate AFP levels one must take into account maternal weight and gestational age. Women with abnormal values should be referred for ultrasonography and amniocentesis. The test should be run by a laboratory familiar with AFP screening and with well-established reference ranges.

II. DISORDERS ASSOCIATED WITH ELEVATED AFP

1. Underestimated gestational age.
2. Open NTDs (meningomyelocele, anencephaly).
3. Fetal nephrosis and cystic hygroma.
4. Fetal GI obstruction, omphalocele, gastroschisis.
5. Prematurity, low birth weight, IUGR.
6. Abdominal pregnancy.
7. Fetal demise.

III. DISORDERS ASSOCIATED WITH LOW AFP LEVELS

1. Overestimated gestational age.
2. Missed abortions.

3. Molar pregnancies.
4. Chromosomal abnormalities (including Down syndrome).

IV. TRISOMY 21

Low estriol, elevated HCG, and low AFP are associated with trisomy 21 (Down syndrome). Many labs now routinely assay for these three in maternal serum drawn at 15 to 20 weeks of gestation.

V. PROJECTED OUTCOME

In the United States, the incidence of NTD is roughly 1 per 1000 live births. In a study of 21,000 nondiabetic women, 249 women (1.2%) had abnormal AFP values. Of these women, 42% had normal infants and 15% had twins. The rest had NTD (8%), fetal death (16.5%), or other abnormalities. Thus, roughly 55% of women with abnormal AFP levels (who have normal infants) will be referred for further testing.

VI. RISKS

Psychologic stress, false positive results, false reassurance, and potential fetal trauma secondary to amniocentesis.

ANTENATAL FETAL SURVEILLANCE

I. OBSTETRIC ULTRASONOGRAPHY

A. Indications.

1. Determine the presence or absence of an intrauterine pregnancy.
2. Determine gestational age.
3. Measure fetal growth and identify intrauterine growth retardation.
4. Identify multiple-gestation pregnancies.
5. Detect fetal anomalies (nearly 100% sensitive for detection of NTD).
6. Detect oligohydramnios or polyhydramnios.
7. Demonstrated placental abnormalities.
8. Identify maternal uterine and pelvic anomalies.

B. Timing. Will depend on the indication for ultrasonography. In general, the earlier ultrasonography is performed in pregnancy, the more accurate is the EDC. Fetal anomalies may not become apparent until after 20 weeks. Amniotic fluid volume and fetal movement, tone, and breathing in conjunction with an NST can be used to calculate scores on biophysical profiles (BPP). This can be helpful in the decision to induce or follow postdated pregnancies, high-risk pregnancies, or diabetic pregnancies.

II. AMNIOCENTESIS: INDICATIONS

1. ***Done at 14 to 18 weeks of gestation to identify selected inherited disorders in the following populations:***

a. Pregnancies in women 35 years of age or older.
b. Previous pregnancy resulting in the birth of a child with a chromosomal abnormality.
c. Down syndrome or other chromosome abnormality in either parent or close family member.
d. Mother is a carrier of any X-linked disease.
e. Neural tube defect in either parent or a first-degree relative.
f. Previous child born with a neural tube defect.
g. Abnormal serum AFP.
h. Either parent is a carrier of a genetically transmitted metabolic disease.
i. Pregnancy after three or more spontaneous abortions.

2. ***Done during late pregnancy to determine fetal lung maturity based on phospholipids.***
   a. *Lecithin-to-sphingomyelin (L/S) ratio.* If L/S >2.0, there is a low risk of respiratory distress secondary to prematurity.
   b. *Phosphatidylglycerol (PG).* PG first appears at 35 weeks of gestation and increases in concentration until 40 weeks. If present, it provides reassurance of fetal lung maturity.
3. ***Detect isoimmunization.***

III. INDICATIONS FOR NONSTRESS TEST AND BIOPHYSICAL PROFILE

1. Hypertension.
2. Diabetes mellitus.
3. Multiple gestation.
4. Suspected oligohydramnios or IUGR.
5. Known placental abnormality.
6. Maternal heart or renal disease.
7. Hemoglobinopathy.
8. Postdated pregnancies.
9. Previous unexplained fetal demise.
10. Maternal perceptions of decreased fetal movement.

IV. NONSTRESS TESTING (NST)

A. Equipment. External fetal heart rate monitor and uterine contraction monitor.

B. Indications. High-risk pregnancies as noted above. Timing should be the earliest point at which an intervention would be performed if a clearly abnormal result is obtained (generally 32 to 34 weeks).

C. Interpretations. A reassuring NST demonstrates three or more fetal movements accompanied by a fetal heart rate acceleration of 15 beats per minute or more lasting at least 15 seconds during a 20-minute period. Lack of fetal movement is nondiagnostic. A repeat NST should be performed after a meal. Lack of movement for short periods of time may be attributable to fetal sleep. However, absence of movement for prolonged periods of time may be ominous. The NST is abnormal when the criteria for a reassuring NST are not met or late or variable decelerations are present. A biophysical profile (BPP) is then indicated.

V. BIOPHYSICAL PROFILE (BPP)

A. Procedural details. Real-time ultrasonography coupled to external fetal heart rate and uterine contraction monitoring.

B. Indications. Same as for NST. May be used as early as 26 to 28 weeks for the surveillance of a complicated or high-risk pregnancy.

C. Interpretation. Five parameters are evaluated:

1. Fetal breathing movements
2. Gross body movements
3. Fetal tone
4. Amniotic fluid volume (look for pocket of amniotic fluid that measures 2 cm in two perpendicular planes)
5. Reactivity of fetal heart rate

Each component of the BPP is given a score of 0 (parameter absent) or 2 (parameter present). The total score ranges from 0 (ominous) to 10 (reassuring; infant at low risk of asphyxia). Further discussion of this topic is beyond the scope of this chapter.

NAUSEA AND VOMITING OF PREGNANCY

I. CAUSE

Unknown. Probably not related to serum HCG levels, but other hormones have been implicated (estradiol, thyroxine). The incidence of hyperemesis gravidarum (severe nausea and vomiting causing ketosis and dehydration requiring hospitalization) is increased in multiple gestation and molar pregnancies, and so ultrasonography is advisable. Exclude organic causes: disorders of GI tract, gallbladder, pancreas, hepatitis, urinary infection. In hyperemesis, elevation of serum transaminase and mild jaundice can be observed to return to normal after adequate hydration and nutrition. Hyperemesis gravidarum has a 26% recurrence rate in subsequent pregnancies.

II. OUTPATIENT MANAGEMENT

A. Reassurance that condition improves with time, usually by end of first trimester.

B. Avoid medications whenever possible.

C. Advise patient to arise slowly and to keep soda crackers at the bedside and eat before rising.

D. Omit iron supplementation until nausea resolves.

E. Eat frequent small meals and protein snacks at night.

F. Antiemetics.

1. Diphenhydramine (Benadryl) 25 to 50 mg PO Q6-8h.

2. Doxylamine succinate (Unisom) 25 mg ½ to 1 tablet PO QA.M. and QP.M.
3. Phosphorylated carbohydrate (Naus-A-Way, Emetrol, Nausetrol) 15 to 30 ml PO on arising and Q3h PRN for nausea.
4. Meclizine 25 to 100 mg PO BID to QID.
5. Pyridoxine (vitamin B_6) 25 mg PO TID.
6. Bendectin (10 mg of doxylamine succinate and 10 mg of pyridoxine) was removed from the market, though large studies have not shown evidence of teratogenicity.

III. INPATIENT MANAGEMENT

For those with severe symptoms, weight loss, dehydration, ketones in urine, or high urine specific gravity.

A. Correct hypovolemia, ketosis, and electrolyte imbalances with IV fluids.

B. Monitor fluid intake and output.

C. Give nothing by mouth for 24 to 48 hours.

D. Antiemetics as above; also consider phenothiazines:
1. Promethazine (Phenergan).
2. Chlorpromazine (Thorazine).
3. Prochlorperazine (Compazine).

E. Parenteral nutrition for prolonged vomiting.

F. Psychotherapeutic measures, stimulus control, biofeedback, and imagery can also be helpful.

DIABETES IN PREGNANCY

I. GESTATIONAL DIABETES MELLITUS (GDM)

A. Evaluation.

1. ***Glucose challenge test (GCT).***
   a. *Timing.* A GCT is frequently performed as a routine screen for GDM in all pregnancies at 24 to 28 weeks of gestation. It should be performed earlier if symptoms are present. Some sources recommend screening at the first prenatal visit if there are risk factors. Repeat at 24 to 28 weeks if previous test is negative.
   b. *Procedure.* A blood glucose level is obtained 1 hour after a 50 g oral glucose load.
   c. *Interpretation.* A level of 140 mg/dl or greater is abnormal. Although values below 140 mg/dl have a high negative predictive value, there are many false positive results. A 3-hour fasting glucose tolerance test should be done if GCT is >130 mg/dl.
2. ***Glucose tolerance test (GTT).***
   a. *Timing.* Follow-up an abnormal GCT result.
   b. *Procedure.* The patient must eat a diet containing at least 150 g of carbohydrate for 2 days. The patient has a serum glucose level obtained after an overnight fast and then ingests 100 g of glucose

solution. Serum glucose levels are then obtained at 1, 2, and 3 hours.

c. *Interpretation* (Table 8-1). If two or more of these readings are abnormal, the patient needs diabetic teaching. If blood glucose cannot be controlled with diet, the patient needs to be prescribed insulin.

B. Potential morbidity.

1. Infants born to diabetic mothers have 5 times the normal risk of respiratory distress syndrome.
2. Macrosomia and associated birth trauma are related to maternal hyperglycemia.
3. Increased incidence of neonatal hypoglycemia, hypocalcemia, and jaundice.
4. The incidence of congenital anomalies is increased with first-trimester hyperglycemia.
5. The mother has an increased incidence of preeclampsia, infection, postpartum bleeding, cesarean section.

C. Management of gestational diabetes.

1. ***Dietary adjustment is the mainstay of therapy.***
   a. Caloric intake should be 30 to 35 kcal/kg/day. Intake should be reduced to 24 kcal/kg/day if patient is obese.
   b. The patient should avoid cakes, candy, and other fast-acting carbohydrates.
   c. Dietary composition should be 50% to 60% carbohydrate, 20% to 25% protein, and 20% fat, with high fiber content.
   d. Exercise has shown added benefit along with dietary therapy.
2. ***Obstetric surveillance.***
   a. Early ultrasonography for accurate gestational dating.
   b. Follow every 2 weeks until 36 weeks and then weekly.
   c. Accucheck QID before meals and at bedtime.
   d. Check fasting blood glucose and review home monitoring at each visit. If fasting glucose levels are >105 mg/dl (or postprandial values are 120 to 130), the patient should be hospitalized to ensure adherence to diet.
   e. If fasting glucose remains >110 mg/dl, insulin therapy is indicated.
   f. Check for ketonuria daily to make sure there has been adequate caloric consumption.

TABLE 8-1
Upper Limits of Normal Serum Glucose Levels (mg/dl) with 3-hour GTT

Fasting	1 hour	2 hours	3 hours
105	190	165	145

g. If macrosomia is suspected, ultrasound examination is performed. If the estimated fetal weight is >4000 g, a cesarean section may be considered at term. Amniocentesis is helpful in documenting fetal lung maturity before cesarean section, since infants of diabetic mothers have delayed lung maturity when compared with infants of nondiabetic mothers of similar gestational ages.
h. Antepartum NST is often initiated on a weekly basis at 34 to 35 weeks of gestation but may be started earlier. If euglycemia can be documented, consider delaying monitoring until 38 weeks. After 40 weeks of gestation, fetal surveillance is initiated, and delivery is recommended if there is any evidence of fetal compromise.
i. Gestational diabetics should have a 75 g oral GTT checked 6 weeks post partum to rule out persistent carbohydrate intolerance. Counsel the patient that she has an approximate 35% risk of developing diabetes at some point in her life.

HYPERTENSION IN PREGNANCY, PREECLAMPSIA, AND ECLAMPSIA

I. PREGNANCY-INDUCED HYPERTENSION (PIH)

A. **Definition.** Hypertension in pregnancy is present when diastolic BP >90 mm Hg, systolic BP >140; systolic BP rises at least 30 mm Hg over baseline value or diastolic BP rises at least 15 mm Hg over baseline value.

B. **Risk factors for PIH.** First pregnancy, multiple gestation, polyhydramnios, hydatidiform mole, malnutrition, positive family history of PIH, underlying vascular disease. Molar pregnancy should be expected if PIH occurs early in gestation.

II. PREECLAMPSIA AND ECLAMPSIA

A. **Preeclampsia.** Defined as the presence of hypertension or PIH accompanied by proteinuria, edema, or both. Preeclampsia is divided into mild and severe forms.

1. ***Criteria for mild preeclampsia.***
   a. Hypertension as defined above but not meeting the criteria for severe preeclampsia.
   b. Proteinuria >300 mg/24 hours.
   c. Mild edema, signaled by weight gain >2 lb/week or >6 lb/month.
   d. Urine output >500 ml/24 hours.
2. ***Criteria for severe preeclampsia.***
   a. The presence of any of the systemic symptoms noted below categorizes the patient as having severe preeclampsia regardless of the blood pressure.
   b. BP >160/110 on 2 occasions at least 6 hours apart with patient on bed rest.

c. Systolic BP rise >60 mm Hg over baseline value.
d. Diastolic BP rise >30 mm Hg over baseline value.
e. Proteinuria >5 g/24 hours or 3+ or 4+ on urine dipstick.
f. Massive edema.
g. Oliguria <400 ml/24 hours.
h. Systemic symptoms including pulmonary edema, headaches, visual changes, right upper quadrant pain, elevated liver enzymes, or thrombocytopenia.
i. Presence of IUGR in fetus.

B. Eclampsia. *Occurrence of a seizure that is not attributable to other causes in a preeclamptic patient.*

III. EVALUATION OF PREGNANCY-INDUCED HYPERTENSION AND PREECLAMPSIA

A. History. Document risk factors and any symptoms outlined above.

B. Physical. Look for evidence of edema (particularly of the hands and face), BP changes, retinal changes, hyperreflexia, clonus, and RUQ tenderness.

C. Initial laboratory studies.

1. ***Blood.*** CBC, electrolytes, BUN and creatinine, uric acid, liver function tests (AST, ALT, LDH), and coagulation studies (PT, PTT, and fibrinogen degradation products). If patient is in labor, send a blood type and screen.
2. ***Urine.*** 24-hour collection for protein and creatinine clearance.
3. ***HELLP syndrome.*** Hemolyis; elevated liver function tests; low platelet count.
4. ***Lab test results that may be abnormal.*** *Uric acid (>5.5 ng/dl) may be elevated before there are other signs or symptoms of preeclampsia,* elevated or normal hemoglobin, creatinine >1.0 ng/dl, BUN >10 ng/dl, or decreased platelet count, hypoalbuminemia, increased LDH or AST, elevated fibrin degradation products, prolonged PT/PTT, schistocytes or helmet cells on peripheral smear (hemolysis).

D. Complications of preeclampsia. Eclamptic seizures, HELLP syndrome, hepatic rupture, DIC, pulmonary edema, acute renal failure, placental abruption, intrauterine fetal demise (IUFD), cerebral hemorrhage, cortical blindness, retinal detachment.

IV. MANAGEMENT OF PIH/PREECLAMPSIA

A. Ambulatory management. For pregnancy-induced hypertension without significant proteinuria, home bed rest is recommended. Home blood pressure monitoring, weight, and urine protein checks are helpful. It is generally recommended that antepartum surveillance (NST) begin early. Ultrasound exams should be performed periodically to ensure adequate amniotic fluid and to monitor for intrauterine growth retardation (IUGR).

B. Hospital management.

1. ***Indications.*** For women with pregnancy-induced hypertension and 2+ or greater proteinuria and for those who fail outpatient management. Bed rest with bathroom privileges is allowed. The goal of IV fluids in severe cases is to replace urine output and insensible losses.
2. ***Laboratory evaluation and weights.*** Performed daily to every other day. Antepartum surveillance including daily fetal movement count, daily NSTs, and weekly amniotic fluid determinations by ultrasonography is essential. Monitor symptoms such as headache, visual disturbances, epigastric pain.
3. ***Delivery is treatment of choice.*** Delivery should be accomplished when the fetus is mature but may be required early if maternal health is in danger or if there is evidence of fetal distress. Delivery is indicated when the patient meets criteria for severe preeclampsia. Betamethasone 12.5 mg IM given twice 24 hours apart to stimulate fetal lung maturation can be repeated weekly if pregnancy is prolonged. Electronic FHR monitoring during labor is indicated.

C. Antihypertensive therapy.

1. Indicated only if BP persistently >160/110.
2. Aim for a diastolic BP 90 to 100 mm Hg. Avoid overcorrection because normal blood pressures can result in placental hypoperfusion.
3. Diuretics are never indicated. These patients are already hypovolemic. ACE inhibitors are also not to be used during pregnancy.
4. Long-term medications (if the fetus is immature) include methyldopa (Aldomet), atenolol, and labetalol.

D. Anticonvulsive therapy.

1. *Seizure prophylaxis* is indicated in all preeclamptic patients during labor and delivery and for a minimum of 24 hours post partum. Some perinatologists continue IV magnesium therapy in preeclamptic patients until the patient begins to diurese. Seizures may occur in the absence of hyperreflexia, and increased DTRs may be present in the normal population; therefore, hyperreflexia is not a useful predictor of risk.
2. *Magnesium sulfate* is the drug of choice.
   a. Loading dose for seizure prophylaxis is 4 to 6 g of magnesium sulfate IV over 20 minutes and continued at 2 g/hour.
   b. *Treatment of seizures.* Magnesium sulfate 1 g/min IV until seizure controlled up to 4 to 6 g maximum. If this fails, see Chapter 1 for management of status epilepticus.

c. *Serum levels.* Therapeutic level is 4 mEq/L (takes 12 to 18 hours to equilibrate). Serum levels of magnesium sulfate are of dubious value, since infusions rarely go longer than 2 days. Monitor urine output (100 ml in 4 hours), presence of deep tendon reflexes.

d. Magnesium toxicity may be signaled by excessive drowsiness and absence of patellar reflexes. At levels of 10 to 12 mEq/L and above, muscle weakness, respiratory paralysis, and cardiac depression can occur. 10 ml of 10% calcium gluconate (or calcium chloride) may be administered IV push in the event of magnesium toxicity, or the infusion can be turned off for 1 to 2 hours.

e. Continue magnesium sulfate therapy at least 24 hours post partum. In 25% of the patients postpartum eclampsia can occur. Monitor urine output and can stop therapy if urine output is >200 ml/hour for 4 consecutive hours. Watch for postpartum hemorrhage because magnesium sulfate can relax the uterus.

E. Prevention. Daily aspirin 81 mg can be given after the first trimester in women with chronic hypertension, previous history or preeclampsia, DM, and SLE. However, the efficacy of aspirin for this indication has been called into question. Several studies show that aspirin makes no difference in maternal or fetal outcomes. A recent meta-analysis indicates that calcium supplementation during pregnancy may reduce the risk of preeclampsia and hypertension during pregnancy. These results will need to be confirmed. However calcium supplementation is innocuous and should be considered.

V. CHRONIC HYPERTENSION

A. Risks.

1. ***Maternal.*** If no superimposed preeclampsia occurs, there is no additional maternal risk. In the presence of superimposed preeclampsia (20%), there is increased maternal mortality, frequently from intracranial hemorrhage.
2. ***Fetal.*** There is an increased incidence of perinatal death, IUGR, and fetal distress.

B. Management.

1. Treatment of chronic hypertension can decrease maternal and, to some extent, fetal morbidity but cannot reduce the risks of superimposed preeclampsia. Appropriate medications include methyldopa, hydralazine, and beta-blockers.
2. During pregnancy, it is not appropriate to use:
   a. Sympathetic ganglion blockers (orthostatic hypotension)
   b. Diuretics (aggravation of volume depletion)
   c. ACE inhibitors (associated with fetal defects and neonatal renal failure)
3. Laboratory evaluation is performed early in pregnancy.

4. Obstetric visits are scheduled every other week at 24 weeks and weekly after 30 weeks.
5. Early ultrasonogram is obtained for dating, and repeated periodically to look for evidence of IUGR.
6. Antenatal surveillance (NSTs) should begin at 34 weeks.
7. The pregnancy should not be allowed to go beyond 40 weeks. Delivery may be required earlier if there is evidence of IUGR or fetal distress or if hypertension cannot be controlled by bed rest and medication.
8. Intrapartum monitoring is required during labor.
9. If there is evidence of IUGR, cesarean section is preferable to a prolonged induction.
10. Complicated cases or women with superimposed preeclampsia should be handled at an appropriate referral center.

EARLY ANTEPARTUM HEMORRHAGE

I. DEFINITION

Vaginal bleeding at <20 weeks of gestation.

II. SPONTANEOUS ABORTION DEFINITIONS

A. **Threatened abortion.** The early symptoms of pregnancy may be present. Mild cramps with bleeding. Cervix long and closed. Uterus appropriate for gestational age. Roughly 50% progress to inevitable abortion.

B. **Inevitable abortion.** Persistent cramps and moderate bleeding. Cervical os is open. (Do not confuse with an incompetent cervix, which is not associated with cramping and is potentially treatable. An incompetent cervix is associated with painless cervical dilatation.)

C. **Incomplete abortion.** As per inevitable abortion but with some retained products of conception in the uterus (blood clots may be mistaken for tissue) or cervical canal, causing ongoing cramping and excessive bleeding. Speculum examination reveals a dilated internal os and tissue present within the endocervical canal or vagina. Bleeding may be heavy.

D. **Complete abortion.** Entire conceptus expelled with decreasing or ceasing of cramps and bleeding. On examination, the uterus is firm, and smaller than one would expect for gestational length of pregnancy.

E. **Missed abortion.** Products of conception retained 3 or more weeks after fetal death. Signs and symptoms of pregnancy abate; pregnancy test becomes negative. Brownish vaginal discharge (rarely frank bleeding) occurs. Cramping rare. Uterus is soft and irregular. Ultrasound exam rules out live pregnancy.,

F. **Septic abortion.** Any of the above scenarios and temperature >38° C without other source of fever may be septic abortion. Associated with IUD or instrumentation during abortion. Abdominal and uterine tenderness are present as well as purulent discharge and possibly shock.

III. INCIDENCE AND CAUSES

A. 15% to 25% of clinically recognized pregnancies, perhaps closer to 50% of all conceptions.

B. Causes. Large proportion of fetal abnormalities incompatible with life (chromosomal and other), defective implantation, maternal infection, uterine and cervical anomalies.

IV. EVALUATION

A. History. Suggestive of pregnancy (missed period or periods, nausea, vomiting, breast tenderness) followed by cramping and spotting or bleeding often with passage of tissue. All patients with bleeding sufficient to soak one pad per hour or symptoms of orthostatic blood pressure drop (dizziness upon standing, faintness) need to be examined. Others may be followed closely by phone. Remember patients must be seen within 48 hours for RhoGAM if indicated.

B. Exam. Including stability of vital signs, orthostatic vital signs, pelvic exam looking for open or closed cervical os, tissue, other causes of vaginal bleeding (such as cervical eversion, polyp, infection, vaginal lesion, ectopic fetus). Size uterus. Check for fetal heart tones with Doppler scanning if 10 to 12 weeks.

C. Lab tests.

1. Pregnancy test positive in 75% of cases, and so negative pregnancy test does not rule out spontaneous abortion.
2. CBC, blood type, and antibody screen in all patients for Rh status. RhoGAM indicated for all Rh-negative, antibody-negative women.
3. Uterine ultrasonography or pathologic exam of tissue if indicated.

V. TREATMENT

A. If orthostatic hypertension, treat with IV normal saline or lactated Ringer's. Consider transfusion if Hg <8 g.

B. Threatened abortion. Bed rest if possible; use acetaminophen for discomfort, nothing in the vagina (no tampons, douches, intercourse), consider ultrasonography for gestational sac, cardiac activity, or to rule out ectopic pregnancy. Positive cardiac activity predictive of continued pregnancy $>90\%$. Consider monitoring quantitative beta-HCG for prognosis with rise $<66\%$ in 48 hours predictive of abortion or ectopic.

C. Incomplete or inevitable abortion.

1. Hospitalize if hypovolemic, anemic, or advanced gestation >12 weeks.

2. Tissue visible in os should be gently removed with ring forceps to allow contraction of uterus but minimizing manipulation to decrease risk of infection.
3. Patients with incomplete abortion (tissue passed with continued bleeding) often require suction curettage or D&C. Consider oxytocin drip as an alternative (20 IU in 1000 ml of crystalloid solution at 50 to 100 ml/hour). If unsuccessful, proceed with D&C.

D. Complete abortion. Discharge home if vital signs stable, Hg documented to be stable, and bleeding decreased. Consider methylergonovine (Methergine) 0.2 mg PO TID for 3 days if diagnosis certain or after uterine evacuation.

E. Missed abortion.

1. Obtain CBC with differential, platelet count, PT and PTT, and DIC panel if indicated.
2. Hospitalize if there are signs of infection, DIC, or if the fetus has been retained longer than 4 weeks.
3. Prepare to perform D&C.
4. Outpatient management may be considered if retained <4 weeks, if weekly fibrinogen levels are obtained, and if the patient is monitored closely for DIC. Fibrinogen levels <150 mg/dl call for immediate evacuation of the uterus.

F. Septic abortion.

1. Obtain CBC, UA, culture of discharge from uterus, blood cultures, chest radiograph for diagnosis of septic emboli, and abdominal radiograph diagnosis of perforation of the uterus (free air) or uterine foreign body. Electrolytes and ABG.
2. Organisms include both anaerobes and aerobes *(Bacteroides, Streptococcus, Enterobacter, Chlamydia, Clostridium).*
3. Hospitalize, treat sepsis, D&C, IV antibiotics:
   a. Doxycycline plus cefoxitin or imipenem or ticarcillin, or
   b. Clindamycin plus third-generation cephalosporin or gentamicin
4. Discharge to home with taking oral doxycycline or clindamycin.

VI. LONG-TERM MANAGEMENT

A. Give RhoGAM to Rh-negative women.

B. Provide emotional support.

C. Traditional but not well-founded recommendation is to wait 3 months before attempting conception. Having a single spontaneous abortion does not increase the risk of aborting the next pregnancy.

D. Evaluate couple for habitual abortion if the woman has had two or more successive spontaneous abortions. If the patient is a habitual aborter, obtain antiphospholipid antibody titers. Obtain tissue for karyotyping if possible.

E. **Ectopic pregnancy.** Vaginal bleeding occurs in 50% to 94% of patients with ectopic pregnancies. Pelvic pain is generally present. Abdominal tenderness is present in 97% of cases. Rebound tenderness may be present. The uterine size is suggestive of early pregnancy, and the cervix is typically tender on motion. An adnexal or cul-de-sac mass can be palpated in 40% of cases. Risk of ectopic pregnancy is increased if there is a history of tubal infection or surgery, endometriosis, or prior infertility problem, or if pregnancy occurred while using a progestin-only BCP or IUD. Serum progesterone levels may be used to differentiate intrauterine pregnancies from ectopic pregnancies and pregnancies destined to go to spontaneous abortion.

F. **Molar pregnancy.** Placenta undergoes trophoblastic proliferation and typically resembles a cluster of grapes. Occurs more often in women <20 or >40 years of age and almost always causes some degree of vaginal bleeding. Hydatidiform moles are associated with hyperemesis gravidarum and the onset of preeclampsia before the third trimester. The uterus is larger than expected for gestational age in 50% of the cases. Ovarian enlargement may occur secondary to thecal lutein cysts. Ultrasonographic findings typically show a “snowstorm” pattern.

LATE ANTEPARTUM HEMORRHAGE

I. DEFINITION

Vaginal bleeding that occurs after 20 weeks of gestation.

II. DIFFERENTIAL DIAGNOSIS

A. **Placenta previa.**

1. ***Incidence.*** Occurs in 1 of 200 deliveries. The diagnosis of placenta previa is very common in the second trimester, but more than 95% of these do not have placenta previa at delivery.
2. ***Classification.*** Placenta previa may be marginal, partial, or total.
3. ***Diagnosis.*** Vaginal bleeding is typically bright red and painless. The blood loss is not massive but tends to recur and become heavier as the pregnancy progresses. Diagnosis may be aided by ultrasonography. The advisability of a speculum exam is debatable. Digital examination is contraindicated other than in a double setup situation when delivery is desirable and can be rapidly accomplished by C-section. Maternal risk factors include increasing age, multiparity, and prior uterine scar. Associated with breech and transverse presentations.

B. **Placental abruption.**

1. ***Incidence.*** Placental abruption occurs in 10% of all deliveries. Severe abruption is rare.

2. ***Classification.***
   a. **Mild.** Slight vaginal bleeding (<100 ml), no FHR abnormalities are present; there is no evidence of shock or coagulopathy.
   b. **Moderate.** Moderate vaginal bleeding (100 to 500 ml) and uterine hypersensitivity with or without elevated tone. Mild shock and fetal distress may be present.
   c. **Severe.** Extensive vaginal bleeding (>500 ml), tetanic uterus, and moderate to profound maternal shock are present. Fetal demise and maternal coagulopathy are characteristic.
3. ***Diagnosis.*** The diagnosis of placental abruption is clinical. Although vaginal bleeding is present in 80% of cases, it may be concealed in the remainder (that is, retroplacental bleeding). Thus, the maternal hemodynamic situation may not be explained by observed blood loss. Pain and increased uterine tone are typically present. Risk factors include prior history of abruption, maternal hypertension, cigarette or cocaine use, increasing maternal age or multiparity. Abruption may be associated with preterm premature rupture of membranes, twin gestation after delivery of first infant and trauma.

C. Uterine rupture. Very rare. May mimic severe abruption. An abdominal film may show free interperitoneal air or an abnormal fetal position. Accompanied by persistent fetal bradycardia. Emergent C-section and hysterectomy are required.

D. Other. Vasa previa (velamentous insertion of the cord). Delivery should be by scheduled C-section. If pregnancy is allowed to progress to term, spontaneous rupture of membrane or amniotomy should be averted because it could lead to fatal bleeding for fetus and possibly mother. Cervical dilation with loss of mucus plug may be confused with other causes of vaginal bleeding or cervical or vaginal lesions (polyps, condylomas).

III. LABORATORY EVALUATION

Laboratory evaluation should include a CBC, type and cross, coagulation studies, urinalysis, and ultrasonography.

IV. MANAGEMENT OF PLACENTA PREVIA AND PLACENTAL ABRUPTION

A. Placenta previa.

1. If pregnancy 37 weeks or greater, or if fetal maturity has been documented, a cesarean section is indicated unless only a minimal degree of placenta previa is present.
2. If bleeding is sufficient to jeopardize the mother or fetus despite transfusion, cesarean section may be indicated regardless of gestation.

3. In the preterm gestation, expectant management is indicated in patients with no observed bleeding, reactive nonstress test, stable hematocrit, who are compliant with instructions. Most patients require inpatient observation. Physical activity is restricted. Nothing is allowed in the vagina, including examining fingers. The hematocrit is maintained at 30% or greater. Preterm labor can be managed with magnesium sulfate. Use of beta-adrenergic agents can cause tachycardia and mask the signs of bleeding. Once 36 to 37 weeks of gestation is reached with fetal maturity demonstrated by amniocentesis, the patient is readied for elective double-setup examination.
4. Check for fetal bleeding: To 5 ml of tap water add 6 drops of 10% KOH in two test tubes. Add 3 drops of maternal blood to one tube and 3 drops of vaginal blood to the other. The maternal blood will turn green yellowish brown after 2 minutes. If fetal red blood cells are present, the solution will turn pink. Immediate delivery is indicated.
5. Remember that placenta accreta may complicate placenta previa in women with history of previous C-section. Hemorrhage can necessitate hysterectomy.

B. Placental abruption.

1. If placental abruption is mild and the fetus is immature, expectant management may be indicated, with fetal heart rate monitoring and serial laboratory and ultrasound examination. Occasionally a small separation occurs without further problem. These patients have no uterine symptoms. Observation is required, but if no fetal distress occurs in the next 2 days, the patient may be sent home.
2. In all other cases, delivery is indicated. A vaginal delivery is preferred when fetal distress is not present or the fetus is no longer viable. A C-section is indicated if fetal distress is present. A C-section is also performed when there is a threat to the mother's life or a failed trial of labor.
3. Shock must be treated with adequate replacement of blood. Fresh whole blood is preferable. While awaiting blood, colloid may be used (1 ml of colloid [that is, albumin, Plasmanate]) for every milliliter of estimated blood loss or 3 ml of crystalloid (that is, NS or LR) per every milliliter of blood. Urine output must be maintained at 25 to 30 ml/hour. A central venous pressure line or Swan-Ganz catheter will assist in monitoring hemodynamic status.
4. Coagulopathy should be treated with fresh whole blood. Fresh frozen plasma is used alternatively. One unit of FFP increases the fibrinogen concentration by 25 mg/dl. Platelet transfusion is required if the count is less than 50,000. Heparin is not used in DIC secondary to placental abruption.

INTRAUTERINE GROWTH RETARDATION (IUGR)

I. DEFINITION

IUGR is a diagnosis that the fetus weighs less than the tenth percentile for its gestational age. *Symmetric IUGR (intrinsic):* normal head circumference–to–abdominal circumference ratio, caused by genetic disease and fetal infection with poor prognosis. *Asymmetric IUGR: (extrinsic):* increased HC/AC ratio, caused by placental insufficiency, good prognosis with appropriate treatment.

II. RISK FACTORS

A. Chronic maternal disease, chronic maternal hypertension, PIH, diabetes, cyanotic heart disease, collagen vascular disease, severe maternal anemia, renal disease, multifetal pregnancy.

B. Fetal genetic disorders or fetal malformations.

C. *Intrauterine infections.* Rubella, herpes, toxoplasmosis, syphilis, CMV.

D. Previous history of small-for-gestational-age baby, smoking, drug, or alcohol abuse.

E. Abnormalities of the placenta or placental blood flow.

III. DIAGNOSIS

One should be suspicious when the fundal height does not exhibit the predicted 1 cm/week growth between 20 and 36 weeks of gestation. A lag in fundal height by 4 cm warrants ultrasonographic evaluation. Serial ultrasonic scanning may confirm the diagnosis.

IV. MANAGEMENT

The development of IUGR makes the pregnancy high risk. Stillbirth, oligohydramnios, and intrapartum fetal acidosis are common antepartum complications. Close antepartum surveillance is required, and the decision on when to deliver the infant is complex. Neonatal complications include persistent fetal circulation, meconium aspiration syndrome, hypoxic ischemic encephalopathy, hypoglycemia, hypocalcemia, hyperviscosity, and defective temperature regulation. These pregnancies should be managed by a perinatologist.

VAGINAL BIRTH AFTER CESAREAN SECTION (VBAC)

I. DEFINITION

Attempted vaginal delivery in a woman who has undergone previous cesarean section.

II. DECISION TO ATTEMPT VBAC

A. Advantages.

1. Overall reduced morbidity and mortality compared with elective C-section.
2. Reduced expense relative to C-section.

3. Rising maternal preference.

B. Disadvantages.

1. Requires closer intrapartum monitoring than a low-risk delivery.
2. If unsuccessful, a C-section after a trial of labor has increased infectious morbidity compared to that of an elective C-section.

C. Contraindications.

1. History of previous classical, T-shaped, or unknown uterine incision.
2. Multiple gestation.
3. Estimated birth weight >4000 g.
4. Nonvertex presentation.
5. Inadequate facilities or personnel for emergency C-section.
6. Patient's refusal to consent.

D. Probability of success. Depends primarily on the indication from the previous C-section. If the primary C-section was for breech position, abruption, placenta previa, cord accident, antepartum hemorrhage, hypertensive disorder, or fetal distress, there is a 74% to 94% rate of success. If the primary C-section was for cephalopelvic disproportion (CPD) or failed induction, there is a 35% to 77% rate of success.

III. RISKS

A. Usual maternal and fetal risks of vaginal delivery.

B. Uterine rupture. Very rare. Incidence increased if prior C-section was classical.

C. Cesarean section. Increased risk of C-section morbidity relative to elective C-section. However, risks comparable to primary C-section.

IV. MANAGEMENT

A. Preparation.

1. Type and screen for 2 units of whole blood; intravenous line should be inserted.
2. The anesthesiologist, surgeon, and physician caring for the newborn infant must be notified in advance and be available.

B. Labor.

1. Electronic fetal monitoring is recommended.,
2. Oxytocin may be cautiously used to augment labor, and close monitoring of uterine contractions (using intrauterine pressure catheter) is necessary. **Oxytocin must be titrated with great care in a VBAC.**
3. The same expectations of normal progression during labor should be applied to patients with a prior C-section.
4. An experienced physician should be in attendance throughout labor and delivery.

C. Post partum. Manual exploration of the uterus after delivery of the placenta is indicated to assess scar integrity.

PRETERM LABOR

I. DEFINITION

Onset between 20 and 37 weeks of gestation of contractions occurring at least every 10 minutes and lasting 30 seconds. Discrimination from "false labor" is difficult unless there is cervical dilatation, which indicates true labor; however, postponement of treatment until this occurs may lower the chances of success.

II. CAUSE

Frequently unknown. Several factors have been associated with preterm labor.

A. Maternal factors. Infections (systemic, vaginal, urinary tract, amnionitis), uterine anomalies, fibroids, retained IUD, cervical incompetence, overdistended uterus (polyhydramnios, multiple gestation), rupture of membranes.

B. Fetal factors. Congenital anomalies, intrauterine death.

III. MANAGEMENT

A. Initial examination.

1. Estimate fetal weight and establish gestational age.
2. Document FHR and uterine activity with external monitoring.
3. Pelvic examination. Attempt to limit to one examiner and use sterile technique. Rule out ruptured membranes by looking for vaginal pooling of amniotic fluid and by nitrazine paper testing (turns blue if amniotic fluid present) and evaluate sample of fluid for ferning. Obtain cervical cultures for group B streptococci and do rapid group B streptococci antigen testing if available. If membranes are ruptured, one can used pooled amniotic fluid to determine fetal maturity by looking at the L/S ratio and PG levels; otherwise amniocentesis may be necessary.
4. Obtain cath UA and culture.
5. Cervix check.
6. U/S for fetal position and anomalies if time.

B. Tocolysis.

1. ***Contraindications.*** Evidence of fetal distress, fetal anomalies, abruptio placentae, placenta previa with heavy bleeding, severe maternal disease.
2. ***Risks of treatment.*** If membranes are ruptured, there is increased risk of cord prolapse and amnionitis. Fetal mortality is increased if labor is suppressed when there is IUGR. Mother may experience tachycardia, nervousness, or pulmonary edema secondary to medication.

3. ***Tocolysis.*** Most likely will be ineffective if labor is well established or if the cervix is dilated to 4 cm or more. Preparation should be made to deliver in the optimal setting. Up to now there have been no large-scale controlled clinical trials demonstrating that tocolytics delay delivery.
4. Experience up to now indicates that beta-adrenergic receptor antagonists may inhibit uterine contractility but only prolong gestation for about 48 hours in PTL. Consequently, some authors state that, to a large extent, the goal of tocolysis is to arrest labor long enough for exogenous steroids to stimulate fetal surfactant production so as to prevent the pulmonary complications of preterm birth.

C. Protocol.

1. Bed rest in left lateral decubitus position. Effective alone in 50% of patients.
2. Sedation (100 mg of *secobarbital* or 50 mg of hydroxyzine).
3. Hydration, but avoid large boluses (should not exceed 500 ml).
4. Antibiotics controversial. Do not use for >2 days, to limit incidence of resistance.
5. FHR and uterine activity monitoring.
6. Steroids accelerate fetal lung maturation (betamethasone or dexamethasone 12.5 mg IM Q24h for 48 hours).
7. Pharmacologic intervention.

D. Sympathomimetics (smooth muscle relaxation).

1. ***Terbutaline.***
   a. *Infusion* should be titrated on an individual basis so as to maximize inhibition of uterine activity and minimize maternal side effects.
   b. *Alternative to infusion:* 0.25 mg SQ Q20-60 min until contractions have subsided.
   c. Continue 2.5 mg PO every 2 to 4 hours. Up to 5.0 mg doses can be used.

E. Magnesium sulfate. $MgSO_4$ also decreases uterine contractility but is not useful long-term. It can be an adjunct to terbutaline.

F. Other. Prostaglandin synthetase inhibitors (such as indomethacin), calcium-channel blockers, aminophylline, and progesterone are under investigation.

IV. PRENATAL CARE FOR PATIENTS AT RISK FOR PRETERM LABOR

Frequent visits during weeks 22 to 32, cervical group B streptococci and urine culture at 24 weeks, vaginal exam for pH and cervical exam, monitor uterine activity, education on nutrition and preterm labor, and reinforce what signs and symptoms to watch for (abdominal cramping, pressure, cramps, backache, increased vaginal discharge, fluid leak, regular uterine contractions).

PREMATURE RUPTURE OF MEMBRANES (PROM)

I. DEFINITIONS

A. "Premature" rupture of membranes occurs if there is a delay of greater than 1 hour until onset of labor.

B. "Preterm premature" rupture of membranes occurs before 37 weeks of gestation.

II. DIAGNOSIS

A. History of fluid gush.

B. Sterile speculum exam.

1. ***Pooling of fluid in vaginal vault.***
2. ***pH determination.*** Amniotic fluid typically turns nitrazine paper blue. Contamination with vaginal-cervical mucus, blood, or urine may lead to false interpretation.
3. ***Fern test.*** Allow a sample of fluid to air dry on a glass or slide. Examination of amniotic fluid under the microscope reveals a classical "fern" pattern.

C. Cervical digital examination increases risk of chorioamnionitis. Evaluate cervix visually with sterile speculum. Avoid digital exams if possible unless patient is in labor and delivery is inevitable. Check for cord prolapse.

III. MANAGEMENT

A. Term PROM. Most sources recommend induction and delivery within a range of 24 to 36 hours after admission.

B. Preterm PROM. Fetal maturity must be considered. Manage expectantly until the fetus is mature unless chorioamnionitis or fetal distress develops, or labor cannot be inhibited with tocolysis (see above). Positive cervical cultures should be treated but do not necessitate induction without other signs of chorioamnionitis or fetal distress. Follow maternal and fetal vital signs, including temperature every 8 hours and WBC counts as indicated. Use of antibiotics for prophylaxis is under investigation.

C. Amnionitis. Signs include maternal or fetal tachycardia, maternal fever, uterine tenderness, foul cervical discharge, uterine contractions, leukocytosis, presence of leukocytes or bacteria in amniotic fluid.

POSTDATE PREGNANCY

I. DEFINITIONS

A. Prolonged pregnancy. Longer than 40 weeks of gestation.

B. Postdate pregnancy. Longer than 42 weeks.

C. Postmature pregnancy. Longer than 42 weeks with evidence of placental dysfunction.

II. ETIOLOGY

A. Most common. Error in estimating EDC.

B. Risk factors. History of prolonged gestation (50% risk), older age, anencephaly, or fetal endocrinopathy.

III. POTENTIAL MORBIDITY

A. Maternal.

1. Birth trauma secondary to macrosomic infant because of shoulder dystocia.
2. Increased incidence of operative delivery, secondary infection, or hemorrhage.

B. Neonatal. Meconium aspiration syndrome, polycythemia, hyperbilirubinemia, hypoglycemia, and anoxic organ damage.

IV. MANAGEMENT

A. Antepartum fetal surveillance with NST and amniotic fluid index assessment should be done at 40 and 41 weeks and twice weekly thereafter.

B. Immediate delivery. Cervix is ripe, decreased amniotic fluid, large fetal size (abdominal circumference), nonreactive NST, and presence of meconium in fluid. Pregnancies complicated by hypertension and diabetes should be induced at or near term.

C. Induction of labor can be preceded by cervical ripening using PGE_2 gel. PGE_2 gel (1 mg placed intracervically) has been shown to decrease both the amount of oxytocin needed to establish labor and the rate of cesarean section in patients induced for medical indications before 41 weeks of gestation. Decreased amniotic fluid leading to variable decelerations and meconium staining may be managed with amnioinfusion. Nasopharyngeal aspiration at the perineum and endotracheal aspiration should be performed once the baby is born to prevent meconium aspiration. Anticipate shoulder dystocia.

EVALUATION OF LABOR

I. HISTORY

A. Defining labor.

1. ***Contractions.*** Onset, frequency, duration, intensity.
2. ***Membranes ruptured or intact.***
3. ***Fetal movement.***

B. Review prenatal course.

1. Accuracy of estimated data of confinement (EDC); usually 40 weeks after LMP. May be modified by other parameters in pregnancy such as dating by ultrasonography.
2. ***Length of gestation.*** Calculated date of labor is compared to EDC, using EDC as "40" weeks.
3. Ask about coexisting medical problems.
4. Calculate weight gain during pregnancy.
5. ***Review laboratory data.*** Blood type, $Rh_0(D)$ immunoglobulin requirements, VDRL test, rubella immunity, hematocrit.

C. **Review previous pregnancies.** Number, gestation, fetal size, duration of labor, complications.

II. PHYSICAL EXAMINATION

A. **General.** Vital signs, funduscopy, thyroid palpation, chest examination, examination of the extremities, brief neurologic exam.

B. **Obstetrical abdominal examination.**

1. Assess fetal position.
2. Fundal height.
3. Estimation of fetal weight.
4. Auscultation of fetal heart tones.

C. **Pelvic examination.**

1. ***Inspection.***
   a. Look for herpetic lesions, condylomas, lacerations.
   b. Speculum examination may reveal pooling of vaginal fluid, consistent with rupture of membranes. A nitrazine paper test or swab of vaginal fluid on a glass slide may be necessary to prove the presence of amniotic fluid in the vagina. The basic pH of this fluid will turn the nitrazine paper blue. Care must be taken to avoid the cervical mucus, which is also basic and may give a false-positive test. If an air-dried sample of fluid reveals a fern-like pattern, the presence of amniotic fluid is confirmed.
2. ***Palpation of the cervix.***
   a. *Dilatation of the cervical os.* Dilatation may range from 0 to 10 cm.
   b. *Effacement.* The degree of thinning of the cervix. The cervix may range from 3 cm long (thick or with no effacement) to paper thin (100% effaced). In nulliparas effacement often precedes dilatation. There is simultaneous effacement and dilatation seen in multiparas.
3. ***Palpation of the presenting part.***
   a. *Identification.* Head, foot, buttock, other.
   b. *Station.* Station is described as the relationship of the fetal presenting part to the level of the ischial spines in the maternal pelvis. Station may range from −3 to +3. Zero station (engagement) occurs when the lower most presenting part is palpable at the level of the ischial spines. Always assess station by both abdominal method and pelvic method to avoid errors caused by caput.
   c. *Position.* Position is described as the orientation of the presenting part in regard to the maternal pelvis. Vertex presentation with the occiput positioned either to the right or left anteriorly is the most common.

LABOR DYSFUNCTION

I. PHASES OF LABOR

A. Latent phase. Slow progress of dilatation. Rate of dilatation <0.6 cm/hour.

B. Active labor.

1. ***Acceleration.*** Dilatation rate >0.6 cm/hour.
2. ***Maximum slope of dilatation.*** Cervix >5 cm or rate >1.2 cm/hour for nullipara and >1.5 cm/hour for multipara.
3. ***Deceleration.*** Cervix >9 cm, not complete.

II. PROLONGED LATENT PHASE.

Defined as >20 hours in nullipara; >14 hours in multipara. *Cause:* unripe cervix, false labor, sedation, uterine inertia. *Management:* observation, need for oxytocin stimulation. Avoid amniotomy. Good prognosis for vaginal delivery.

III. PROTRACTED ACTIVE PHASE.

Rate of dilatation: <1.2 cm/hour in nullipara; <1.5 cm/hour in multipara. *Cause:* fetal malpositions (occiput posterior), CPD, hypotonic uterine contractions, and anesthesia. *Management:* oxytocin stimulation. 70% require C-section.

IV. SECONDARY ARREST OF CERVICAL DILATATION

Cessation of dilatation for >2 hours. High incidence of CPD: guarded prognosis.

V. FAILURE OF DESCENT

Arrest of descent during second stage. High incidence of CPD: guarded prognosis.

VI. PROTRACTED DESCENT

Nullipara <1 cm/hour; multipara <2 cm/hour. CPD, macrosomia. Inadequate pushing because of anesthesia can also cause this disorder.

VII. PRECIPITOUS LABOR

>5 cm/hour dilatation in nullipara; >10 cm/hour in multipara. *Complications:* trauma to birth canal, fetal distress, and postpartum hemorrhage.

INTRAPARTUM MONITORING AND MANAGEMENT

I. FETAL HEART RATE

Electronic fetal heart rate monitoring may be performed by means of external Doppler, or direct scalp lead when membranes are ruptured.

A. Indications. Meconium staining, use of oxytocin; delivery of an anticipated premature, postmature, Rh-sensitized, or growth-retarded infant; medical complications associated with uteroplacental insufficiency (hypertension, diabetes, severe anemia, heart disease, renal disease), presence of abnormal FHR by Doppler scanning, VBAC, other intrapartum obstetrical complications (failure to progress, excessive vaginal bleeding).

B. Fetal heart rate tracing interpretation.

1. ***Baseline fetal heart rate.***
   a. Normal 120 to 160 bpm.
   b. Tachycardia >160 bpm. *Cause:* fetal hypoxia, maternal fever, maternal hyperthyroidism, parasympatholytic or sympathomimetic drugs.
   c. Bradycardia <120 bpm. *Cause:* fetal asphyxia, anesthetics, fetal cardiac conduction defect. Usually benign if good variability is present.
2. ***Variability.***
   a. *Short-term variability.* Beat-to-beat variation is normally 5 to 10 bpm.
   b. *Long-term variability.* Waviness of the FHR tracing, which normally has a frequency of 3 to 10 cycles/min and an amplitude of 10 to 25 bpm.
   c. *Decreased variability.* Variability may be decreased by fetal sleep cycles, CNS depression secondary to hypoxia or drugs, parasympatholytic agents, extreme prematurity, or congenital anomalies. Loss of variability is associated with a high incidence of fetal acidosis and low Apgar scores.
3. ***Common periodic patterns.***
   a. *Accelerations.* Reassuring if associated with fetal movement. May be compensatory before or after deceleration.
   b. *Early decelerations.* Occur coincidentally with uterine contractions and are associated with fetal head compression. These are vagally mediated and not ominous when they occur late in labor. These start early in the contraction phase, reach their lowest point at the peak of the contraction, and return to baseline levels as the contraction finishes. The FHR does not fall below 100 bpm.
   c. *Late decelerations.* Transient but repetitive deceleration of the FHR observed to occur late in the contraction phase. Reaches its lowest point after the acme of the contraction and returns to baseline rate once the contraction is over. Late decelerations result from fetal hypoxia, indicate uteroplacental insufficiency, and are always considered ominous.
   d. *Variable decelerations.* Characterized by variable duration, timing in relation to contraction and intensity. This is a reflex pattern, typically secondary to umbilical cord compression. Poor prognostic signs are:
      (1) Association with poor FHR baseline variability.
      (2) Lack of predeceleration and postdeceleration accelerations.

(3) Slow return to baseline.
(4) Biphasic shape (W = knot in cord).
(5) Failure to return to baseline rate.

e. *Prolonged decelerations.* Isolated decelerations >120 seconds can be seen with maternal hypotension, maternal hypoxia, tetanic contractions, prolapsed umbilical cord, fetal scalp procedures (vagal), and paracervical or epidural anesthesia. A prolonged deceleration after severe variable deceleration may signal impending fetal demise.

C. Management of abnormal FHR pattern or fetal distress.

1. Turn patient onto side to alleviate vena cava compression.
2. Discontinue intravenous oxytocin.
3. Apply 100% oxygen to mother by face mask.
4. Correct maternal hypertension.
5. Vaginal examination to rule out prolapsed cord.
6. Consider fetal scalp blood sampling for pH determination (see Table 8-2).
7. With decreased variability, consider fetal scalp stimulation. The return of variability is reassuring. If tracing maintains poor variability, consider points 1 to 6 above.
8. With prolonged bradycardia unresponsive to other maneuvers or late decelerations with worsening fetal acidosis (pH <7.20), consider delivery by C-section.

II. UTERINE ACTIVITY

May be determined by an indirect (external) pressure monitor, or by an intrauterine pressure transducer when more accurate estimations are required.

A. Contractility. Effective contractions should have an amplitude of 50 to 75 mm Hg, duration of 45 to 90 seconds, and frequency of every 3 to 5 minutes.

B. Resting tone. Spontaneous labor 5 to 10 mm Hg. Induced labor 15 to 20 mm Hg.

TABLE 8-2
Interpretation of fetal scalp pH

Fetal scalp blood pH	Interpretation	Management
>7.25	Normal	Continue FHR monitoring and resample if appropriate.
7.20-7.24	Preacidotic	Consider resampling and continue FHR monitoring.
< 7.19	Fetal acidosis	Resample in 5 to 10 minutes and prepare for immediate delivery if low scalp pH is confirmed.

C. Rhythmicity. Presence of coupling or tripling may represent hyperstimulation.

D. Configuration. Typically bell shaped. May become rectangular during pushing. The area under the curve when an internal transducer is used may be calculated to determine the adequacy of uterine contractions.

III. FETAL STIMULATION

When the scalp is stimulated and there is an acceleration of 15 bpm lasting 15 seconds, it denotes fetal pH value of 7.22 or greater. Reverse is not true. Obtain baseline fetal scalp pH in meconium staining. Draw maternal venous blood simultaneously for comparison. In the case of maternal fever do not rely on fetal scalp pH because fetal compromise can occur with normal values.

AMNIOINFUSION

I. DEFINITION

Amnioinfusion (AI) is a procedure in which a physiologic solution (such as normal saline) is infused into the uterine cavity to replace the amniotic fluid.

II. INDICATIONS

A. Correcting variable decelerations because of cord compression.

B. Reduce fetal distress caused by meconium staining of fluid (rule out concurrent signs of fetal stress).

C. Correction of oligohydramnios.

III. TECHNIQUE

A. Catheter. Double-lumen catheter: expensive but helps monitor uterine contractions.

B. Infusate. Normal saline, lactated Ringer's (like amniotic fluid).

C. Temperature. Room temperature can cause fetal bradycardia if infused rapidly. Body temperature is more physiologic.

D. Methods. Continuous infusion by gravity drainage or by infusion pump 10 to 15 ml/min or intermittent infusion by gravity drainage (1 liter over 20 to 30 minutes, repeat Q6h).

E. Small risk of uterine rupture if efflux of infusate blocked.

IV. EFFICACY

A. Oligohydramnios. Lower rate of C-section for fetal distress and higher umbilical artery pHs at birth compared to those in patients not receiving AI.

B. Moderate to thick meconium. Decreased rate of operative delivery, increased average 1-minute Apgar scores, less meconium aspirated from below neonate's vocal cords, and a lower incidence of meconium aspiration syndrome compared to that in patients not treated with AI.

INDUCTION OF LABOR

I. INDICATIONS AND CONTRAINDICATIONS

A. Indications. Pregnancy-induced hypertension, premature rupture of membranes, chorioamnionitis, postdate pregancy, isoimmunization, other evidence of hostile intrauterine environment, diabetes mellitus, other selected maternal diseases, fetal demise.

B. Contraindications. Placenta previa, cord presentation, floating presenting part, abnormal fetal lie, active genital herpes, invasive cervical carcinoma, pelvic structural deformities, prior classical uterine incision. Oxytocin stimulation would be relatively contraindicated in conditions that predispose to uterine rupture (high parity, advanced maternal age, fetopelvic disproportion, uterine overdistension, prior uterine scar).

II. RISKS

A. Amniotomy.

1. ***Cord prolapse.*** Make sure presenting part well applied to cervix.
2. ***Injury to fetal part (unlikely with blunt instruments).***

B. Oxytocin.

1. ***Hyperstimulation.*** Greater than 5 contractions in 10 minutes, diastole less than 1 minute, or contractions lasting greater than 90 seconds.
2. ***Uterine rupture.***
3. ***Water intoxication.*** Hyponatremia may result if excessive oxytocin is administered with large volumes of non–electrolyte containing IV fluids.
4. ***Hypotension.*** Large IV bolus of oxytocin should be followed by rapid hydration to maintain blood pressure.

C. Prostaglandin E_2. Hyperstimulation and uterine rupture.

III. METHODS

A. Determine indications for induction of labor, weighing the relative contraindications and risks.

B. Assess the inducibility of the cervix using Bishop score (see Table 8-3).

C. Decide whether to use amniotomy alone or combined with oxytocin. Amniotomy in the face of a high Bishop score often leads to successful induction of labor. Oxytocin is indicated in arrest disorders of active labor if inadequate uterine activity is the cause rather than CPD. Oxytocin is also indicated for a prolonged latent phase, along with complicating factors such as premature rupture of membranes or a postdate pregnancy. Oxytocin should not be used in CPD.

TABLE 8-3
Bishop Scoring System

Cervix	Score			
	0	1	2	3
Position	Posterior	Midposition	Anterior	—
Consistency	Firm	Medium	Soft	—
Effacement (%)	0-30	40-50	60-70	>80
Dilatation (cm)	Closed	1-2	3-4	>5
Station	−3	−2	−1	+1, +2

A Bishop score of >9 indicates induction should be successful.

Modified from Romney S et al, editors: *Gynecology and obstetrics: the health care of women,* ed 2, New York, 1981, McGraw-Hill.

D. Guidelines for amniotomy.
1. Cervix should be dilated enough to allow reaching the membranes with the amniotomy hook.
2. The fetus should be vertex (unless breech delivery is planned) with the presenting part well engaged and well applied to the cervix.
3. The umbilical cord should not be palpable.
4. Membranes are hooked, and a gentle tug should cause release of amnionic fluid.
5. Assess fluid for presence of meconium.
6. Monitor fetal heart tones before and after the procedure.

E. Guidelines for oxytocin administration.
1. Close monitoring of the parturient and fetus is essential. Most hospitals have written protocols available.
   a. Place 10 units of oxytocin in 1000 ml of D_5NS or D_5LR.
   b. Begin with a low dose of oxytocin: 0.5 to 2 milliunits per minute. (Each milliliter of the above solution contains 10 mU.)
   c. Various protocols exist regarding the rate for increasing the dose and the maximum dose. If little uterine response is observed, the dose can be increased by 1 to 2 mU/min every 30 minutes. Most patients respond to rates of 20 mU/min or less. The faster the increase, the more likely the risk of hyperstimulation. The rate of administration is held steady when a good labor pattern (contractions every 2 to 3 minutes lasting 60 to 90 seconds with an intrauterine pressure of 50 to 60 mm Hg and a resting tone of 10 to 15 mm Hg) is achieved.
   d. Ideally you want 150 to 250 Montevideo units. Montevideo units = Number of contractions/10 min × (Average peak of contraction − Average baseline of contraction).

2. If at any point the fetal heart rate indicates distress, the patient should be placed on her left side, oxygen administered, and oxytocin discontinued. Reinstatement of oxytocin drip requires reassessment of the situation.

OBSTETRIC ANESTHESIA AND ANALGESIA

I. Pain during first stage of labor is attributable to uterine contractions and cervical dilatation. During the second stage, pain occurs from distension and stretching of pelvic structures and the perineum. Pain is conducted along the paracervical and inferior hypogastric plexus.

II. SYSTEMIC NARCOTICS

Meperidine 25 mg IV and nalbuphine (Nubain) 10 mg IV are given early during labor. Usually avoided at or near delivery. *Maternal complications:* nausea, vomiting, decreased gastric motility, respiratory depression. *Fetal complications:* respiratory depression, CNS depression, and impaired temperature regulation. Naloxone (0.01 mg/kg) can be administered to depressed newborn as IV bolus for counteracting the effect of narcotics.

III. LOCAL ANESTHESIA

A. Pudendal block. Provides analgesia to vaginal introitus and perineum. Usually used in second stage of labor. Insert a needle through guide into the vagina. Identify ischial spines. Direct the needle laterally and posteriorly to the ischial spine. Feel loss of resistance when you pass through the sacrospinous ligament and enter pudendal canal with pudendal vessels and nerves. Aspirate for blood and instill 5 ml of anesthetic solution. Advance the needle to a range of 0.5 to 1 cm and inject another 5 ml of 1% lidocaine after aspirating for blood. Repeat the same on other side. Takes 10 minutes for anesthesia to establish itself. Infection at the injection site is the major potential complication.

B. Paracervical block. Provides analgesia during active phase of labor. Blocks pain caused by uterine contractions. Insert a needle through the guard and identify the 4- and 8-o'clock positions of the cervicovaginal junction. Instill 6 ml of 1% lidocaine superficially under the vaginal mucosa on either site.

C. Lumbar epidural anesthesia.

Contraindications. Patient refusal, maternal fever, preexisting CNS disease, severe hypertension, hypotension, hypovolemia, blood coagulopathy. Epidural anesthesia is associated with prolonged labor and an increased risk of chorioamnionitis.

IV. PSYCHOLOGIC METHODS OF PAIN RELIEF

Lamaze classes aid in preparation; hypnosis, acupuncture, and biofeedback are also used.

VAGINAL DELIVERY

I. NORMAL SPONTANEOUS VAGINAL DELIVERY

A. Cardinal movements (for vertex presentation).

1. ***Engagement.*** Occurs late in pregnancy for primigravida, at the onset of labor for multigravida.
2. ***Flexion.*** Of the neck so that the smallest diameter possible presents. If the neck does not flex, it may actually extend during labor, producing a brow or face presentation.
3. ***Descent.*** Progressive with thinning of the cervix and lower uterine segment. Depends on the force of contractions and on pelvic and presenting part configuration.
4. ***Internal rotation.*** Occurs during descent. Vertex rotates from transverse to either posterior or anterior position to pass the ischial spines.
5. ***Extension.*** Occurs as the head distends the perineum and the occiput passes beneath the symphysis.
6. ***External rotation.*** Occurs after delivery of the head with the head rotating back to a transverse position as the shoulders internally rotate to an anteroposterior position.

B. Management of vertex delivery.

1. ***Preparations for delivery.*** Should be made when the presenting part begins to distend the perineum, sooner for multigravida. (Local or pudendal anesthesia should be administered at this time.) Episiotomy is not performed until delivery is imminent.
2. ***Delivery of the head.***
   a. Controlled so that there is no forceful, sudden expulsion (which may produce injury to mother or baby). As the vertex appears beneath the symphysis, the perineum is supported by direct pressure from a draped hand over the coccygeal region (Ritgen's maneuver). This will protect the perineum and assist in extension of the head as the vertex passes the symphysis.
   b. As the head is delivered, it will rotate to a transverse position, at which time the baby should be checked for the presence of umbilical cord about the neck. If present, it should be gently slipped over the infant's head (or double clamped and cut if this cannot be done easily).
   c. The mouth and nose should be cleared of secretions with a bulb syringe or DeLee suction trap.
3. ***Delivery of the shoulders.*** Shoulders should be rotated to an AP position in the pelvic outlet as the head externally rotates. Gentle traction downward on the head will assist in bringing the anterior shoulder beneath the symphysis. Gentle elevation of the infant head toward the symphysis will release the posterior shoulder.

4. ***Delivery of the body.*** The rest of the body will generally deliver spontaneously and quickly after delivery of the shoulders. Care must be taken to control the delivery of the body to prevent unnecessary injury.
5. ***Immediate care of the infant.*** Includes double clamping and cutting of the umbilical cord. The clamp closest to the umbilicus should be just distal to the skin reflection or longer if anticipate a need for an umbilical line. A clear airway must be assured and body temperature maintained by drying and wrapping or placing under a radiant heater.

II. FORCEPS DELIVERY

Forceps are generally used to shorten the second stage of labor when in the best interest of the mother or the fetus. A fully dilated cervix and experienced physician are required. Advantages must be weighed against the increased risk of maternal lacerations.

A. Indications.

1. ***Prolonged second stage.***
   a. Primigravida with regional anesthesia >3 hours.
   b. Primigravida without regional anesthesia >2 hours.
   c. Multigravida with regional anesthesia >2 hours.
   d. Multigravida without regional anesthesia >1 hour.
2. ***Fetal distress.***
3. ***Maternal exhaustion.***

B. Requirements.

1. Fetal head engaged and in vertex-face presentation.
2. Position of head known exactly.
3. Membranes ruptured.
4. Cervix fully dilated.
5. No clinical evidence of cephalopelvic disproportion.

C. Definitions.

1. ***Outlet forceps.*** The fetal scalp is visible at the introitus. The head is at or on the perineum, and the sagittal suture is in the AP plane or rotated up to 45 degrees.
2. ***Low forceps.*** The leading point of the skull is at least at +2 station.
3. ***Midforceps.*** The leading point of the skull is engaged but is above +2 station. (Midforceps delivery should be attempted only in extreme situations while simultaneously preparing for C-section.)

D. Selection of forceps.

1. ***Simpson.*** Good for primigravida with prolonged second stage (molded fetal head).
2. ***Elliot.*** Better if multigravida and if less molded fetal head.
3. ***Tucker-McLane.*** Has sliding lock, good for asynclitic fetal head.
4. ***Kielland.*** Has minimal pelvic curve, often used for rotation.
5. ***Piper.*** Used in breech extractions.

III. VACUUM EXTRACTION

A safe, effective alternative to forceps delivery. A term, vertex fetus is required. Delivery should not be one that will require rotation or excessive traction. Prior scalp sampling is a contraindication.

A. Advantages.

1. Simpler to apply, with fewer mistakes in application.
2. Less force applied to fetal head.
3. Less anesthesia necessary (local anesthetic may suffice).
4. No increase in diameter of presenting head.
5. Less maternal soft-tissue injury.
6. Less fetal injury.
7. Less parental concern.

B. Disadvantages.

1. Traction applied only during contractions.
2. Proper traction necessary to avoid losing vacuum.
3. Possible longer delivery than with forceps.
4. Small increase in incidence of cephalohematomas.

C. Technique.

1. Ascertain that the cervix is fully dilated and the vertex is in low or outlet position.
2. The vertex is then wiped clean, the labia are spread, and the cup is compressed and inserted. Pressure is applied inward and downward until contact is made with the fetal scalp. The cup should be placed over the posterior fontanelle.
3. A finger is swept around the cup to make sure no maternal tissue is within the cup. Suction pressure is raised to 100 mm Hg, and the location of the cup is rechecked.
4. With the onset of a contraction, suction pressure is raised to a range of 380 to 580 mm Hg. (Negative pressure should not exceed 600 mm Hg.) Traction is applied perpendicularly to the cup, in line with the maternal axis.
5. Should the cup be dislodged, the fetal scalp is to be checked before the cup is reapplied.
6. When the contraction subsides, the suction pressure is reduced to 100 mm Hg.
7. The sequence is repeated with each contraction. More than three good attempts are not recommended unless progress is being made.
8. As the head crowns, an episiotomy may be cut. Traction is then changed to a 45-degree angle upward as the vertex clears the symphysis.
9. Suction is released and the cup removed after delivery of the fetal head.
10. The procedure should be discontinued if one fails to achieve extraction after 10 minutes at maximal pressure,

extraction is not achieved within 30 minutes of initiation, the cup disengages three times, fetal scalp trauma is sustained, or no progress is made after three pulls.

BREECH DELIVERY

I. OVERVIEW

A. **Incidence.** 25% of all pregnancies <28 weeks of gestation, 3% to 4% of all pregnancies at or beyond 34 weeks of gestation.

B. **Cause.** Low birth weight, placenta previa, uterine and fetal anomalies, contracted pelvis, multiple fetuses all contribute to breech presentations.

II. TYPES OF BREECH

A. **Frank.** Thighs and hips flexed, knees extended. 65% of cases are frank.

B. **Complete.** Thighs and hips flexed, one or both knees flexed. 10% of cases.

C. **Incomplete or footling.** One or both thighs extended, one or both knees below the buttocks. 25% of cases.

III. BREECH DELIVERY—BUTTOCKS, EXTREMITIES, AND SHOULDERS: CRITERIA FOR VAGINAL DELIVERY OF BREECH PRESENTATION

1. Frank breech presentation.
2. Fetal weight 2500 to 3800 g.
3. Fetal head flexed.
4. Gestational age at or beyond 36 weeks.
5. Adequate maternal pelvis.
6. No other maternal or fetal indicator for C-section.

EPISIOTOMY

A deliberate incision in the perineum used to facilitate vaginal delivery.

I. MIDLINE

Good anatomic results, easy repair, low incidence of postpartum pain or dyspareunia. However, increases the risk of a third or fourth degree laceration compared to patients without an episiotomy.

II. MEDIOLATERAL

Less likely to extend through the sphincter, but more likely to cause pain during healing, dyspareunia, or excessive blood loss. Good anatomic results are more difficult to obtain.

SHOULDER DYSTOCIA

I. INCIDENCE

Directly related to fetal size: >2500 g 0.15%; >4000 g 1.7%; >4500 g 10.0%.

II. DIAGNOSIS

Suspect shoulder dystocia if there is reason to suspect macrosomia (gestational diabetes, history of large infants, large maternal size, prolonged gestation), or if second stage is prolonged. Consider C-section. In vaginal deliveries, suspect dystocia if the head pulls back against the perineum after delivery, and external rotation is difficult.

III. MANAGEMENT

A. Ensure adequate maternal anesthesia and cut a very generous episiotomy.

B. Attempt McRobert's maneuver. The mother's thighs are hyperflexed, bringing her feet "to her ears." Have an assistant apply suprapubic pressure This causes the shoulder to move under the symphysis pubis. Attempt delivery with gentle downward traction.

C. Attempt the Wood's screw maneuver. Gently rotate the posterior shoulder by pushing on the posterior scapula until the shoulder passes under the symphysis and can be delivered as the anterior shoulder.

D. If this is unsuccessful, try delivering the posterior arm first and then rotating the anterior shoulder into the oblique position for delivery.

E. If all else fails, one may attempt deliberate fracture of the clavicle of the impacted shoulder. The thumb and forefinger are used to push the clavicle outward to avoid a pneumothorax. Although the fracture will heal, damage to cervical nerve roots may occur and cause permanent sequelae.

GROUP B STREPTOCOCCAL INFECTION

A. Risk factors for neonatal sepsis. Intrapartum chorioamnionitis, maternal group B streptococcal (GBS) colonization in the rectum or vagina, prolonged rupture of membranes, and prolonged monitoring with an internal pressure catheter or fetal scalp lead.

B. Vertical transmission of GBS. Number one cause of neonatal sepsis and meningitis in the U.S. Infection occurs in 2 or 3 neonates per 1000 live births. Maternal colonization can be transient, and 20% to 25% of pregnant females are carriers at any given time. In addition to threatening the life of a neonate, GBS is also an important risk factor for the development of chorioamnionitis in the mother, thereby increasing morbidity and the rate of intrapartum complications.

C. The CDC recommends 2 options for dealing with GBS.

1. ***Option 1.***
   a. *Culture all women (rectal and vaginal) at 35-37 weeks.* If the patient's rectal or vaginal cultures are positive for GBS, she should be offered intrapartum antibiotic prophylaxis.
   b. Treatment. Oral antibiotics are ineffective. The following regimens may be used:
      (1) Penicillin G 5 million units IV and then 2.5 million units Q4h until delivery. Penicillin G is the preferred antibiotic because of its narrow spectrum, thereby making it less likely to select for antibiotic-resistant bacteria.
      (2) Ampicillin 2 g IV followed by 1 g Q4h until delivery.
      (3) If the patient has a penicillin allergy, either clindamycin 900 mg IV Q8h or erythromycin 500 mg IV Q6h may be given until delivery.
2. ***Option 2.*** Screening cultures are not done, but antibiotic prophylaxis is given if any of the following risk factors are present:
   a. Previously delivered neonate who developed GBS infection.
   b. The patient had GBS bacteriuria during the current pregnancy.
   c. Labor and delivery occur at less than 37 weeks of gestation (attack rates for preterm infants are higher).
   d. Membranes have been ruptured for >18 hours.
   e. Intrapartum temperature ≥38.0° C (100.4° F).

D. If PROM occurs at <37 weeks of gestation and the patient is not yet laboring, GBS cultures should be collected as above. Either of the following regimens may then be used:

1. Give IV antibiotics until culture results are known, or
2. Initiate antibiotic therapy only when culture result confirms presence of GBS.

E. Care of the infant of a mother who has had GBS prophylaxis.

1. Any infant with symptoms or signs of GBS disease must have a full work-up (CBC, blood culture, CXR for pulmonary symptoms, LP if indicated) as should all infants born at <35 weeks.
2. For those >35 weeks without symptoms, approach is stratified based on duration of labor *after the administration of antibiotics.*
   a. If duration of labor *after antibiotics is <4 hours,* infant should have CBC, blood culture, and 48 hours of observation.
   b. If duration of labor *after antibiotics is >4 hours,* observation for 48 hours is indicated.

CESAREAN SECTION

I. INDICATIONS

A. Maternal and fetal. Cephalopelvic disproportion, failed induction or progression of labor, abnormal uterine contraction pattern.

B. Maternal.

1. ***Maternal diseases.*** Eclampsia or preeclampsia with noninducible cervix, diabetes mellitus (if macrosomic infant precludes vaginal delivery), cardiac disease, cervical cancer, active herpes genitalis. One double-blind clinical trial showed that acyclovir suppression (400 mg PO TID) given after 36 weeks of gestation significantly reduces the need for cesarean section by preventing a herpetic outbreak at term.
2. ***Previous uterine surgery.*** Classic cesarean section, previous uterine rupture, full-thickness myomectomy. If there is any question about the type of incision made during a previous cesarean section, the operative report for that delivery must be obtained so that incisional type can be known with certainty.
3. ***Obstruction to the birth canal.*** Fibroids, ovarian tumors.

C. Fetal. Fetal distress, cord prolapse, fetal malpresentations.

D. Placental.

1. Placenta previa (unless marginal).
2. Abruptio placentae.

II. RISKS

A. Maternal. Infection, hemorrhage, injury to urinary tract, adverse reactions to anesthesia, prolonged recovery.

B. Fetal. Depend on gestational age and indications for C-section. Less birth trauma, though injury can be sustained during operative delivery. May have increased incidence of respiratory distress syndrome.

POSTPARTUM CARE

I. EXAMPLES OF ORDERS AFTER ROUTINE VAGINAL DELIVERY

A. Immediately post partum.

1. Pitocin 10 units IM.
2. Bed rest, and vitals Q15 min for 1 hour post partum.
3. Consider NPO for 1 to 2 hours post partum.
4. Ice pack to perineum immediately post partum.

B. Thereafter.

1. Ambulate as tolerated when stable.
2. ***Diet.*** General or other.
3. ***Vital signs.*** Q4h.
4. Tucks to perineum PRN.
5. Sitz baths TID and HS PRN.
6. ***IV (if present).*** Discontinue when vital signs are stable and uterine bleeding is normal.

7. Urethral catheterization if unable to void in 6 to 8 hours.
8. Breast binder if not nursing.
9. CBC postpartum day 2.
10. Type and cross for Rh_o(D) immunoglobulin if indicated.
11. ***Medications.***
    a. *Vitamins.* Continue prenatal vitamins; additional $FeSO_4$ if anemic.
    b. *Pain.* Acetaminophen 650 mg PO Q4-6h PRN or ibuprofen 400 to 600 mg PO Q4-6h for cramping pain.
    c. *Bowels.* Docusate sodium 100 mg PO BID; milk of magnesia 30 ml PO QD PRN; bisacodyl 10 mg PO or PR PRN.

II. HOSPITAL CARE

A. Physical examination.

1. Monitor uterine changes. The fundus should be firm and at or below the umbilicus. Gradual involution occurs over the next 6 weeks.
2. Lochia (uterine drainage) is initially red or bloody, gradually becoming serosanguinous. By 2 to 3 weeks it should be white. Tampons are contraindicated.
3. Breasts are examined for signs of infection and presence of milk. Colostrum is present initially. Milk production should occur by the third to fifth day in primiparas, sooner in multiparas. Breast feeding should not be allowed for greater than 15 minutes on each side per feeding initially to help prevent soreness.
4. Legs should be examined for evidence of thrombophlebitis.

B. Parental education.

1. Newborn care.
2. Breast feeding if applicable.
3. Prevention of lactation or engorgement if applicable.

III. DISCHARGE

A. Discharge instructions.

1. Rubella vaccination, if indicated, before discharge.
2. Instruct regarding signs of puerperal infection, postpartum hemorrhage, mastitis.
3. Counsel on avoidance of intercourse and tampons for 4 weeks.
4. Contraception (barrier methods versus oral contraception). OCPs can be started early, if desired. Low-dose or progestin-only pills have less influence on lactation.
5. Nutrition. Especially if breast feeding.
6. Medications. Vitamins, iron, stool softener, when appropriate. Counsel on medications to avoid during breast feeding (see Chapter 10).
7. Discuss need for rest, possible stresses that can occur with new infant at home.

B. Follow-up exam.

1. Postpartum check at 4 to 6 weeks.
2. Newborn checkup typically at 1 to 2 weeks.

POSTPARTUM HEMORRHAGE

I. DEFINITION

Postpartum hemorrhage is most often defined as a blood loss greater than 500 ml in the first 24 hours after delivery. However, blood loss after spontaneous vaginal delivery is frequently up to 600 ml and between 1 and 1.5 liters after instrumental or operative delivery. Therefore, clinical experience is necessary to determine when bleeding is occurring too rapidly or at the wrong time or is unresponsive to appropriate treatment. Blood loss will be less well tolerated if the patient has not had the normal expansion of blood volume during pregnancy, as in cases of preeclampsia.

II. DIAGNOSIS

A. Risk factors. Multiparity (>5 babies), previous postpartum hemorrhage, manual removal of the placenta, placental abruption or placenta previa, polyhydramnios, prolonged labor, precipitant labor, difficult forceps delivery, prolonged oxytocin administration, breech extraction.

B. Etiology.

1. Uterine atony accounts for most cases.
2. Other causes include retained placenta, cervical or vaginal tear, coagulopathy.

C. Physical examination.

1. Vital signs (BP and pulse may underestimate the degree of blood loss).
2. Uterus should be palpated for evidence of atony, tenderness, or lack of involution.
3. Vaginal exam may reveal evidence of laceration (generally bright red blood) or atony (darker blood). Bimanual exam may reveal mass (suggestive of broad ligament or paravaginal hematoma).
4. A hematocrit is helpful only in comparison to the value before delivery. It will not adequately reflect acute blood loss.

III. MANAGEMENT

A. Evaluate promptly once excessive bleeding is detected. Reliable IV access must be obtained with 2 large-bore IVs. Monitor vital signs and maintain circulatory status with fluids. If the patient shows evidence of symptomatic hypovolemia, blood should be sent for type and cross. Coagulation profile should also be obtained.

B. Review clinical course for probable cause (see predisposing factors listed above).

C. Perform bimanual examination in recovery area or delivery room.

1. If uterus is found to be boggy, initiate stimulation with massage or oxytocin (40 units in 1000 ml of crystalloid, infused at 200 ml/hr or 10 units of oxytocin IM).
2. If placental fragments are detected within uterus on exploration or by ultrasonography, return to delivery room for curettage.
3. Laceration or hematoma should be repaired in delivery room.

D. If cause is not identified or fails to respond to the above measures, notify obstetric physicians, anesthesia, and operating room personnel of potential need for surgical intervention.

E. Inform patient of the problem and what measures are being taken to correct it. Get an appreciation of her desires regarding further childbearing and hysterectomy.

F. If hemorrhage is unresponsive to the above measures, administration of prostaglandins should be considered. Prostaglandin E_2 vaginal suppositories (Prostin E_2 = 20 mg) have been used.

G. If uterine bleeding persists, surgery must be considered. Packing is a temporary measure and is rarely effective. Surgical alternatives include uterine artery and hypogastric artery ligation. Hysterectomy is the treatment of last resort when the patient desires future fertility but may be preferred if sterility is desired.

PUERPERAL FEVER

I. DEFINITION

Temperature >38.4° C in first 24 hours or >38.0° C for 2 consecutive days in the following 9 days post partum.

II. DIFFERENTIAL DIAGNOSIS

A. Endometritis.

1. ***Etiology.***
   a. *Infection.* Polymicrobial with a mixture of aerobic and anaerobic organisms. In particular, high fever within the first 25 hours after delivery may be caused by gram-negative sepsis, group B streptococcal disease, clostridial sepsis, or toxic shock syndrome.
   b. *Risk factors.* C-section (20 times greater than vaginal delivery), chorioamnionitis, prolonged rupture of membranes or premature labor, multiple vaginal exams, retained products, low socioeconomic status.
2. ***Treatment.***
   a. Cultures of the cervix and blood may help identify the causative organism, but treatment is often started empirically.

b. There is no consensus on the safest and most effective antibiotic regimens, only that it must have a broad spectrum. Antibiotics are usually continued for 4 or 5 days and for 24 to 48 hours after defervescence.
c. "Gold standard" = Gentamicin (2 mg/kg IV loading dose, followed by 1.5 mg/kg IV Q8h) + Clindamycin (900 mg IV Q8h).
d. Newer single-agent regimens (second- or third-generation cephalosporins, semisynthetic penicillins).
   a. Cefoxitin 1 to 2 g IV Q6-8h.
   b. Ampicillin 2 g IV Q4-6h.
e. If no response (maximum temperature not dropping within 48 hours of initiation of therapy), start triple-agent therapy: ampicillin and gentamicin and clindamycin.

B. **Pelvic abscess.** Suspect if patient develops a pelvic mass or has persistent fever and pain despite therapy for aerobic bacteria. Frequently develops 5 or more days after delivery. Must add therapy for anaerobic bacteria and consider surgical or percutaneous drainage.

C. **Septic pelvic thrombophlebitis.** Symptoms include spiking fevers with or without pain despite antibiotic therapy. The patient may have a tender palpable mass. May have a diagnostic response with improvement of symptoms after beginning intravenous heparin.

D. **Wound infection.** Presentation includes fever; a tender, erythematous, or fluctuant incision; drainange of pus or blood. Usually occurs after the fifth postoperative day. Risk factors include having an intrapartum cesarean section; emergent abdominal delivery, use of electrocautery, placement of open drains, obesity, and diabetes.

E. **Pulmonary atelectasis.** Fever usually begins within 48 hours. Patients may have poor inspiratory effort, dullness to percussion, rales, or decreased breath sounds. Observe increased frequency in patients who receive general anesthetics or have abdominal delivery. Narcotic analgesics may also predispose to atelectasis.

F. **Deep vein thrombosis.** Symptoms include fever and lower extremity pain, swelling, and pallor. Traumatic delivery, cesarean section, delay in the resumption of ambulation, and varicose veins all increase likelihood for DVT formation.

G. **Pyelonephritis.** Often accompanied by fever, malaise, flank pain, costovertebral angle tenderness, and pyuria. Risk factors include occult bacteriuria, bladder trauma, and Foley catheterization.

H. **Mastitis.** Suggested by fever and swollen, tender breast. Typically occurs 3 to 4 weeks after delivery. Breast feeding and contact with a carrier of *Staphylococcus aureus* are the two prime risk factors.

BIBLIOGRAPHY

Antepartum fetal surveillance, *ACOG Techn Bull,* No 107, Aug 1987 (American College of Obstetricians and Gynecologists, Washington, D.C.).

Benson M: *Obstetrical P*E*A*R*L*S,* Philadelphia, 1989, FA Davis Co.

Besinger RE, Niebyl JR: The safety and efficacy of tocolytic agents for the treatment of preterm labor, *Obstet Gynecol Surg* 45(7):415, 1990.

Board PJ et al: Gestational diabetes: definition, diagnosis, and treatment strategies in practical diabetology, *Practical Diabetol* 5(6):1, 1980.

Campbell TL: Maternal serum alpha-fetoprotein screening: benefits, risks and costs, *J Fam Pract* 25(5):461, 1987.

Centers for Disease Control and Prevention: Prevention of perinatal group B streptococcal disease: a public health perspective, *MMWR* 45(RR-7):16, 1996.

Clark SL et al: Effect of indication for previous cesarean section on subsequent delivery outcome in patients undergoing a trial of labor, *J Reprod Med* 19(1):22, 1984.

Cox SM, Gilstrap LC: Postpartum endometritis, *Obstet Gynecol North Am* 16(2): 363, 1989.

Creasy RK, Resnik R, editors: *Maternal-fetal medicine: principles and practice,* Philadelphia, 1984, Saunders.

Cruikshank DP: Genetic diagnosis by amniocentesis, *Iowa Perinatal Letter* 1(5), July/Aug 1980.

Darroca RJ et al: Prostaglandin E_2 gel for cervical ripening in patients with an indication for delivery, *Obstet Gynecol* 87:228, 1996.

Deutschman M: The problematic first-trimester pregnancy, *Amer Fam Physician* 39(1):185, 1989.

Driscoll CE et al, editors: *Handbook of family practice,* St. Louis, 1986, Mosby.

Eggelston MK: Management of preterm labor and delivery, *Clin Obstet Gynecol* 29(2):230, 1986.

Epperly TD, Bretinger ER: Vacuum extraction, *Am Fam Physician* 38(3):205, 1988.

Evans MI et al: The variation in maternal serum alpha-fetoprotein reports in one metropolitan area: concerns for the quality of prenatal testing, *Obstet Gynecol* 72:342, 1988.

Flamm BL: Vaginal birth after cesarean section: controversies old and new, *Clin Obstet Gynecol* 18(4):735, 1985.

Freeman RK et al, editors: *Fetal heart rate monitoring,* ed 2, Baltimore, 1991, Williams & Wilkins.

Gabbe SG et al, editors: *Obstetrics: normal and problem pregnancies,* ed 2, New York, 1991, Churchhill Livingstone.

Gonik B, Creasy RK: Preterm labor: its diagnosis and management, *Am J Obstet Gynecol* 154:3, 1986.

Goplerud, CP: The proper use of RH immoglobulin, *Iowa Perinatal Letter* 1(3), May/June 1980.

Hacker N, Moore JG, editors: *Essentials of obstetrics and gynecology,* Philadelphia, 1986, Saunders.

Hahlin H et al: Single progesterone assay for early recognition of abnormal pregnancy, *Hum Reprod* 5(5):622, 1990.

Harris BA Jr: Shoulder dystocia, *Clin Obstet Gynecol* 27(1):106, 1984.

Hauth JC et al: Reduced incidence of preterm delivery with metronidazole and erythromycin in women with bacterial vaginosis, *N Engl J Med* 333:1732, 1995.

Herbert WNP, Cefalo RC: Management of postpartum hemorrhage, *Clin Obstet Gynecol* 27(1):139, 1984.

Higby K et al: Do tocolytic agents stop preterm labor? A critical and comprehensive review of efficacy and safety, *Am J Obstet Gynecol* 168:1247, 1993.

Hillier SL et al: Association between bacterial vaginosis and preterm delivery of a low-birth-weight infant, *N Engl J Med* 333:1737, 1995.

Induction and augmentation of labor, *ACOG Techn Bull,* No 110, Nov 1987 (American College of Obstetricians and Gynecologists, Washington, D.C.).

Jack BW et al: Routine obstetric ultrasound, *Am Fam Physician* 35(5):173, 1987.
Johnson CA: Prenatal screening, *Am Fam Physician* 37(5):175, 1988.
Johnson SR: Postpartum hemorrhage, *Iowa Perinatal Letter* 7(2), 1986.
Johnson SR: Puerperal infections, *Iowa Perinatal Letter* 5(1), 1984.
Klavan M et al: *Clinical concepts of fetal heart rate monitoring,* Andover, Mass., 1977, Hewlett-Packard Co, Medical Products Group.
Krebs AB et al: Intrapartum fetal heart rate monitoring. I. Classification and prognosis of fetal heart rate patterns, *Am J Obstet Gynecol* 133(7): 762, 1979.
Kruse J: Alcohol use during pregnancy, *Am Fam Physician,* 29(4):199, 1984.
Kuller JA, Laifer SA: Contemporary approaches to prenatal diagnosis, *Am Fam Physician* 52:2277, 1995.
Laurence C: Vaginal birth after cesarean delivery, *Am Fam Physician* 37(6):167, 1988.
Lavin JP et al: Vaginal delivery in patients with a prior cesarean section, *Obstet Gynecol* 59(2):135, 1982.
Lee CY: Shoulder dystocia, *Clin Obstet Gynecol* 30(1):77, 1987.
Losh DP, Dutring JL: Management of the postdate pregnancy, *Am Fam Physician* 36(2):184, 1987.
McDonald HM et al: Bacterial vaginosis in pregnancy and efficacy of short-course oral metronidazole treatment: a randomized controlled triak, *Obstet Gynecol* 84:343, 1994.
Mills JL et al: Moderate caffeine use and the risk of spontaneous abortion and intrauterine growth retardation, *JAMA* 269:593, 1993.
Milunsky A, Haddow JE: Cautions about maternal serum alpha-fetoprotein screening [Letter], *N Engl J Med* 313:694, 1985.
Nagey DA, Saller DN: An analysis of the decisions in the management of premature rupture of the membranes, *Clin Obstet Gynecol* 29(4):826, 1986.
National Diabetes Data Group: Classification and diagnosis of diabetes mellitus in other categories of glucose intolerance, *Diabetes* 28:1039, 1979.
Nielsen TF: Cesarean section: a controversial feature of modern obstetric practice, *Gynecol Obstet Invest* 21(2):57, 1986.
Niswander KR, editor: *Manual of obstetrics: diagnosis and therapy,* ed 3, Boston, 1987, Little, Brown & Co.
Norman CA, Karp LE: Biophysical profile and antepartum fetal assessment, *Am Fam Physician* 34(4):83, 1986.
Paisley JE, Mellion MB: Exercise during pregnancy, *Am Fam Physician* 38(5):143, 1988.
Peter G: Childhood immunizations, *N Eng J Med* 327(25):1794, 1992.
Pickles CJ et al: *Br J Obstet Gynaecol* 99:964, 1992.
Pritchard JA et al, editors: *Williams obstetrics,* ed 17, Norwalk, Conn., 1985, Appleton-Century-Crofts.
Ramin SM et al: Randomized trial of epidural versus intravenous analgesia during labor, *Obstet Gynecol* 86(5):783, 1995.
Rayburn WF, Lavin JP, editors: *Obstetrics for the house officer,* Baltimore, 1984, Williams & Wilkins.
Rouse DJ et al: Screening and treatment of asymptomatic bacteriuria of pregnancy to prevent pyelonephritis: a cost-effectiveness and cost benefit analysis, *Obstet Gynecol* 86:119, 1995.
Rubin PC: Hypertension in pregnancy, *J Hypertension* 5 (suppl 3):357, 1987.
Sabakian V et al: Vitamin B_6 is effective therapy for nausea and vomiting of pregnancy: a randomized double blind placebo controlled study, *Obstet gynecol* 78:33, 1991.
Schwager EJ, Weiss BD: Prenatal testing for maternal serum alpha-fetoprotein, *Am Fam Physician* 35(4):169, 1987.
Scott LL et al: Acyclovir suppression to prevent cesarean delivery after first-episode genital herpes, *Obstet Gynecol* 87:69, 1996.
Stovall TG et al: Improved sensitivity and specificity of a single measurement of serum progesterone over serial quantitative beta-human chorionic gonadotrophin in screening for ectopic pregnancy, *Hum Reprod* 7(5):723, 1992.

Usta IM et al: The impact of a policy of amnioinfusion for meconium-stained amniotic fluid, *Obstet Gynecol* 85:237, 1995.
Varner MW: Third-trimester bleeding, *Iowa Perinatal Letter* 5(6), Nov-Dec 1987.
Varner MW: Hypertension in pregnancy, *Iowa Perinatal Letter* 7(6), Nov/Dec 1986.
Walbroehl GS: Sexuality during pregnancy, *Am Fam Physician* 29(5):273, 1984.
Weiner CP: The diagnosis and management of gestational diabetes, *Iowa Perinatal Letter* 3(5), Sept-Oct 1987.
Wenstrom K et al: Amnioinfusion survey: prevalence, protocols, and complications, *Obstet Gynecol* 86:572-576, 1995.
Williamson R: Maternal alpha-fetoprotein screening, *Iowa Perinatal Letter* 7(1), Jan-Feb 1986.
Yancey MK et al: Peripartum infection associated with vaginal group B streptococcal colonization, *Obstet Gynecol* 84:816, 1994.
Yancey MK et al: Risk factors for neonatal sepsis, *Obstet Gynecol* 87:188, 1996.

9

General Surgery

Mark A. Graber

WOUND MANAGEMENT

I. GENERAL PRINCIPLES

The goal of wound management is primarily restoration of function, which requires minimizing risk of infection and repair of injured tissue with a minimum of cosmetic deformity. *Be sure to maintain universal precautions.*

II. SIGNIFICANT HISTORY

A. Mechanism of injury.

1. ***Blunt trauma.*** Split or crush type of injuries will swell more and tend to have more devitalized tissue and a higher risk of infection.
2. ***Sharp trauma.*** Clean edges, low cellular injury, and risk of infection.
3. ***Bite injury.*** See p. 58.

B. Contaminants. Wound contact with manure, rust, dirt, etc., will increase risk of infection. Wounds sustained in barnyards or stables are considered contaminated. *Clostridium tetani* is indigenous in manure.

C. Time of injury. After 3 hours, the bacterial count in a wound increases dramatically. Wounds may be closed primarily up to 18 hours out; clean well and use clinical judgment when choosing which wounds to close. Wounds up to 24 hours old on the face may be closed after good cleaning. The blood supply in this area is much better and the risk of infection therefore much less. The risk of infection may be reduced in wounds by use of tape closures (such as Steri-Strip tape).

D. Tetanus status (Table 9-1).

E. Other medical illnesses. Diabetes, chemotherapy, steroids, peripheral vascular disease, and malnutrition may delay wound healing and increase the risk of infection.

III. PHYSICAL EXAM

A. Vascular injury. Direct pressure is the first choice for controlling bleeding. If a fracture is involved, immobilization will help control bleeding. Do not clamp vascular structures until it is determined if it is a significant vessel needing repair. If the anatomy is suspicious for injury to major vascular structures, obtain angiogram and consider surgical consult (see Chapter 1). Capillary refill should be checked distally. Bleeding on the scalp is best controlled by suturing of the wound. For extremities, inflating a blood pressure cuff above systolic pressure assists in wound inspection and repair. *However, be careful not to cause ischemic injury to the extremity.*

B. Neurologic injury. Check distal muscle strength and sensation. Always check sensation before administering anesthesia. For hand and finger lacerations check 2-point discrimination, which should be less than 1 cm at the fingertips. A crush injury may also decrease 2-point discrimination. This may take several months to recover. A lacerated nerve may be repaired immediately or have repair delayed. Loss of sensation may be the first sign of a developing compartment syndrome. See p. 44 for full discussion of compartment syndrome.

C. Tendons. Can be evaluated by inspection, but individual muscles must also be tested for full range of motion and full strength.

D. Bones. Check for open fracture or associated fractures. X-ray if any question. An open fracture is an indication for surgical débridement and repair except in the case of a distal phalanx fracture where copious irrigation and oral antibiotics are acceptable treatment if the injury can be watched carefully for infection.

E. Foreign bodies. Inspect and x-ray the area. Remember that wood or low-lead glass may not show on radiograph. Wound markers can be used during radiographing, and views obtained in two planes can help localize the object for recovery. Glass may penetrate at an angle and be buried deeper than it appears to be. Ultrasonography is very sensitive at picking up foreign bodies if radiograph is questionable or there is strong clinical suspicion.

IV. REPAIR

A. Wound healing.

1. ***Collagen formation.*** Peaks at day 7. Wound has 15% to 20% of full strength at 3 weeks, 60% full strength at 4 months. Ephithelialization occurs in 48 hours under optimal conditions. The wound is then completely sealed.
2. ***Scar formation.*** Requires 6 to 12 months for a mature scar. The smallest scar will be formed when the wound is not under tension. Scars should not be revised until 12

TABLE 9-1
Tetanus Status

Last tetanus booster	Clean wound	Dirty wound
Unknown or never immunized	0.5 ml of tetanus toxoid Repeat 6 weeks and 6 months to 1 year	0.5 ml of tetanus toxoid Repeat at 6 weeks and 6 months to 1 year 250 U of human tetanus immune globulin
>5 years to <10 years	None (consider 0.5 ml of tetanus toxoid)	0.5 ml of tetanus toxoid
10 years	0.5 ml of tetanus toxoid	0.5 ml of tetanus toxoid

months have passed. Contractures can develop when a scar intersects perpendicularly to a joint crease.

B. Anesthesia.

1. ***Topical anesthesia.*** LAT and TAC can be used alone or can be used to greatly decrease the pain of infiltration.
   a. *LAT.* 4% lidocaine, 1:2000 epinephrine (also known as adrenaline), and 0.5% tetracaine. 5 ml on cotton ball and placed in wound.
      (1) Works well as TAC and does not need to be locked up as controlled substance.
      (2) Takes 10 to 30 minutes to work.
      (3) Cheaper than TAC ($3.00 versus $35.00 per dose).
      (4) *Precautions.* Avoid use on face or near mucous membranes (absorption through mucous membranes may cause seizures). Avoid LAT in areas where epinephrine would be contraindicated, as on distal digits, tip of nose, ears, penis.
   b. *TAC.* (0.5% tetracaine, 1:2000 epinephrine (also known as adrenaline), 11.8% cocaine); requires approximately 30 minutes for onset of action. Put 5 ml on a cotton ball and then place in wound. Same precautions as with LAT.
   c. *Both TAC and LAT* can be combined with hydroxyethylcellulose to make a gel that can be applied to the wound.
2. ***Local.*** Use 27- or 30-gauge needle and infiltrate slowly and through the open wound edge avoiding the intact skin. This decreases the pain of infiltration. The addition of bicarbonate to lidocaine before infiltration has been shown to significantly decrease the pain of injection (9 ml of lidocaine and 1 ml of bicarbonate) and warming lidocaine to body temperature may help as well.

a. *Lidocaine* (0.5% to 2%) most frequently used with onset 2 to 5 minutes, duration 60 minutes. Can use 3 to 5 mg/kg with not more than 300 mg total (in adults). Avoid using lidocaine with epinephrine on distal extremities such as the ears, fingers, toes, and penis.
b. *Mepivacaine* (Carbocaine) has onset 3 to 5 minutes, duration of 90 to 120 minutes.
c. *Bupivacaine* (Marcaine) has onset 5 to 10 minutes, duration of hours; longest lasting of the local anesthetics. Intravenous administration may cause serious arrhythmias.
d. *For "caine" allergies*, use diphenhydramine diluted to 1%. Mix 5% diphenhydramine 1:4 ml with normal saline to make a 1% solution. Onset of anesthesia takes longer and does not last so long as with lidocaine. Stronger solutions may cause tissue necrosis.

3. ***Regional anesthesia.*** Especially good for fingers, hands, feet, toes, mouth, and face. See Chapter 17 for common blocks.

C. Wound prep.

1. ***Débridement.*** Using aseptic technique, devitalized tissue should be removed; avoid taking healthy tissue. High-pressure irrigation is the most effective means of cleansing a wound. Can use a 35 ml syringe with a 19-gauge needle and normal saline. Scrubbing does not cleanse the wound as well and using any disinfectant in the wound damages healthy cells needed for healing.
2. ***Skin disinfection.*** Can be performed with povidone-iodine solution or chlorhexidine. Avoid getting these solutions in the wound because they impede wound healing. Shaving the area increases the risk of infection. Hair can be clipped in the area if necessary. Never shave eyebrows because they are needed for alignment of the wound and may not grow back.

D. Wound closure.

1. Avoid primary closure of infected and inflamed wounds, dirty wounds, human and animal bites, neglected and severe crush wounds.
2. ***Tape closure (with Steri-Strips or others).*** Strips carry a lower risk of infection than suturing does and may be a consideration for higher-risk wounds.
3. ***Open wound care.*** Saline wet to dry dressings with gauze will keep the tissue moist and help débride, Gentle washing of the wound 2 to 3 times per day will remove bacterially contaminated secretions (showers are appropriate for this). Avoid iodine dressings because they damage healthy tissue and will slow granulation. When clean granulation tissue is apparent, secondary

closure may be considered or can change to dry, sterile, packing material.

4. ***Suturing.*** Sutures are of two types: (1) absorbable and (2) nonabsorbable. Precision-point cutting needles, and small-sized suture (5-0 or 6-0) should be chosen for skin when a cosmetic closure is important as on the face. Conventional cutting needle is used for routine skin closure. 4-0 or 3-0 nylon may be used on extremities. Noncutting needle should be used for subcutaneous tissue. Extensor tendons are slow healing and should have permanent suture of small size chosen (such as polypropylene). Depending on your practice situation, a surgical consultation should be considered. The majority of subcutaneous or dermal suturing may be performed with an intermediate-duration absorbable suture. However, some wounds require permanent sutures (such as stainless steel wires in sternotomy). See Table 9-2.
5. ***Staples.*** Can be used on the scalp and abdomen with good result. However, avoid use on face, hand, or other areas where structures such as tendons and nerves may become incorporated into the staples.
6. ***Dressings.*** Consider antibiotic ointment on face and torso. Antibiotic ointment should be avoided on distal extremities for more than 24 to 48 hours because it may lead to maceration and delayed wound healing. Immobilize if motion of a joint is going to increase skin tension. Keep the wound dry for 24 hours, after which time most wounds do not require a dressing.
7. Facial wounds should have crusts soaked off and bacitracin or other ointment applied QID × 5 days to reduce scar formation.
8. ***Antibiotics.*** There is no medical indication for using prophylactic antibiotics in routine, noncontaminated, skin wounds.
   a. Consider antibiotic use for patients prone to endocarditis, patients with hip prostheses, lymphedema, contaminated foot wound in diabetics, or others with peripheral vascular disease.
   b. See Chapter 1 for antibiotic choices for bite wounds, p. 58.

V. FOLLOW-UP CARE

A. Risk of infection highest 24 to 48 hours, and so all wounds should be rechecked.

B. General guidelines for suture removal.

- *Face,* 3 to 5 days with tape reinforcement after suture removal.
- *Scalp,* 7 to 10 days; *trunk,* 7 to 10 days; *arms,* 7 to 10 days; *legs,* 10 to 14 days; *joints, dorsal surface,* 14 days.

TABLE 9-2
Suture Materials and Characteristics

Suture	Strength	Inflammatory reaction	Ease of use	Infection resistance	Notes
NONABSORBABLE SUTURES					
Nylon monofilament	+++	++	+++	+++	Good for skin closure Use two throws on the first knot
Polypropylene (Prolene) monofilament	++++	+	+	++++	Good for skin More difficult to use than nylon
Silk	+	++++	++++	++	Has fallen out of favor Used mostly intraorally
ABSORBABLE SUTURES					
Gut or chromic gut	++	+++	++	+	Rarely used Can almost always be replaced by Dexon or Vicryl
Dexon (polyglycolic acid braided polymer)	++++	+	++++	++++	A good choice for subcutaneous and intraoral sutures
Vicryl (polyglactin 910 braided polymer)	++++	+	++++	+++	Same as above

Adapted from Barkin R, Rosen P, editors: *Emergency pediatrics,* St. Louis, 1986, Mosby.

- Increase length for diabetics or steroid-dependent patients who may require several weeks to heal.

PREOPERATIVE CARDIAC RISK ASSESSMENT

There are currently 8 million surgeries in the United States on patients with known or suspected cardiac disease. Preoperative evaluation can help stratify risk. Several methods of assessing risk are available.

A. **The Goldman index.** Useful in predicting cardiac events in an unselected, random group of patients. However, it does not work well when applied to subgroups, such as all those with known heart disease. The type and extent of surgery anticipated needs to be taken into account when one is interpreting the results of the Goldman index. See Table 9-3 for Goldman index and Table 9-4 for risk and preoperative characteristics.

TABLE 9-3
Goldman Index

Factor	Definition	Number of points
Ischemic heart disease	MI within 6 months	10
Congestive heart failure	S_3 gallop, JVD	11
Cardiac rhythm	Rhythm other than sinus or premature atrial contractions on last preoperative ECG *or* >5 premature ventricular contractions per minute at anytime before surgery	7 7
Valvular heart disease	Significant aortic stenosis	3
General medical status	Po_2 <60 mm Hg, Pco_2 >50 mm Hg, K <3.0 mmol/L, bicarbonate <20 mmol/L, BUN >50 mg/dl, creatinine >3.0 mg/dl, abnormal AST, signs of chronic liver disease, patient bedridden from noncardiac causes	3
Age	>70	5
Type of surgery	Intraperitoneal, intrathoracic, aortic or emergency operation	3 4

Class I, 0-5 points; *class II*, 6-12 points; *class III*, 13-25 points; *class IV*, >25

Modified from Mangano DT, Goldman L: *N Engl J Med* 333(26):1750, 1995.

TABLE 9-4

Risk of Major Cardiac Complications of Different Patient Groups Using the Goldman Index

Goldman index class	Unselected patients over 40 years of age (%)	Patients with known coronary disease or other high-risk patients (%)	Patients undergoing minor surgery (all patients) (%)
I	1.2	3	0.3
II	3.0	11	1
III	12	30	about 2.8
IV	48	75	about 19

Modified from Mangano DT, Goldman L: *N Engl J Med* 333(26):1750, 1995.

B. **Functional status.** If patient can walk up stairs while carrying a load (functional status class I and II) and has a low Goldman index, no known cardiac disease, there is a very low risk of cardiac complications.

C. **Electrocardiography.**
   1. Ischemia on a resting ECG is suggestive of a worse outcome.
   2. Exercise tolerance appears to be more important than ECG changes, and so if functional status is good (class I or II), GXT need not be done. GXT should be reserved for those with recent-onset chest pain and in those whose functional status is unclear.

D. **Echocardiography.** Should be reserved for those who would need an echocardiogram even if they were not having surgery, this is, those with murmurs that have not been previously evaluated and those with CHF of unknown cause (diastolic versus systolic versus valvular, etc.). Preliminary data on stress echocardiography indicate that those with wall-motion abnormalities at a low heart rate may be at higher surgical risk. If used, this modality should be reserved for those with known cardiac disease. Further data are needed, however, before this can be recommended.

E. **Radionuclide ventriculography determined ejection fraction.** Has not been shown to be useful in determining risk for infarction. Note, however, that this type of datum is taken into account with clinical measures in the Goldman index (S_3 gallop, JVD) and in functional status (class).

F. **Thallium scanning.** Seems to be highly sensitive at selecting those who will have postoperative cardiac problems. Specificity is a problem (53% to 80%) unless restricted to a high-risk group. The use of thallium scanning should be restricted to those individuals who cannot exercise (therefore cannot determine functional status) and those whose risk cannot be determined by clinical criteria.

G. **History of MI.** <3 weeks has 25% mortality; urgent procedure only. At 3 months 10% mortality; semiurgent procedures. At 6 months 5% mortality: elective. At 1 year, same risk as asymptomatic patient with cardiac disease.

H. See Tables 9-2 to 9-5 for approach suggested by D.T. Mangano and L. Goldman: *N Engl J Med* 333(26):1750, 1995.

I. Recent data indicate that in those patients undergoing noncardiac surgery who have known coronary artery disease or a high risk of coronary artery disease (2 or more risk factors) atenolol started preoperatively and continued until discharge from the hospital may decrease overall mortality at 2 years. Most of the lower mortality is attributable to lower cardiac mortality in the 6 to 8 months after surgery. (See Mangano DT et al: *N Engl J Med* 335:1713-1720, 1996.)

TABLE 9-5
Patient Characteristics and Preoperative Testing Required

Characteristics of patient	Preoperative diagnostic testing	Special perioperative treatment
No known cardiac disease, good functional status, class I or II on the Goldman index	None except routine ECG and CXR if indicated	None
Known stable coronary artery disease and good functional statue (function class I or early class II)	None except routine ECG and CXR if indicated	Conservative treatment*
Known coronary artery disease, functional status unclear	Noninvasive testing‡	If test is *negative,* conservative treatment.* If test is *positive,* aggressive medical therapy or angiography†; then retest. If test is *positive,* aggressive medical treatment† including medication intensification and addressing risk factors (such as smoking) and repeat test. If now *negative,* use conservative treatment.* If still *positive,* consider more aggressive treatment and repeat noninvasive test. If still *positive,* consider coronary angiography and revascularization (such as PTCA) if indicated.

Continued

TABLE 9-5
Patient Characteristics and Preoperative Testing Required—cont'd

Characteristics of patient	Preoperative diagnostic testing	Special perioperative treatment
Known coronary artery disease, poor cardiac functional status	None	Aggressive medical treatment or angiography if indicated.‡
Poor *noncardiac* functional status, no known coronary artery disease or status unclear		
1. No or few risk factors§	1. If no or few risk factors, none.	1. If no or few risk factors, none.
2. Multiple risk factors§	2. If multiple risk factors, noninvasive testing.‡	2. If multiple risk factors and test is *negative*, conservative treatment.* If test is *positive*, aggressive medical treatment or angiography.†
Coronary artery disease and either class III or IV on Goldman cardiac risk index	None	Aggressive medical treatment or angiography.†

Modified from Mangano DT, Goldman L: *N Engl J Med* 333(26):1750, 1995.
**Conservative treatment:* Continue cardiac medications, postoperative ECG day 1, after any suspicious perioperative events, and before discharge.
†*Aggressive medical therapy:* Aggressive medical treatment including medication intensification and addressing risk factors (i.e., smoking) followed by repeat noninvasive testing.
‡*Noninvasive testing:* Exercise stress testing if patient can exercise. If patient cannot exercise, use stress echocardiogram, dipyridamole-thallium scan, or ambulatory monitor for ischemia.
§Risk factors include age >70 years, diabetes mellitus, CHF, important arrhythmias, known vascular disease, need for aortic, abdominal, or thoracic surgery.
Functional class I or II: Can walk up steps carrying groceries or similar load.

PREOPERATIVE LAB EVALUATION

A complete history and physical examination will uncover most abnormalities and preoperative lab testing can be targeted to those in whom it is indicated. One guideline from Mayo clinic suggests that the minimal preoperative test requirements are (1) an ECG and determination of creatinine and glucose in apparently healthy patients 40 to 59 years of age; (2) an ECG, chest radiograph, and determination of the CBC, creatinine, and glucose in patients 60 years of age or older; and (3) no testing for apparently healthy patients below 40 years. Other recommendations are below. Your surgeon and institution may require certain preoperative tests, and these guidelines should be followed. However, the literature would suggest the following approach in the healthy patient who is having an elective procedure:

A. **Coagulation studies (PT/INR, PTT).** Routine use is not indicated. Should be performed on those with stigmas of liver disease, history of coagulopathy, those in whom DIC is suspected, those receiving anticoagulation, those with alcohol abuse, etc.
B. **CBC.** Routine use is not indicated. Useful only in those who are expected to have significant blood loss during surgery or when hematologic or infectious processes are believed to be present.
C. **Electrolytes.** Routine use is not indicated. Indicated only in those patients using diuretics, who have renal or cardiac disease, or who may be dehydrated secondary to fluid loss.
D. **Glucose.** Routine use is not indicated. Indicated only in those diabetic, obese, or undergoing vascular procedures or have another reason to have an elevated glucose such as steroid use.
E. **BUN and creatinine.** Routine use is not indicated. Should be obtained in those over 60 years of age and those with a history of renal disease, cardiac disease, or peripheral vascular disease.
F. **Urinalysis.** Routine use is not indicated. Indicated in those patients who have a symptomatic UTI or who are diabetic.
G. **Pregnancy test.** If indicated by history.
H. **Liver enzymes.** Routine use not indicated. Use only when historical or physical evidence of liver disease.
I. **ECG and CXR.** As indicated by history or physical exam.

PREOPERATIVE CARE AND EVALUATION

I. ADMIT ORDERS

A. **Admit to ward or primary physician.**
B. **Diagnosis and planned procedure.**
C. **Condition.**
D. **Vital signs.** For elective procedure every shift. For emergency procedure as dictated by condition.
E. **Allergies.** Medications (especially antibiotics), foods, dressing materials (such as tape), etc.

F. **Activity.** Bed rest if unstable vital signs or other indication; otherwise encourage activity to avoid DVT, muscle atrophy, pneumonia.

G. **Nursing.** Neurologic checks, monitoring lines (CVP, Swan-Ganz), preoperative teaching, PCA pump, pulmonary toilet, etc.

H. **Diet.** Determined by rest of medical history and the preparation required for surgery. Period of NPO before surgery dependent on age of patient (infants may have clear liquids up to 4 hours before surgery; adults should be NPO at least 6 to 8 hours).

I. **Intake and output.** Fluids for rehydration (NS or LR), maintenance and correction of electrolyte imbalance. Blood products if needed. Monitoring of fluids and fluid status (CVP/Swan-Ganz, Foley).

J. **Special tests.** As indicated by diagnosis (such as endoscopy before colorectal surgery for cancer).

K. **Special medications.**

1. Patient's routine medications; change medications to IM or IV as needed.
2. Increased steroids preoperatively if steroid dependent.
3. Pain medications as needed. There is some evidence that treating pain with morphine preoperatively reduces postoperative pain.
4. Antibiotics as indicated for infection and sepsis or prophylaxis of endocarditis, indwelling hardware or graft placement.
   a. Preoperative antibiotics are most effective when given within 2 hours before surgery. Cefotaxime 1 g IV or cefoxitin 2 g IV have been shown to reduce infection rates for intra-abdominal surgery and should be used.
   b. There is no evidence that continuing "prophylactic" antibiotics postoperatively is helpful. However, antibiotics should be continued if there is active infection or contamination.
   c. For cardiac valvular disease, history artificial valve, etc, use additional prophylactic antibiotics as recommended by the American Heart Association (see Chapter 2).
5. ***Prep for surgery.*** Bowel preps, DVT (see p. 397 for DVT prophylaxis recommendations), and antiseptic shower and hair clipping if indicated.
6. Premedication by anesthesia to lower anxiety, lower secretions, and interact with narcotics for sedation.

L. **Lab tests.** See p. 391 for suggested routine lab tests.

II. MEDICAL HISTORY OF MAJOR IMPORTANCE

A. **Neurologic disorders.** For seizures some anticonvulsants are oral only. May need to change medications if patient will be NPO for long period of time.

B. Hematologic disorders.

1. ***Positive sickle cell screen.*** Needs Hb electrophoresis. If majority is Hb S will need partial exchange transfusion before surgical procedure.
2. ***Clotting disorders.*** May need evaluation, treatment (see Chapter 5).
3. ***Anemia.*** Ideally HCT >30%, with Hb >10 g by time of surgery though there is no evidence that anemia contributes to surgical morbidity in the well-hydrated patient with a Hb >7.0 g.

C. Integument disorders. If possible, avoid operating when there are active skin infections present. Chronic skin disorders should be optimally controlled for postoperative healing. For those who are keloid formers may need to consider different closure techniques.

D. Nutritional status.

1. For elective or semielective surgery consider optimizing nutritional status if patient has chronic disease.
2. ***Obesity.*** Weight loss to improve cardiopulmonary status and decrease problems with healing.

E. Cardiac. For congestive heart failure, optimize myocardial function and fluid balance. Consider preoperative Swan-Ganz catheter. Also consider pacemaker if indicated. However, Swan-Ganz monitoring may adversely affect outcome.

F. Pulmonary.

1. ***COPD.*** Optimize pulmonary toilet and use incentive spirometry to encourage lung expansion. Check for any change in sputum production or color indicating active infection; delay elective or semiurgent procedures until pulmonary reserve maximized.
2. ***Baseline spirometry and ABGs.*** May help with postoperative management.

III. OPERATIVE NOTE

A. Preoperative diagnosis.
B. Postoperative diagnosis.
C. Procedure or operation performed.
D. Surgeon, assistants.
E. Anesthesia. General endotracheal, general mask, spinal, epidural, regional block, local, etc.; include specific agent used.
F. Findings.
G. Specimen. Frozen section if obtained, pathologic and microscopic characteristics, etc.
H. Estimated blood loss.
I. Intraoperative fluids and blood products administered.
J. Drains and tubes placed.
K. Complications.
L. Patient's condition and disposition.

POSTOPERATIVE CARE

I. ORDERS

A. Admit to ward, ICU, or recovery room.

B. Diagnosis. Operation.

C. Vital signs. Every 30 minutes for first few hours and then reduce as stable.

D. Allergies.

E. Activity. Bedrest until fully awake; up walking that night or next morning depending on surgery. Up to chair QID if unable to ambulate.

F. Diet. NPO until nausea resolves or resumption of bowel activity as determined by bowel sounds, passing gas, or having bowel movement. Start with clear liquids and advance as tolerated.

G. Intake and output.

1. Record I&O every shift or more frequently if patient's condition is unstable.
2. ***IV fluids.*** With surgeries involving third spacing replace with isotonic solutions or colloid for first 24 hours. NG losses should be replaced with 0.45 NS, and if in exceptionally large amounts, replace losses milliliter for milliliter. Maintenance fluids should generally be 0.2 NS or 5% dextrose in 0.45 NS. Potassium is normally included in replacement solutions but is excluded from maintenance solutions until normal renal function is established. See below for evaluation of postoperative oliguria.
3. Instructions for care of all tubes and drains including a Foley catheter and nasogastric tube. NG tube should be connected to low intermittent suction and irrigated frequently to ensure patency. *Remove Foley and other tubes as soon as possible. Prolonged indwelling catheters predispose to infection.*

H. Nursing.

1. Encourage turning, coughing, deep breathing, and incentive spirometry. Deep breathing has been shown to significantly reduce the rate of respiratory complications such as pneumonia.
2. Dressing changes.
3. Parameters to notify doctor such as urine output (<0.5 ml/kg/hour), fever, hypertension or hypotension, tachycardia or bradycardia, inability to void within 8 hours of beginning surgery, or unusual drainage on dressings, tachypnea, or bleeding.
4. Specify neurologic or vascular checks.

I. Medications.

1. ***Pain medications.*** Oral or IV (by PCA or injection). PCA provides better analgesia, and patients generally require less narcotic than with IM treatment; there is little indication for IM pain medications. Adequate doses improve mobility. High doses lead to hypoventilation and atelectasis.

2. There is little or no evidence that hydroxyzine or promethazine HCl (Phenergan) have an opiate-sparing effect. In fact, Phenergan may have an antianalgesic effect. They are, however, sedatives.
3. Tramadol (Ultram) has not been shown to be effective in postoperative pain.
4. Propoxyphene-acetaminophen combinations have not been shown to be any better than acetaminophen alone.
5. Hydrocodone combinations (such as Lortab, Vicodin) are as effective as or more effective than codeine combinations (Tylenol 3 and others) and have fewer GI and CNS side effects. Oxycodone (Percodan and others) may also be effective.
6. ***Patient-controlled analgesia.***
   a. *Morphine.* Bolus with 2 to 10 mg over 20 to 30 minutes. Use PCA pump that delivers 1.0 mg aliquots with an initial lockout time of about 5 to 15 minutes (therefore 4 to 12 mg/hour). Generally start at 10-minute lockout and adjust from there.
   b. *Meperidine.* Bolus 20 to 100 mg over 20 to 30 minutes and then PCA pump that delivers 10 mg aliquots with a lockout time of 5 to 20 minutes. Generally start at 10-minute lockout and adjust from there.
7. ***If using IM.***
   a. *Morphine:* 0.1 mg/kg IM Q3-6h.
   b. *Meperidine:* 10 mg/kg IM Q3-6h.
8. ***Antiemetics.*** First consider if medications may be causing nausea, if NG tube is plugged, or if this is post-anesthetic nausea. Some options are:
   a. *Prochlorperazine* (Compazine and others) 5 to 10 mg IV Q6h. May cause hypotension and dystonic reactions.
   b. *Metoclopramide* (Reglan and others) 5 to 10 mg or more (up to 30 mg) IV Q6h. May cause dystonic reactions.
   c. *Droperidol* (Inapsine) 1.25 to 2.5 mg IV. May be sedating.
   d. *Ondansetron* (Zofran) 4 mg IV over 15 minutes (good but expensive). Does not cause dystonia.
   e. Watch for dystonic reactions and confusion with first three (a, b, c). Diphenhydramine 25 to 50 mg or benztropine 1 mg can be used to counteract dystonia.
9. Antibiotics. For infection.
10. Routine medications that need to be renewed.
11. PRN medications such as laxatives, sleeping medications, and antacids.

J. Special test such as follow-up CXRs or serial ECGs. ECG should be performed on postoperative day 1 for high-risk patients.

K. **Laboratory.** Follow-up CBC for possibility of hemorrhage or for large amount of blood loss. If patient continues on IV fluid, check daily electrolytes.

L. See below for postoperative DVT prophylaxis.

II. POSTOPERATIVE FEVERS BY ORGAN SYSTEM

A. Respiratory.

1. Initial may be secondary to aspiration.
2. 24 to 48 hours postoperatively most commonly blamed on atelectasis but recent data has called this association into question. Do not ignore an emerging pneumonia.
3. After 48 hours most likely is a developing pneumonia.

B. Wound infections.

1. First 24 hours suggestive of *Clostridium*.
2. 48 to 72 hours most commonly caused by streptococci.
3. 4 days consider enteric aerobes and anaerobes and staphylococci.

C. Thrombophlebitis. Occurs intraoperatively, and fever usually begins after 24 hours.

D. Urinary tract infections. Usually related to instrumentation or indwelling Foley catheter and occurs after 24 hours.

E. Less common causes of perioperative fever.

1. ***Transfusion reaction.*** Immediate (see hematology).
2. ***Malignant hyperthermia.*** Starts intraoperatively and is generally secondary to anesthetic drugs (see Chapter 1).
3. Drug reaction.
4. Endocrine, such as thyroid storm.
5. Thrombophlebitis from IV site.
6. Intra-abdominal abscess.

III. POSTOPERATIVE OLIGURIA

See also renal failure in Chapter 11.

A. Oliguria is defined as urine output less than 30 ml/hour or 1ml/kg/hour in children. Postoperative oliguria can be divided into:

1. ***Prerenal azotemia*** (that is, hypovolemia). Caused by decreased glomerular filtration rate secondary to hypovolemia or hypotension. This can occur with hemorrhage, GI loss, excessive renal loss, and sequestered loss (that is, third spacing loss).
2. ***Acute tubular necrosis*** (renal failure). Postoperatively it often develops when there is either preexisting renal disease, long periods of hypotension, use of nephrotoxic agents, septicemia, or hemolysis. (See Chapter 11 for detailed discussion of diagnosis and management.)
3. ***Other causes.***
   a. Reflex spasm of voluntary sphincter because of pain or anxiety.
   b. Medications such as anticholinergics and narcotics.
   c. Detrusor atony as result of surgery and manipulation (especially after retroperitoneal or pelvic surgery).
   d. Preexisting partial bladder outlet obstruction such as an enlarged prostate.

e. Mechanical obstruction such as an expanding hematoma or fluid collection, or occluded Foley catheter.

B. Diagnosis. Look for signs of hypovolemia such as decreased skin turgor or dry mucous membranes, tachycardia, hypotension. If patient cannot or has no desire to urinate after several hours postoperatively, consider oliguria secondary to hypovolemia. A palpable bladder is a sign of urinary retention.

C. Treatment. Relieve pain. If condition permits, perhaps standing or sitting may facilitate voiding.

1. ***Hypovolemia.*** Treat hypovolemia if present with a bolus of normal saline (250 ml aliquots) until maintaining urine output at 30 to 60 ml/hour in adults and 0.5 to 1 ml/kg/hour in children. Diuretics will worsen prerenal azotemia.
2. ***Mechanical obstruction.*** If mechanical obstruction, such as enlarged prostate, consider intermittent catheterization. If the patient already has a Foley catheter, irrigate it to assess for obstruction.

IV. POSTOPERATIVE DVT PROPHYLAXIS

A. 40% to 50% of those with hip surgery will develop a DVT postoperatively; 16% will develop DVT even with the best prophylaxis. If not given prophylaxis, 15% to 30% of those with abdominal surgery will develop a DVT; DVT prophylaxis after surgery is cost effective and reduces the incidence of DVT and PE. Early ambulation is important. Enoxaparin is approved for post–hip surgery prophylaxis; dalteparin is approved for post–abdominal surgery prophylaxis.

B. Options for DVT prophylaxis.

1. ***Enoxaparin.*** 30 mg SQ BID. Subcutaneous low-molecular-weight heparin is the most effective form of prophylaxis and has fewer complications than unfractionated heparin has. Start postoperatively within 24 hours and continue until patient is ambulatory. It is approved for this indication in the United States. It also may be cost effective because no need to monitor PTT and reduced incidence of bleeding compared to other prophylactic measures. Can also be used for DVT prophylaxis after other surgery, such as abdominal surgery. May have delayed excretion with renal failure.
2. ***Dalteparin.*** 2500 anti–factor Xa IU SQ QD starting 1 to 2 hours before abdominal surgery and continuing for 5 to 10 days postoperatively. Must be adjusted for renal function. No good evidence that it is better than unfractionated heparin and is more expensive and so is not suggested. Use with caution in renal and hepatic disease.
3. ***Heparin (unfractionated).*** 5000 units SQ Q12h.
4. ***Graded compression stockings.*** Effective and have few side effects.

5. ***Warfarin.*** Less effective than low-molecular-weight heparin and has greater bleeding complications.
6. ***Aspirin.*** Not very effective in postsurgical DVT prophylaxis, and other choices, especially enoxaparin, are preferred.
7. Only low-molecular-weight heparin and graded compression stockings have been shown to reduce the incidence of pulmonary embolism.

ABDOMINAL PAIN

Although classic surgical teaching has been that pain medication may confuse the diagnosis of abdominal pain in the emergency setting, this is not supported by the literature. In fact, if anything, the diagnosis may be clarified by pain relief resulting in fewer unnecessary surgeries. Clearly we need to work with our surgical colleagues and should discuss this with them before the need arises.

I. HISTORY

A. The area of the pain, including its origin and pattern of radiation, time of onset, nature, and associated symptoms will frequently make the diagnosis. A menstrual history should be obtained (Table 9-6).

B. Associated symptoms.

1. Weight loss, which might indicate malignancy or malabsorption.
2. Vomiting as with a small bowel obstruction or volvulus (obstruction especially if fecal).
3. Diarrhea and constipation, which might indicate inflammatory bowel disease, cancer, obstipation, malabsorption.
4. Melena or blood per rectum: check with Hemoccult. If negative consider foods (Kool-Aid, beets) or medicines (iron).

C. Jaundice. Consider pancreatic cancer (painless), hepatitis, hemolysis (sickle cell, G6PD deficiency, transfusion reaction), alcoholic hepatitis, choledocholithiasis, primary biliary cirrhosis, etc.

D. Urinary symptoms. Dysuria, frequency, urgency, hematuria. Renal problems often present as a complaint of abdominal pain. Consider urolithiasis, UTI, testicular torsion, etc.

E. Sexual activity, last period, birth control, history of venereal disease, vaginal discharge, spotting or bleeding. Consider ectopic pregnancy, PID, ovarian torsion, ruptured ovarian cyst, etc.

F. Past medical history including other major illnesses, prior surgeries, prior studies performed for evaluation of abdominal problems, family history of any similar complaints.

G. Medications. Especially digoxin, theophylline, steroids, tetracycline (esophageal ulcers), analgesics, antipyretics, antiemetics, barbiturates, diuretics, alendronate (esophageal ulcers).

TABLE 9-6
Abdominal Pain by Main Location

Diagnosis	Usual pain location	Diagnostic studies	Pain radiates to and comments
Hepatitis, subphrenic abscess, hepatic abscess	RUQ	Ultrasonography, CT	Right shoulder, elevated liver enzymes, jaundice
Cholecystitis, cholelithiasis, and cholangitis	RUQ	Ultrasonography	Back, right scapula, midepigastric, sudden onset with associated nausea
Fitz-Hugh-Curtis syndrome	RUQ and signs of PID	Perihepatitis: elevated liver enzymes, associated pelvic disease	Right shoulder and back
Pancreatitis	Midepigastric region	Elevated amylase, lipase, WBC May have normal amylase and lipase if chronic pancreatitis CT scan or U/S will show edema	Radiates to back, may have peritonitis
Cardiac disease	May present as epigastric pain	ECG and enzymes to rule out cardiac disease	May be confused with esophageal reflux
Duodenal ulcer or gastric ulcer	Midepigastric/LUQ pain	UGI or endoscopy Usually historical (see Chapter 4)	Radiation to back if posterior ulcer, peritonitis with perforation

TABLE 9-6
Abdominal Pain by Main Location—cont'd

Diagnosis	Usual pain location	Diagnostic studies	Pain radiates to and comments
Splenic hematoma or enlargement	LUQ pain	U/S or CT	Hypotension, peritonitis if ruptured
Aortic aneurysm	Periumbilical especially into back flanks May be colicky	U/S or CT	May present as epigastric or back pain, flank, hip pain Rule this out in the proper age group if history suggestive of renal stones Hypotension if ruptured
Appendicitis	Early periumbilical Late RLQ	CT or U/S may show abscess, enlarged appendix	May present with peritoneal signs
Cecal volvulus	RLQ pain	Seen on flat plate radiograph as RUQ distended bowel	May be generalized with persistent obstruction Generally elderly patients
Crohn's disease or ulcerative colitis	RLQ but may be LLQ	Sedimentation rate, ANCA, endoscopy (see Chapter 4)	Diarrhea (bloody in ulcerative colitis), cramps, elevated sedimentation rate
Mesenteric adenitis	RLQ	Diagnosis of exclusion	Pain secondary to enlarged mesenteric nodes from streptococcal pharyngitis
Pneumonia	May mimic appendicitis	CXR	Cough, etc.

Diverticulitis	Generally LLQ, very rarely RLQ	Clinical diagnosis (LLQ pain, diarrhea, vomiting, fever), CT scan most sensitive test	May be generalized
Gynecologic disease including ovarian cyst, ovarian torsion, ectopic pregnancy, *Mittelschmerz,* PID	Pain in pelvis, either adnexal area	Pregnancy test, cervical cultures, U/S	Radiation to groin, may radiate to right shoulder if free intraperitoneal bleeding
Urolithiasis or nephrolithiasis	Either flank	IVP but CT also Can do single post-CT flat plate to examine ureters	May radiate to labia or testicles
Cystitis	Suprapubic pain	UA	
Spontaneous bacterial peritonitis	Generalized with peritoneal signs	Paracentesis	Usually in alcoholics or those with indwelling dialysis catheters
Mesenteric thrombosis	Severe generalized abdominal pain without peritoneal signs and out of proportion to physical finding	May have elevated serum phosphate, serum lactate CT scan	
Intussusception	Cramping abdominal pain with asymptomatic periods Mental status changes are common and may have periods of lethargy Bloody "currant jelly" stools are a late sign Few have palpable sausage-shaped mass in RLQ	Air enema (has replaced barium for this indication) is often curative (see text)	Generally 2 weeks to 2 years old

Continued

TABLE 9-6
Abdominal Pain by Main Location—cont'd

Diagnosis	Usual pain location	Diagnostic studies	Pain radiates to and comments
Metabolic disease such as diabetic ketoacidosis, Addison's disease	Pain may be diffuse with associated nausea, vomiting, may have guarding		
Superior mesenteric artery syndrome	Midepigastric pain, especially after eating	Upper GI may show duodenal outlet obstruction	Usually thin individuals with a midepigastric bruit
Acute intermittent porphyria	Diffuse and especially into back	24-hour urine for ALA, PGB (porphobilinogen), porphyrins Screening urine for PGB is also available	Colicky abdominal pain that is intermittent may be associated with dark urine Have associated psychiatric or neurologic symptoms including sensory changes, paresthesias, psychosis Exacerbated by medications (especially estrogens, alcohol, sulfonamides), menstruation, weight loss May have photosensitivity
Hemolysis	Back and CVA pain	Reticulocyte count, serum free hemoglobin, LDH	G6PD deficiency, transfusion reactions, paroxysmal nocturnal hemoglobinuria
Meckel's diverticulum	Below or left of umbilicus		May be recurrent with rectal bleeding or intestinal obstruction

II. PHYSICAL EXAMINATION

A. Vital signs. Observe for signs of shock, elevated temperature.

B. Signs of dehydration noted with dry mucous membranes and decreased skin turgor.

C. Abdominal exam.

1. ***Inspection.*** Scaphoid appearance or distension, point of most severe pain, hernia, scars.
2. ***Ausculation.*** High-pitched bowel sounds are suggestive of an obstructive process. Absent bowel sounds are suggestive of an ileus.
3. ***Palpation and percussion.*** Muscle rigidity (voluntary/involuntary), localized tenderness, masses, pulsation, hernias, peritoneal irritation (rebound: cough or jumping also may elicit "rebound"), involuntary guarding, obturator sign (pain on internal and external rotation of hip), psoas sign (pain on straight leg raising by using obturator muscle, may indicate abscess, etc.), Murphy's sign (RUQ pain when breathing in and pressing over the liver), liver dimension and spleen dimension.
4. ***CVA tenderness.***
5. ***Pelvic exam in women.***
6. ***Rectal exam.*** To rule out GI bleeding, prostatitis, etc. The absence of rectal tenderness does not preclude the diagnosis of appendicitis nor does it make the diagnosis of appendicitis. The rectal examination should be used to add to your entire clinical picture.

III. LABORATORY

A. CBC with differential, platelet count, and urinalysis routinely done on most cases of abdominal pain.

B. Electrolytes with vomiting or diarrhea.

C. Liver function tests and liver enzymes; amylase and lipase for upper abdominal pain.

D. Other studies as indicated: chest radiograph (upright) for pneumonia or free air (best radiograph for free air). Abdominal flat plate and upright for bowel obstruction, ileus, free air, abnormal calcification. Ultrasonography to look for peritoneal fluid. ECG for acute MI, ischemia, or arrhythmias. Paracentesis may be important with fluid in the abdomen or in evaluation of abdominal trauma. Culdocentesis (nonclotting blood for ruptured ectopic pregnancy).

E. Pregnancy test on **all reproductive-age females** unless status post hysterectomy. Sexual history is often unreliable in the emergency setting.

IV. INITIAL TREATMENT

A. Decide whether to admit and observe, discharge, operate. Serial exams may clarify the diagnosis.

B. Keep NPO until diagnosis is clear.
C. IV fluids: Decide on expected fluid losses and current level of hydration.
D. NG tube for vomiting, bleeding. or obstruction.
E. Foley catheter to monitor fluids.
F. Pain medications will often help clarify the diagnosis.
G. Serial labs may be helpful, especially CBC, cardiac enzymes.

APPENDICITIS

I. OVERVIEW

Appendicitis is a common cause of abdominal pain. However, the presentation is not always classical and a high index of suspicion is necessary. Affects any age group but is rare in infants, most common in adolescence and young adult years. Generally occurs from obstruction of the appendiceal lumen by lymphoid hyperplasia or a fecalith.

II. CLINICAL PRESENTATION

A. **History.** Classic history is that of periumbilical or epigastric pain that migrates to right lower quadrant. Anorexia, nausea, and vomiting occur after the onset of pain. Anorexia is less likely to be present in children. Presentation is more likely to be atypical in very young, very old, and pregnant patients. Maintain a high index of suspicion in any patient with abdominal pain.

B. **Physical exam.** Low-grade temperature is common. High temperature is not common unless perforation has occurred. Abdominal exam should reveal right lower quadrant pain, possibly with rebound or guarding. Psoas sign (pain on active elevation of the legs) may be present as may be the obturator sign (pain on internal and external rotation of the hip). Rectal exam may reveal localized tenderness but cannot be used to differentiate between those with and those without appendicitis. Pelvic exam should be performed to rule out other illness (such as PID).

C. **Lab tests.** CBC with differential, UA, and pregnancy test (women only) should be obtained on all patients with lower abdominal pain. Obtain cervical or urethral culture if indicated. Mild to moderately elevated WBC with left shift is typical but rarely may be normal. UA may show ketonuria or a few RBCs or WBCs, but the presence of significant hematuria or pyuria is suggestive of urinary tract as source of pain.

III. MANAGEMENT

A. **Classical presentation.** Consultation with surgeon for appendectomy. Pain relief may help clarify the situation. Patient should be kept NPO after arrival at emergency department or clinic and hydrated IV.

B. If going to the operating room, patient should receive IV antibiotics within 2 hours of procedure (such as cefoxitin; see above).

C. Unclear presentation. In general, the history and physical exam are more reliable indicators of appendicitis than the WBC is. Surgeon should be consulted for suspected appendicitis if history and exam suggest the diagnosis. If minimal findings are present on exam, consider observation for several hours with repeated exams (including vital signs and temperature), differential CBC Q4h during observation period. Ultrasonography of appendix may be helpful if positive.

GALLBLADDER DISEASE

I. OVERVIEW

Asymptomatic cholelithiasis, choledocholithiasis, biliary colic, and acute cholecystitis are very common with cholelithiasis being found in 10% of the population. The incidence of cholelithiasis increases with age and is more common in women. Other predisposing factors include obesity, pregnancy, diabetes, chronic hemolytic states.

II. ASYMPTOMATIC CHOLELITHIASIS

A. 80% of gallstones are asymptomatic, with a small percentage becoming symptomatic each year (10% at 5 years, 15% at 10 years, 18% at 15 years). Stones are composed of bile salts, cholesterol (80% in the United States are cholesterol stones), phospholipids, or unconjugated bilirubin. Calcification may occur and results in about 15% of the stones becoming radiopaque.

B. Management. Asymptomatic patients do not require surgery. Previously diabetes was considered an indication for cholecystectomy in the asymptomatic patient, but this recommendation has recently been changed. Consider surgery for those asymptomatic individuals with calcified gallbladder, those with particularly large stones (>3 cm), and those who are at a high risk for gallbladder cancer (Pima Indians and others). See p. 407 for medical management.

III. EVALUATION OF THE GALLBLADDER

A. Lab tests including liver function tests, amylase for evidence of pancreatic damage, WBC if symptoms acutely present. An elevated alkaline phosphatase is possibly the most sensitive but not specific indicator of biliary disease.

B. Plain radiographs may help, since about 15% of stones are radiopaque, but need not be done if other modalities available.

C. Ultrasonography should be the initial exam used to evaluate for cholelithiasis. Can visualize stones, evaluate biliary ducts and pancreas. Obesity and overlying abdominal gas decrease the quality of the exam. Overall sensitivity is 90%, specificity 85%.

D. Oral cholecystogram is performed by having patient ingest 3 g of iopanoic acid about 12 hours before study. Failure of the gallbladder to opacify indicates gallbladder disease. Is not reliable in setting of significant hyperbilirubinemia or acute cholecystitis and has been replaced by ultrasonography.

E. Radionuclide hepatobiliary scan can be used in the setting of moderately elevated bilirubin and acute cholecystitis. Failure of gallbladder to visualize with presence of radioisotope in common bile duct 4 hours after injection indicates dysfunction of the gallbladder (that is, cholecystitis) or outlet obstruction (such as tumor, choledocholithiasis).

F. ERCP (endoscopic retrograde cholangiopancreatography) may also be used to define the anatomy of the biliary tree and may be a better choice than radionuclide scanning in many situations.

G. **Endoscope-guided ultrasonography.** Not commonly available but sensitive at picking up common duct stones.

IV. BILIARY COLIC

A. Caused by intermittent obstruction of the cystic duct by gallstones. History will generally include episodes of epigastric and RUQ pain, which may radiate to back. Pain is usually constant, is abrupt in onset, and subsides slowly. Nausea is commonly associated. Attacks may be precipitated by ingestion of fatty foods.

B. Consider also choledocholithiasis (stone in common duct).

C. Physical exam will reveal absence of fever, possible RUQ or midepigastric tenderness without rebound. Gallbladder may be palpable and may have a positive Murphy's sign (sudden increase in pain with palpation of RUQ during deep inspiration).

D. **Laboratory evaluation.** CBC with differential should be obtained and consider amylase and lipase. WBC should not be significantly elevated. LFTs may be normal or slightly elevated.

E. **Treatment.** Analgesics and antiemetics (prochlorperazine, metoclopramide) should be provided acutely. Morphine may increase biliary pressure and is contraindicated. Ketorolac 30 to 60 mg IM or 15 to 30 mg IV is especially useful in this condition. Meperidine IV in 25 mg aliquots may be used to supplement the ketorolac. If pain resolves, further evaluation may be obtained as convenient in the next few days with the patient instructed to avoid fatty foods. Cholecystectomy should be performed electively.

V. ACUTE CHOLECYSTITIS

A. 95% of those with cholecystitis will have cholelithiasis.

B. Presentation is similar to biliary colic (nausea, vomiting, abdominal pain, RUQ tenderness) with the additional features of fever, leukocytosis, mild elevation of bilirubin, elevated alkaline phosphatase. Murphy's sign may be present.

C. Treatment. Consultation with surgeon is required. Antibiotics are indicated for acute cholecystitis. A third-generation cephalosporin and metronidazole or ampicillin-sulbactam (Unasyn) will cover the most common organisms. There are advantages and disadvantages to early or delayed surgery, though early surgery appears to generally result in lower morbidity and shorter hospitalizations. Surgeon will ultimately need to decide based upon the particular features of the case.

VI. MEDICAL MANAGEMENT OF CHOLELITHIASIS

A. Generally a surgical therapy is considered the treatment of choice for cholelithiasis. However, in patients in whom this is not practical, other modalities may be used.

B. Cholesterol stones may be dissolved using ursodeoxycholic acid. About 70% of cholesterol stones will respond. However, stones tend to recur when ursodeoxycholic acid is discontinued.

C. Lithotripsy can be used to fragment stones, which are then passed spontaneously. ERCP may help with stone removal, and use of ursodeoxycholic acid may prevent recurrence.

D. ERCP with sphincterotomy may assist in passing stones.

INTESTINAL OBSTRUCTION

I. CLASSIFICATION

A. Mechanical obstruction. Complete or partial physical blockage of intestinal lumen (Table 9-7).

B. Simple obstruction. Implies one obstruction point.

C. Closed-loop obstruction. Blockage at two or more points.

TABLE 9-7
Causes of Mechanical Intestinal Obstruction in Adults

Site of obstruction	Cause	Relative incidence (%)
SMALL INTESTINE (85%)	Adhesions	60
	External hernia	15
	Neoplasm	15
	Miscellaneous	10
LARGE INTESTINE (15%)	Carcinoma of colon	65
	Diverticulitis	20
	Volvulus	5
	Miscellaneous	10

D. **Paralytic (adynamic) ileus.** Impairment of muscle function (such as after abdominal surgery, trauma, peritonitis, spinal injury, pneumonia, hypokalemia, uremia, pancreatitis, etc.).

E. **Strangulating obstruction.** When obstructing mechanism occludes mesenteric blood supply on wall of lumen. Necrosis occurs in 3 to 4 hours. Difficult to diagnose preoperatively.

F. Think of GI neoplasm, hypokalemia, intra-abdominal process such as irritation from free blood (as from an ovarian cyst rupture), localized inflammatory process (pancreatitis, pneumonia, PID), toxic megacolon, adhesions, intussusception (see next page), peritonitis, etc.

II. SMALL BOWEL OBSTRUCTION

A. Clinical manifestations.

1. ***Cramping abdominal pain.*** Crescendo-decrescendo pattern. Continuous pain is suggestive of strangulation.
2. ***Vomiting.*** Earlier in high obstruction. Feculent vomiting, caused by bacterial overgrowth, may be seen especially with distal obstruction.
3. ***Distension.*** More in lower obstruction.
4. ***Obstipation.***
5. ***High-pitched bowel sounds.***
6. ***Secondary electrolyte abnormalities.***

B. Work-up.

1. CBC with differential, electrolytes.
2. Supine and upright abdominal radiographs with stepladder pattern of air-fluid levels and no colonic gas are suggestive of obstruction.
3. History and physical examination may point to a particular cause such as adhesions or obstipation.

C. Treatment.

1. Fluid and electrolyte resuscitation and supportive care.
2. If partial obstruction with patient passing gas may treat with NG tube. This may relieve vomiting and decompress distension.
3. Surgical intervention is indicated if obstruction does not resolve with conservative treatment.

III. LARGE BOWEL OBSTRUCTION

A. Clinical manifestations.

1. Cramping pain.
2. Little vomiting (less with competent ileocecal valve, vomitus rarely feculent).
3. Constipation and obstipation.
4. Distension (severe).
5. Loud borborygmi.
6. Little loss of electrolytes.

B. Work-up.

1. Electrolytes and CBC.
2. Colonoscopy or flexible sigmoidoscopy may reveal obstructive lesion.
3. Radiograph will reveal gas-filled colon with absence of gas beyond obstruction.

C. Treatment.

1. Nasogastric tube.
2. IV fluids, monitoring, with or without antibiotics.
3. Sigmoidoscopy may reduce a sigmoid volvulus.
4. Surgical intervention if above measures not successful in relieving obstruction.

IV. INTUSSUSCEPTION

A. General.

1. Intussusception is the most common cause of bowel obstruction in those 3 months to 6 years of age. Rare under 3 months and most commonly occurs between 4 and 12 months.
2. Less than 10% have a "lead point" but may be secondary to polyp, sarcoma, Henoch-Schönlein purpura, etc.
3. Ileocecal valve area is the most commonly involved.
4. Male to female ratio is 4:1.

B. Clinically.

1. Main presenting symptom is intermittent, inconsolable crying with asymptomatic periods. *Frequently have mental status changes with lethargy between episodes of abdominal colic.*
2. Vomiting will develop 6 to 12 hours after onset of colicky pain. Eventually will vomit bilious material.
3. "Currant jelly" stools are late finding after venous stasis and bowel wall necrosis. Generally pale and shocky by this point.
4. Abdominal exam may be negative. "Sausage-shaped mass" in only two thirds.
5. Rule out other causes of pain such as bone injury, hairs around fingers, toes, penis, otitis media.

C. Diagnosis.

1. Ultrasonography has been used successfully.
2. Plain film may be negative.
3. Early lab test data are not helpful. Fever and elevated white blood cell count are late findings.
4. Only about 70% have guaiac-positive stool.
5. Barium or air enema diagnostic and therapeutic.

D. Treatment.

1. Barium or air enema successful in 75% if caught early. 25% successful if has been over 1 or 2 days. Air enema preferred because of risk of barium peritonitis if perforation.
2. Surgical intervention if this doesn't work
3. Admit for 24 hours if reduced with enema. About 25% will recur.

BIBLIOGRAPHY

Attard AR et al: Safety of early pain relief for acute abdominal pain, *Br Med J* 305:554, 1992.

Bland KI, Love N: Evaluation of common breast masses, *Postgrad Med* 92:5, 1992.

Brogan GX et al: Comparison of plain, warmed, and buffered lidocaine for anesthesia of traumatic wounds, *Ann Emerg Med* 26(2):121, 1995.

Clark R et al: Breast imaging, *Postgrad Med* 92:5, 1992.

Classen DC et al: The timing of prophylactic administration of antibiotics and the risk of surgical wound infections, *N Engl J Med* 326(5):281, 1992.

Condon RE, Nyhus LM, editors: *Manual of surgical therapeutics,* ed 4, Boston, 1978, Little, Brown & Co.

Cummings P et al: Antibiotics to prevent infection of simple wounds: a meta-analysis of randomized studies, *Am J Emerg Med* 13(4):396, 1995.

Daneman A et al: Perforation during attempted intussusception reduction in children–a comparison of perforation with barium and air, *Pediatr Radiol* 25(2):81-88, 1995.

Dickson AR et al: Rectal examination and acute appendicitis, *Arch Dis Child* 60(7):666, 1985.

Dire DJ et al: Prospective evaluation of topical antibiotics for preventing infections in uncomplicated soft-tissue wounds repaired in the ED, *Acad Emerg Med* 2(1):4, 1995.

Dixon JM et al: Rectal examination in patients with pain in the right lower quadrant of the abdomen, *Br Med J* 302(6773):386, 1991.

Dushoff IM: A stitch in time, *Emerg Med*, pp 1-16, Jan 1973.

Edlich RF et al: Principles of emergency wound management, *Ann Emerg Med* 17(12):1284, 1988.

Engoren M: Lack of association between atelectasis and fever, *Chest* 107(1):81, 1995.

Ernst AA et al: LAT (lidocaine-adrenaline-tetracycline) versus TAC (tetracaine-adrenaline-cocaine) for topical anesthesia in face and scalp lacerations, *Am J Emerg Med* 13(2):151, 1995.

Forbes JA et al: Evaluation of two opioid-acetaminophen combinations and placebo in postoperative oral surgery pain, *Pharmacotherapy* 14(2):139-146, 1994.

Glazier HS: Potentiation of pain relief with hydroxyzine: a therapeutic myth? *Ann Pharmacother* 24:484, 1990.

Goldstein EJ, Richwald GA: Human and animal bite wounds, *Am Fam Physician* 36(10):101, 1987.

Goswick CB: Ibuprofen versus propoxyphene hydrochloride and placebo in acute musculoskeletal trauma, *Curr Ther Res* 34(4):685, 1983.

Gracie WA, Ransohoff DF: The natural history of silent gallstones: the innocent gallstone is not a myth, *N Engl J Med* 307:798, 1982.

Hall JC et al: Prevention of respiratory complications after abdominal surgery: a randomised clinical trial, *Br Med J* 312(7024):148-152, 1996.

Houry S et al: A prospective multicenter evaluation of preoperative hemostatic screening tests, *Am J Surg* 170(1):19, 1995.

Kattlove H et al: Benefits and costs of screening and treatment for early breast cancer: development of a basic benefit package, *JAMA* 273(2):142, 1995.

Katz M et al: Gas enema for the reduction of intussusception: relationship between clinical signs and symptoms and outcome, *Am J Roentgenol* 160(2):363-366, 1993.

Kirks DR: Air intussusception reduction: "the winds of change" [Review], *Pediatr Radiol* 25(2):89-91, 1995.

Lim JH et al: Determining the site and causes of colonic obstruction with sonography, *Am J Roentgenol* 163(5):1113-1117, 1994.

Mangano DT, Goldman L: Preoperative assessment of patients with known or suspected coronary disease, *N Engl J Med* 333(26):1750, 1995.

Mangano DT et al: Effect of atenolol on mortality and cardiovascular morbidity after noncardiac surgery, *N Engl J Med* 335:1713-1720, 1996.

Narr BJ et al: Preoperative laboratory screening in healthy Mayo patients: cost effective elimination of tests and unchanged outcomes, *Mayo Clin Proc* 66(2):155, 1991.

Nussbaum MS, editor: *The Mont Reid handbook,* St. Louis, 1987, Mosby.

Ramoska EA et al: Reliability of patient history in determining the possibility of pregnancy, *Ann Emerg Med* 18(1):48, 1989.

Ransohoff DF, Gracie WA: Treatment of gallstones, *Ann Intern Med* 119(7 Pt 1):606-619, 1993.

Schrock TR, editor: *Handbook of surgery,* ed 9, Greenbrae, Calif., 1989, Jones Medical Publications.

Simon B, editor: *Emergency medicine–concepts and clinical practice,* St. Louis, 1988, Mosby.

Stubhaug A et al: Lack of analgesic effect of 50 and 100 mg oral tramadol after orthopaedic surgery: a randomized, double-blind, placebo and standard active drug comparison, *Pain* 62(1):111, 1995.

Sunshine A et al: Analgesic oral efficacy of tramadol hydrochloride in postoperative pain, *Clin Pharmacol Ther* 51(6):740-746, 1992.

Wade DS et al: Accuracy of ultrasound in the diagnosis of acute appendicitis compared with the surgeon's clinical impression, *Arch Surg* 128(9):1039, 1993.

Williams S et al: Aspirin-acetaminophen combination vs propoxyphene-APC combination: a double blind study of analgesic efficacy and safety, *Curr Ther Res* 29(2):275, 1981.

10

Pediatrics

Viviana Martínez-Bianchi, Michelle Rejman-Peterson and Mark A. Graber

NEONATAL RESUSCITATION

We strongly recommend that any family physician who will be caring for neonates in the delivery room or nursery be certified through the American Heart Association and American Academy of Pediatrics Neonatal Resuscitation Program.

1. Good prenatal care can prevent the need for neonatal resuscitation.
2. Apgar score at 1 minute of <5 indicates intrapartum asphyxia, 5 to 7 mild asphyxia, and >8 normal. Reassess every 5 minutes until >7.
3. See Fig. 10-1 and Table 10-1 for details of neonatal resuscitation.

NEWBORN NURSERY

I. HISTORY AND PHYSICAL EXAMINATION

II. NORMAL BODY TEMPERATURE

Observe and maintain a normal body temperature. Hyperthermia or hypothermia warrants further investigation:

1. Rectal temperatures provide the only accurate noninvasive method of measuring temperature.
2. If hyperthermia, consider sepsis or intracranial bleed.
3. If hypothermia, consider sepsis, hypoglycemia, hypothyroidism, and heat loss caused by environmental conditions.

III. INITIAL GASTROINTESTINAL AND GENITOURINARY FUNCTION

1. Approximately 70% of newborns pass meconium and urine in the first 12 hours of life, 25% in 24 hours, and the remainder by 2 days.

2. If meconium is delayed, look for meconium plug, sepsis, narcotic exposure, Hirschsprung's disease, hypothyroidism, cystic fibrosis, or imperforate anus.
3. If infant is anuric or oliguric, think about dehydration, sepsis, renal abnormalities, or obstruction.
   a. *Monitor weight and head circumference.* Weight initially drops (not >10%) and is usually regained by 1 week. Head circumference may decrease or increase (not >1 cm) as a result of initial trauma or molding of labor, or both.
   b. *Red reflex.* The pupil should be black on direct examination, and red when examined through an ophthalmoscope. If the red reflex looks pale or white, suspect retinoblastoma.

IV. NEWBORN PROPHYLAXIS

A. Eyes. Erythromycin 0.5% ointment to prevent gonorrheal conjunctivitis or *Chlamydia trachomatis* ophthalmia neonatorum.

B. Vitamin K. 0.5 to 1 mg IM to prevent hemorrhagic disease. Avoid products containing benzyl alcohol because they can be toxic to the newborn.

C. Hepatitis.

1. ***For those born of a hepatitis B–negative mother.*** Give hepatitis B vaccine 10 µg IM routinely at birth and at 1 and 6 months.
2. ***If mother hepatitis B positive (positive HBsAg).***
   a. Clean newborn of hepatitis BsAg-positive mother thoroughly (use alcohol).
   b. Give hepatitis B globulin 0.5 ml IM and hepatitis B vaccine 10 µg IM, ASAP.
   c. Repeat hepatitis B vaccine 10 µg IM at 1 and 6 months.
   d. Do a hepatitis B screen at 9 months; if negative, give fourth dose of vaccine; if positive, monitor for chronic active or carrier state.

D. AIDS. *See Chapter 16 for information about diagnosis, treatment, and prophylaxis of the newborn born to an HIV-positive mother.*

1. HIV testing should be offered to all pregnant women to determine which infants are at risk for infection. If positive, treatment with AZT should then be offered. This measure has been shown to decrease the rate of infection in the neonate.
2. All infants born to HIV-infected women should be started ASAP on AZT and given PCP prophylaxis starting at 4 to 6 weeks. See Chapter 16 for details.

E. Bathing. Once the body temperature is stabilized, the infant may be bathed with warm standing water. Avoid running water to avoid burns. Immersion above the umbilicus should be avoided until the umbilical stump has fallen off.

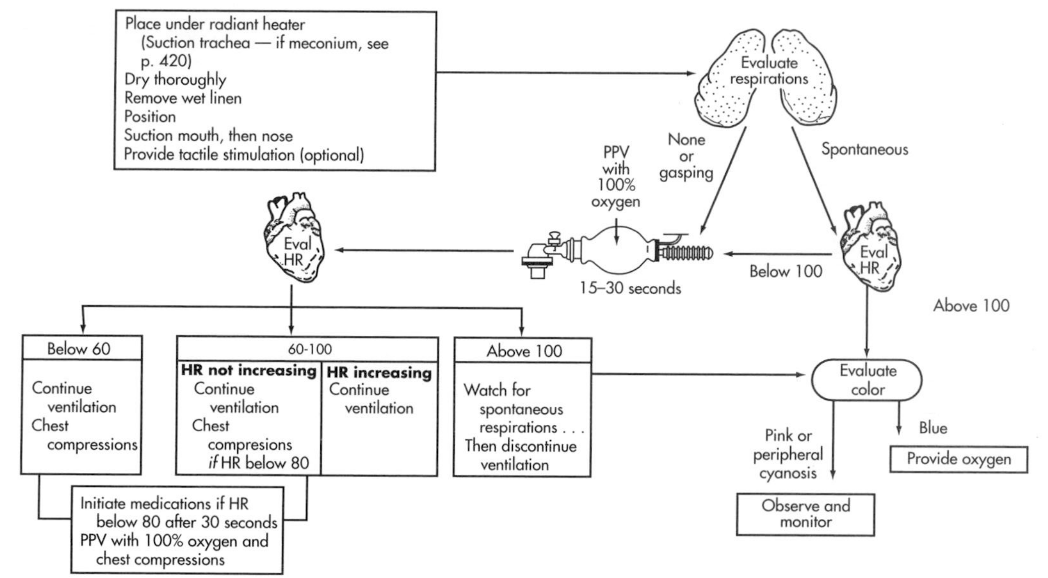

FIG. 10-1 Overview of resuscitatioı. in the delivery room. *EVAL*, Evaluate; *HR*, heart rate; *PPV*, positive pressure ventilation. (Data from American Heart Association: *Textbook of Neonatal Resuscitation*, Dallas, 1994, the Association.)

TABLE 10-1
Medications for Neonatal Resuscitation

Medication	Concentration to administer	Preparation	Dosage/route	Total dose/infant			Rate/precautions
				Weight	**Total ml**		
Epinephrine	1:10 000	1 ml	0.1-0.3 ml/kg IV or ET	1 kg	0.1-0.3 ml		Give rapidly
				2 kg	0.2-0.6 ml		May dilute with normal saline to 1-2 ml if giving ET
				3 kg	0.3-0.9 ml		
				4 kg	0.4-1.2 ml		
				Weight	**Total ml**		
Volume expanders	Whole blood 5% Albumin-saline Normal saline Lactated Ringer's	40 ml	10 ml/kg IV	1 kg	10 ml		Give over 5-10 minutes
				2 kg	20 ml		
				3 kg	30 ml		
				4 kg	40 ml		
				Weight	**Total dose**	**Total ml**	
Sodium bicarbonate	0.5 mEq/ml (4.2% solution)	20 ml or two 10 ml prefilled syringes	2 mEq/kg IV	1 kg	2 mEq	4 ml	Give *slowly*, over at least 2 minutes
				2 kg	4 mEq	8 ml	Give only if infant is being effectively ventilated
				3 kg	6 mEq	12 ml	
				4 kg	8 mEq	16 ml	

Continued

TABLE 10-1
Medications for Neonatal Resuscitation—cont'd

Medication	Concentration to administer	Preparation	Dosage/route	Total dose/infant			Rate/precautions
				Weight	**Total dose**	**Total ml**	
Naloxone hydrochloride	0.4 mg/ml	1 ml	0.1 mg/kg (0.25 ml/kg) IV, ET, IM, SQ	1 kg	0.1 mg	0.25 ml	Give rapidly IV, ET preferred IM, SQ acceptable
				2 kg	0.2 mg	0.50 ml	
				3 kg	0.3 mg	0.75 ml	
				4 kg	0.4 mg	1.00 ml	
	1.0 mg/ml	1 ml	0.1 ml/kg (0.1 ml/kg) IV, ET, IM, SQ	1 kg	0.1 mg	0.1 ml	
				2 kg	0.2 mg	0.2 ml	
				3 kg	0.3 mg	0.3 ml	
				4 kg	0.4 mg	0.4 ml	
				Weight		**Total μg/min**	
Dopamine	$\frac{6 \times \text{Weight (kg)} \times \text{Desired dose (μg/kg/min)}}{\text{Desired fluid (ml/h)}} =$	mg of dopamine per 100 ml of solution	Begin at 5 μg/kg/min (may increase to 20 μg/kg/min if necessary) IV	1 kg		5-20 μg/min	Give as a continuous infusion using an infusion pump Monitor heart rate and blood pressure closely Seek consultation
				2 kg		10-40 μg/min	
				3 kg		15-60 μg/min	
				4 kg		20-80 μg/min	

From American Heart Association: *Textbook of neonatal resuscitation,* Dallas, 1994, the Association.
ET, Endotracheal; *IM*, intramuscular; IV, intravenous; *SQ*, subcutaneous.

F. Umbilical cord care. Keep dry. Apply an antiseptic agent such as triple dye (Brilliant Green, Crystal Violet, and proflavine hemisulfate) or alcohol to avoid colonization and infection with *Streptococcus, Staphylococcus,* and *Clostridium* species and coliforms. Generally separates by the end of second week but may not occur until the third week of life. Delayed separation may be normal or may be attributable to sepsis or poorly functioning leukocytes.

G. Screening laboratory tests.

1. ***Metabolic.*** Should be done at 24 hours of age or later. Phenylketonuria, hypothyroidism, galactosemia, etc. as required by state law or indicated (such as cystic fibrosis if no meconium stool). If screening is done before 24 hours of age, may miss some diseases, and screening should be repeated at 1 week to 10 days. Antibiotics may also interfere with screening, and screening should be repeated when patient is no longer using antibiotics.
2. ***Hematologic.*** Hemoglobin and hematocrit at birth and at 12 months, glucose-6-phosphate dehydrogenase deficiency, sickle cell screening in blacks, thalassemia in those of Mediterranean descent.
3. ***Urinary and meconium drug screening.*** If there is maternal history of drug abuse.
4. ***Glucose screening at birth and at 2 and 6 hours of age.*** Repeat regularly until stable (>40 mg/dl). Warm the infant's heel, and draw capillary blood samples from the side of the heel using finger stick test strips for glucose. See section on hypoglycemia, p. 428, for further information on diagnosis and management.
5. ***Bilirubin.*** Transcutaneous bilirubinometry should be used for screening suspect neonates for jaundice. If value is above 17 mg/dl, serum bilirubin should be measured. The transcutaneous jaundice meter is affected by factors such as gestational age, birth weight, and skin pigmentation.
6. ***ABO incompatibility.*** Perform blood type and direct Coombs' test (use cord blood) on every infant born to a mother with type O blood or those with Rh-negative mothers.
7. ***Neonatal nutrition.*** See section on pediatric wellness, p. 434.

JAUNDICE

I. Jaundice is visible when a baby has a serum bilirubin level that exceeds 5 mg/dl. Generally jaundice is visible first on the head and progresses to the feet. It resolves with the opposite pattern, the feet clearing first.

II. PHYSIOLOGIC HYPERBILIRUBINEMIA

1. Usually not present in first 24 hours.

2. Rarely increases by more than 5 mg/dl in 1 day.
3. Peaks at 48 to 72 hours in full-term infants and 4 to 5 days in the premature ones.
4. Serum bilirubin does not exceed 13 mg/dl in the full-term infant and 15 mg/dl in the preterm infant.
5. Direct bilirubin fraction is generally <2 mg/dl.
6. Physiologic jaundice disappears by 1 week in full-term infants and by 2 weeks in premature infants.

Any infant that does not meet the above description has nonphysiologic hyperbilirubinemia and should be worked up.

III. NONPHYSIOLOGIC HYPERBILIRUBINEMIA

A. Those with primarily elevated direct bilirubin. Direct bilirubin >15% of total and therefore conjugated by the liver.

1. Infections including sepsis, perinatally acquired viral infections including hepatitis, and intrauterine viral infections (hepatitis B, TORCHS).
2. Metabolic abnormalities including Rotor syndrome and Dubin-Johnson syndrome.
3. Anatomic abnormalities including biliary atresia and obstructions as with a choledochal cyst.
4. Cholestasis from CVN/TPN antibiotics (especially ceftriaxone).
5. Galactosemia, tyrosinosis, cystic fibrosis, hereditary fructose intolerance.

B. Those with primarily elevated indirect bilirubin. Therefore not conjugated by liver. Two basic mechanisms:

1. ***From increased production of bilirubin (therefore hemolysis or hematoma breakdown).***
   a. *With positive direct Coombs' test (mother's antibodies on child's cells).* Isoimmunization (Rh, ABO, minor blood group), erythroblastosis fetalis.
   b. *With negative Coombs' test and RBC morphologic abnormalities.* Spherocytosis, thalassemias, G6PD deficiency, elliptocytosis, etc.
   c. *Extravascular blood.* Cephalohematoma, severe bruising, cerebral and pulmonary hemorrhage.
   d. DIC, other hemolytic anemia
   e. Polycythemia resulting from delayed clamping of cord, twin-twin transfusion, maternal-fetal transfusion.
2. ***From delayed excretion of bilirubin.***
   a. Inherited disorders of bilirubin metabolism including Crigler-Najjar syndrome, Gilbert's disease, Dubin-Johnson syndrome, Rotor syndrome.
   b. Hypothyroidism and prematurity.

IV. BREAST MILK JAUNDICE

Progressive increase in bilirubin from day 4, peaks at 10 to 15 days of life in breast-fed infant.

V. See algorithm, neonatal jaundice (Fig. 10-2).

VI. TREATMENT

1. Treat the underlying disorder.
2. Ensure adequate hydration, caloric intake, stooling.
3. Phototherapy is not indicated in those with liver disease or jaundice secondary to obstruction.
4. ***Prophylactic phototherapy.*** Indicated for infants showing a rapid rise in bilirubin (>1 mg/dl per hour) and as a temporizing measure when one is contemplating exchange transfusion.
5. ***Phototherapy.*** Serum bilirubin usually decreases by 2.5 to 3 mg/dl per day. Bilirubin level should be followed every 12 hours. Phototherapy should be discontinued when the bilirubin reaches levels of about 13 mg/dl. Bilirubin levels should be rechecked again 12 hours after discontinuation, to assess for recurrence.
6. ***Exchange transfusions.*** Needed when bilirubin level rises to 25 mg/dl or more in nonhemolytic jaundice, >20 mg/dl in hemolytic jaundice, or unresponsiveness to phototherapy.

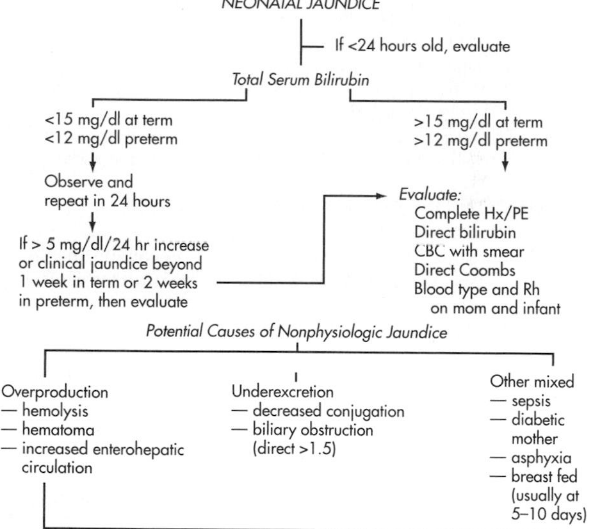

FIG. 10-2 Algorithm of neonatal jaundice. *CBC*, Complete blood count; *Hx/PE*, history/physical examination.

RESPIRATORY DISORDERS IN THE NEWBORN

I. RESPIRATORY DISTRESS SYNDROME AND HYALINE MEMBRANE DISEASE

A. Characteristics.

1. Most common in preterm infants because of surfactant deficiency. Higher incidence with maternal diabetes, acute asphyxia, second twin.
2. Prevention and diagnosis of preterm labor is paramount; steroids can be used if delivery is imminent to hasten lung maturity (betamethasone or dexamethasone 12.5 mg IM Q24h for 48 hours). Resuscitate promptly at delivery.

B. Clinical findings.

1. ***Shortly after birth.*** Tachypnea, grunting, retractions, and cyanosis.
2. ***Radiographs.*** Ground-glass reticulogranular appearance, air bronchogram.

C. Treatment.

1. Rule out infection; use antibiotics as needed.
2. Respiratory support (endotracheal intubation, mechanical ventilatory support) and metabolic support.
3. Exogenous surfactant (doses differ by preparation).

II. TRANSIENT TACHYPNEA OF THE NEWBORN

A. Characteristics. Diagnosis of exclusion. More common in C-section deliveries.

B. Presentation.

1. Tachypnea, minimal respiratory distress.
2. ***Radiographs.*** Fluid in fissures, pleural effusion, streaky parenchymal changes.

C. Management. Short-term oxygen supplementation. This is a self-limited illness that will resolve spontaneously.

III. MECONIUM ASPIRATION SYNDROME

A. Characteristics.

1. Caused by the presence of thick meconium in the distal airways, causing a valvelike mechanism that obstructs air movement.
2. Meconium aspiration can occur in a stressed neonate in utero or at the time of delivery. Deep fetal gasping causes the aspiration of the meconium-mixed amniotic fluid into the lungs.
3. ***Radiographs.*** Thick infiltrates, air entrapment, pneumothorax.

B. Preventive management.

1. At the delivery of the head, the airway should be cleared by DeLee suctioning.
2. Tracheal visualization and suctioning should then follow. If meconium is at or below the vocal cords, intubation must be repeatedly performed until suctioning returns clear fluid.

C. Treatment.

1. Management is complex, and a neonatology physician should be consulted.
2. Treatment requires pulmonary support, as well as management of asphyxia-related effects on CNS, cardiovascular system, renal and GI systems. High-frequency ventilation, nitrous oxide, ECMO, are being used with good results.

IV. SPONTANEOUS PNEUMOTHORAX

A. Spontaneous pneumothorax occurs in 1% to 2% of live births. Only symptomatic in 1:1500 live births.

B. When symptoms occur, they include tachypnea, minimal retractions, grunting, nasal flaring, cyanosis. May notice diminished air entry on effected side, shifting of cardiac impulse, muffled heart tones.

C. Radiographs. Diagnostic.

D. Treatment. Supportive, spontaneous resolution is common. If not resolving, consider chest tube.

V. BRADYCARDIA AND APNEA SPELLS

A. Types. Bradycardia may be a primary cardiac event. The following refers *only* to noncardiogenic bradycardia and apnea spells.

1. ***Central.*** No respiratory effort for 15 seconds because of arrest of respiratory drive. May have secondary bradycardia. May be secondary to CNS disorder.
2. ***Obstructive.*** Cessation of gas exchange in the lungs because of obstruction to air flow. May be infectious, functional (poor tone or coordination of pharyngeal muscles), or structural.

B. Causes. Prematurity, hypoxia, idiopathic, anatomic abnormalities (choanal atresia), maternal drugs (especially narcotics), infections, metabolic imbalances, temperature instability, seizures, hematologic, cardiovascular, genetic, and CNS disorders. GE reflux or trouble coordinating swallow and palate malformations can all contribute to apnea. In the older child consider breath-holding spells.

C. Clinical characteristics, work-up, and treatment.

1. Document the duration, frequency, state of consciousness, temporal relationship to feeding, sleep, stooling, seizure activity as well as obstetric history (such as maternal fever, meconium). Gestational age is especially important.
2. Physical exam should include temperature, BP, gestational age, eye position (as an indication of a CNS disorder), pupillary dilatation, muscle tone, dysmorphic features, respiratory effort, murmur, skin changes.
3. ***Lab tests.*** Blood glucose, electrolytes, differential CBC, drug levels, T_4, TSH, sepsis work-up, CXR, ABGs, head ultrasonogram (for CNS bleed), EEG.

D. Treatment.

1. ***Apnea monitor and addressing underlying factor.*** Teach CPR to parents and caregivers. Any individual spell will generally resolve with stimulation.
2. ***For neonatal apnea.*** Caffeine citrate 20 mg/kg PO (10 mg caffeine/10 mg citrate) followed by 5 mg/kg QD started 24 hours after first dose. May also be compounded at same dose for IV. Maintain serum levels at 5 to 25 µg/ml. Theophylline has also been used, but caffeine is preferred.

NEONATAL INFECTIONS

I. THRUSH

Oral candidiasis; peaks at 14 days of life.

A. Clinically. White plaques on erythematous base over oral mucosa, tongue.

B. Treatment. Nystatin suspension 100,000 to 200,000 U PO QID for 7 days. Mycostatin cream to maternal areola and nipple if breast-fed infant.

II. NEONATAL BACTERIAL SEPSIS

A. General comments. Neonatal bacterial sepsis is associated with 10% to 40% mortality and significant morbidity, especially neurologic sequelae of meningitis. Infants <1 month old are immunologically deficient and are predisposed to serious infections.

B. Predisposing factors. Premature rupture of membranes (>24 hours), premature labor, maternal fever, UTI, foul lochia, chorioamnionitis, IV catheters (in infant), intrapartum asphyxia, and intrauterine monitoring (pressure catheter or scalp electrode).

C. Organisms.

1. ***Early infection (0 to 4 days of age).*** Group B streptococci and *Escherichia coli* 60% to 70% of infections. Also *Listeria* (rare in United States), *Klebsiella, Enterococcus, Staphylococcus aureus* (uncommon), *Streptococcus pneumoniae*, group A streptococci.
2. ***Late infection (>5 days of age).*** *Staph. aureus,* group B streptococci, *E. coli, Klebsiella, Pseudomonas, Serratia, Staph. epidermidis, Haemophilus influenzae.*

D. Signs and symptoms. Presentation may be subtle; thus any febrile neonate must have a septic work-up. Fever may be absent; so watch for symptoms below.

1. The presentation may include irritability, vomiting, poor feeding, poor temperature control, lethargy, apneic spells.
2. May progress to respiratory distress, poor perfusion, abdominal distension, jaundice, bleeding, petechiae, or seizures.
3. Bulging fontanel is a very late sign of neonatal meningitis, and Brudzinski's sign or Kernig's sign is rarely found.

E. Work-up.

1. Include LP for cell count, protein, glucose, and culture.
2. UA, CBC (remember neutropenia or thrombocytopenia are also suggestive of infection) and repeat in 5 hours, CXR and C-reactive protein.
3. Cultures of blood, urine, and any other site as indicated. Latex agglutination test for pneumococcus, *E. coli, H. influenzae,* group B streptococci, and meningococcus in blood, urine, and CSF is done even though the usefulness is questionable. Negative latex agglutination tests do not rule out infection, but positive results may help guide therapy.

F. Associated lab findings. Hypocalcemia, hypoglycemia, hyponatremia, and DIC.

G. Treatment.

1. Should be tailored to age of onset, clinical setting, and initial findings.
2. ***There should be NO DELAY in antibiotic therapy.*** Begin empiric therapy after cultures are obtained or before cultures if any delay is anticipated.
   a. *Empiric early (0 to 4 days old).* Ampicillin 50 mg/kg/day (100 mg/kg/day in meningitis) divided 12 hours IV and gentamicin 5 mg/kg/day divided 12 hours IV.
   b. *Empiric late (>5 days old).* Depends on cause (for example, methicillin-resistant *Staph. aureus* outbreak requires vancomycin) ampicillin 100 to 200 mg/kg/day divided Q8h plus (ceftriaxone 100 mg/kg/day IV Q12h or cefotaxime 150 mg/kg/day IV Q8h), or ampicillin-gentamicin as above usually adequate.
   c. *Repeat cultures in 24 to 48 hours.* In meningitis, repeat LP every day until clear.
   d. *There are isolates of* Streptococcus pneumoniae *that are resistant to penicillin and cephalosporins. Depending on your institution, vancomycin plus rifampin should be added to the above regimens until sensitivities are known.*
   e. *Other.* Hemodynamic, respiratory, hematologic, metabolic, and nutritional support and surveillance are critical. Shock may require volume expansion (FFP preferred) or respiratory depression may require supplemental oxygen or artificial ventilation (see Chapter 1 section on shock, p. 48).

CONGENITAL INFECTIONS: TORCHS, HIV

I. MATERNAL DIAGNOSTIC SCREENING

Screen early for antibody to rubella, syphilis, and hepatitis B. Offer HIV testing to all pregnant women. Serologic tests as indicated for HSV, CMV, HIV. Viral cultures as indicated for HSV, rubella, CMV, enterovirus.

II. CONGENITAL INFECTIONS

Congenital infections should be suspected in those infants who are premature or have IUGR, failure to thrive, hepatomegaly (elevated direct bilirubin), lethargy, thrombocytopenia, anemia, rashes, or seizures. See specific entities below.

III. LABORATORY STUDIES FOR SUSPECTED CONGENITAL INFECTIONS

1. TORCHS (toxoplasmosis, rubella, cytomegalovirus, herpes simplex, syphilis) titers on baby and mother (draw serum before any blood transfusion).
2. Obtain IgM antibodies from baby as well as acute and convalescent IgG titers from baby and mother. IgM does not cross the placenta and therefore indicates a reaction of the infant to infection.
3. Viral cultures (HSV, rubella, CMV, enterovirus). Culture of CSF or PCR may be useful in HSV.
4. Tzanck test of vesicles in HSV (infant or mother).
5. Urine cytology and culture for CMV.
6. Dark-field exam of lesions or umbilical cord scraping in syphilis.
7. Send placenta to pathology lab for culture and microscopy.
8. General lab screen including liver function tests, electrolytes, glucose, CBC and clotting studies.

IV. SPECIFIC AGENTS

A. Toxoplasmosis.

1. ***Epidemiology.*** Caused by *Toxoplasma gondii.* Fetus is infected by transplacental passage during maternal parasitemia. Infection occurs through ingestion of sporulated oocysts in cat feces or ingestion of poorly cooked meat. 50% of the infants born to mothers who seroconvert during pregnancy will become infected.
2. ***Postnatal diagnosis.*** Isolation of organism from placenta. ELISA to detect specific IgG and IgM; comparison with mother's serum is necessary, since maternal IgG will cross the placenta.
3. ***Clinical findings.***
   a. Only 10% are symptomatic. Most of those who acquire toxoplasma in utero are asymptomatic.
   b. Maculopapular rash, generalized lymphadenopathy, hepatosplenomegaly, thrombocytopenia, signs of active central nervous system infection (such as CSF pleocytosis, CSF hypoglycemia, elevated CSF protein, and, in some instances, microcephaly, cerebral calcifications, seizures, and motor abnormalities), chorioretinitis, and pneumonitis. Infants with untreated congenital toxoplasmosis and generalized or neurologic abnormalities at presentation almost uniformly develop mental retardation, seizures, and spasticity.

4. ***Prevention and treatment.***
    a. Avoid changing cat litter and eating raw and poorly cooked meat during pregnancy.
    b. Treat infant for clinically, serologically, or maternally apparent disease with pyrimethamine and sulfadiazine for 1 year. Folinic acid should be given to prevent bone marrow suppression. Recent evidence indicates that those treated for greater than 1 month have better neurologic and developmental outcomes than those left untreated or those treated for only 1 month. A pediatric infectious disease (ID) consultation should be obtained.
    c. Corticosteroid for ocular disease, jaundice, high level of CSF protein.

B. Cytomegalovirus (CMV).

1. ***Epidemiology.***
    a. Most common congenital infection (up to 2.5% incidence) with 95% asymptomatic.
    b. Vertical transmission (from maternal primary or reactivated disease) may be acquired transplacentally or at birth in the genital tract. CMV may also be acquired postnatally by ingestion of CMV-positive breast milk. Infected infants are contagious.
2. ***Clinical findings.***
    a. Sensorineural deafness, mental retardation.
    b. "Cytomegalic inclusion disease" with jaundice, hepatosplenomegaly, petechial-purpuric rash, microcephaly, and cerebral calcifications.
3. ***Diagnostic tests.*** Virus isolated from urine, pharynx, WBC, CSF, human milk, cervical secretions. CMV-IgM titers. PCR has been used to detect virus as well.
4. ***Treatment.*** Recent evidence indicates that ganciclovir given postnatally may reduce incidence of retardation and other sequelae. Consider a pediatric infectious disease or neurology consultation.

C. Herpes simplex.

1. ***Epidemiology.*** Mostly HSV type 2 transmission occurs at birth through direct contact (5% transmission in recurrent lesion, 50% in primary). Probably 20% or more of women have had HSV-2 and carry the virus. Many women are asymptomatic shedders at the time of delivery, and these account for most of the neonatal infections.
2. ***Clinical findings.***
    a. Average incubation 6 days; can be up to 20.
    b. Disseminated disease may mimic fulminate sepsis with seizures, jaundice, hepatitis, encephalitis, DIC, or pneumonia. If untreated, up to 90% mortality.
    c. Local mucocutaneous disease may be mild. Conjunctivitis, keratitis, or chorioretinitis can result in vision loss and blindness.

3. ***Prevention and treatment.***
   a. Any active lesions during pregnancy should be cultured to confirm disease. Active disease at delivery mandates C-section. Routine use of PCR to identify asymptomatic shedders is not yet standard of care.
   b. If vaginal delivery occurs over active lesions or ROM >4 hours, begin acyclovir 30 mg/kg/day IV Q8h for 14 days. Infected mother and infant should be kept in contact isolation.

D. Rubella.

1. ***Epidemiology.*** Nonvaccinated or rubella-susceptible mother acquires infection while pregnant. Teratogenicity is the greatest in the first trimester, less in second, none in third. Infants may be contagious.
2. ***Presentation.*** Retinopathy, cataracts, patent ductus arteriosus, pulmonary artery stenosis, deafness, thrombocytopenia with "blueberry-muffin" skin lesions.
3. ***Treatment.*** Supportive only. Immunize children and nonpregnant women of childbearing age. Immune globulin given to mother does not prevent prenatal infection.

E. Syphilis.

1. ***Epidemiology.*** High probability that infected mother will transmit the disease. Treponemes cross placenta in all trimesters.
2. ***Presentation.***
   a. 50% asymptomatic. Clinical picture can be benign to fatal.
   b. Findings include SGA, jaundice, recurring rashes, anemia, hepatosplenomegaly, "snuffles" (a serous rhinitis), meningitis, condylomata lata, osteochondritis usually of humerus or of tibia.
3. ***Diagnosis and treatment.***
   a. Suspect strongly in infants of mothers who are seropositive and (1) are untreated or inadequately treated, (2) had no decrease in antibody titers after treatment, (3) had poor follow-up during pregnancy, etc.
   b. Evaluate with physical exam, VDRL, RPR, FTA-ABS, CSF analysis, dark-field microscopy of fluids of vesicular lesions or of condylomata lata, long bone radiographs.
   c. *Treat if there is* a fourfold greater titer of antibody in the infant than in the mother, abnormal CSF (reactive VDRL, cells in the CSF, elevated CSF protein), evidence of active disease by exam (such as rash) or radiologic evidence of disease.
   d. *Treatment.* Procaine penicillin G 50,000 units/kg IM QD × 14 days or aqueous penicillin G 50,000 units/kg IV Q8-12h × 14 days.
   e. *Follow-up titers.* At 1, 2, 3, 6, 12 months to ensure that they are falling. Titer should revert to negative at 6 months. HIV testing should be considered.

F. HIV. See treatment of newborn at beginning of this chapter and Chapter 16.

G. Enterovirus.

1. ***Characteristics.*** Enteroviruses (coxsackievirus, hepatitis A virus, echovirus, poliovirus), prevalent during warmer months and in transplacental or postpartum transmission.
2. ***Treatment.*** Supportive measures for enterovirus infection. Hepatitis A immunoglobulin 0.5 ml at birth if appropriate.

H. Gonorrhea and chlamydia.

1. ***Prevention.*** Diagnosis and treatment of GC and chlamydial infections will prevent most neonatal infections. Both infections are transmitted intra partum by direct contact. Culture endocervix initially and at 36 weeks if indicated.
2. ***Clinical findings.*** Both can cause conjunctivitis at 2 to 12 days. Obtain chlamydial, viral, and bacterial cultures of any purulent conjunctival discharge with Gram stain and Giemsa stain of conjunctival scraping for *Chlamydia.* For documented disease obtain blood and CSF cultures and treat for systemic disease.
   a. *Disseminated gonorrhea* typically involves arthritis and meningitis. Treat all infants of culture-positive mothers with a single dose of ceftriaxone 50 mg/kg IM (maximum of 125 mg). If evidence of disease or positive culture of blood or CSF, then ceftriaxone 25 to 50 mg/kg/day single IM × 7 to 10 days (75 mg/kg/day × 10 to 14 days for meningitis).
   b. *Chlamydia* may produce pneumonia at about 3 weeks with the insidious onset of tachypnea, cough, and no fever. Conjunctivitis is often present. Interstitial infiltrate and hyperinflation may be present on CXR. Diagnose *Chlamydia* with nasopharyngeal culture or seropositivity. Topical treatment has minimal efficacy even for isolated conjunctival disease because of colonization of other sites. Treat with oral erythromycin 40 to 50 mg/kg/day Q6h × 2 to 3 weeks. Trials with azithromycin are currently underway.

NEONATAL HEMATOLOGIC DISORDERS

I. POLYCYTHEMIA

Hyperviscous blood from increased HCT, which can cause stasis resulting in venous congestion or thrombosis. Increased incidence with IUGR, Down syndrome and other chromosomal abnormalities, congenital hypothyroidism or congenital adrenal hyperplasia, diabetic mothers, or heavy smokers. May also be response to chronic in utero hypoxia with secondary increase in RBC mass. Finally, it may be caused by increased blood volume from cord milking or twin-to-twin transfusion.

A. **Clinical diagnosis.** Usually presents by 2 to 72 hours with plethora, acrocyanosis, poor peripheral perfusion, respiratory distress or irritability. May be confused with cyanotic congenital heart disease.

B. **Lab diagnosis.** Venous HCT >65% (capillary is usually 4% to 7% higher); thrombocytopenia may occur.

C. **Complications.** Majority do well; stroke is usually the only lasting complication, but there can be CHF, oliguria, gangrene, or necrotizing enterocolitis.

D. **Treatment.**
   1. Observe if HCT 65% to 70% and asymptomatic.
   2. If HCT >70% or symptomatic, then partial exchange transfusion through umbilical vein using FFP or 5% albumin in saline with volume of exchange =

$$\frac{(90 \times \text{Weight in kg}) \times (\text{Measured HCT} - 50)}{\text{Measured HCT}}$$

   3. ***Do not merely phlebotomize!*** This can cause shock and worsen the situation. Watch for hypoglycemia or hypocalcemia.

NEONATAL METABOLIC DISORDERS

I. HYPOGLYCEMIA

Defined as serum glucose <40 mg/dl at term, <30 mg/dl premature. Recommend using level of 40 mg/dl to begin looking for cause and treating.

A. **Causes.** Neonatal gluconeogenesis is underdeveloped and is easily disrupted. Be aware of hypoglycemia in small-for-gestational-age and postdate infants and infants with a history of asphyxia, hypothermia, sepsis, prematurity, hypermetabolism (such as erythroblastosis), if mother diabetic (hyperinsulinism) or maternal ingestion of oral hypoglycemics or of beta-agonists. May also be secondary to sepsis.

B. **Diagnosis.** Have a high index of suspicion. *Clinical signs*: pale, cool, irritable, jittery, poor feeding, apnea, seizures, or may be asymptomatic. Routinely screen as described in the section on newborn nursery (p. 417) and recheck if any clinical suspicion of hypoglycemia.

C. **Treatment** should be given for 48 hours before tapering with frequent monitoring as follows:
   1. ***Stable and >34 weeks, blood glucose >30 mg/dl:*** 15 to 30 ml D_5W PO or IV and then advance to breast feeding or formula. Check glucose Q2-3h until 3 normal.
   2. ***Unstable, <34 weeks or blood glucose <30 mg/dl:*** $D_{10}W$ 5 ml/kg or $D_{25}W$ 2 ml/kg IV over 10 minutes and then 2 to 4 ml/kg/hour IV. Advance to PO while continuing IV, follow serial glucose level and taper off IV.
   3. If no IV access attainable, glucagon 0.1 mg/kg IM SQ IV for <10 kg (up to 1 mg) Q30 min will raise glucose for 2

to 3 hours but depletes glycogen stores and is not effective when stores are not present (such as SGA). NG feeding is another option.

II. HYPOCALCEMIA

Serum calcium <8 mg/dl associated with asphyxia, SGA, premature infant, or diabetic mother. Usually is transient.

A. Diagnosis. Hypotonia, apnea, poor feeding, jitters, seizures, serum calcium <8 mg/dl.

B. Treatment. Usually resolves in a couple of days; no need to treat asymptomatic infant.

1. ***If asymptomatic and wish to treat.*** Give 5 to 10 ml/kg/24h of 10% solution of *calcium gluconate* either PO in feedings or by continuous IV over 24 hours.
2. ***If symptomatic.*** Give 1.0 to 1.5 ml/kg of *calcium gluconate* 10% IV with a maximum of 5 ml in premature infants or 10 ml in a full-term infant. Should get a maximum of 1 ml/min. Can repeat if still symptomatic and then initiate treatment as in (1) above.
3. Consider low magnesium level or congenital hypoparathyroidism if persistent.

III. NEONATAL-WITHDRAWAL SYNDROME

Passive addiction of drugs by maternal use. Estimated 10% of urban births. Narcotics, and stimulants (such as cocaine) most common. Increased risk of SIDS.

A. Diagnosis.

1. ***Narcotics.*** Jittery, irritable, large appetite, vomiting, hypertonicity, and sneezing.
2. ***Cocaine.*** Lethargy, hypotonia, and poor feeding. Look for IUGR and cerebral infarctions.

B. Treatment. For both, swaddling and frequent high caloric feedings. For narcotics use tincture of opium (10 mg/ml morphine) diluted 1:25 in water, 2 drops/kg Q4-6h to control symptoms, monitor closely. Alternatively, may use phenobarbital 5 mg/kg/day divided Q8 or 12 hours IV, IM, or PO. Taper either regiment gradually over 1 to 3 weeks.

NEONATAL GASTROINTESTINAL DISORDERS

I. VOMITING AND REGURGITATION

A. General Comments. Regurgitation of the first few feedings is common. 80% infants <3 months of age regurgitate formula at least once a day. Bilious vomiting usually represents a surgical case of obstruction.

B. Cause.

1. ***Nonbilious.*** Benign overfeeding, infection, reflux, necrotizing enterocolitis, CNS lesion with increased intracranial pressure, pyloric stenosis, metabolic or electrolyte disorders, drugs, sepsis, other entities discussed elsewhere.

2. ***Bilious.*** Malrotation, atresia, stenosis, or other congenial anomalies.

C. Evaluation.

1. ***History.*** In infants need to determine how much is being fed (overfeeding), relation to position (reflux), choking or coughing with feeding (achalasia, tracheoesophageal fistula).
2. ***Exam and lab tests.*** Evaluate state of hydration (see section on dehydration, p. 466). Look for site of infection. Abdominal and rectal exam for obstruction or imperforate anus. Radiologic studies as indicated.
3. If child less than 2 months, consider ultrasonograpy for pyloric stenosis.
4. If neonatal, consider congenital abnormalities such as duodenal or esophageal atresia, Hirschsprung's disease, volvulus, malformation.
5. ***Reye's syndrome.*** Generally occurs after viral illness and presents with intractable vomiting, elevated liver enzymes, decreased mental status, prolonged PT, and elevated serum ammonia. See p. 461.
6. Consider elevated intracranial pressure as a cause of isolated vomiting.

D. Treatment. See dehydration section, p. 466. Also consider antiemetics such as promethazine or trimethobenzamide if cause is benign.

II. MECONIUM PLUG SYNDROME

A. General comments. Obstruction of the colon with meconium or mucus. More common in premature, infants of diabetic mothers, acute illness. Can be early presentation of cystic fibrosis or Hirschsprung's disease.

B. Signs and symptoms. Difficulty passing stools, normal rectal exam.

C. Management. Rectal stimulation with digital exam or glycerin suppository. See constipation, p. 471.

III. NECROTIZING ENTEROCOLITIS

A. Causes. Unclear, more common in premature babies (80%), SGA, maternal preeclampsia, cyanosis, exchange transfusions, umbilical catheterization, polycythemia. Precipitated by enteral feeding, ischemia, bacteria. *Prognosis*: mortality of 20% to 40%.

B. Signs and symptoms. Baby has abdominal distension, lethargy, bloody stools, ileus, vomiting. It can progress to DIC, apnea, shock, perforation. Onset may be gradual or fulminant.

C. Diagnosis. Abdominal radiograph will show distended loops of bowel, air fluid levels, pneumatosis intestinalis, free air. Requires full sepsis work-up including stool and CSF cultures, CBC, electrolytes, and enzymes. INR/PTT, ABG, etc.

D. Treatment.

1. Supportive treatment of acidosis, shock.

2. Surgery indicated if perforation, peritonitis, acidosis.
3. Begin broad-spectrum antibiotics (such as ampicillin and gentamicin) after cultures done. If resistant organisms known in hospital, cover with other antibiotics as required.

FEEDING AND SUPPLEMENTATIONS

I. BREAST FEEDING

A. Breast feeding should be recommended to all pregnant and postpartum mothers (except those who are HIV positive) and should provide adequate nutrition for the first 5 to 9 months. Human colostrum immediately after delivery is the optimal first feeding. Normal, term babies are born fully hydrated, and supplementation of the first breast feeding is not required.

B. Information and encouragement must be provided. References such as those to the local chapter of La Leche League may prove to be valuable.

C. Feeding on demand should be encouraged, with recognition that there is a large variety in normal feeding patterns. Typically, infant feeding intervals average every 2 to 3 hours in the first few weeks. Newborns should not go longer than 4 to 5 hours between feedings.

D. The supply of breast milk is adequate if the infant is satisfied after each nursing period, has 6 to 8 wet diapers a day, sleeps 2- to 4-hour intervals, and gains weight according to the growth chart.

E. Attention to sore nipples should be provided early before severe pain with cracking and abrasions occur. Exposing nipples to air and varying the infant feeding position are recommended; avoid drying soaps. Check the infant for thrush and treat both mother's nipples and infant if present.

F. Engorgement can be very uncomfortable for the mother. The mother should be encouraged to nurse or pump often, every 2 to 3 hours. If engorgement is severe, it can cause difficulty with the infant latching on. In this case, recommend manual expression before feeding.

G. Maternal fatigue and psychosocial factors should be addressed. Mothers should be encouraged to sleep when their infant sleeps.

H. **Mastitis.** Mastitis is an infection of the breast usually secondary to a blocked milk duct.

1. ***Exam.*** Reveals a hot, swollen, tender, and erythematous breast; mastitis is most commonly secondary to *Staphylococcus aureus.*
2. ***Treatment.***
   a. Treatment is by use of antistaphylococcal antibiotics such as dicloxacillin, erythromycin, or amoxicillin-clavulanate. Mastitis can usually be treated in an outpatient setting. However, if patient has fever or looks ill, consider admission for IV antibiotics.

b. The mother should continue to breast feed or use a breast pump. This is critical and will help resolve the infection.
c. Local care including hot packs may be helpful.

I. Drugs and breast milk. Drugs concentrated in breast milk tend to be weak bases (such as metronidazole, antihistamines, erythromycin, or antipsychotics and antidepressants).

1. ***Drugs absolutely contraindicated in breast feeding.*** Chemotherapeutic or cytotoxic agents, all drugs used recreationally (including alcohol and nicotine), radioactive nuclear medicine tracers, lithium carbonate, chloramphenicol, phenylbutazone, atropine, thiouracil, iodides, ergotamine and derivatives, and mercurials.
2. ***Drugs to strongly avoid or consider bottle feeding.*** Antipsychotics, antidepressants, metronidazole, tetracycline, sulfonamides, diazepam, salicylates, corticosteroids, phenytoin, phenobarbital, or warfarin.
3. ***Drugs safe to use in normal doses.*** Acetaminophen, insulin, diuretics, digoxin, beta-blockers, penicillins, cephalosporins, erythromycin, birth control pills, OTC cold preparations, and narcotic analgesics (short term in normal doses).
4. ***Lactation-suppressing drugs.*** Levodopa, anticholinergics, bromocriptine, trazodone, and large-dose estradiol birth control pills.

J. Failure to thrive in the breast-fed infant.

1. Infant causes include inadequate intake or increased caloric need.
2. Maternal causes include poor milk production because of inadequate diet (especially fluids), illness and fatigue, or poor letdown because of smoking, drugs, or psychologic reasons.

II. FORMULA FEEDING

Recent data indicate that a linkage of formula feeding with an increase in IDDM is doubtful.

1. In cases of preference or inability to breast feed, commercial infant formulas are able to provide adequate nutrition. Most are cow's milk based and contain lactose. Lactose-free soybean-based formulas are available for infants with primary lactase deficiency (watery, guaiac-negative stools, gas), galactosemia, cow's milk protein allergy (generally have diarrhea with blood and failure to thrive), and secondary lactase deficiency from GI insult (such as viral gastroenteritis).
2. Most formulas contain 20 kcal/oz, osmolality of 300 to 400 mOsm, and calorie breakdown of 7.2% to 18% protein, 30% to 54% fat, and 40% to 50% carbohydrate.
3. An on-demand schedule of feeding should be encouraged. Most newborns will typically take 2 to 3 ounces every 2 to 3 hours and should not be allowed to go greater than 5 hours between feedings. It is important to inform the parents to avoid overfeeding by being aware of satiety clues from the infant.

4. Reflux or occasional diarrhea are not in themselves indications for switching formula.

III. DIETARY ADVANCEMENT

1. Solids may begin to be added between months 4 and 6, typically occurring when the infant's hunger is no longer satisfied by milk alone or it is convenient in the family's schedule.
2. New foods should generally be introduced at the rate of one a week to give the child time to adjust to each new change.
3. Generally, cereal is started first, followed by fruits and vegetables and then meats. Infants typically show an interest in self-feeding at 6 to 8 months of age. Zwieback toast and crackers are typically offered first. A spoon can typically be introduced between 10 and 12 months. By the end of the second year of life, infants should not require assistance.
4. The introduction of cow's milk should be delayed until 12 months of age. Cow's milk given as primary food source before 12 months of age is associated with an increased incidence of iron-deficiency anemia believed to be secondary to GI blood loss. Additionally, there is some thought that earlier introduction may contribute to the development of diabetes.

IV. TODDLER FEEDING

Toddlers typically eat three meals as well as one or two snacks a day. Many toddlers will resist eating certain foods or insist on eating one or two favorite foods for long periods of time. It is advisable to avoid struggles and offer a variety of foods and leave the choices to the child. Vitamin supplements are rarely necessary.

V. VITAMIN SUPPLEMENTATION

A. Iron.

1. Iron supplementation in breast-fed infants is indicated for infants not receiving formula supplementation between 4 and 6 months of age.
2. Ferrous sulfate drops may be added at a dose of 1 to 2 mg/kg/day. An alternative is iron-fortified cereals, particularly when mixed with juice, since the vitamin C enhances iron absorption.
3. Premature infants should have supplementation with ferrous sulfate drops at a dose of 2 mg/kg/day at 2 months of age.
4. Bottle-fed infants should use an iron-fortified formula throughout the first year of life. Constipation should not be an indication to switch to a low-iron formula because there is no evidence that there is a causal relationship.

B. Vitamin D. Vitamin D is needed only when the breast-fed infant's mother's diet is deficient or the infant has limited sun exposure.

C. Vitamin B_{12}. Be aware of vitamin B_{12} deficiency in the children of strict vegetarian mothers.

TABLE 10-2
Recommended Supplemental Fluoride Dosage Schedule (in milligrams of fluoride per day)

	Parts per million of fluoride in water supply		
Age of child (years)	<0.3	0.3 to 0.7	>0.7
Birth to 2*	0.25	0	0
2 to 3	0.50	0.25	0
3 to 13*	1.00	0.50	0

*Recommended by the Council on Dental Therapeutics of the American Dental Association and the Committee on Nutrition of the American Academy of Pediatrics. The American Academy of Pediatrics recommends providing supplementation from 2 weeks of age through at least 16 years of age.

D. Fluoride.

1. Dietary fluoride supplements are recommended by the American Academy of Pediatrics and American Dental Association for infants and young children without access to optimally fluoridated water. The following dosage schedule based on age and water fluoride level has been recommended since 1979 (Table 10-2).
2. Recent international conferences have focused on appropriate use of fluorides in light of declining rates of dental caries and increasing rates of dental fluorosis. It was recommended that dietary fluoride supplements should be used more conservatively in the United States because ingestion of too much fluoride from supplements and other sources has been associated with increased prevalence of fluorosis, whereas substantial caries prevention can be achieved with the use of topical forms of fluoride such as fluoride toothpaste. Although a new dosage schedule and guidelines have not been agreed upon, there now is a general consensus that breast-fed infants in areas with fluoridated water usually do not need fluoride supplementation, in part because very few infants are exclusively breast fed for extended periods of time.

PEDIATRIC WELLNESS

I. IMMUNIZATIONS

Recent evidence proves that the measles-mumps-rubella (MMR) vaccine is safe in those with egg allergies and should not be withheld in this group.

A. Recommended vaccinations. See Fig. 10-3. An afebrile URI is not a contraindication to vaccination. Antibody conversion rates are the same in this population as in the well population.

B. If a patient misses a vaccination, start up where the patient left off. For example, if a patient had a diphtheria-pertussis-tetanus (DPT) vaccine at 2 months but missed subsequent doses and shows up at 2 years of age, start at what would have been the fourth-month dose and continue the series from there. Therefore, the patient would get a fourth-month, sixth-month, fifteenth-month, and 4- to 6-year dose for a total of 5 doses by 6 years of age.

C. Immunization side effects.

1. ***DTP vaccine.*** Local reaction common with erythema, tenderness, swelling. Mild systemic symptoms may occur, including low-grade fever, listlessness. Few children develop high fever. The relationship between DPT vaccine and neurologic symptoms has not been substantiated when cases are looked at critically. In any case, the acellular pertussis vaccine should allay any fears.
2. ***MMR vaccine.*** May have local reaction. Fever may occur and may be delayed with onset between 5 and 7 days. A morbilliform rash may occur at the same time.
3. ***Haemophilus influenzae vaccine.*** Minimal reaction including local reaction and low-grade fever.
4. ***Poliomyelitis vaccine.*** Adults may develop polio if given oral immunization as may the immunosuppressed.

II. GROWTH AND DEVELOPMENT

1. The caloric requirements for full-term infants are 80 to 120 kcal/kg/day for the first few months of life and 100 kcal/kg to the twelfth month of life. There is significant individual variation.
2. The newborn infant can be expected to lose up to 10% of body weight in the neonatal period. The birth weight should be regained by 10 days of life. The full-term infant generally doubles its birth weight by 5 months of age and triples it by 1 year.
3. ***Fontanelles and sutures.*** Principle sutures should fuse by fifth to sixth month. Premature closure is termed "craniosynostosis" and may lead to neurologic abnormalities. Lateral fontanelle closes by week 6 of life and posterior by 4 months of age. Anterior fontanelle should start to shrink after 6 months of life and closes by 9 to 16 months.
4. ***Sinuses.*** Maxillary and ethmoid sinuses present at birth and enlarge during childhood, Sphenoid sinuses develop by 1 to 2 years and continue to enlarge during childhood, frontal sinuses by 2 to 6 years.

III. DEVELOPMENTAL SCREENING (Table 10-3)

IV. DEVELOPMENTAL MILESTONES

See growth charts (Figs. 10-4 to 10-10 and Tables 10-4 and 10-5).

Text continued on p. 450.

Recommended Childhood Immunization Schedule
United States, January - December 1997

Vaccines[1] are listed under the routinely recommended ages. Bars indicate range of acceptable ages for vaccination. Shaded bars indicate *catch-up vaccination:* at 11-12 years of age, hepatitis B vaccine should be administered to children not previously vaccinated, and varicella vaccine should be administered to children not previously vaccinated who lack a reliable history of chickenpox.

<table>
<tr><th>Age ➤
Vaccine ▼</th><th>Birth</th><th>1 mo</th><th>2 mos</th><th>4 mos</th><th>6 mos</th><th>12 mos</th><th>15 mos</th><th>18 mos</th><th>4-6 yrs</th><th>11-12 yrs</th><th>14-16 yrs</th></tr>
<tr><td rowspan="2">Hepatitis B[2,3]</td><td colspan="3">Hep B-1</td><td></td><td></td><td></td><td></td><td></td><td></td><td></td><td></td></tr>
<tr><td></td><td colspan="3">Hep B-2</td><td colspan="4">Hep B-3</td><td></td><td>Hep B[3] (shaded)</td><td></td></tr>
<tr><td>Diphtheria, tetanus, pertussis[4]</td><td></td><td></td><td>DTaP or DTP</td><td>DTaP or DTP</td><td>DTaP or DTP</td><td></td><td colspan="2">DTaP or DTP[4]</td><td>DTaP or DTP</td><td colspan="2">Td</td></tr>
<tr><td>H. influenzae type b[5]</td><td></td><td></td><td>Hib</td><td>Hib</td><td>Hib[5]</td><td colspan="2">Hib[5]</td><td></td><td></td><td></td><td></td></tr>
<tr><td>Polio[6]</td><td></td><td></td><td>Polio[6]</td><td>Polio</td><td></td><td colspan="3">Polio[6]</td><td>Polio</td><td></td><td></td></tr>
<tr><td>Measles, mumps, rubella[7]</td><td></td><td></td><td></td><td></td><td></td><td colspan="2">MMR</td><td></td><td colspan="2">MMR[7] or MMR[7]</td><td></td></tr>
<tr><td>Varicella[8]</td><td></td><td></td><td></td><td></td><td></td><td colspan="3">Var</td><td></td><td>Var[8] (shaded)</td><td></td></tr>
</table>

Approved by the Advisory Committee on Immunization Practices (ACIP), the American Academy of Pediatrics (AAP), and the American Academy of Family Physicians (AAFP).

FIG. 19-2 (From *MMWR* 46[2]:35-40, 1997.)

[1]This schedule indicates the recommended age for routine administration of currently licensed childhood vaccines. Some combination vaccines are available and may be used whenever administration of all components of the vaccine is indicated. Providers should consult the manufacturers' package inserts for detailed recommendations.

[2]Infants born to HBsAg-negative mothers should receive 2.5 μg of Merck vaccine (Recombivax HB) or 10 μg of SmithKline Beecham (SB) vaccine (Engerix-B). The 2nd dose should be administered ≥1 mo after the 1st dose. Infants born to HBsAg-positive mothers should receive 0.5 ml hepatitis B immune globulin (HBIG) within 12 hrs of birth, and either 5 μg of Merck vaccine (Recombivax HB) or 10 μg of SB vaccine (Engerix-B) at a separate site. The 2nd dose is recommended at 1-2 mos of age and the 3rd dose at 6 mos of age.
Infants born to mothers whose HBsAg status is unknown should receive either 5 μg of Merck vaccine (Recombivax HB) or 10 μg of SB vaccine (Engerix-B) within 12 hrs of birth. The 2nd dose of vaccine is recommended at 1 mo of age and the 3rd dose at 6 mos of age. Blood should be drawn at the time of delivery to determine the mother's HBsAg status; if it is positive, the infant should receive HBIG as soon as possible (no later than 1 wk of age). The dosage and timing of subsequent vaccine doses should be based upon the mother's HBsAg status.

[3]Children and adolescents who have not been vaccinated against hepatitis B in infancy may begin the series during any childhood visit. Those who have not previously received 3 doses of hepatitis B vaccine should initiate or complete the series during the 11-12 year-old visit. The 2nd dose should be administered at least 1 mo after the 1st dose, and the 3rd dose should be administered at least 4 mos after the 1st dose and at least 2 mos after the 2nd dose.

[4]DTaP (diphtheria and tetanus toxoids and acellular pertussis vaccine) is the preferred vaccine for all doses in the vaccination series, including completion of the series in children who have received ≥1 dose of whole-cell DTP vaccine. Whole-cell DTP is an acceptable alternative to DTaP. The 4th dose of DTaP may be administered as early as 12 months of age, provided 6 months have elapsed since the 3rd dose and if the child is considered unlikely to return at 15-18 mos of age. Td (tetanus and diphtheria toxoids, absorbed, for adult use) is recommended at 11-12 years of age if at least 5 years have elapsed since the last dose of DTP, DTaP, or DT. Subsequent routine Td boosters are recommended every 10 years.

[5]Three *H. influenzae* type b (Hib) conjugate vaccines are licensed for infant use. If PRP-OMP (Pedvaxhib [Merck]) is administered at 2 and 4 mos of age, a dose at 6 mos is not required. After completing the primary series, any Hib conjugate vaccine may be used as a booster.

[6]Two poliovirus vaccines are currently licensed in the US: inactivated poliovirus vaccine (IPV) and oral poliovirus vaccine (OPV). The following schedules are all acceptable by the ACIP, the AAP, and the AAFP, and parents and providers may choose among them:

1. IPV at 2 and 4 mos; OPV at 12-18 mos and 4-6 yrs
2. IPV at 2, 4, 12-18 mos, and 4-6 yrs
3. OPV at 2, 4, 6-18 mos, and 4-6 yrs

The ACIP routinely recommends schedule 1. IPV is the only poliovirus vaccine recommended for immunocompromised persons and their household contacts.

[7]The 2nd dose of MMR is routinely recommended at 4-6 yrs of age or at 11-12 yrs of age but may be administered during any visit, provided at least 1 month has elapsed since receipt of the 1st dose and that both doses are administered at or after 12 months of age.

[8]Susceptible children may receive varicella vaccine (Var) at any visit after the first birthday, and those who lack a reliable history of chickenpox should be immunized during the 11-12 year-old visit. Children ≥13 years of age should receive 2 doses, at least 1 month apart.

TABLE 10-3
Developmental Milestones/Language Skills

Age	Gross motor	Visual motor	Language	Social
1 mo	Raises head slightly from prone, makes crawling movements, lifts chin up	Has tight grasp, follows to midline	Alerts to sound (e.g., by blinking, moving, startling)	Regards face
2 mo	Holds head in midline, lifts chest off table	No longer clenches fist tightly, follows object past midline	Smiles after being stroked or talked to	Recognizes parent
3 mo	Supports on forearms in prone, holds head up steadily	Holds hands open at rest, follows in circular fashion	Coos (produces long vowel sounds in musical fashion)	Reaches for familiar people or objects, anticipates feeding
4–5 mo	Rolls front to back, back to front, sits well when propped, supports on wrists and shifts weight	Moves arms in unison to grasp, touches cube placed on table	Orients to voice; *5 mo*—orients to bell (localized laterally), says "ahgoo," razzes	Enjoys looking around environment
6 mo	Sits well unsupported, puts feet in mouth in supine position	Reaches with either hand, transfers, uses raking grasp	Babbles; *7 mo*— orients to bell (localizes indirectly); *8 mo*—"dada/mama" indiscriminately	Recognizes strangers
9 mo	Creeps, crawls, cruises, pulls to stand, pivots when sitting	Uses pincer grasp, probes with forefinger, holds bottle, finger-feeds	Understands "no," waves bye-bye; *10 mo*—"dada/mama" discriminately; *11 mo*—one word other than "dada/mama"	Starts to explore environment, plays pat-a-cake
12 mo	Walks alone	Throws objects, lets go of toys, hand release, uses mature pincer grasp	Follows one-step command with gesture, uses 2 words other than "dada/mama"; *14 mo*—uses 3 words	Imitates actions, comes when called, cooperates with dressing

15 mo	Creeps upstairs, walks backward	Builds tower of 2 blocks in imitation of examiner, scribbles in imitation	Follows one-step command without gesture, uses 4 to 6 words and immature jargon (runs several unintelligible words together)	
18 mo	Runs, throws toy from standing without falling	Turns 2 or 3 pages at a time, fills spoon and feeds self	Knows 7 to 20 words, knows 1 body part, uses mature jargon (includes intelligible words in jargon)	Copies parent in tasks (e.g., sweeping, dusting), plays in company of other children
21 mo	Squats in play, goes up steps	Builds tower of 5 blocks, drinks well from cup	Points to 3 body parts, uses 2-word combinations, has 2-word vocabulary	Asks to have food and to go to toilet
24 mo	Walks up and down steps without help	Turns pages one at a time, removes shoes, pants, etc., imitates stroke	Uses 50 words, 2-word sentences, uses pronouns (I, you, me) inappropriately, points to 5 body parts, understands 2-step command	Parallel play
30 mo	Jumps with both feet off floor, throws ball overhand	Unbuttons, holds pencil in adult fashion, differentiates horizontal and vertical line	Uses pronouns (I, you, me) appropriately, understands concept of "one," repeats 2 digits forward	Tells first and last names when asked, gets drink without help

Continued

TABLE 10-3
Developmental Milestones/Language Skills—cont'd

Age	Gross motor	Visual motor	Language	Social
3 yr	Pedals tricycle, can alternate feet when going up steps	Dresses and undresses partially, dries hands if reminded, draws a circle	Uses 3-word sentences, plurals, and past tense. Knows all pronouns. Minimum of 250 words, understands concept of "two"	Group play, shares toys, takes turns, plays well with others, knows full name, age, sex
4 yr	Hops, skips, alternates feet going downstairs	Buttons clothing fully, catches ball	Knows colors, says song or poem from memory, asks questions	Tells "tall tales", plays cooperatively with a group of children
5 yr	Skips, alternating feet, jumps over low obstacles	Ties shoes, spreads with knife	Prints first name, asks what a word means	Plays competitive games, abides by rules, likes to help in household tasks

TABLE 10-4
Normal Values—Hematology

Age	Hb (g/dl), mean (−2 SD)	HCT (%), mean (−2 SD)	MCV (fl), mean (−2 SD)	MCHC, mean (−2 SD)	Reticulocytes (%)	WBC/mm^3 ×100, mean (−2 SD)	Platelets (10^3/mm^3), mean ±2 SD)
26-30 WK gestation*	13.4 (11)	41.5 (34.9)	118.2 (106.7)	37.9 (30.6)	—	4.4 (2.7)	254 (180-327)
26 wks	14.5	45	120	31	(5-10)	—	275
32 wks	15.0	47	118	32	(3-10)	—	290
TERM†							
Cord	16.5 (13.5)	51 (42)	108 (98)	33 (30)	(3-7)	18.1 (9-30)‡	290
1-3 days	18.5 (14.5)	56 (45)	108 (95)	33 (30)	(3-7)	18.1 (9-30)‡	290
2 wk	16.6 (13.4)	53 (41)	105 (88)	31.4 (28.1)		11.4 (5-20)	252
1 mo	13.9 (10.7)	44 (33)	101 (91)	31.8 (28.1)	(0.1-1.7)	10.8 (5-19.5)	
2 mo	11.2 (9.4)	35 (28)	95 (84)	31.8 (28.3)			
6 mo	12.6 (11.1)	36 (31)	76 (68)	35 (32.7)	(0.7-2.3)	11.9 (6-17.5)	
6 mo-2 yr	12 (10.5)	36 (33)	78 (70)	33 (30)		10.6 (6-17)	(150-350)
2-6 yr	12.5 (11.5)	37 (34)	81 (75)	34 (31)	(0.5-1.0)	8.5 (5-15.5)	(150-350)
6-12 yr	13.5 (11.5)	40 (35)	86 (77)	34 (31)	(0.5-1.0)	8.1 (4.5-13.5)	(150-350)

Continued

TABLE 10-4
Normal Values—Hematology—cont'd

Age	Hb (g/dl), mean (−2 SD)	HCT (%), mean (−2 SD)	MCV (fl), mean (−2 SD)	MCHC, mean (−2 SD)	Reticulocytes (%)	WBC/mm^3 ×100, mean (−2 SD)	Platelets (10^3/mm^3), mean ±2 SD)
12-18 YR							
Male	14.5 (13)	43 (36)	88 (78)	34 (31)	(0.5-1.0)	7.8 (4.5-13.5)	(150-350)
Female	13 (12)	41 (37)	90 (78)	34 (31)	(0.5-1.0)	7.8 (4.5-13.5)	(150-350)
ADULT							
Male	15.5 (13.5)	47 (41)	90 (80)	34 (31)	(0.8-2.5)	7.4 (4.5-11)	(150-350)
Female	14 (12)	41 (36)	90 (80)	34 (31)	(0.8-4.1)	7.4 (4.5-11)	(150-350)

MCHC, Mean corpuscular hemoglobin concentration; *MCV,* mean corpuscular volume.
*Values are from fetal samplings.
†Under 1 month, capillary hemoglobin exceeds venous: 1 hour, 3.6 g difference; 5 days, 2.2 g difference; 3 weeks, 1 g difference.
‡Mean (95% confidence limits).

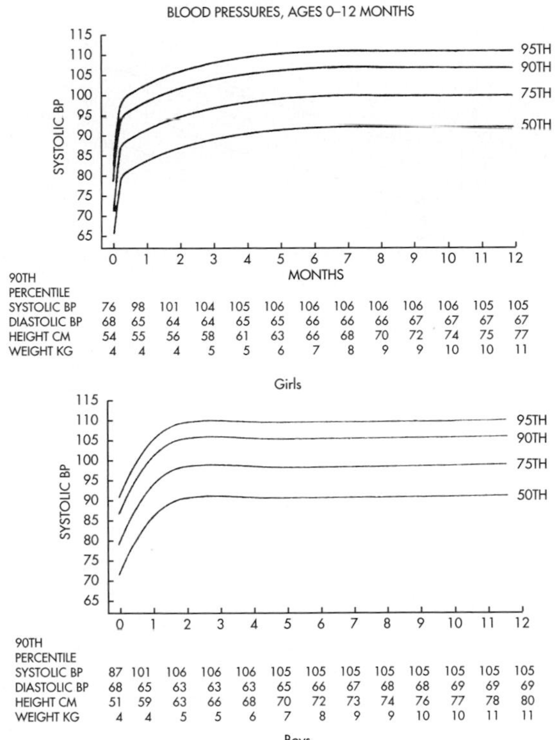

Girls

90TH PERCENTILE	0	1	2	3	4	5	6	7	8	9	10	11	12
SYSTOLIC BP	76	98	101	104	105	106	106	106	106	106	106	105	105
DIASTOLIC BP	68	65	64	64	65	65	66	66	66	67	67	67	67
HEIGHT CM	54	55	56	58	61	63	66	68	70	72	74	75	77
WEIGHT KG	4	4	4	5	5	6	7	8	9	9	10	10	11

Boys

90TH PERCENTILE	0	1	2	3	4	5	6	7	8	9	10	11	12
SYSTOLIC BP	87	101	106	106	106	105	105	105	105	105	105	105	105
DIASTOLIC BP	68	65	63	63	63	65	66	67	68	68	69	69	69
HEIGHT CM	51	59	63	66	68	70	72	73	74	76	77	78	80
WEIGHT KG	4	4	5	5	6	7	8	9	9	10	10	11	11

FIG. 10-4 Blood pressures, ages from birth to 12 months. (From Horan MJ: *Pediatrics* 79:1, 1987.)

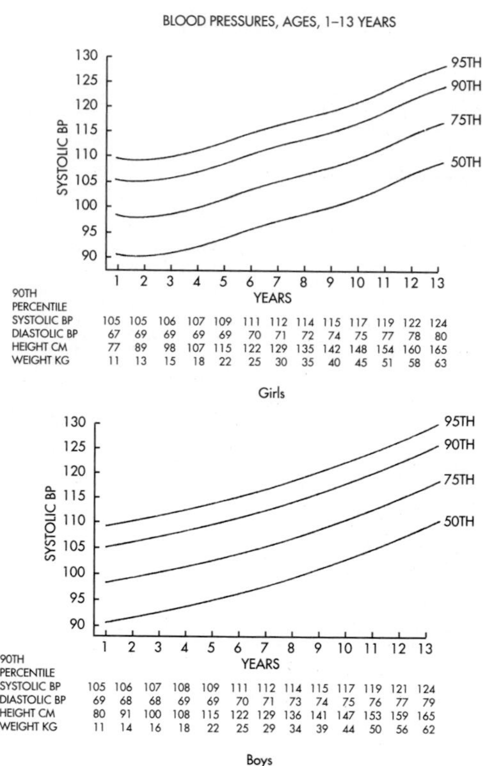

90TH PERCENTILE	1	2	3	4	5	6	7	8	9	10	11	12	13
SYSTOLIC BP	105	105	106	107	109	111	112	114	115	117	119	122	124
DIASTOLIC BP	67	69	69	69	69	70	71	72	74	75	77	78	80
HEIGHT CM	77	89	98	107	115	122	129	135	142	148	154	160	165
WEIGHT KG	11	13	15	18	22	25	30	35	40	45	51	58	63

Girls

90TH PERCENTILE	1	2	3	4	5	6	7	8	9	10	11	12	13
SYSTOLIC BP	105	106	107	108	109	111	112	114	115	117	119	121	124
DIASTOLIC BP	69	68	68	69	69	70	71	73	74	75	76	77	79
HEIGHT CM	80	91	100	108	115	122	129	136	141	147	153	159	165
WEIGHT KG	11	14	16	18	22	25	29	34	39	44	50	56	62

Boys

FIG. 10-5 Blood pressures, ages 1 to 13 years. (From Horan MJ: *Pediatrics* 79:1, 1987.)

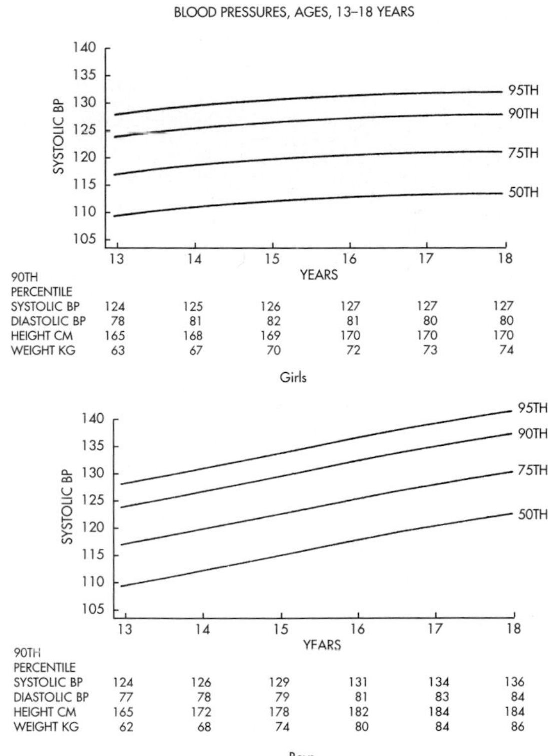

Girls

90TH PERCENTILE	13	14	15	16	17	18
SYSTOLIC BP	124	125	126	127	127	127
DIASTOLIC BP	78	81	82	81	80	80
HEIGHT CM	165	168	169	170	170	170
WEIGHT KG	63	67	70	72	73	74

Boys

90TH PERCENTILE	13	14	15	16	17	18
SYSTOLIC BP	124	126	129	131	134	136
DIASTOLIC BP	77	78	79	81	83	84
HEIGHT CM	165	172	178	182	184	184
WEIGHT KG	62	68	74	80	84	86

FIG. 10-6 Blood pressures, ages 13 to 18 years. (From Horan MJ: *Pediatrics* 79:1, 1987.)

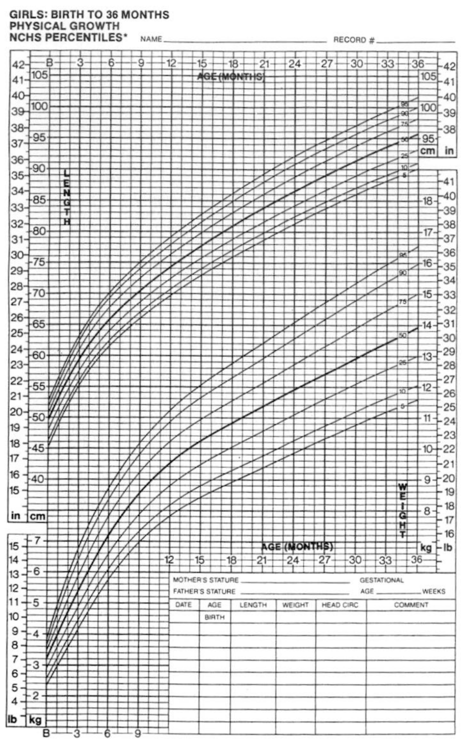

FIG. 10-7 Length and weight of girls from birth to 36 months. (Adapted from Hamill PVV et al: Physical growth: National Center for Health Statistics percentiles, *Am J Clin Nutr* 32:607-629, 1979. Data from the Fels Longitudinal Study, Wright State University School of Medicine, Yellow Springs, Ohio.)

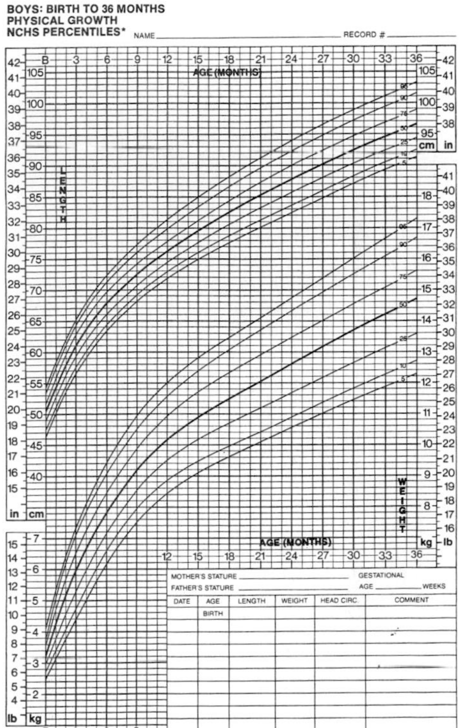

FIG. 10-8 Length and weight of boys from birth to 36 months. (Adapted from Hamill PVV et al: Physical growth: National Center for Health Statistics percentiles, *Am J Clin Nutr* 32:607-629, 1979. Data from the Fels Longitudinal Study, Wright State University School of Medicine, Yellow Springs, Ohio.)

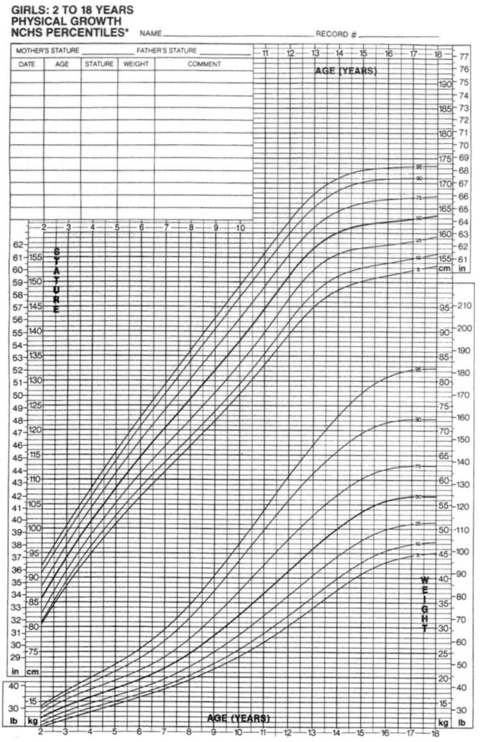

FIG. 10-9 Stature and weight of girls from 2 to 18 years. (Adapted from Hamill PVV et al: Physical growth: National Center for Health Statistics percentiles, *Am J Clin Nutr* 32:607-629, 1979. Data from the National Center for Health Statistics [NCHS], Hyattsville, Md.)

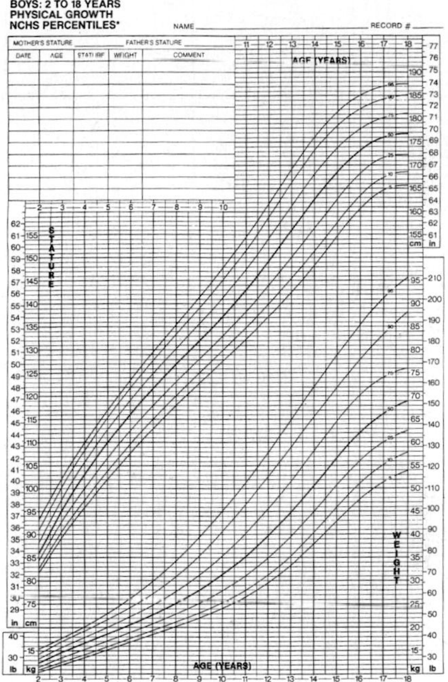

FIG. 10-10 Stature and weight of boys from 2 to 18 years. (Adapted from Hamill PVV et al: Physical growth: National Center for Health Statistics percentiles, *Am J Clin Nutr* 32:607-629, 1979. Data from the National Center for Health Statistics [NCHS], Hyattsville, Md.)

TABLE 10-5
Dental Development

	Deciduous teeth				Permanent teeth	
	Eruption		Shedding		Eruption	
	MAXILLARY	**MANDIBULAR**	**MAXILLARY**	**MANDIBULAR**	**MAXILLARY**	**MANDIBULAR**
CENTRAL INCISORS	6-8 mo	5-7 mo	7-8 yr	6-7 yr	7-8 yr	6-7 yr
LATERAL INCISORS	8-11 mo	7-10 mo	8-9 yr	7-8 yr	8-9 yr	7-8 yr
CUSPIDS	16-20 mo	16-20 mo	11-12 yr	9-11 yr	11-12 yr	9-11 yr
1ST PREMOLAR	—	—	—	—	10-11 yr	10-12 yr

2ND PREMOLAR	—	—	—	—	10-12 yr	11-13 yr
1ST MOLARS	10-16 mo	10-16 mo	10-11 yr	10-12 yr	6-7 yr	6-7 yr
2ND MOLARS	20-30 mo	20-30 mo	10-12 yr	11-13 yr	12-13 yr	12-13 yr
3RD MOLARS	—	—	—	—	17-22 yr	12-22 yr

Sexes are combined although girls tend to be slightly more advanced than boys. Averages are approximate values derived from various studies.
Adapted from Driscoll CE et al: *The family practice desk reference*, ed 3, St. Louis, 1996, Mosby.

FAILURE TO THRIVE

I. GENERAL COMMENTS

Failure to thrive is a general term used to describe a child who is failing to maintain growth above the third percentile for weight or height. Typically weight for height is the first parameter affected and later height and head circumference are affected. Psychosocial and parental are the most common causes, but many disease states can also prevent adequate growth. There are three major patterns of inadequate growth when one is comparing age to height, weight, and head circumference.

A. *Decreased weight in proportion to height with a normal head circumference* is the pattern most commonly seen. In the majority of these cases, there is inadequate caloric intake for social, economic, or physical reasons. Malabsorption and metabolic abnormalities can also be the cause.

B. *A moderate decrease in weight compared to height with a normal or enlarged head circumference* can signal a structural dystrophy, endocrine disorder, or other congenital reason for low weight and short stature.

C. *Small head circumference with low weight for height* may indicate a CNS defect or IUGR.

II. EVALUATION

A. A thorough history and physical exam focusing on diet, feedings, mother-child interaction, signs of neglect, signs of physical abuse, or obvious physical illness such as diarrhea or chronic infection; a complete calorie count should be done.

B. Initial screening lab tests include CBC, UA, electrolytes, sedimentation rate, serum glucose, stool for ova and parasites and for guaiac test. Depending on the clinical situation, serum lead levels, thyroid functions, and evaluation for adrenal disease may be important.

C. The hallmark of evaluation is a period of time (1 to 2 weeks) under careful observation, with appropriate physical stimulation and adequate caloric intake while growth parameters are being monitored. This typically requires hospitalization but may be accomplished elsewhere if close observation with objective data collection is possible. Usually this cannot be accomplished at home. *To determine dietary need:* Caloric requirements = 120 kcal/kg (actual weight)/day × (Ideal weight/Actual weight). Consulting a dietitian may be helpful.

D. An approach to evaluating a period of observation is found in Table 10-6.

SHORT STATURE

A. Definition. Subnormal height (usually less that third to fifth percentile) relative to other children of the same sex, age,

TABLE 10-6
Possible Approaches for Failure to Thrive

Adequate Intake?	Weight gain?	Most likely diagnoses	Treatment plan
Yes	Yes	1. Feeding problem 2. Neglect 3. Inability to purchase food	1. Counseling and information 2. Social services help
Yes	No	1. Malabsorption, cystic fibrosis, celiac sprue, parasitic infection, milk allergy 2. Hypermetabolic, chronic infection, malignancy, hyperthyroid 3. Metabolic dysfunction, renal acidosis, hypercalcemia, diabetes, others such as inborn errors of metabolism	Stool: culture O&P, pH, reducing substances, 72-hour stool fat, D-xylose test Thyroid function tests, CBC, sedimentation rate, C-reactive protein, liver function tests Serum pH, electrolytes, glucose, calcium, UA
No	No	Sucking or swallowing difficulties caused by neurologic disease, congenital anomaly Regurgitation: GI obstruction (such as pyloric stenosis), CSF pressure elevation, chronic metabolic disease	If nonorganic cause is definitely ruled out, begin to do further work-up and appropriate consultation Neurologic work-up: head CT, consultation GI work-up: barium swallow, consultation Endocrine work-up: TSH, T_4, etc.

and ethnicity. This contrasts with growth failure, which is a slow rate of growth irrespective of stature.

B. Short stature should be defined with parents' height being taken into account. If child is on the growth curve to reach projected height based on parents' heights, it is not considered short stature.

1. ***For girls.*** *Approximate* projected adult height = (Mother's height + [Father's height − 5"])/2
2. ***For boys.*** *Approximate* projected adult height = ([Mother's height + 5"] + Father's height)/2

C. **Causes.** May be a variation of normal (familial or constitutional); endocrine disorders including growth hormone deficiency, diabetes, and hypothyroidism; skeletal dysplasias; genetic syndromes including Turner's syndrome and Prader-Willi syndrome; malnutrition; chronic disease; lysosomal storage disorders; and psychosocial deprivation. Precocious puberty or elevated levels of androgens and estrogens will prematurely mature bones causing epiphyseal closure and short stature.

D. **History.** Should include a family history (parental heights, relatives with short stature, genetic syndromes), perinatal insults, hypopituitarism, social and nutritional components. Review of systems should include respiratory and gastrointestinal systems.

E. **Physical exam.** Should include examination of sexual development, nutritional status, disproportionate body segments (seen in chondromalacias), and observation for stigmata of genetic syndromes.

F. **Laboratory tests.** Should be considered in those more than 3 standard deviations below the mean and whose history and physical do not reveal a cause. Consider CBC for evidence of anemia, inflammation, infection, malignancy, and bone marrow suppression; electrolytes, BUN, UA to assess renal status; ESR to screen for inflammatory bowel disease and other chronic inflammatory disorders; karyotype, particularly in girls to evaluate for Turner's syndrome; thyroid studies and calcium, phosphorus, and alkaline phosphatase to screen for rickets.

G. **To assess growth hormone.** Draw insulin-like growth factor I and II (IGF-I, IGF-II) and IGF-binding protein (IGF-BP). Additional studies may include insulin infusion and induced hypoglycemia, which should lead to an increase in serum growth hormone if system is functioning properly. This test should generally be done under the supervision of an endocrinologist.

H. **Hand and wrist radiographs to determine bone age.** Delay is seen in hypopituitarism, constitutional delay, chronic disease, Turner's syndrome, and hypothyroidism. It may also be delayed in psychosocial dwarfism, gonadal dysgenesis, and primordial dwarfism. The bone age is normal in cases of familial short stature. Delayed bone age is hopeful, since growth potential is still maintained and child may still reach normal adult stature with resolution of the underlying cause.

CRYING AND COLIC

I. GENERAL COMMENTS

About one fifth of infants are described as having colic. This is described as inconsolable crying often accompanied by drawing up of the legs and gaseous distension of the abdomen. It may occur around the clock but more commonly occurs at a predictable time in the evening. Colic starts by 3 weeks of age, and the peak occurs by 6 weeks of age and may include about 3 hours of crying a day. The severity declines and by 3 months of age "normal" patterns are reestablished.

II. CONTRIBUTING FACTORS

Contributing factors may include formula, aerophagia, too small a hole in a bottle nipple, various foods in the diet of breast-fed infants.

III. TREATMENT

1. After an exam to rule out other causes for irritability and crying (especially otitis, another infections cause, intussusception, hairs around the penis, fingers, or toes, etc.) the parents should be advised on the anticipated course and management. The importance of never shaking a baby should be stressed. An alternative caregiver should be identified if the parents feel at the limit of their ability to cope. Additionally there is good evidence that behavioral interventions (beyond simple emotional support) can be of benefit (Wolke et al: *Pediatrics* 94(3):322-332, 1994).
2. Rocking the child or using a child swing may be beneficial. Elimination of cruciferous vegetables and chocolate from a breast-feeding mother's diet may be helpful but has not been proved in a blinded study. Changing formulas to soybean milk or a hydrolzyed milk formula may help in some cases.
3. *There is no evidence that either simethicone or dicyclomine work for infant colic.*

SAFETY AND ACCIDENT PREVENTION

SIDS prevention. SIDS is the leading cause of death in infants 1 to 12 months of age. To reduce risk, infants should be placed to sleep on their back or side on a firm surface with no pillows or other compressible objects in the bed. Avoiding smoking in the house may also be helpful.

PEDIATRIC INFECTIONS AND INFESTATIONS

I. APPROACH TO THE FEBRILE CHILD

Fever may be a marker of sepsis, localized infection, occult bacteremia, or benign illness.

A. General considerations.

1. *Temperature should be taken rectally.* Axillary and tympanic temperatures are not adequate in the small child.

2. The degree of elevation of the temperature does correlate with the likelihood of bacteremia, especially if >40° C. However, those with a low-grade fever can be septic, and those with high temperatures can have a benign course.
3. The response to antipyretics cannot be used as a guide to differentiate septic children from those with viral illnesses. Responders to antipyretics may be septic, whereas those who do not respond may have a mild illness.
4. In those greater than 2 to 3 months of age, clinical appearance is the best indicator of severity of illness. Children less than 3 months of age may not manifest signs of systemic illness. However, children 3 months to 2 years may not manifest the "typical" symptoms of their underlying illness (that is, no meningeal signs with meningitis).
5. Blood cultures are of limited usefulness in determining which patients should be treated, since results are delayed 48 to 72 hours. A single blood culture may miss up to 50% of bacteremic children, and if cultures are appropriate, two cultures should be done with the largest volume of blood possible (at least 6 ml total). Additionally, most bacteremic children will clear the bacteremia spontaneously.
6. Teething is related to fever, but look for other sources in the ill-appearing child.
7. Fever may be treated with acetaminophen 10 to 15 mg/kg Q4-6h or ibuprofen 10 mg/kg Q6-8h or both. Tepid bathing does not add much to the efficacy of these drugs. Aspirin should be avoided because of the risk of Reye's syndrome.

B. History. Should focus on the duration and height of the fever; associated symptoms such as vomiting and diarrhea, rash (especially petechiae), and behavioral changes; and parental estimation of the degree of illness. Known exposures should be reviewed as well as an immunization and travel history.

C. Physical exam. Should begin with a careful consideration of the general appearance. Careful observation and analysis of the vital signs, state of hydration, and peripheral perfusion are required. Attention should be paid to tachypnea out of proportion to fever, which may indicate pneumonia. A complete exam should be performed including a musculoskeletal exam for septic arthritis and osteomyelitis, neurologic exam, and skin exam.

D. Approach to the febrile child without an obvious source of infection varies with age:

1. ***For a child <3 months of age with any degree of fever >38° Celsius (100.4° F).***
   a. The exam and clinical signs and symptoms do not correlate well with seriousness of illness in these children and are an unreliable indicator of severity of disease. 3% to 10% of febrile children in this age group will have a serious bacterial illness.

b. Any febrile child of this age without an identifiable focus of disease should have a complete septic work-up including CBC, blood cultures, LP with CSF Gram stain, culture, glucose and cell count, UA, and C&S. The white count is an insensitive indicator of bacterial illness but can be used to separate febrile children into "high-risk" and "low-risk" categories. Those with a WBC count of <5000 or >15,000 are in the "high-risk" group. Some authors suggest a CXR as well, but in a child without pulmonary or respiratory symptoms the yield is very low. However, 12% of those with isolated rhinorrhea will have a positive CXR.

c. *Decide if patient has a high risk or a low risk.* A "low-risk" infant is considered:
   (1) 28 to 90 days old and previously healthy.
   (2) Nontoxic appearing.
   (3) No apparent site of focal bacterial infection, except for otitis.
   (4) Good social situation.
   (5) WBC count of 5,000 to 15,000 with a band count below 1,500.
   (6) Normal urinalysis with fewer than 5 WBCs/HPF.
   (7) If diarrhea is present, there should be fewer than 5 WBCs/HPF in the stool.

d. Admit all patients who look toxic or ill or are less than 28 days of age and cover with ceftriaxone (50 to 75 mg/kg Q24h not >2 g) until cultures available.

e. Admit and treat patients with an identifiable illness requiring hospitalization such as meningitis, pneumonia, or UTI (see specific section for treatments). Admit all "high-risk" infants (WBC count of >15,000 or <5000/mm^3, inability to follow up for social reasons, abnormal UA, WBCs in stool) even if no source evident and treat as for sepsis with ceftriaxone while awaiting cultures.

f. Patients who are at low risk (see c above) *and* appear well can be treated as an outpatient while awaiting culture results with ceftriaxone 75 mg/kg IM (not >2 g) and should be followed up in 24 hours. If cultures positive, treat as appropriate. If cultures are negative and patient is afebrile and looks well, can follow up closely. If remains febrile, cover with ceftriaxone until cultures final.

2. ***Children 3 months to 2 years.***

a. Many authors will treat children up to 3 months of age as above.

b. 4% of febrile children in this age group will have occult bacteremia with *Streptococcus pneumoniae* or *Haemophilus influenzae,* though most of these children will clear the bacteremia spontaneously and have no sequelae.

c. Those with a WBC count of >15,000 or <5000 are at a higher risk of sepsis, but this should not be used as an absolute guide, since children with any WBC count can be septic.
d. Non–toxic appearing children with a temperature of <39° C may be observed with laboratory testing addressed to the clinical picture.
e. For those who are toxic appearing, a complete physical exam should be done and lab examination should be addressed to findings. Blood cultures should be done in those considered at high risk for sepsis (generally look ill). Do not forget a UA.
f. Those with a temperature of >39° C should have a CBC, blood culture, urinalysis, and urine culture. If WBC >15,000 or <5000, cover with ceftriaxone 50 to 75 mg/kg IM (not >2 g) and see patient back the next day.

II. BACTERIAL MENINGITIS

A. Bacterial meningitis must be suspected in any febrile child or any child with mental status changes. Prompt diagnosis and treatment are paramount to successful outcome. Viral (or aseptic) meningitis is more common, seldom needs more than supportive care, and rarely causes significant sequelae.

B. Epidemiology. There is an increased frequency among rural, African-American and Native-American populations.

1. **<1 month** = Group B strep, *E. coli, Listeria.*
2. **>1 month** = *H. influenzae,* type B (especially in toddlers), *Neisseria meningitidis, Streptococcus pneumoniae.*
3. *H. influenzae, N. meningitidis,* and *Strep. pneumoniae* are respiratory tract–borne pathogens, *Listeria* species is most commonly food borne.

C. Clinical signs and symptoms.

1. Triad of nuchal rigidity (may be absent in <2 years of age), headache, and fever. Kernig's sign is pain caused by leg extension, and Brudzinski's sign is neck flexion causing flexion of hips and knees.
2. Nonspecific signs of irritability, lethargy, poor feeding, nausea, and vomiting are more commonly the presentation in younger children. Check for bulging fontanelle in the neonate.
3. Most common neurologic sign is altered mental status. Focal neurologic deficits are uncommon.
4. Generalized signs include erythematous (early) or petechial (later) rash and endotoxin-mediated hypotension in meningococcal sepsis.

D. Laboratory findings.

1. *Do not delay LP and CSF examination to do a CT scan unless focal neurologic signs or papilledema suggestive of increased*

intracranial pressure are present. If any of these is present, get a head CT first (but start antibiotics before CT). Send CSF for CBC, glucose, protein, culture, and Gram stain. Look for leukocytosis, high protein, and low glucose. See Table 10-7 for interpretation of CSF fluid analysis.

2. General sepsis work-up including CBC, UA, CXR (if indicated) should be done. Perform latex agglutination on serum and urine and send blood, CSF, and urine cultures. However, a negative latex agglutination does not rule out an infectious disease and should be used only to guide the choice of antibiotics.
3. Monitor electrolytes, oxygen saturation, serum glucose, C-reactive protein, serum osmolality, and INR/PTT.

E. Treatment.

1. Stabilize with proper airway management (if needed) and IV access. Evaluate and institute needed therapy for dehydration, hypotension, hypoxia, electrolyte abnormalities, SIADH, hypoglycemia, or DIC.

TABLE 10-7
Cerebrospinal Fluid

Component	Normal values
Cell count (WBCs/mm^3)	
Preterm mean	9.0 (0-25.4), 57% PMNs
Term mean	8.2 (0-22.4), 61% PMNs
>1 mo	0-7, 0% PMNs
Glucose (mg/dl)	
Preterm	24-63 (mean, 50)
Term	34-119 (mean, 52)
Child	40-80
CSF glucose/blood glucose (%)	
Preterm	55-105
Term	44-128
Child	50
Lactic acid dehydrogenase: mean, 20 units/ml (range, 5-30 units/ml)	
Myelin basic protein: <4 ng/ml	
Pressure: initial LP (mm H_2O)	
Newborn	80-110 (<110)
Infant/child	<200 (lateral recumbent position)
Respiratory movements	5-10
Protein (mg/dl)	
Preterm	65-150 (mean, 115)
Term	20-170 (mean, 90)
Children	5-15, ventricular 5-25, cisternal 5-40, lumbar

2. Give empiric IV antibiotics immediately according to most likely organism for age. Do not await culture results. *However, changing antibiotics to reflect sensitivities once available is prudent.*
3. Although the data are contradictory, dexamethasone 0.15 mg/kg Q6h for 4 days may improve outcome when given together with antibiotics especially in *H. influenzae* meningitis. To be effective, however, steroids should be started before or just after first dose of antibiotics.
   a. *<7 days.* Ampicillin 100 mg/kg/day divided Q12h plus gentamicin 5 mg/kg/day Q12h, or ampicillin plus ceftriaxone 100 mg/kg/day either as a single dose or divided Q12h.
   b. *>7 days.* Ampicillin 150 mg/kg/day divided Q8h plus gentamicin 7.5 mg/kg/day divided Q8h, or ampicillin plus cefotaxime 150 mg/kg/day divided Q8h or ceftriaxone 100 mg/kg/day either as a single dose or divided Q12h.
   c. *1 to 3 months.* Ampicillin 300 mg/kg/day divided Q6h plus cefotaxime 200 mg/kg/day divided Q6h, or ceftriaxone 100 mg/kg as a single dose or divided Q12h.
   d. *>3 months.* Cefotaxime 200 mg/kg/day divided Q6h, or ceftriaxone 100 mg/kg/day as a single dose or divided Q12h, or ampicillin 300 mg/kg/day divided Q6h plus chloramphenicol 100 mg/kg/day divided Q6h.
   e. *>6 years.* Ceftriaxone 100 mg/kg/day as a single dose or divided Q12h.
4. ***Duration of therapy.*** 14 to 21 days for group B streptococci or gram-negative bacteria; 10 days for others.
5. *An increasing number of* Streptococcus pneumoniae *isolates are resistant to penicillins and cephalosporins. Depending on the epidemiologic procedures in your institution, initial treatment of meningitis including vancomycin and rifampin may be indicated until sensitivities are available.*

F. Prophylaxis.

1. ***Neisseria meningitidis.*** Vaccine available for acute outbreak; consult local public health organization. Rifampin 20 mg/kg/day PO >1 month (not >600 mg) divided Q12h for 2 days is indicated for all intimate contacts, including household members of patient. Other options for adults include ciprofloxacin 500 mg PO or ceftriaxone 250 mg IM. For children less than 15 years of age ceftriaxone 125 mg IM can be used.
2. ***Haemophilus influenzae.*** Active immunization recommended, given as 3-dose vaccination at 2, 4, and 6 months with a booster at 15 months. When there are other children in the home, rifampin 20 mg/kg/day as single oral dose for 4 days is recommended for all household contacts including adults.

III. PARASITIC INFESTATION BY PINWORMS

A. Presentation. *Enterobius vermicularis* is a small 2 to 5 mm yellow-white worm that inhabits the lower GI tract and migrates out the anus at night causing pruritus, vulvitis, and restless sleep. May present as acute nocturnal vaginal pain in girls. Often whole families are affected.

B. Examination. Sometimes worms can be seen in the perianal area about an hour after the child goes to sleep. The definitive diagnostic test is to stick cellophane tape onto the perianal area in the morning before bathing. Then place the tape on a slide and examine under a microscope for the characteristic oval ova. Ask the patient to obtain specimens over 3 to 5 mornings and store them in the refrigerator before bringing them to the office.

C. Treatment. All members of the household should be treated simultaneously along with daily laundering of the affected child's underclothes and bedding.

1. *Mebendazole* (Vermox) 100 mg PO in 1 dose for adults and children >2 years. Repeat in 2 weeks.
2. *Pyrantel pamoate* (Antiminth) 11 mg/kg (up to 1 g PO in 1 dose. Repeat in 2 weeks.

D. Prevention. Good hand washing, keeping affected child's fingernails short, and tight-fitting pajamas to prevent perianal scratching.

IV. COMMON PEDIATRIC INFECTIOUS DISEASES

(Table 10-8)

VOMITING, DIARRHEA, AND DEHYDRATION

I. VOMITING

A. Overview. Forceful ejection of gastric contents as opposed to passive reflux. Most common cause is gastroenteritis. In infants consider gastroesophageal reflux, overfeeding, anatomic obstruction, and systemic infection. In children, consider systemic infection, toxic ingestion, appendicitis, Reye's syndrome, and pertussis. Consider elevated intracranial pressure as a cause of isolated vomiting.

B. Evaluation.

1. ***History.*** Assess pattern and severity as well as accompanying dehydration/malnutrition. If neonatal, consider congenital abnormalities such as duodenal or esophageal atresia, Hirschsprung's disease, volvulus, malformation. In infants, assess how much is being fed (overfeeding), relation to position (reflux), choking or coughing with feeding (achalasia, tracheosophageal fistula).
2. ***Reye's syndrome.*** Reye's syndrome generally occurs after viral illness and presents with intractable vomiting,

TABLE 10-8
Common Pediatric Infectious Diseases and Exanthems

Disease	Etiologic agent	Incubation	Prodrome	Signs and symptoms	Isolation	Treatment and comments
Chickenpox (varicella)	Varicella	10-21 days	Minimal	Mixture of macules, papules,vesicles in all stages of development; spreads from trunk to extremities for 5-20 days	Until all lesions are crusted Infectious 2 days before appearance	Symptomatic or acyclovir*
Fifth disease (erythema infectiosum)	Parvovirus B19	6-14 days	None	Maculopapular rash on face with circumoral pallor (slapped cheek) and spreading to extremities; rash lasts a few days to a few weeks and is brought out by warmth	Not needed but avoid in pregnant women	None
Herpangina	Coxsackievirus, herpesvirus	?	None	High fever, vomiting, ulcers of oral mucosa for 5-6 days	2-6 days	Symptomatic
Kawasaki disease (mucocutaneous aneurysms lymph node	Probable infectious agent not yet discovered	?	Unknown	Fever, adenopathy, inflamed mucosa (pharyngitis, cracked lips, etc.), polymorphous	?	May have cardiac involvement with artery Aspirin and IgG are used for

				Most common below 1 year		
Meningococcal meningitis	*Neisseria meningitidis*	1-7 days	URI, fever, headache, diarrhea	Meningitis; purpuric or petechial rash; septic arthritis	Until 24 hours after first antibiotic dose	See section on meningitis
Mononucleosis	Epstein-Barr virus, CMV, toxoplasmosis, primary HIV	2-8 weeks	None	Fatigue, anorexia, exudative tonsillitis, lymphadenopathy, splenomegaly Macular rash not unusual with amoxicillin use	Avoid saliva contact for 3 months	See section on mononucleosis in Chapter 19
Roseola infantum (exanthema subitum)	Human herpesvirus type 6 and type 7	1-15 days	3-4 days of sustained high fever; child generally looks well	Fine pink rash begins at fever defervescence and lasts 2 days; seen from 6 months to 3 years of age	Unknown	Fever control, may have aseptic meningitis
Rubella, German measles, 3-day measles	Rubivirus	14-21 days	Lymphadenopathy, fever, headache, malaise	Maculopapular discrete rash appears on face and rapidly spreads to trunk and proximal extremities, lasting 1-3 days; postauricular and suboccipital lymphadenopathy	Communicable from 7 days before until 5 days after rash appears	None

Continued

TABLE 10-8
Common Pediatric Infectious Diseases and Exanthems—cont'd

Disease	Etiologic agent	Incubation	Prodrome	Signs and symptoms	Isolation	Treatment and comments
Rubeola (measles)	Rubeola virus	10-12 days	High fever, cough, coryza, and conjunctivitis for 3 days	Koplik spots appear 1 or 2 days before maculopapular rash; rash is confluent and spreads from hairline to face and then body; lasts 4-5 days	From fifth day of incubation to fifth day after rash appears	Symptomatic care of cough, coryza, conjunctivitis
Whooping cough (pertussis)	*Bordetella pertussis*	5-10 days; 21 days maximum	1-3 weeks of cough, coryza, and occasional emesis	Short paroxysmal cough ending with inspiratory "whoop"	5-10 days with treatment	Erythromycin Culture nasopharynx

**Chickenpox:* Some authors would treat the second and subsequent children in a family who develop chickenpox with acyclovir. The second and subsequent cases in a family tend to be more severe than the first case because of a higher initial viral load. Acyclovir reduces duration of illness by 24 to 48 hours and must be started within the first 24 hours of the illness to be effective. Adults and adolescents with chickenpox may be better candidates for acyclovir, since they tend to have more consequences.

Adapted from Driscoll CE et al: *The family practice desk reference,* ed 3, St. Louis, 1996, Mosby.

elevated liver enzymes (but normal bilirubin), decreased mental status (encephalopathy), prolonged PT/INR, and elevated serum ammonia and hypoglycemia. Treatment includes glucose (at least 0.4 mg/kg/hour) to maintain normal serum glucose, fluid and electrolytes at one half maintenance (correct shock first), neomycin 100 mg/kg/day PO Q6h, vitamin K 5 to 10 mg IV for coagulopathy or FFP for acute bleeding, and management of elevated intracranial pressure. Some would add lactulose to this regimen.

3. ***Pyloric stenosis.*** Occurs at <2 months of age and presents with intractable vomiting after feeds. Most common in first-born males, may have severe electrolyte disturbance depending on duration. Diagnosis is by ultrasonography (best modality) or "string sign" on upper GI film (barium passing through a narrowed pylorus). Treatment is surgical though recent studies indicate that nitric oxide may be helpful.

C. Exam and lab tests. Evaluate state of hydration (see section on dehydration, p. 466). Look for site of infection. Abdominal and rectal exam for obstruction or imperforate anus. Radiologic studies as indicated. If child less than 2 months, consider ultrasonography for pyloric stenosis.

D. Treatment. See dehydration and oral rehydration sections, pp. 466 and 467. Also consider antiemetics such as promethazine, prochlorperazine (Compazine and others), trimethobenzamide (see Chapter 20 for dosing).

II. DIARRHEA

A. Overview. There are numerous causes of acute and chronic diarrhea. Infectious causes include viruses (rotavirus most common), bacteria *(Salmonella, Shigella, Campylobacter* most common), parasites *(Giardia* and *Cryptosporidium* most common), localized infection elsewhere, antibiotic-associated (antibiotic side effect as well as *Clostridium difficile),* and food poisoning. Noninfectious causes include overfeeding (particularly of fruit juices), irritable bowel syndrome, celiac disease, milk protein intolerance, lactose intolerance after infectious diarrhea, cystic fibrosis, and inflammatory bowel.

B. Evaluation.

1. ***History.*** Acute versus chronic. Volume, frequency, character of stools, presence of blood or mucus. Associated symptoms (vomiting, fever, malaise, etc.). Epidemiologic data (travel, day care, family history).
2. ***Exam.*** Estimate dehydration (see section on dehydration, p. 466). Examine for other infectious process or source. Determine if nutritional status is compromised. Neurologic symptoms, mental status changes or seizures, suggest *Shigella* or *Rotavirus.*

3. ***Lab tests.*** Culture may be indicated for acute bloody diarrhea. Fecal leukocytes and RBCs not sensitive or specific enough to be useful except to suggest need for further work-up. O&P for prolonged diarrhea or as indicated. Studies for chronic disease as appropriate. An ELISA test is available for *Rotavirus* (Rotazyme). See Chapter 4 for further information about diarrhea.

C. Treatment.

1. Acute diarrhea with dehydration in the absence of vomiting is treated with large amounts of osmotically bal-anced clear liquids such as Pedialyte, Ricelyte, or the WHO rehydration formula until rehydration is complete. See dehydration and oral rehydration section below for details.
2. There is abundant evidence that early reinstitution of a lactose-free general diet will decrease the duration and severity of diarrhea. Therefore the foods provided should be the same as those in the child's normal diet with the exclusion of high-sugar foods such as apple juice, which may cause an osmotic diarrhea, and milk products with lactose. Breast-fed infants should continue to nurse without restrictions. Lactose-free soybean formulas may be used in those who are bottle fed.
3. Avoid the use of antiperistaltic agents in infants and children.
4. Most episodes of diarrhea do not benefit from antimicrobial therapy. Bacterial diarrhea should be treated appropriately after culture results are available. Caution should be used in the treatment of diarrhea caused by *Salmonella* species because this may prolong the carrier state. However, antibiotics should be used for *Salmonella* in infants <3 months old, patients with symptoms of toxicity, patients with metastatic foci, or with *Salmonella typhi.* See Chapter 4 for further details.
5. Diarrhea with vomiting is treated as for vomiting until patient is able to tolerate oral feedings.

III. DEHYDRATION

A. Clinical Assessment.

1. ***Clinical observation.*** See Table 10-9. Clinical signs and symptoms are neither sensitive nor specific.
2. ***In hypotonic dehydration*** (Na^+ <130 mEq/L) all manifestations appear with less fluid deficit, whereas in hypertonic dehydration (Na^+ >150 mEq/L) the circulating volume is relatively preserved, and so circulatory disturbances are seen later.

B. Calculation of electrolyte deficits. See section V.

IV. ORAL REHYDRATION

There is no role for weak tea, flat soda, Jell-O (gelatin), water, etc.

TABLE 10-9
Clinical Signs Associated with Various Degrees of Dehydration

Dehydration (%)	Clinical observation
5-6	Heart rate (10% to 15% above baseline value) Slightly dry mucous membranes Concentration of the urine Poor tear production*
7-8	Increased severity of above Decreased skin turgor Oliguria Sunken eyeballs* Sunken anterior fontanelle*
>9	Pronounced severity of above signs Decreased blood pressure Delayed capillary refill (>2 seconds) Acidosis (large base deficit)

*These signs may be less sensitive indicators of dehydration than the others are.

TABLE 10-10
Intracellular and Extracellular Fluid Composition

Ion	Intracellular (mEq/L)	Extracellular (mEq/L)
Na^+	20	145
K^+	150	3-5
Cl^-	—	110
HCO_3^-	10	20-25
PO_4^-	110-115	5
Protein	75	10

Dehydration for <3 days: 80% extracellular fluid and 20% intracellular fluid losses. Dehydration for >3 days: 60% ECF and 40% ICF losses.

A. Concept of "gut rest," that is, stopping oral intake for several hours before refeeding, has been found to have several negative effects, such as increased intestinal permeability and worsening of starvation and dehydration. Studies have shown that stool production is actually less with rapid refeeding.

B. Oral rehydration is appropriate in most cases of mild to moderate dehydration.

C. Currently only two fluids meet the recommendations of the World Health Organization (WHO) and the American Academy of Pediatrics for the rehydration phase of the treatment of diarrhea–Rehydralyte. (Ross) and the WHO-ORS product (oral rehydration solution). These are the only two products that contain the 75 to 90 mEq/L of sodium recommended for rehydration. A simple alternative for making a rehydration solution is to mix half a teaspoon of table salt and 8 teaspoons of sugar in 1 liter of water. However, this solution neither replaces potassium nor contains bicarbonate to hasten the resolution of acidosis. One also needs to be sure that the parent is able to mix the solution properly. One can make a more complicated but more complete solution by adding 8 teaspoons of table sugar, half a teaspoon of salt, half a teaspoon of sodium bicarbonate (baking soda), and a third of a teaspoon of potassium chloride to 1 liter of water.

D. Oral rehydration should be accomplished over 4 hours. The dose for mild dehydration is 50 ml/kg, or 100 ml/kg for moderate dehydration. If vomiting is occurring, the child may be given frequent small doses of the rehydration fluid and then subsequent maintenance fluids by using a teaspoon or a small oral syringe to provide a rate of approximately 5 ml/min.

E. For replacement of ongoing losses, it is recommended that a fluid with a lower sodium content than the rehydration fluid be used. Pedialyte (Ross) or Ricelyte (Mead Johnson) are examples of appropriate maintenance fluids. *Other solutions such as weak tea, dilute or full-strength soft drinks, Jell-O (gelatin), water, tap water, apple juice, etc. are contraindicated and may lead to hyponatremia.* Alternatively, the rehydration fluid may be given along with other low-sodium fluids, such as water, breast milk, or formula. Replacement of ongoing losses is advised at a rate of 10 ml/kg or ½ to 1 cup of ORS for each diarrheal stool.

V. INTRAVENOUS REHYDRATION

A. Formulas for calculating electrolyte deficits.

1. Sodium deficit (mEq total) = (125 [or Desired serum sodium] − Current serum sodium) × 0.6 × Weight (kg).
2. Potassium deficit (mEq total) = (Desired serum K [mEq/liter] − Measured serum K) × 0.25 × Weight (kg).
3. Chloride deficit (mEq total) = (Desired serum chloride [mEq/liter] − Measured serum Cl) × 0.45 × Weight (kg).

B. Correction of free water deficit in hypernatremic dehydration. Free water deficit = 4 ml/kg for every mEq that the serum Na exceeds 145 mEq/L.

C. Maintenance requirements for fluids and electrolytes.

1. ***Fluid maintenance.***

   Weight <10 kg: 100 ml/kg/day

   Weight 11 to 20 kg: 1000 ml + 50 ml/kg/day for every kg over 10 kg

   Weight >20 kg: 1500 ml + 20 ml/kg/day for every kg over 20 kg

Adult: 2000 to 2400 ml/day

2. ***Total body water.*** 60% of body weight.
3. ***Maintenance electrolyte requirements.***
   Na^+: 3 mEq/kg/day, or 3 mEq/100 ml of H_2O
   K^+: 2 mEq/kg/day or 2 mEq/100 ml of H_2O (adult: 50 mEq/day)
   Cl^-: 3 mEq/100 ml of H_2O
   Glucose: 5 g/100 ml of H_2O

D. Replacement of ongoing losses.

1. See Table 10-11 for composition of various body fluids.
2. NG losses usually replaced with D_5 ½NS with 20 mEq/L of KCl.
3. Diarrhea usually replaced with D_5 ¼NS with 40 mEq/L of KCl.

E. General principles in treating dehydration.

1. Weigh the child.
2. Be sure to add ongoing losses to maintenance + deficit fluids and electrolytes.
3. If moderately or severely dehydrated, give an initial fluid bolus of 20 ml/kg LR or NS over 20 minutes. Repeat bolus if response is inadequate. If poor response after three fluid boluses, that is, poor perfusion, no urine output, abnormal vital signs, may need CVP or PCWP to guide fluid resuscitation.
4. In hypotonic or isotonic dehydration, calculate the total fluids and electrolytes (maintenance + deficit replacement) for the first 24 hours, give half over the first 8 hours and the other half over the next 16 hours. In hypertonic dehydration, correct the fluid and electrolyte deficits slowly over about 48 hours.
5. Do not add potassium to IV line until urine output established. Diabetic ketoacidosis may be an exception, where correction of hyperglycemia and acidosis may lead to rapid development of hypokalemia.

TABLE 10-11
Electrolyte Composition of Various Body Fluids

Fluid	Na (mEq/L)	K (mEq/L)	Cl (mEq/L)	Protein (g/dl)
Gastric	20-80	5-20	100-150	—
Pancreatic	120-140	5-15	40-80	—
Small bowel	100-140	5-15	90-130	—
Bile	120-140	5-15	80-120	—
Ileostomy	45-135	3-15	20-115	—
Diarrhea	10-90	10-80	10-110	—
Burns	140	5	110	3-5

6. Increase maintenance fluids by 12% for each Celsius degree of fever (Table 10-12).

F. Hypotonic dehydration (Na <125 mEq/L).

1. Symptomatic earlier than in isotonic or hyertonic dehydration. Therefore use weight loss of 3% = mild, 6% = moderate, and 9% = severe dehydration as a guide.
2. Hypotonic dehydration usually results from replacing losses (vomiting and diarrhea) with low-solute fluids, such as dilute juice, cola, weak tea.
3. Lethargy and irritability are common, and vascular collapse can occur early.
4. ***Therapy.*** Calculate total fluid and electrolyte needs according to the maintenance and deficit replacement formulas in sections B to D above. Do not try to raise serum Na in more than 10 mEq/L increments (that is, if the current serum sodium is 125, use 135 as the desired serum Na level in the calculation). To calculate the milliequivalents of Na needed in each liter during the first 24 hours of therapy: mEq of Na per liter of IV fluid = total sodium needed in the first 24 hours divided by total volume of fluid needed. (Normal saline = 154 mEq of Na/liter). Usually D_5 ½NS or D_5 NS is used. Potassium can be added after urine

TABLE 10-12
Temperature Conversion Scale

Fahrenheit	Celsius	Fahrenheit	Celsius
104	40	100.2	37.9
103.8	39.9	100	37.8
103.6	39.8	99.9	37.7
103.5	39.7	99.7	37.6
103.3	39.6	99.5	37.5
103.1	39.5	99.3	37.4
102.8	39.4	99.1	37.3
102.7	39.3	99	37.2
102.6	39.2	98.8	37.1
102.4	39.1	98.6	37
102.2	39	98.4	36.9
102	38.9	98.2	36.8
101.8	38.8	98	36.7
101.6	38.7	97.9	36.6
101.5	38.6	97.7	36.5
101.3	38.5	97.5	36.4
101.1	38.4	97.3	36.3
100.9	38.3	97.2	36.2
100.8	38.2	97	36.1
100.6	38.1	96.8	36
100.4	38		

output is established. Give half of the calculated total fluid and electrolyte requirements for the first 24 hours over the first 8 hours and the other half over the next 16 hours.

G. Severe, symptomatic hyponatremia. (See Chapter 5.)

H. Isotonic dehydration (Na = 130 to 150 mEq/L).

1. Symptoms are less dramatic than in hypotonic dehydration.
2. Use estimate (loss of weight) 5% = mild, 10% = moderate, 15% = severe dehydration.
3. Calculate total maintenance + deficit replacement fluids and electrolytes for first 24 hours.
4. Treatment is similar to treatment for hypotonic dehydration: give half of first 24 hours needs in first 8 hours, and give the remaining half over the next 16 hours.
5. Usually can use D_5 ¼NS or D_5 ½NS; may add potassium after urine output established.
6. Remember to estimate and replace ongoing losses.

I. Hypertonic dehydration.

1. Usually occurs as a result of using inappropriately high solute load as replacement, renal concentrating defect with large free-water losses, heat exposure with large insensible losses, etc.
2. Typical symptoms include thick, doughy texture to skin (tenting is uncommon), shrill cry, weakness, tachypnea, intense thirst.
3. Shock is a very late manifestation. If severe dehydration or shock is present, the patient may need an initial fluid bolus of 20 ml/kg NS over the first 20 to 30 minutes.
4. Free-water deficit (ml) is estimated to be 4 ml/kg × (Actual serum Na (mEq/L) − 145 mEq/L).
5. Replace the free-water deficit *slowly* over 48 hours. Aim to decrease the serum sodium by about 10 mEq/L/day. Reducing serum sodium more rapidly can have severe repercussions, such as cerebral and pulmonary edema.
6. Usual replacement fluid is D_5 ¼NS or D_5 ½NS.
7. If Na >180, may need dialysis.

CONSTIPATION AND ENCOPRESIS

I. OVERVIEW

Infrequent passage of dry, hard stools. Causes can be organic (Hirschsprung's disease, anal stenosis, anal stricture, drugs, dehydration, neuromuscular disease) or functional (voluntary withholding). Beyond the neonatal period 90% to 95% of constipation is functional.

II. CAUSES

A. *In newborn* must rule out anatomic and cogenital causes such as rectal or colonic atresia, myelomeningocele, absent abdominal muscles, cystic fibrosis, Hirschsprung's disease.

B. *In older* children, functional or dietary.

1. ***Dietary.*** Lack of dietary bulk, excessive intake of cow's milk, early introduction of cow's milk.
2. ***Stool retention.*** Painful defecation caused by fissure, rectal abscess, etc., or conflicts in toilet training. Voluntary withholding results in decreased rectal sensation and rectal distension and subsequent loss of defecation urge. Stooling around impaction with soiling is known as "encopresis" if noted after normal toilet training age of 4 to 5 years.
3. ***Other causes of constipation.*** Narcotics, antidepressants and other anticholinergics, overuse of laxatives, hypothyroidism, hypokalemia.

III. EVALUATION

A. History. Age of onset. Parent expectation of stool pattern. Stool consistency, size, frequency, soiling, abdominal pain, anorexia, tenesmus. Infants should pass meconium in first 24 hours.

B. Exam. Palpable abdominal mass. Rectal exam reveals hard stool present with dilated ampulla. Anal fissure may be present.

C. Lab tests.

Abdominal flat plate will show stool filling the colon. Barium enema to demonstrate atresia. Rectal biopsy for Hirschsprung's. Thyroid functions and electrolytes and calcium as indicated.

IV. TREATMENT

A. *Simple constipation in infants* treated with lactulose 2.5 to 10 ml/24 hours, divided TID or QID. Add fruit and fruit juices to diet if older than 4 months. Avoid karo syrup and honey because of possible infant botulism. A glycerin suppository may stimulate the passage of a stool. Changing to Carnation Good Start formula may be helpful with constipation.

B. *In older children,* clear impaction using pediatric enema or cathartic (such as bisacodyl suppositories). Polyethylene glycol (Golitely) may also be used. Give 40 ml/kg over 6 hours. Increase dietary fiber (prunes, figs, raisins, beans, bran, fresh fruits, and vegetables) or use a psyllium supplement. Limit milk if excessive by history. Avoid hypotonic and phosphate enemas, which can cause electrolyte abnormalities and seizures.

C. *Encopresis* (soiling with impaction).

1. Usually starts as a functional voluntary withholding but progresses to decreased urge to defecate because of rectal enlargement and loss of sensation of full rectum.
2. Counseling of patient and parents on cause of soiling. Outline plan to help patient resolve problem.
3. Clear rectum of impaction before starting treatment.
4. Start milk of magnesia (<1 year = 5 ml; >1 year = 7.5 to 30 ml), or mineral oil 5 to 30 ml, and increase until having soft stools. Mineral oil should not be used in those <5

years of age. Continue treatment for 2 to 6 months while rectal size and sensation return to normal.

5. When decreasing dose of laxative start toilet-sitting regimen, that is, sitting for 15 minutes after each meal. Consider reward system appropriate to age.
6. Implement dietary changes as above.

GI BLEEDING IN CHILDHOOD

I. SURGICAL CAUSES

A. If less than 1 year of age, think of:
Anal fissure (43%), intussusception (39%), duodenal-gastric ulcer (15%), gangrenous bowel (9%), Meckel's diverticulum (3.8%).

B. If more than 1 year, think of:
Polyps (50%), ulcers (14%), anal fissure (12.5%), esophageal varices (10.5%), intussusception (9%), hemorrhoids (0.8%).

II. MEDICAL CAUSES

A. Hematologic abnormalities. Hemophilia, iron deficiency, thrombocytopenia, vitamin K deficiency.

B. Systemic causes. Milk allergy, infectious diarrhea, Henoch-Schönlein purpura, scurvy, uremia, etc.

C. Drugs. NSAIDs, iron poisoning.

D. Swallowed blood. From nose bleed, maternal blood from breast feeding, etc.

E. To differentiate swallowed maternal blood (from breast feeding, etc.) from neonatal blood. Take vomitus, stool, etc., and mix with 5 to 10 parts of water. Centrifuge to remove debris and decant the pink supernatant (if not pink, won't work). Mix 1 ml of 0.25N (1%) sodium hydroxide with 5 ml of supernatant. Read color change in 2 minutes. If remains pink, blood is of fetal origin. If turns brown-yellow, blood is of adult origin. It is helpful to run a control of the infant's blood.

STRIDOR AND DYSPNEA (Table 10-13)

I. EPIGLOTTITIS

A. Definition. Infection of the epiglottis and of the aryepiglottic folds and surrounding soft tissues. Becoming less common since use of *H. influenzae* vaccine.

B. Cause. Almost always by *H. influenzae* type B. Other causes: beta-hemolytic streptococci, *Staphylococcus aureus,* and *Streptococcus pneumoniae.*

C. Clinical presentation. May occur at any age, with a peak incidence at 2 to 7 years. Presents with sudden onset of high fever, respiratory distress, severe dysphagia, drooling, muffled voice, and a toxic appearance. Stridor, if present, may be mild

TABLE 10-13
Differential Diagnosis of Stridor and Dyspnea

	Viral laryngotracheitis	Bacterial tracheitis	Retropharyngeal abscess	Epiglottitis
Cause	Parainfluenza Influenza RSV	Viral prodrome + Staphylococci Streptococci *Haemophilus influenzae* Enteric pathogens	Beta-hemolytic streptococci anaerobes	*H. influenzae* Staphylococci Streptococci
Age	3 months to 3 years	3 months to 3 years	6 months to 3 years	2 to 7 years
Clinical characteristics	Low-grade fever Coryza Barking cough Hoarse voice Winter/spring peak	Improving croup then sudden increase: temperature, work of breathing, stridor *No drooling* Fall/winter peak	Initial URI Dysphagia, refusal to feed Drooling, toxic appearance, stridor	Sudden onset of high fever, dysphagia, stridor, drooling. *No cough*
Radiograph	Unnecessary (steeple sign unreliable)	Detached pseudomembrane may give soft-tissue shadow	Radiograph shows retropharyngeal soft-tissue density and air-fluid level	Unnecessary (thumb sign)
Treatment	Cool mist, epinephrine, steroids	Intubation, antibiotics	Surgical drainage, antibiotics	Intubation, antibiotics

in comparison to croup. Often there is little or no coughing. Child typically prefers being upright in "sniffing" position.

D. Lab tests. Invasive procedures and examinations should be avoided until after airway is secured. CBC and blood and epiglottic cultures may then be obtained. Radiographs of lateral area of neck shows characteristic swollen epiglottis (thumb sign). **Never send a child suspected of having epiglottitis to be radiographed unaccompanied by someone who can emergently manage airway.**

E. Treatment.

1. **Do not move, upset, or lay child down unless prepared to manage obstructed airway.**
2. ***Airway.*** *In an emergency, a bag, valve, or mask can buy time. Consider a needle cricothyrotomy.* Controlled intubation by an experienced operator is preferred. Tracheostomy is acceptable if unable to intubate. Usually safely extubated in 48 to 72 hours after appropriate antibiotics are started. *Airway must be secure.*
3. ***Antibiotics.*** Initiated once artificial airway secure. Cefotaxime 50 to 200 mg/kg/24 hours divided Q6h or ceftriaxone 75 mg/kg Q24h are the first-line drugs with TMP/SMX as a second-line agent.
4. ***Admission to ICU.*** Use proper sedation and restraints during period of intubation. Antibiotics should be continued for 7 to 10 days after extubation.

II. CROUP (LARYNGOTRACHEOBRONCHITIS)

A. Definition. A syndrome of airway swelling in the glottic and subglottic area of viral origin.

B. Causes. Parainfluenza virus types 1 and 3 responsible for majority of cases; remainder respiratory syncytial virus, influenza virus, and adenovirus.

C. Clinical presentation. Age usually 6 months to 6 years. Common cold symptoms usually precede onset. Brassy cough (seal bark), hoarseness, and inspiratory stridor are characteristic. If severe may include retractions, decreased air entry, and cyanosis. Usually benign course but can progress to obstruction.

D. May be resolved by presentation to office or ED from exposure to cool air.

E. Must differentiate from epiglottitis and bacterial tracheitis, which require emergent management. See Table 10-13.

F. Classification.

1. ***Very mild.*** Intermittent stridor, present when awake or excited, goes away when sleeping.
2. ***Mild.*** Continuous stridor when awake or asleep not audible without stethoscope.
3. ***Moderate.*** Continuous stridor audible without stethoscope and may be accompanied be sternal retractions.

4. ***Severe.*** Continuous stridor with evidence of respiratory failure, that is, cyanosis, altered mental status.

G. Lab tests. Usually not indicated and may induce further agitation with respiratory compromise. If in doubt and no need for emergent airway management, AP radiograph of neck may show subglottic narrowing (steeple sign).

H. Management.

1. Calm the child on the parent's lap and provide cool, humidified air.
2. Oxygen if saturation <95%.
3. Reassess status after 15 to 30 minutes.
4. If mild classification, consider discharge with instructions for cool mist humidifier.
5. ***If moderate classification.***
   a. The traditional treatment has been nebulized racemic epinephrine, 2.25% solution, 0.5 ml diluted in 3 ml of saline.
   b. *Recently, nebulized epinephrine,* of 5 ml of 1:1000, has been shown to be as safe as, at least as good as, and perhaps superior to racemic epinephrine. May repeat PRN.
   c. There is no "rebound effect" from epinephrine, but patients may return to their pretreatment state.
   d. *Steroids.* Generally those who need nebulized epinephrine should also be treated with dexamethasone 0.6 mg/kg/dose IM or PO up to 10 mg. Although not standard of care, nebulized budesonide 1 mg given twice at 30-minute intervals is effective in mild to moderate croup and may prevent the need for systemic steroids. However, up to now, it has not been compared to dexamethasone in any trial.
   e. Continuation of cool, humidified air may also be helpful.
   f. *Disposition.* Although not yet universally accepted, the literature indicates that patients may be discharged with instructions for cool mist humidifier if, after 3 to 6 hours of observation, they require no further treatment with epinephrine and their croup is mild. If patient remains in the moderate classification, hospitalization with epinephrine or racemic epinephrine PRN and dexamethasone 0.25 to 0.5 mg/kg/dose Q6h.
   g. If in severe classification, the decision to intubate should be left to experienced personnel and, when feasible, be performed in the operating room. Management is as above while awaiting trained personnel for sedation and intubation.

III. FOREIGN-BODY ASPIRATION

A. Clinical presentation. Majority 3 months to 6 years. Have triphasic history:

1. Initial cough, choking, gagging, stridor, wheeze.

2. FB then passes into smaller airways and have silent phase.
3. Then have recurrent pneumonia, wheezing, abscess, bronchiectasis.
4. A third not witnessed or not remembered by caregiver.

B. Radiographs. Can show air trapping on exhalation but one fourth have normal radiograph. Radiography is only 50% specific. Do CXR with patient lying on affected side. Dependent lung will not deflate normally.

C. Bronchoscopy. Diagnostic procedure of choice if there is any question.

D. Treatment.

1. ***Without respiratory distress.*** Refer for removal by bronchoscopy.
2. ***Respiratory distress present.***
   a. If the patient is breathing, do not interfere; allow the child's efforts to attempt to clear the foreign body.
   b. If not moving air, American Heart Association obstructed airway maneuvers should be employed. For infants, 4 interscapular back blows with the child's head lower than the chest, alternating with 4 chest compressions. In older children, Heimlich maneuver. ACLS protocol should be initiated if necessary.
   c. Bag-valve-mask ventilations can convert a total obstruction to a partial one by pushing foreign body into a main bronchus.
   d. Immediate direct laryngoscopy and removal with Magill forceps should be performed.
   e. If unsuccessful, cricothyrotomy or intubation if needed.

E. Prevention. Infants and young children should not eat nuts, popcorn, hot dogs, uncooked carrots, whole grapes, or hard candies. *Balloons are especially dangerous for young children.* Dice food. Avoid small toys. Educate parents.

IV. BRONCHIOLITIS

A. Epidemiology. Illness of young children and infants. Most serious in first 2 years of life. Respiratory syncytial virus (RSV) principal agent. Also associated with parainfluenza, adenovirus, influenzavirus, rhinovirus. Majority occur during winter but can occur any season.

B. Clinical presentation. Rhinorrhea, sneezing, coughing, low-grade fever. Onset of rapid breathing and wheezing. Signs of respiratory distress in severe cases: nasal flaring, tachypnea, prolonged expiratory phase, retractions.

C. Lab tests. CBC usually within normal limits. Blood gas, O_2 saturation levels, as appropriate. Nasal wash for RSV culture and antigen assay. CXR can be normal but occasionally shows air trapping and peribronchial thickening.

D. Treatment.

1. ***Indications for hospitalization.*** Use clinical judgment. Some suggested criteria include <6 months old, resting

respirations >50 to 60, Po_2, <60 mm Hg, pulse oximetry <93% to 95%, apnea, unable to tolerate oral feedings.

2. ***Supportive measures.*** Antipyretics, IV fluids, humidified O_2, nebulized bronchodilators, such as albuterol 2.5 mg in 3 ml of NS; this can be repeated PRN. Oral albuterol can be used (0.1 mg/kg Q8h up to 12 mg) but is much less effective. *Epinephrine, 5 ml of 1:1000 by nebulizer is safe and effective and is an alternative.* Only one study up to now demonstrates the efficacy of steroids for this condition (inhaled budesonide 500 µg BID for 8 weeks followed by 250 mg BID for 8 weeks). However, they continue to be widely used in doses similar to those for asthma.
3. ***Ribavirin aerosol.*** If croup or bronchiolitis secondary to RSV, consider use of ribavirin in:
   a. High-risk groups.
      - Congenital heart disease
      - Chronic lung disease (such as bronchopulmonary dysplasia)
      - Infants <6 weeks of age
      - Neurologic disorders
      - Immunosuppressed

   b. Severely ill infants.
      - Pao_2 <65 mm Hg or Sao_2 <90%
      - Increasing Pco_2

   c. The efficacy of ribavirin has recently been called into question. The use of ribavirin even in severely ill patients is at the discretion of the physician.
4. Intubation and mechanical ventilation as indicated.
5. Respiratory syncytial virus immunoglobulin (RSV-IGIV) 750 mg/kg IV Q30 days can prevent RSV infection and hospitalization in those children with severe underlying illness such as bronchopulmonary dysplasia or prematurity.

LIMP AND JOINT PAIN

I. JOINT PAIN

1. Will have pain on weight bearing or refusal to bear weight. Pain on passive motion of joints involved with arthritis.
2. Determine if true arthritis by exam, presence of fever, number of joints involved.

II. LIMP

1. Pain from hip often felt as knee pain in children.
2. Examine shoes and feet (look for tiny pebble in shoe bottom, etc.).
3. General approach to the child with a limp.
   A conservative approach indicated, since very few children without systemic symptoms or true arthritis have any significant disorder. If pain persists or you suspect an acute arthritis, diagnostic evaluations can include a CBC, with

differential ESR, anti–streptolysin O titer, rheumatoid factor, throat and urine cultures, ultrasonography for joint effusion, and radiographic studies of the hips. A joint tap should be done when there is clinical suspicion of a septic joint and an effusion by U/S.

III. DIFFERENTIAL DIAGNOSIS AND APPROACH

A. Transient tenosynovitis (irritable hip).

1. Most common cause of limp (well over 90% in some series).
2. Frequently follows URI or streptococcal infection.
3. May have joint effusion but not true arthritis.
4. Generally resolves within 24 to 48 hours with rest and ibuprofen-acetaminophen.

B. Septic hip joint. A true emergency (see also Chapter 6).

1. Generally febrile with elevated ESR, WBC >18,000/mm^3, but lab values may be normal and may overlap with those of other illnesses.
2. Will generally look sick and hold hip in flexion and external rotation.
3. Effusion present on ultrasonography but may also have effusion with transient tenosynovitis (71%). Tap is diagnostic.
4. Relatively sudden onset and rapid course.
5. Treat with antistaphylococcal antibiotics. Requires orthopedic consultation and surgical intervention.

C. Legg-Calvé-Perthes disease (aseptic necrosis of the femoral capital head).

1. Most common between 5 and 10 years of age.
2. Slow insidious onset of limp and hip pain, which is progressive. Have limitation of motion of the hip.
3. Diagnosis by radiography of affected hip (see lucency of femoral head and eventually sclerosis and destruction of femoral head). Bone scan may reveal abnormalities earlier than radiograph would show.
4. Treatment requires consultation with orthopedics staff and includes rest, anti-inflammatories, and casting for more severe cases.

D. Slipped femoral epiphysis.

1. Generally seen in overweight teenagers, especially boys.
2. May have insidious onset of pain but can also follow acute trauma.
3. May be pain with passive motion.
4. Diagnosis by frog-legged radiographs of both hips.
5. Treatment is by orthopedic referral and surgical fixation.

E. Osgood-Schlatter disease.

1. Characterized by pain over the tibial tubercle, which is usually unilateral.
2. Usually occurs in active children between 10 and 15 years of age.
3. Treatment is rest and NSAIDs.

F. Diskitis.

1. An inflammatory process of the disk or disks (usually L3 to L5), which may be infectious in cause (staphylococcal primarily).
2. Presents with refusal to walk or limp, low-grade fever, and "tripod posturing"–leaning back with back extended onto outstretched arms when sitting.
3. Generally have pain over involved disk area but may also have pain on straight-leg raising, hip motion.
4. Sedimentation rate almost always elevated, but CBC may be normal. Disk space may be narrowed on radiograph. Bone scan will show inflammatory focus.
5. Treatment is generally supportive with anti-inflammatories but may need antibiotics. Orthopedic consultation recommended.

G. Juvenile rheumatoid arthritis.

1. Defined as presentation of rheumatoid arthritis before 16 years of age.
2. See Chapter 6 for course.
3. 20% have "Still's disease," which is JRA plus fever, thrombocytopenia, splenomegaly, generalized adenopathy.
4. 40% have onset in one or a few joints.
5. 40% have polyarticular onset similar to adult onset.
6. 75% have complete remissions.
7. See Chapter 6 for work-up.

H. Rheumatic fever. (See Chapter 2 for details.) Must meet one or two major Jones's criteria (arthritis, chorea, carditis, subcutaneous nodules, erythema marginatum) and have evidence of recent group A streptococcal infection and minor manifestations such as fever, elevated ESR, elevated WBC count.

I. Sickle cell crisis in appropriate populations.

J. Other arthritides including manifestation of ulcerative colitis, Crohn's disease, etc. Diagnosis by looking for and, finding symptom complex.

NOCTURNAL ENURESIS

I. DEFINITION

Involuntary loss of urine during sleep. Nocturnal enuresis is a disorder of delayed maturation and generally cannot be officially diagnosed until the child is at least 5 years old.

A. Primary enuresis. Wetting that proceeds more or less continuously for at least 1 year without prior dry spells.

B. Secondary enuresis. The child has been dry at least for 1 year before wetting the bed.

II. EPIDEMIOLOGY

Most often primary, affects 10% to 20% of children 5 to 6 years of age. Tends to be familial; affects the child's self-esteem. Only

1% to 4% are attributable to uropathies. *Etiology theories:* "Organic" (deficiency in the nocturnal production of ADH, obstructive sleep apnea, need to rule out other organic causes), "psychologic," "sleep stage," and "failure to learn control." The definite cause is yet undetermined.

III. EVALUATION

History: developmental milestones (assess delay in neurologic development), voiding history, toilet training, social history, child rearing, family milestones. Obtain history of UTI, medical and surgical problems, medications, diet. Gait, posture, spine exam may be important in diagnosing neurologic abnormalities. Abdominal mass, bladder size, UA, and culture to look for urinary tract infection, obstruction with overflow. If child is diurnal and nocturnal wetter, a renal and bladder ultrasonogram should be done. If there is history of UTI should do VCUG.

IV. MANAGEMENT

Motivate the child to establish control!

- **A. Pharmacotherapy.** DDAVP 1 or 2 sniffs QHS. Oxybutynin 1 to 5 mg QHS (used in daytime also for day wetting); imipramine less effective (25 to 50 mg QHS 6 to 12 years, 50 to 75 mg QHS >12 years).
- **B. Behavioral** (most successful). Self-monitoring, motivation and responsibility training, charting of success and failure nights, bladder training, enuresis alarms, nocturnal awakenings, avoid diapers.
- **C. Diet.** Avoid caffeine, liquids before bedtime. May use DDAVP on sleep-overs, travel.

BIBLIOGRAPHY

Adcock PM et al: Effect of urine latex agglutination tests on the treatment of children at risk for invasive bacterial infection, *Pediatrics* 96(5):951, 1995.

Allen UD: Cow's milk versus soy-based formula in mild and moderate diarrhea: a randomized, controlled trial, *Acta Paediatr* 83(2):183, 1994.

American Academy of Pediatrics, Council on Nutrition: Fluoride supplementation, *Pediatrics* 77:758-761, 1986.

American Dental Association, Council on Dental Therapeutics: *Dental therapeutics,* ed 40, Chicago, 1984, the Association.

Avery ME et al: Oral therapy for acute diarrhea: the underused simple solution, *N Engl J Med* 323(13):891, 1990.

Baker MD et al: Failure of infant observation scales in detecting serious illness in febrile, 4- to 8-week-old infants, *Pediatrics* 85(6)1040, 1990.

Balfour HH et al: Acyclovir treatment of varicella in otherwise healthy adolescents, *J Pediatr* 120(4 Part 1):627, 1992.

Baraff LJ et al: Probability of bacterial infections in febrile infants less than three months of age: a meta-analysis, *Pediatr Infect Dis* 11(4):257-264, 1992.

Baraff LJ et al: Practice guideline for the management of infants and children 0 to 36 months of age with fever without source, *Ann Emerg Med* 22(7):1198, 1993.

Baskin MN et al: Outpatient treatment of febrile infants 28 to 89 days of age with intramuscular administration of ceftriaxone, *J Pediatr* 120(1):22, 1992.

Bawden JW et al: Changing patterns of fluoride intake. Proceedings of the workshop, *J Dent* Res 71:1212-1227, 1992.

Behrmann RD, Kliegman R, editors: *Nelson essentials of pediatrics,* Philadelphia, 1990, Saunders.

Bickerstaff DR et al: An investigation into the etiology of irritable hip, *Clin Pediatr* 30(6):353, 1991.

Blatt SD et al: Diagnostic utility of lower extremity radiographs of young children with gait disturbance, *Pediatrics* 87(2):138, 1991.

Blumberg DA et al: Severe reactions associated with diphtheria-tetanus-pertussis vaccine: detailed study of children with seizures, hypotonic-hyporesponsive episodes, high fevers, and persistent crying, *Pediatrics* 91(6):1158, 1993.

Bonadio WA et al: Relationship of temperature pattern and serious bacterial infections in infants 4 to 8 weeks old 24 to 48 hours after antibiotic treatment, *Ann Emerg Med* 20(9):1006, 1991.

Bond T, Welch V, Mikula P: *Overview and management of sleep enuresis in children.* AUA Update Series, lesson 16, vol XV, Baltimore, 1996, American Urological Association, Inc.

Bramson RT et al: The futility of the chest radiograph in the febrile infant without respiratory symptoms, *Pediatrics* 92(4):524, 1993.

Breiman RF et al: Emergence of drug-resistant pneumococcal infections in the United States, *JAMA* 271(23):1831, 1994.

Brown PJ et al: Taking an infant's temperature: axillary or rectal thermometer? *N Z Med J* 105(939):309, 1992.

Brown KH: Dietary management of acute childhood diarrhea: optimal timing of feeding and appropriate use of milks and mixed diets, *J Pediatr* 118(4 Part 2):S92-S98, 1991.

Chesney PJ et al: Penicillin-and cephalosporin-resistant strains of *Streptococcus pneumoniae* causing sepsis and meningitis in children with sickle cell disease, *J Pediatr* 127(4)526-532, 1995.

Chiodo F et al: Varicella in immunocompetent children in the first two years of life: role of treatment with oral acyclovir, *J Chemother* 7(1):62, 1995.

Crain EF: Is a chest radiograph necessary in the evaluation of every febrile infant less than 8 weeks of age? *Pediatrics* 88(4):821, 1991.

Cushing AH: Diskitis in children, *Clin Infect Dis* 17(1):1, 1993.

Driscoll CE et al, editors: *The family practice desk reference,* ed 2, St. Louis, 1991, Mosby.

Dunkle LM et al: A controlled trial of acyclovir for chickenpox in normal children, *N Engl J Med* 325(22):1539, 1991.

Fasano MB et al: Egg hypersensitivity and adverse reactions to measles, mumps and rubella vaccine, *J Pediatr* 120(6):878-881, 1992.

Fox R et al: Acute gastroenteritis in infants under six months old, *Arch Dis Child* 65:936, 1990.

Greene MG, editor: *The Harriet Lane handbook,* ed 12, St. Louis, 1991, Mosby.

Hoeve LJ et al: Foreign body aspiration in children: the diagnostic value of signs, symptoms and preoperative examination, *Clin Otolaryngol* 18(1):55, 1993.

Huicho L et al: Occult blood and fecal leukocytes as screening tests in childhood infectious diarrhea: an old problem revisited, *Pediatr Infect Dis J* 12(6):474, 1993.

Husby S et al: Treatment of croup with nebulized steroid (budesonide): a double blind placebo controlled study, *Arch Dis Child* 68(3):352, 1993.

Jaber L et al: Fever associated with teething, *Arch Dis Child* 67(2):233, 1992.

James JM et al: Safe administration of the measles vaccine to children allergic to eggs, *N Engl J Med* 332(19):1262-1266, 1995.

Kempe CH et al: *Current pediatric diagnosis and treatment,* ed 9, Norwalk, Conn., 1987, Appleton & Lange.

Klassen TP et al: Nebulized budesonide for children with mild-to-moderate croup, *N Engl J Med* 331(5):285, 1994.

Kristjansson S et al: Nebulized racemic adrenaline in the treatment of acute bronchiolitis in infants and toddlers, *Arch Dis Child* 69(6):2, 1993.

Larsen PB et al: Aminophylline versus caffeine citrate for apnea and bradycardia prophylaxis in premature neonates, *Acta Paediatr* 84(4):360-364, 1995.

Levy SM, Muchow G: Provider compliance with recommended dietary fluoride supplement protocol, *Am J Public Health* 82:281-283, 1992.

Levy SM: A review of fluoride exposers and ingestion, *Community Dent Oral Epidemiol* 22(3):173-180. 1994.

Lieu TA et al: Clinical and cost-effectiveness of outpatient strategies for management of febrile infants, *Pediatrics* 89(6):1135, 1992.

Lust KD et al: Maternal intake of cruciferous vegetables and other foods and colic symptoms in exclusively breast-fed infants, *Am Diet Assoc* 96(1):46-48, 1996.

Martínez JC et al: Hyperbilirubinemia in the breast-fed newborn: a controlled trial of four interventions, *Pediatrics* 91(2):470-473, 1993.

Maximum access to diagnosis and therapy, Boston, 1996, Electronic Library of Medicine, Little, Brown & Co.

McMillin JA et al: *The whole pediatrician catalog*, Philadelphia, 1977, Saunders.

Menon K et al: A randomized trial comparing the efficacy of epinephrine with salbutamol in the treatment of acute bronchiolitis, *J Pediatr* 126(6):1004, 1995.

Metcalf TJ et al: Simethicone in the treatment of infant colic: a randomized, placebo-controlled, multicenter trial, *Pediatrics* 94(1)29-34, 1994.

Mu L et al: The causes and complications of late diagnosis of foreign body aspiration in children, *Arch Otolaryngol Head Neck Surg* 117:876, 1991.

Muñoz M et al: Appearance of resistance to beta-lactam antibiotics during therapy for *Streptococcus pneumoniae* meningitis, *J Pediatr* 127(1):98-99, 1995.

Nanulescu M et al: Early re-feeding in the management of acute diarrhoea in infants of 0-1 year of age, *Acta Paediatr* 84(9):1002, 1995.

Nigro G et al: Ganciclovir therapy for symptomatic congenital cytomegalovirus infection in infants: a two-regimen experience, *J Pediatr* 124(2):318-322, 1994.

Nutman J et al: Racemic versus *l*-epinephrine aerosol in the treatment of postextubation laryngeal edema: results from a prospective, randomized, double-blind study, *Crit Care Med* 22(10):1591, 1994.

Oggero R et al: Dietary modifications versus dicyclomine hydrochloride in the treatment of severe infantile colics, *Acta Paediatr* 83(2):222-225, 1994.

Pascoe DJ, Grossman M: *Pediatric emergencies*, ed 2, Philadelphia, 1978, Lippincott.

Pendrys DG: Dental fluorosis in perspective, *J Am Dent Assoc* 122:63-66, 1991.

Prasad K et al: Dexamethasone treatment for acute bacterial meningitis: how strong is the evidence for routine use? *J Neurol Neurosurg Psychiatry* 59(1):31, 1995.

Ratnam S et al: Measles and rubella antibody response after measles-mumps-rubella vaccination in children with afebrile upper respiratory tract infection, *J Pediatr* 127(3):432, 1995.

Rimell FL et al: Characteristics of objects that cause choking in children, *JAMA* 274(22):1763, 1995.

Roizen N et al: Neurologic and developmental outcome in treated congenital toxoplasmosis, *Pediatrics* 95(1):11-20, 1995.

Romagnoli C et al: Effectiveness and side effects of two different doses of caffeine in preventing apnea in premature infants, *Therapeutic Drug Monitoring* 14(1):14-19, 1992.

Rudolph AM: *Rudolph's pediatrics*, ed 19, Norwalk, Conn., 1991, Appleton & Lange.

Sanford JP: Guide to antimicrobial therapy 1996, Dallas, 1996, Antimicrobial Therapy, Inc.

Schaad UB et al: Dexamethasone therapy for bacterial meningitis in children, *Lancet* 342(8869):457. 1993.

Seidel H et al: *Primary care of the newborn*, St. Louis, 1993, Mosby.

Szpunar SM, Burt A: Fluoride supplements: evaluation of appropriate use in the United States, *Community Dent Oral Epidemiol* 20:148-154. 1992.
Waisman Y et al: Prospective randomized double-blind study comparing *l*-epinephrine and racemic epinephrine aerosols in the treatment of laryngo-tracheitis (croup), *Pediatrics* 89(2):302, 1992.
Wald ER et al: Cautionary note on the use of empiric ceftriaxone for suspected bacteremia, *Am J Dis Child* 145(12):1359, 1991.
Wald ER et al: Dexamethasone therapy for children with bacterial meningitis, *Pediatrics* 95(1):21, 1995.
Wolke D et al: Excessive infant crying: a controlled study of mothers helping mothers, *Pediatrics* 94(3):322-332, 1994.

11

Genitourinary and Renal Disease

MARK A. GRABER AND VIVIANA MARTÍNEZ-BIANCHI

URINARY TRACT INFECTIONS: FEMALES

I. ACUTE CYSTITIS

A. Signs and symptoms. Dysuria, frequency, nocturia, enuresis, incontinence, urethral pain, suprapubic pain, low back pain, hematuria. Significant fever is unusual. The onset frequently follows intercourse ("honeymoon cystitis"). Urinary frequency and urgency can be caused by UTI, diuretic use, caffeine, tea, drugs (such as theophylline), interstitial cystitis, vaginitis, pregnancy, pelvic mass, etc.

B. Cause. Colonization by fecal flora, usually *Escherichia coli* (75% to 95%). Other organisms include *Klebsiella (5%), Enterobacter, Proteus, Pseudomonas,* etc.

C. Laboratory findings.

1. ***Urinalysis findings*** (from clean catch midstream).
   a. *Positive leukocyte esterase, or pyuria.* Usually >5 WBCs per high-power field (HPF). However, a patient may have typical UTI symptoms and a false-negative urinalysis and still have a bacterial cystitis.
   b. *Bacteriuria.* 2 organisms per HPF by microscopy. By culture, 10^5 organisms per milliliter has classically been considered as a UTI. However, 10^2 organisms/ml is more predictive of symptoms of a UTI.
   c. Positive dipstick result for nitrates.
   d. May have gross or microscopic hematuria.
2. ***Culture and sensitivity.*** Not needed in simple UTI. Should culture if recurrent UTIs, pyelonephritis.

D. Treatment.

1. ***Deciding who to treat.*** The presence of pyuria correlates poorly with the definitive diagnosis of UTI. Pyuria may be present in the absence of UTI and vice versa. Classic symptoms in a patient who has had a previous documented

UTI is about 70% predictive of a UTI, and so one can consider treatment even in absence of positive urine findings. However, also consider other causes as listed above in "signs and symptoms," especially vaginitis.

2. ***Antibiotics.*** Can be used in a 3-day regimen (preferred over single dose; decreases relapse without increase in side effects), or a standard oral regimen lasting 7 to 10 days. A 7- to 10-day course of antibiotics should be used in pregnant patients, those who have "complicated" urinary tract infections such as the elderly, those with recurrent UTI, diabetic patients, etc.
3. All the drugs below can be used in a 3-day or 7- to 10-day course. *Failure of a short course of antibiotics generally indicates an upper tract infection and requires 10 to 14 days of antibiotics.*
   a. *TMP/SMX DS:* PO BID. This is generally the preferred treatment, since it is inexpensive and has a cure rate superior to cephalosporins and amoxicillin.
   b. *Fluoroquinolone.* Ciprofloxacin 250 to 500 mg PO BID or ofloxacin 200 mg PO BID.
   c. *Oral cephalosporin.* Cephalexin 250 to 500 mg QID. Not so efficacious as TMP/SMX.
   d. *Nitrofurantoin.* 50 to 100 mg PO QID with meals and at bedtime. Absorption increased when taken with food.
   e. *Other antibiotics used.* Doxycycline 100 mg PO BID for 7 days; amoxicillin-clavulanic acid; amoxicillin has a lower cure rate than other drugs.
3. If culture done and organism is resistant to the drug prescribed, a change in antibiotics is indicated only if the patient is still symptomatic. Many drugs reach such high levels in the urine that standard sensitivity testing may not reflect in vivo activity.
4. ***Other measures.***
   a. Consider a bladder anesthetic, such as phenazopyridine hydrochloride (Pyridium) 200 mg three times daily for 2 days will promptly relieve symptoms. Inform the patient that this will produce an orange tinge in tears and urine. Warn the patient not to wear contact lenses because they may become discolored.
   b. Instruct patient to increase fluid intake. See below for other measures.

II. CHRONIC CYSTITIS

Unresolved, recurrent, or persistent bladder infection.

A. Symptoms. Similar to simple cystitis but variable in severity.

B. Laboratory findings. UA shows a significant bacteriuria and may have any degree of pyuria. Urine culture will be positive, with *Escherichia coli* most common. Pyuria without bacteriuria should be suggestive of: *Mycobacterium tuberculosis* (TB), or *Chlamydia* infection.

C. Radiographs. Unless associated with other GU tract disease; radiographic studies are normal. Excretory and retrograde urograms and voiding cystograms may demonstrate associated conditions: obstructive uropathy, vesicoureteral reflux, atrophic pyelonephritis, vesicoenteric or vesicovaginal fistulas.

D. Treatment. Antibiotic directed to the causative organism, based on susceptibility testing.

E. Addressing causative factors is important.

1. If cystitis develops in relationship to intercourse, use TMP/SMX DS, 1 tablet after coitus may prevent UTIs. A single dose of a fluoroquinolone may also be used but is second line. Patients should void immediately after intercourse.
2. The use of a diaphragm for birth control may exacerbate recurrent UTIs secondary to incomplete voiding. Additionally the use of nonoxynol-9 is associated with an increased incidence of bacteriuria.
3. Cranberry juice has been proved to reduce pyuria and bacteruria by preventing *E. coli* adherence to cells. Increasing fluids in general may be helpful as well.
4. Vaginal estrogen cream (0.5 to 2 g intravaginally daily) diminishes the incidence of UTIs for postmenopausal women.
5. Women should be instructed to wipe from front to back after a bowel movement to avoid bringing infective organisms toward the urethra.
6. Long-term preventive therapy is with TMP/SMX 1 single-strength tablet daily, nitrofurantoin 50 to 100 mg daily, or methenamine and an acidifier may prove necessary in those with recurrent UTIs not related to intercourse.
7. There is no evidence that avoiding baths reduces the incidence of cystitis. However, if irritating soaps are used in the bath, these should be eliminated.
8. Pneumaturia is suggestive of an enterovesical fistula (especially secondary to diverticular disease) or infection caused by gas-forming pathogens (most often in diabetics).

III. INTERSTITIAL CYSTITIS

A. Signs and symptoms. Frequency, urgency, and rarely urge incontinence with periurethral and suprapubic pain on bladder filling that is improved by voiding. May have terminal hematuria.

B. Cause. Unclear; possible autoimmune or allergic process.

C. Treatment. Refer to a urologist for cystoscopy and possible biopsy. Unable to diagnose without cystoscopy under anesthesia.

D. May respond symptomatically to Pyridium.

IV. RADIATION CYSTITIS

Symptoms may develop months after cessation of treatment with history based on exposure to radiation. Urine may or may not be sterile.

V. NONINFECTIOUS HEMORRHAGIC CYSTITIS

Noninfectious hemorrhagic cystitis can occur after radiation therapy or treatment with cyclophosphamide. There is often serious vesical hemorrhage. Urgent consultation with a urologist should be sought.

VI. URETHRITIS

A. Patient may have UTI symptoms, pyuria, but negative cultures.

B. Causes. Infections with a low colony count, *Chlamydia, Neisseria gonorrhoeae, Trichomonas*, or vaginitis.

C. Treatment. Treat as *Chlamydia* and gonorrhea in Table 11-1.

VII. ASYMPTOMATIC BACTERIURIA

A. Diagnosis requires >100,000 CFU/ml of urine of *same* organism in 2 clean-catch specimens *or* >100 organisms on a single catheterized specimen.

B. Must be distinguished from contamination from vaginal or urethral organisms attributable to poor technique in specimen collection. Treat based on C&S, not empirically.

C. The only patients who should be treated for asymptomatic bacteriuria include those who (1) are pregnant, (2) are past a urologic procedure, (3) are past a removal of an indwelling catheter, (4) have diabetes mellitus, or (5) are children. Asymptomatic bacteriuria is not an indication for treatment with antibiotics in the elderly, since treatment does not affect the outcome in these patients.

URINARY TRACT INFECTION: CHILDREN

I. CLINICAL PRESENTATION

Differs from adults in that symptoms may include only fever, new incontinence of a previously toilet-trained youngster, abdominal pain, diarrhea, vomiting, or lethargy. UTI is a common cause of fever in the neonatal period. Uncircumcised males <8 weeks of age are more prone to UTIs than circumcised males or females are.

II. DIAGNOSTIC CRITERIA

Same as for cystitis in females above. However, fever may cause pyuria; therefore culture is indicated. Quick catheterization should be considered; "bag" urines generally yield poor specimens for culture because of contamination.

TABLE 11-1
Treatment of Sexually Transmitted Diseases

Type and location	Drug of choice	Alternatives
***Chlamydia trachomatis* diseases**		
Urethritis, proctitis (Treat also for gonorrhea)	Doxycycline 100 mg PO BID × 7 days Azithromycin 1 g as single dose	Tetracycline 500 mg PO QID × 7 days Erythromycin 500 mg PO QID × 7 days (preferred in pregnancy)
Lymphogranuloma venereum	Doxycycline 100 mg PO BID × 21 days	Erythromycin 500 mg PO QID × 21 days Sulfisoxazole 500 mg PO QID × 21 days
***Neisseria gonorrhoeae*—gonorrhea**		
Urethritis, proctitis, pharyngitis (Treat also for *Chlamydia*)	Ceftriaxone 250 mg IM Azithromycin 2 g PO as single dose (also covers *Chlamydia*)	Ofloxacin 400 mg or ciprofloxacin 500 mg or cefixime 400 mg All single dose
Disseminated	Ceftriaxone 1 g IV or IM Q24h until asymptomatic followed by cefixime 400 mg BID or ciprofloxacin 500 mg BID for total of 7-day course	Spectinomycin 2.0 g Q12h IM

Continued

TABLE 11-1
Treatment of Sexually Transmitted Diseases—cont'd

Type and location	Drug of choice	Alternatives
Epididymo-orchitis		
<35 years of age	Treat for gonorrhea and *Chlamydia*	
>35 years or insertive partner in anal intercourse	Ciprofloxacin 500 mg PO BID or 400 mg IV BID or ofloxacin 200 mg PO or IV BID × 10 to 14 days	Ampicillin/sulbactam or third-generation cephalosporin
***Trichomonas* urethritis or vaginitis**	Metronidazole 2 g PO in single dose; *contraindicated in pregnancy*. If treatment failure, give 2 g/day as single dose × 5 days	Clindamycin 300 mg PO BID × 7 days

Granuloma inguinale	Doxycycline 100 mg PO BID × 1 to 4 weeks	TMP/SMX DS 1 tablet PO BID × 14 to 30 days
Chancroid	Ceftriaxone 250 mg IM once or azithromycin 1 g PO in single dose or erythromycin 500 mg PO QID × 7 days	Ciprofloxacin 500 mg PO BID × 3 days or TMP/SMX DS 1 PO BID × 7 days
Herpes simplex		
Initial episode	Acyclovir 400 mg PO TID × 10 days or famciclovir 250 to 500 mg PO BID × 10 days	Valacyclovir 1000 mg PO BID × 10 days
Recurrent	Acyclovir 400 mg PO TID × 5 days or famciclovir 125 mg PO BID × 5 days	Valacyclovir 500 mg PO BID × 5 days
Chronic suppression	Acyclovir 400 mg PO TID	

Modified from *The Medical Letter,* 37(964):119, 1995.
If treating for either a *Neisseria gonorrhoeae* or *Chlamydia trachomatis*, treat for both organisms, since patients frequently have concurrent infections. *Always treat a sexual partner or partners as well when treating any of these infections!*

III. MANAGEMENT

All children with UTIs need a repeat culture 1 to 2 weeks after completing treatment. All children <3 months of age should be admitted for IV antibiotics as should children who look ill (same antibiotic choices as in pyelonephritis section below). An older child with simple, uncomplicated UTI can be treated as an outpatient. A 10- to 14-day course of antibiotics is generally prescribed for UTI in children.

IV. EVALUATION

Radiologic evaluation for anatomic abnormality (IVP, U/S, voiding cystourethrogram) should be obtained on all girls less than 5 years of age, all boys regardless of age, children with evidence of pyelonephritis, and any female >5 years of age with recurrent UTIs. Some authors would not work up first cystitis in a girl but would defer work-up until there is a second infection.

LOWER UROGENITAL INFECTIONS: MALES

I. OVERVIEW

- **A. Cause.** Ascending infection from the urethra most common; reflux of infected urine into prostatic ducts and then into the posterior urethra likely an important cause of prostatitis. Hematogenous, lymphatic spread or extension from adjacent organs also possible. *Pathogens: Escherichia coli* (80% to 91%), *Proteus, Enterobacter, Pseudomonas, Serratia, Streptococcus faecalis,* and *Staphylococcus* species are the most common.
- **B. Localization of infection.** Divided urine collection may help localize the infection: Urethra represented by first voided 10 ml, bladder represented by midstream collection, and prostate represented by the last 10 ml of voided urine. Prostatic massage before the last voided 10 ml will increase the yield.

II. URETHRITIS

- **A. Presentation.** Generally complain of a urethral discharge (watery to purulent), with or without urethral burning or itching, and burning on urination. May not note discharge but may have spotting in underwear.
- **B. Cause.** *Neisseria gonorrhoeae* and *Chlamydia trachomatis* (causes 80% of non-GC) most common, followed by *Ureaplasma urealyticum, Mycoplasma hominis, Trichomonas vaginalis, Candida,* and herpesviruses.
- **C. History.** Ask about first onset of symptoms, recent sexual contacts, prior history of STDs.
- **D. Work-up.** Examination should be performed at least 1 hour after the last void. *Notice character of discharge*: watery and thin are suggestive of *Chlamydia,* whereas a purulent-looking

discharge is suggestive of gonorrhea. Obtain a specimen by inserting a Calginate (calcium alginate) swab 2 to 3 cm within the urethra (a drop of the discharge is not acceptable because *Chlamydia* organisms are intracellular and urethral cellular material is required for culture).

E. Laboratory findings. Gram stain of urethral discharge should show >4 WBCs per HPF. Demonstration of intracellular gram-negative diplococci within PMNs is strong evidence of gonorrhea. Absence of gram-negative cocci is strong evidence of nongonococcal urethritis (such as *Chlamydia*). However, Gram stain only 95% sensitive for GC. Culture on modified Thayer-Martin medium for gonorrhea (<100% sensitive) and send for immunofluorescent testing and PCR, or culture for *Chlamydia.*

F. Treatment. See Table 11-1. Be sure to treat for both *Chlamydia* and *N. gonorrhoeae* and to treat partner.

III. BACTERIAL CYSTITIS

A. Signs and symptoms. Similar to those in females (see above). Also examine urethra for discharge (urethritis), prostate, and epididymis for tenderness to rule out other disorders.

B. Laboratory findings. UA shows pyuria, bacteriuria, no casts, occasionally gross or microscopic hematuria. *C&S should be done in males with history consistent with UTI.*

C. Treatment. Treat 10 to 14 days and then obtain follow-up culture. Antibiotic choices are similar to those for female UTI. After successful treatment (urine is sterile), consider intravenous pyelography (IVP) or cystoscopy to rule out structural obstruction to outflow.

IV. INFECTIONS OF THE PROSTATE GLAND

A. Acute bacterial prostatitis.

1. ***Signs and symptoms.*** Acute febrile illness, chills, malaise, lower back pain, perineal pain, urinary urgency or frequency, nocturia, or dysuria. Varying degrees of urinary retention, tenesmus, or pain with bowel movement. The prostate is very tender, boggy, and warm to touch. (Do not massage because of risk of bacteremia.)
2. ***Laboratory findings.*** Leukocytosis with left shift, bacteriuria, hematuria, pyuria. C&S required.
3. ***Therapy.***
   a. Hospitalization for IV antibiotics if sepsis suspected. Start gentamycin or tobramycin 3 to 5 mg/kg/day divided every 8 hours and ampicillin 2 g every 6 hours pending culture results.
   b. If hospitalization is not necessary (no fever; patient not toxic), prescribe TMP/SMX DS twice daily for 10 to 14 days, ciprofloxacin 500 BID, or ofloxacin 300 mg BID for 10 to 14 days. In young, sexually active men,

treat for gonorrhea and *Chlamydia* infections for 14 days as well.

c. Continuing oral antibiotics for 1 month after an episode of acute prostatitis may reduce recurrence and reduce transformation into chronic prostatitis.

d. Avoid urethral catheterization if possible.

e. After completion of successful therapy, the patient should be followed for at least 4 months with periodic examinations and cultures of prostatic fluids to ensure cure.

B. Chronic bacterial prostatitis.

1. ***Signs and symptoms.*** Low back and perineal discomfort; voiding symptoms similar to those of acute bacterial prostatitis but with a more insidious onset. No systemic signs; rarely painful ejaculation. Prostate may feel normal, boggy, or focally indurated. Chronic prostatitis is the most common cause of recurrent UTIs in men.
2. ***Laboratory tests.*** UA and cultures should be done. Prostatic secretions reveal inflammatory cells, with macrophages containing oval fat bodies. UA will show WBCs and bacteriuria if secondary cystitis is present. Causative agents are usually *E. coli* or *Pseudomonas*.
3. ***Treatment.*** Ciprofloxacin 500 mg orally, or norfloxacin 400 mg orally, twice daily for 4 to 6 weeks. This yields about an 80% cure rate. TMP/SMX DS twice daily for 3 months cures about one third of cases and improves symptoms in about three fourths. Failure of therapy may indicate the need for IV antibiotics or the presence of infected prostatic calculi. Chronic suppression with TMP/SMX or a quinolone at nighttime may be helpful.

C. Nonbacterial prostatitis.

1. ***Cause.*** Unknown. It is a diagnosis of exclusion. *Chlamydia*, *Ureaplasma*, and *Mycoplasma* infection and autoimmune processes are suspected but not proved. Consider also tuberculosis, mycotic infections, viral infections, or *Cryptococcus* infection in AIDS patients.
2. ***Signs and symptoms.*** Same as for chronic bacterial prostatitis.
3. ***Laboratory findings.*** Prostatic secretions reveal inflammatory *cells* but no bacteria. Never able to document UTI.
4. ***Therapy.***

    a. A clinical trial of antibiotic therapy directed to abovementioned organisms is recommended: doxycycline 100 mg twice daily, erythromycin 500 mg 4 times daily, or ofloxacin 300 mg twice daily should be tried for at least 4 weeks. Since nonbacterial prostatitis usually does not respond to antibiotics, their continued empirical use is not justified.

b. Symptomatic flare-ups often respond to anti-inflammatory agents, such as ibuprofen 400 to 600 mg PO Q4-6h.
c. Alpha-andrenergic receptor blocking agent may help: prazosin 2 to 4 mg orally twice daily, or terazosin 5 to 10 mg orally twice daily.
d. Other measures: hot sitz baths, reassurance. The recurrent symptoms can often cause significant emotional stress, anxiety, and depression resulting in significant morbidity.

D. Prostatodynia.

1. Symptoms suggestive of prostatitis (prostatic or pelvic pain) but without infection or inflammation and negative labs and cultures.
2. It is a syndrome of variable cause.
   a. In some men urodynamic testing discloses voiding dysfunction associated with apparent functional obstruction of the bladder neck and urethra. This "spasm" may result in intraprostatic reflux and chemical irritation of the prostate by urine. In such cases there is a favorable response to an alpha-blocker such as prazosin 2 to 4 mg orally twice daily or terazosin 5 to 10 mg orally once daily.
   b. In other cases there is tension myalgia of the pelvic floor, which may respond to diathermy, muscle relaxants, and physiotherapy with or without the use of diazepam 5 mg orally TID.

V. EPIDIDYMITIS

A. Causes.

1. Sexually transmitted form associated with urethritis and commonly caused by *Chlamydia* or *N. gonorrhoeae* or both.
2. Non–sexually transmitted form associated with UTI or prostatitis, commonly caused by *Enterobacter* or *Pseudomonas* organisms.
3. Causes such as trauma, tuberculosis, urine reflux, or as a complication of TURP or systemic infection are less common.

B. Signs and symptoms. Similar to urethritis, prostatitis or cystitis. Epididymis is painful, and swelling and tenderness may extend to groin, lower abdomen, or flank. Fever, urethral discharge, and reactive hydrocele are common but may not be present in traumatic epididymitis.

C. Laboratory findings. White count may be normal or elevated with left shift. UA may show pyuria or bacteriuria. C&S is indicated.

D. Differential diagnosis. Mumps orchitis, tumor, testicular abscess, torsion, and trauma must be considered.

E. Therapy.

1. ***General measures.*** Bed rest, scrotal elevation and support, analgesics, ice (early), heat (late), and spermatic cord block with lidocaine may be used.
2. ***Antibiotics.*** If patient <35 years of age, treat for gonorrhea and then follow with treatment for nongonococcal urethritis (Table 11-1). If patient >35 years of age, treat with TMP/SMX or fluoroquinolone for 10 to 14 days. If severe disease, can consider amoxicillin clavulanate, ampicillin-sulbactam, or imipenem-cilastatin.
3. ***NSAIDs.*** Effective for inflammatory component.

UPPER URINARY TRACT INFECTION: MALES AND FEMALES

I. ACUTE PYELONEPHRITIS

A. Definition. Infection of the parenchyma and pelvis of the kidney, which may affect one or occasionally both kidneys.

B. Causes. Aerobic gram-negative bacterium, most commonly *E. coli.* All *Proteus* species are specially important because they produce urease, which causes alkaline urine and favors formation of struvite and apatite stones. Coagulase-negative staphylococci *(S. epidermidis* and *S. saprophyticus),* *S. aureus,* and group D streptococci (enterococci) occasionally cause pyelonephritis. Staphylococci may infect by hematogenous route and cause renal abscesses.

C. Clinical findings. Abrupt onset of shaking chills and fever >38.5° C, flank pain, malaise, urinary frequency and burning. Often nausea, vomiting, and diarrhea as well. Generally have CVA tenderness. May be in septic shock. Children may complain of abdominal pain.

D. Laboratory findings. Leukocytosis with left shift. UA will show pyuria, white blood cell casts, hematuria, and mild proteinuria. C&S of urine and blood are mandatory. BUN and creatinine usually remain normal in uncomplicated pyelonephritis.

E. In uncomplicated acute pyelonephritis, radiologic examinations are not required. IVP is indicated in recurrent episodes to screen for stones or obstructive uropathy. CT scanning is the most sensitive method for differentiating between acute pyelonephritis and a renal or perinephric abscess in a patient who is not responding to therapy.

F. Treatment.

1. **Hospitalize.** If the patient is a child, is an infant, is pregnant, has a high fever, is dehydrated, appears "acutely ill," or is septic. Recent data indicate that "healthy-looking" pregnant patients can be treated as an outpatient, but this is not yet the standard of care. Treat empirically

with IV third-generation cephalosporin with or without gentamicin, IV fluoroquinolone, gentamicin and ampicillin, ampicillin-sulbactam, or ticarcillin–clavulanic acid pending culture and sensitivity results. Avoid gentamicin and fluoroquinolones in pregnant patients. Treat IV for about 48 to 72 hours or more according to clinical response. Continue oral antibiotics and then complete with oral antibiotics for 2 to 6 more weeks. Medication should be given for pain, fever, and nausea. Ensure adequate hydration and maintenance of good urine output with either IV or oral fluids. See also septic shock in Chapter 18.

2. **If the patient is not acutely ill,** treat as outpatient for 10 days to 6 weeks with TMP/SMX, fluoroquinolone (that is, ciprofloxacin 500 mg PO BID), amoxicillin–clavulanic acid, or a cephalosporin. A good option is to give 1 to 2 g of ceftriaxone IV or IM at the time of diagnosis and then follow up the patient the next day. If required, an additional dose of ceftriaxone can be given at the follow-up exam if the patient warrants more than oral antibiotics but does not require hospitalization. Ensure good communication in case of worsening condition and establish follow-up care.
3. **If the patient is not improving,** infected stones or obstruction must be considered early and dealt with effectively to avoid complications. Consider IVP or VCUG after resolution of UTI in all children and males or in females with frequent recurrences or unusual symptoms. If the patient is not responding to antibiotics and the organism is known to be sensitive to the current antibiotics, consider emphysematous pyelonephritis or abscess formation. CT scan will identify these patients.
4. **Follow-up study.** Urine culture should be done 1 to 2 weeks after therapy in pregnant patients, children, patients who remain symptomatic, and those for whom suppression therapy is being considered. Follow-up cultures are optional for others.

II. CHRONIC PYELONEPHRITIS

A. Caused by repeated acute attacks that result in renal scarring. This may lead to renal insufficiency and hypertension. Patients with recurrent or chronic pyelonephritis need a full evaluation, including IVP and voiding cystourethrogram, to search for predisposing factors.

B. Surgical treatment includes correction of anatomic defects or nephrectomy for renin-mediated hypertension associated with unilateral atrophic pyelonephritis.

C. Prophylactic antibiotic therapy may be used to prevent infection recurrence.

SEXUALLY TRANSMITTED DISEASES

I. SYPHILIS

Caused by the spirochete *Treponema pallidum*.

A. Primary syphilis.

1. ***Clinical presentation.*** Characteristic sign is the chancre, a painless sore that usually presents 2 to 4 weeks after exposure. These are 1 to 2 cm in diameter, may be multiple, appear as shallow ulcerations with noninflamed margins, and occur most commonly on mucous membranes abraded during sexual contact. Chancres heal spontaneously and slowly without scarring in 2 to 12 weeks. Unilateral or bilateral inguinal lymphadenopathy may be present.
2. ***Laboratory findings.*** Dark-field exam of suspicious lesions will reveal spirochetes. VDRL test or RPR test is initially positive in 50% of patients but may remain negative for up to 3 weeks after the appearance of the chancre. FTA-ABS is the quickest, least expensive, and most specific and sensitive examination.
3. ***Therapy.*** See below. Patients may experience fever, chills, arthralgias, myalgias, and nausea several hours after treatment (the Jarisch-Herxheimer reaction), usually subside within 24 hours. VDRL titers usually return to nonreactive within 1 year of treatment.

B. Secondary syphilis.

1. Clinical presentation. Widespread, symmetric rash, often involving palms or soles (80%). Rash is usually erythematous but is otherwise variable in appearance (such as morbilliform, similar to pityriasis rosea, etc.) and normally occurs 4 to 8 weeks after chancre. Condylomata lata, oral or genital mucous patches (superficial mucosal erosions), systemic symptoms (50%), and symmetric adenopathy also occur. The lesions of secondary syphilis resolve with or without treatment in 2 to 10 weeks.
2. ***Laboratory findings.*** Dark-field exam of condylomata lata is often positive. VDRL test is highly reactive in 90% but should be confirmed with FTA-ABS.
3. ***Therapy.*** See below.

C. Tertiary syphilis. May have gumma formation, tabes dorsalis (sensory loss in legs secondary to dorsal column changes), lymphocytic meningitis as well as aortic insufficiency, and dementia.

D. Therapy. Treat based on duration of infection.

1. ***Early (primary, secondary, or early latent).*** Benzathine penicillin 2.4 million units IM once, doxycycline 100 mg PO BID for 14 days, erythromycin 500 mg PO QID for 14 days, or ceftriaxone 250 mg IM QD for 10 days.
2. ***Late (latent, gummas, or cardiovascular).*** Benzathine penicillin 2.4 million units IM weekly × 3 doses or doxycycline 100 mg PO BID for 4 weeks.

3. ***CNS syphilis.*** Aqueous penicillin 12 million units/day for 10 days followed by benzathine penicillin G 2.4 million units IM weekly × 3 doses.

E. Follow the VDRL test at 3, 6, and 12 months in all patients with syphilis. If the treatment is adequate, the VDRL test results should become negative.

II. GONORRHEA

Caused by gram-negative diplococcus *Neisseria gonorrhoeae.* (For discussion of gonococcal disease in the male, see previous section on urethritis.)

A. Signs and symptoms. The primary site of infection is the endocervix with secondary infection of the rectum or urethra. Yellow-white discharge may be present, but the infection is frequently asymptomatic. Findings may include friable cervix, yellow-green cervical discharge, sterile pyuria, positive cultures, or other evidence of gonorrhea. Other infections include proctitis, pharyngitis, salpingitis, and disseminated disease (pustulovesicular lesions with arthralgias and arthritis).

B. Laboratory findings. Gram stain of a vaginal smear reveals gram-negative intracellular diplococci (only 30% to 70%). Culture on Thayer-Martin (chocolate agar) medium to grow *Neisseria* organisms.

C. Therapy. See Table 11-1. Repeat cultures should be obtained 3 to 7 days after treatment to assure adequate treatment. Sexual partner or partners should also be treated.

III. CHANCROID

Caused by a gram-negative rod, *Haemophilus ducreyi.*

A. Signs and symptoms. A papule that becomes a pustule that ulcerates. In distinction to syphilis, the ulcers of chancroid are painful. Lesions are deep with flat, ragged erythematous borders that may extend into subcutaneous tissue. Adenopathy is common; systemic signs of fever, headache, and malaise occur in 50%.

B. Laboratory findings. Smear reveals gram-negative rods in chains ("school of fish"). Culture on enriched chocolate agar with vancomycin may be positive; biopsy specimen is diagnostic.

C. Therapy. See Table 11-1.

IV. LYMPHOGRANULOMA VENEREUM

Caused by a very virulent strain of *Chlamydia trachomatis.*

A. Signs and symptoms. A papule or pustule that appears 5 to 21 days after exposure and ulcerates. This lesion often goes unnoticed. Painful adenopathy (usually unilateral) occurs 1 to 2 weeks later. May form buboes, become fluctuant, or form chronic draining sinuses. Generally have fever, chills, or rash. Rectal strictures from anorectal node involvement can be seen.

B. Laboratory findings. Complement fixation titers should show a fourfold increase after 4 weeks. Culture of aspirate for *C. trachomatis* is a diagnostic but is positive in only 20% to 30%.

C. Therapy. See Table 11-1. I&D of nodes is rarely indicated.

V. HERPES SIMPLEX GENITALIS

Caused by herpes simplex virus type II (occasionally type I).

A. Signs and symptoms. Often asymptomatic. Incubation is 2 to 10 days. Primary lesion is manifest by grouped painful vesicles on an erythematous base that ulcerate and heal without scarring. Fever and adenopathy are common. Secondary lesions are similar to primary lesions except that the duration and severity are less and accompanying fever and adenopathy are rare.

B. Laboratory findings. Tzanck smear of a base of a fresh vesicle (Giemsa stain) reveals multinucleated giant cells. Culture requires 48 to 72 hours; rapid antigen test is available. Serologic tests are available for *Herpesvirus* but are generally negative during a primary disease and do not reliably differentiate type I from type II *Herpesvirus.*

C. Therapy. See Table 11-I.

VI. CONDYLOMA ACUMINATUM

Caused by human papillomavirus.

A. Signs and symptoms. Soft, flesh-colored, verrucous lesions in genital area. Is associated with an increased risk of cervical dysplasia and cancer.

B. Laboratory findings. Serologic studies may be necessary to rule out condyloma latum of secondary syphilis. Biopsy specimen (rarely necessary) is diagnostic.

C. Therapy.

1. ***Podophyllin (10% to 25% in tincture of benzoin).*** Applied and then thoroughly washed off in 1 to 4 hours. Alternatively, home therapy with the preparation Podofilox 0.5% can be tried. Warts are treated twice daily for 3 days; an area of no more than 10 cm^2 should be treated. No further applications should be made for 4 days. This cycle can be repeated 3 times (a total of 4 cycles of 3 days of treatment over a 4-week period). If a poor or no response is noted, another therapeutic modality should be tried.
2. ***Trichloroacetic acid.*** Can be applied cautiously to lesions. It is quite caustic and will injure normal skin.
3. ***Intravaginal 5-FU.*** Has been used. Use 5% 5-fluorouracil cream and apply one fourth of applicator full QHS for 1 week and then once a week for 10 weeks. Alternatively the cream can be used 2 times per week for 10 weeks. Many women will not tolerate these regimens because of erosion of vaginal mucosa.

4. ***Alternative therapies.*** Cryotherapy, electrosurgery, excision, laser vaporization, or intralesional interferon. Imoquimod will soon be approved for use in the United States. It is an immune modulator that is used 3 times per week and is 73% successful in women after 16 weeks of treatment. Its efficacy is only 30% to 40% in men.

D. Condylomas. Will tend to recur in 7.5% to 80%.

VII. MOLLUSCUM CONTAGIOSUM

Caused by a poxvirus.

A. Signs and symptoms. Dome-shaped papules, 2 to 6 mm with central umbilication.

B. Laboratory findings. Incision of a papule reveals white waxy core. Smear of contents reveals swollen epithelial cells. Biopsy specimen is diagnostic.

C. Therapy. Curettage, cryosurgery, or electrodesiccation.

VIII. CANDIDIASIS

Yeast infection caused by *Candida albicans.*

A. Signs and symptoms. In the male, red erythematous pruritic skin with peripheral pustules. In the female, pruritic vaginal mucosa and profuse creamy white discharge. More common in diabetics or patients using long-term antibiotics.

B. Laboratory findings. Smear or culture reveals *C. albicans.*

C. Therapy. Good hygiene and antifungal creams or suppositories. (See Table 11-1.) Evaluate for diabetes or immunosuppression in those with recurrent candidal infection.

IX. TRICHOMONIASIS

Caused by protozoon *Trichomonas vaginalis.* See Chapter 7 for details of trichomoniasis in the female.

A. Signs and symptoms. Often asymptomatic. Vaginal and urethral discharge or pruritus are the most common complaints.

B. Laboratory findings. *Trichomonas vaginalis* is motile and best seen under low power.

C. Therapy. See Table 11-1. Be sure to treat partner or partners.

X. CHLAMYDIA

Caused by *Chlamydia trachomatis.* See Chapter 7 for details of *Chlamydia* in the female patient.

A. Signs and symptoms. Generally asymptomatic but may have vaginal discharge, dysuria, pelvic pain, or dyspareunia.

B. Laboratory findings. May have purulent cervical discharge that after Gram staining is notable for the absence of gonococci. Can also detect using immunologic studies or by culture of the organism.

C. Therapy. See Table 11-1. All persons with *Chlamydia* should be treated for gonorrhea and the reverse holds true as well.

XI. BACTERIAL VAGINOSIS

May present as malodorous vaginal discharge. See Chapter 7 for details. See Table 11-1 for treatment.

BENIGN PROSTATIC HYPERTROPHY (BPH)

I. CAUSE

The cause for BPH is still unclear. It rarely affects men <40 years of age, with symptoms generally beginning between 60 to 65 years of age. Three components are responsible for the symptoms of BPH: (1) fixed mechanical obstruction from structural changes, (2) dynamic obstruction related to tone of muscle fibers, or (3) detrusor response with detrusor hypertrophy and decreased bladder compliance and functional capacity.

II. CLINICAL PRESENTATION

A. **Signs and symptoms.** Enlargement occurs silently; only when bladder outlet obstruction occurs do symptoms present. These include decreased force and caliber of urinary stream, hesitancy, retention, postmicturition dribbling, double voiding, (patient voids and is able to void again in 5 to 10 minutes), and overflow urinary incontinence (on staining or coughing). Irritative symptoms such as dysuria, frequency, nocturia, urgency, hematuria, and incontinence occur frequently. Flank pain during micturition, suprapubic pain, and azotemic symptoms occur less commonly.

B. **Exam.** The bladder may be distended, and the prostate is enlarged, smooth, and symmetric. The prostate gland may be soft or firm and possibly nodular. However, the nodules lack the stony-hard consistency associated with carcinoma.

C. **Laboratory findings.** UA may reveal signs of infection. If the obstruction has been severe enough to impair renal function, BUN and creatinine may be elevated. PSA may be elevated.

D. **Radiographic findings.** IVP may show upper tract or bladder changes secondary to obstruction (hydroureteronephrosis, bladder trabeculation and thickening, bladder diverticula or calculi). VCUG may be indicated. Postvoid catheterization will reveal residual urine. Order an ultrasonogram with rectal probe and biopsies if indicated, to rule out carcinoma. Cystoscopy if indicated.

III. TREATMENT

A. An indwelling Foley catheter may help acute episodes but is only a temporary measure.

B. Surgical measures, most commonly transurethral prostatectomy (TURP), are the preferred and definitive therapy.

C. Antibiotics should be used to control infection when indicated.

D. Terazosin 1 to 2 mg/day is often very helpful in relieving symptoms.

E. Finasteride (Proscar) 5 mg PO QD. Blocks transformation of testosterone to 5α-dihydrotestosterone. Shrinks prostate tissue but may take 6 to 12 months to have a clinical effect. Hypertrophy reoccurs on stopping drug. Recent data indicate that finasteride may be no better than placebo at relieving symptoms of benign prostatic hypertrophy.

F. If exam reveals nodularity of the gland, referral to a urologist is indicated.

HEMATURIA

I. DEFINITION

Hematuria is defined as >3 to 5 RBC/HPF. Hematuria in the anticoagulated patient has the same significance as that in the "normal" patient and should not be ignored. Hematuria is relatively common, occurring in from 13% to 40% of individuals depending on the population studied.

II. CAUSE

A. Possible causes include trauma, tumor, kidney stones, bladder infection, prostatitis, pyelonephritis, glomerulonephritis, urethral structure or foreign body, and systemic disorders that produce vasculitis (Wegener's granulomatosis, lupus, etc.). Additionally, one must consider "malignant" hypertension, bacterial endocarditis, or interstitial cystitis. Crystalluria may cause hematuria as can familial thin basement membrane disease and traumatic exercise such as running. Parasites such as schistosomiasis should be considered in the proper population. In the proper population, consider sickle cell disease.

B. If dipstick is positive for blood but microscopic exam is negative for cells, consider hemoglobinuria or myoglobinuria.

III. EVALUATION (for trauma-related hematuria, see Chapter 1).

A. History. Will often provide evidence for cause with symptoms of infection (fever, dysuria), urolithiasis (pain), etc.

B. Physical exam. May provide evidence to indicate cause (that is, prostate may be tender, suprapubic region tender, CVA tenderness, trauma to perineum or urethra [including sexual trauma]). Catheterization will often cause hematuria.

C. Laboratory and Radiologic Investigation.

1. ***Urinalysis.*** Document hematuria, assess for possible infection as indicated by WBCs, possible WBC casts, or bacteria. Presence of red blood cell casts or proteinuria is suggestive of glomerulonephritis. Culture if indicated. Renal function studies if indicated.
2. ***Different strategies have been suggested.*** This is the strategy suggested by Panzer R et al, editors: *Diagnostic*

strategies for common medical problems, (Philadelphia, 1991, American College of Physicians):

a. All patients over 50 years of age *or* with risk factors for urologic malignancy (smoking, dye exposure, chemical, textile, leather or rubber industry work, cyclophosphamide history, use of phenacetin-containing products) should be evaluated with urine cytologic analysis, IVP, and cystoscopy unless cause is clear (such as hemorrhagic cystitis).
b. All individuals with a history consistent with a significant underlying cause (such as weight loss, fevers) should be investigated as appropriate.
c. For those <50 years of age without any risk factors, the incidence of a significant underlying cause for hematuria in the absence of any other signs or symptoms is <1%. A minimal work-up of creatinine and a flat-plate radiograph of abdomen should be done. A renal ultrasonogram may be more useful than a flat-plate radiograph of the abdomen. If these are normal, a follow-up exam with recheck of the urine can be done. If hematuria is persistent and no other cause is evident (such as running), it seems prudent to work up the patient.
d. *Other authors argue for a full work-up of all patients with hematuria.* If one chooses watchful waiting, discussion with the patient of pros and cons of work-up versus waiting must be documented.
e. *All children with unexplained hematuria need a complete work-up including radiologic examination.*

IV. TREATMENT

Address underlying cause.

UROLITHIASIS

I. OVERVIEW

Urinary tract stones are a common cause of both hematuria and abdominal, flank, or groin pain affecting about 4% to 5% of the population at some point in their life. Of these, 50% will have a second stone within 5 years and 60% within 9 years. Development of stones is related to decreased urine volume or increased excretion of stone-forming components. Stones can be composed of calcium, oxalate, urate, cystine, xanthine, phosphate, or all of these. Stones form in the renal pelvis, and their size ranges from microscopic to the size of the entire renal pelvis.

II. CLINICAL PRESENTATION

A. History. Commonly a past history of stone. Pain is usually of sudden onset, severe and colicky, not improved by position, radiating from the back, down flank, and into groin. Hematuria may be noted. Nausea and vomiting are common.

Predisposing factors may be present: recent reduction in fluid intake, medications that predispose to hyperuricemia, history of gout, increased exercise with dehydration. Children <16 years of age make up 7% of those with stones and may present with only painless hematuria.

B. Physical examination. May reveal costovertebral-angle tenderness. Tachycardia may be present, or the patient may have bradycardia from a vasovagal reaction. Vitals are usually stable, and the abdomen may be benign.

C. Laboratory findings. Urinalysis will demonstrate gross or microscopic hematuria in 75% to 90% of patients with stones. In the other 10% to 25% the urine may be normal. *A normal urinalysis does not rule out kidney stones.* Urine culture should be obtained, and a fresh urine sample should be examined for crystals. WBC may be increased on CBC count secondary to pain and demargination. BUN and creatinine should be obtained.

D. Differential diagnosis. Abdominal aortic aneurysm dissection and bowel ischemia can mimic urolithiasis and must be ruled out before IVP. Also consider other causes of abdominal pain (see Chapter 9).

E. Imaging studies. IVP is the gold standard and should be obtained in most patients with suspected kidney stone. If the diagnosis is clear (a patient with past history of documented kidney stones and typical symptoms and findings on history, physical, and laboratory), IVP is not necessary for acute conditions but should be done if pain persists to determine the degree of obstruction. In all other cases, an IVP should be obtained to evaluate renal anatomy, to rule out obstruction, and to document stones in urinary tract. If the patient is elderly or has poor renal function, ultrasonography or CT is an alternative though U/S will miss some stones of <5 mm.

F. Initial treatment. Analgesia, adequate hydration, and obtaining a urine specimen for analysis. Antibiotics as indicated for pyelonephritis or concurrent UTI.

1. *Toradol 15 to 30 mg IV or narcotics* (such as morphine 2 to 10 mg or more IV) are usually required for analgesia. NSAIDs are as effective as if not more effective for renal colic than narcotics are. However, they should be used as supplements to IV narcotics. There is no indication for IM medications in treating renal colic.
2. *IV fluids* should be used to maintain hydration. However, the use of large volumes of fluid is controversial and may increase pain in the patient with an obstructed ureter by increasing hydrostatic pressure behind the stone.
3. The majority of stones will pass spontaneously within 48 hours. However, those 6 mm or greater will pass spontaneously only 10% of the time and those 4 to 6 mm 50% of the time. If pain persists or the stone does not pass, consideration of nephrostomy stent placement and urologic intervention (such as basket removal of stone) is suggested.

Renal injury from obstruction generally does not occur for at least 72 hours.

4. ***Hospital admission is required.*** If parenteral analgesics are required, if persistent vomiting prevents adequate oral hydration, if pyelonephritis is suspected, or if patient has elevated BUN and creatinine, oliguria or anuria.
5. ***Discharge.*** If the patient is discharged, he or she should be sent home with indomethacin suppositories or other NSAID (reduces need for narcotics, decreases return visits to ED) and oral narcotics (such as hydrocodone). All urine should be strained, and any stones found brought for analysis.

III. CONTINUING CARE

All patients with kidney stones should increase their daily fluid intake regardless of the composition of the stones. Analysis of the stones may identify specific preventive measures. There is good evidence that reducing the dietary intake of animal protein can reduce stone formation.

A. **Uric acid stones.** Represent 10% of stones. Should evaluate for hyperuricosuria. Allopurinol 200 to 300 mg/day inhibits uric acid synthesis and can reduce stone formation. Purines in the diet should be limited. Alkalinization of urine (oral bicarbonate 1.0 to 1.5 mEq/kg/day) will also be of some benefit.

B. **Calcium oxalate stones.** Represent 75% of all stones. Hypercalciuria is often idiopathic, but it may occur in hyperparathyroidism, sarcoidosis, and type I renal tubular acidosis (have associated non–anion gap acidosis, alkaline urine pH). Reducing sodium intake in diet can reduce hypercalciuria and stone formation. Despite "common wisdom," it is clear that *increasing and not decreasing calcium intake* leads to a reduction in stone formation by reducing oxalate absorption. Thiazide diuretics (25 to 100 mg/day) decrease calcium excretion and lead to a reduction in stone formation within 1 to 2 years. Potassium phosphate also reduces stone formation but is falling out of favor because of need for QID administration.

C. **Magnesium ammonium phosphate stones (struvite stones).** Represent 10% of all stones. Occur in the setting of high urinary pH seen in chronic urinary infections with urease-producing organisms. Antibiotics and acidification of the urine are indicated. Lithotripsy should be used to remove all visible stones from the urinary tract.

ACUTE SCROTAL PAIN AND SCROTAL MASSES

I. ACUTE SCROTAL PAIN

A. **Cause.** Generally history will indicate likely cause. Differential diagnosis includes trauma, orchitis, epididymitis, hernia, urolithiasis, or torsion of the testicle.

B. **Evaluation.**

1. ***History.*** Inquire about trauma; nature, location, and duration of pain; associated symptoms; or recent infection of urethra, bladder, prostate.
2. ***Examination.*** Localization of the painful structure is important for diagnosis. Assess for inguinal hernia, urethritis, or possible prostatitis.
3. ***Lab tests.*** Will be directed by findings on history and physical. Urinalysis should be obtained to assess for hematuria, or evidence of infection.

C. Causes.

1. ***Trauma.*** May be difficult to get accurate history if unusual sexual practices involved. Ultrasonography of scrotum and testicles can be quite useful in assessing trauma.
2. ***Urolithiasis.*** Indicated by hematuria. Often there is or has been associated flank pain. Examination will reveal normal scrotal contents.
3. ***Hernia.*** Incarcerated hernia may cause only scrotal pain. Examination may reveal the presence of bowel sounds in the scrotum. Signs of intestinal obstruction may be present. Ultrasonogram is diagnostic.
4. ***Epididymitis.*** Often a history of prior urethral symptoms. Commonly occurs in sexually active men. Culture urethral discharge and urine. Will be swelling and tenderness of the epididymis. The pain of epididymitis is often lessened by elevation of the scrotum. See Table 11-1 for treatment.
5. ***Torsion of the testicle.*** Urologic emergency, torsion present for longer than 4 to 6 hours will result in loss of the testicle. Generally present in young males after physical activity. Frequently complain of abdominal pain and nausea and may not initially notice testicular pain. Exam may be remarkable for localized tenderness of the testicle. If torsion has been present for some time, epididymis will also be swollen and tender, complicating differentiation. Cremasteric reflex will generally be absent on the affected side. Doppler scanning may be used to assess for presence of testicular artery pulses. Ultrasonography also may be useful as radionuclide scanning may. *However, in no case should urgent consultation with a urologist be delayed if torsion is clinically suspected.* Manual detorsion may be attempted (if immediate surgical evaluation is not possible) by infiltrating the spermatic cord near the external ring with 5 ml of 2% lidocaine and counterrotating the affected testicle. Viewed from below the patient's scrotum, the *patient's* right testicle would be detorsed by counterclockwise rotation, the *patient's* left by clockwise rotation.

II. PAINLESS SCROTAL MASSES

Possible causes include tumors of the testicle or spermatic cord, spermatoceles, hydroceles, varicoceles, hernias, or lipomas.

Most are painless or associated with only mild pain. Acute, severe pain should prompt evaluation, as discussed above. Occasionally tumors will have acute pain, possibly caused by hemorrhage.

A. **Varicocele.** Very common. Usual clinical presentation is adolescent or young adult male with incidentally noted swelling in left scrotum. Physical examination is generally diagnostic with varicosities palpated above and separate from testicle. Varicosities enlarge with Valsalva maneuver.
   1. ***Treatment.*** Firm scrotal support if symptomatic.
   2. ***Further evaluation and referral indicated for the following:***
      a. Large or bilateral varicocele in young adolescent. May result in inhibited growth of left or both testicles, possibly resulting in decreased function (testosterone production, spermatogenesis).
      b. Adult male who is a member of an infertile couple.
      c. New-onset varicocele in male older than 30 years (may indicate intra-abdominal process that is impeding blood return).
      d. Right-sided varicocele without concomitant left-sided varicocele.

B. **Hydrocele.** Typically presents as a gradually enlarging painless cystic structure. Can be transilluminated. Ultrasonography may be advisable because a hydrocele can be secondary to tumor.

C. **Spermatocele.** Usually asymptomatic. Firm but somewhat compressible mass located superior to and separate from the testicle in the spermatic cord. Ultrasonography can aid in diagnosis. Requires no treatment.

D. **Testicular tumor.** Generally presents in a young adult. Usually painless. Firm, nontender mass will be found on the testicle. Cannot be transilluminated. Ultrasonography will confirm location of mass. Urologic consultation required for evaluation.

RENAL FAILURE

I. ACUTE RENAL FAILURE

Sudden loss of renal function as evidenced by oliguria or anuria, increase in BUN or serum creatinine.

A. **Cause.** 75% of cases of acute renal failure are secondary to diminished renal perfusion (prerenal causes) or ATN.
   1. ***Prerenal cause:*** Diminished renal perfusion because of volume depletion, inadequate cardiac output, or volume redistribution ("third spacing" from cirrhosis, burns, nephrotic syndrome, etc.). Kidney retains sodium and fluid in attempt to increase circulating volume (and therefore renal perfusion). BUN to creatinine ratio generally >20:1.
   2. ***Renal cause.*** Glomerular (rapidly progressive glomerulonephritis), vascular (renal artery or vein thrombosis, vasculitis), or tubulointerstitial (ATN most common, see below).

3. ***Postrenal cause.*** Obstruction of the urinary tract from prostate disease, or retroperitoneal disease.

B. Diagnosis. May have urine output less than 400 ml/24 hours, elevated BUN and creatinine, or decreased creatinine clearance. A progressive daily increase in serum creatinine is diagnostic of acute renal failure.

Estimated creatinine clearance =

$$\frac{(140 - \text{Age [yr]})(\text{Body weight [kg]})}{72\ (\text{Serum creatinine [mg/dl]})}$$

1. For women, multiply this figure by 0.85.
2. May not reflect early renal damage because of compensatory hypertrophy of remaining glomeruli.
3. Normal for healthy adult is 94 to 140 ml/min for men and 72 to 110 ml/min for women.
4. The creatinine clearance normally decreases with age.

C. Differentiating the causes of renal failure.

1. ***Prerenal azotemia.*** U/P osmolality = 1 to 1.5; urine Na >40; FE_{Na} >0.04; RFI >2.
2. ***Renal azotemia (ATN).*** U/P osm >1.5; urine Na <20; FE_{Na} <0.01; RFI <1 (90% of cases).
3. ***Postrenal azotemia.*** U/P osm = 1 to 1.5; urine Na >40; FE_{Na} >0.02; RFI >2 (>90% of cases).
4. ***Glomerulonephritis.*** U/P osm 1 to 1.5; urine Na <30; FE_{Na} <0.01; RFI <1.

U/P = Urine osmolality to plasma osmolality ratio

FE_{Na} = Fractional excretion of Na = $U/P_{Na}/U/P_{creatinine}$

RFI = Renal failure index = Urine Na (mmol/L)/$U/P_{creatinine}$

These formulas apply best when there is oliguria (<500 ml/day). Factors such as diuretic use may invalidate their results.

D. Urinalysis in renal failure. If prerenal cause, generally normal UA with only hyaline casts. If ATN, may have smoky urine with dark granular casts (however, 20% may be normal). In glomerulonephritis, hematuria and proteinuria will be present.

II. ACUTE TUBULAR NECROSIS (ATN)

A. Acute renal failure resulting from renal ischemia (hypoperfusion from cardiac arrest, surgical procedures) or renal damage from toxic insults (radiocontrast material, rhabdomyolysis, aminoglycosides, etc.). Renal function generally returns to adequate level if patient survives acute phase, which usually lasts 1 to 2 weeks. Sepsis is a major cause of death in renal failure.

B. May progress from oliguric renal failure (urine output <400 ml/day) to nonoliguric renal failure, which may be manifest by massive urine output. The duration of renal failure is generally 1 day to 6 weeks (average 10 to 14 days). There is no prognostic difference; however, nonoliguric renal failure is easier to manage because of less need for stringent fluid restriction.

C. Laboratory findings. Progressive hyponatremia, hyperkalemia, azotemia (creatinine increase by 0.5 to 2.5 mg/dl/day) and acidosis.

D. Causes of ATN.

1. **Ischemic and hypoperfusion injury.** Shock, sepsis, hypoxia, hypotension, or surgery.
2. **Toxic sources.** Radiologic contrast media, heavy metals, aminoglycosides, myoglobinuria from burns, trauma, polymyositis, cisplatin, IV acyclovir, and many other drugs.

E. Evaluation. Diagnosis often apparent because of clinical history. Rule out obstructive process (ultrasonography of kidneys and ureters helpful).

1. Urinalysis may reveal renal epithelial cells, cellular casts, or may be normal.
2. See section IC above for differentiation from other causes.

F. Treatment. Maintain fluid balance and blood pressure. Dopamine, mannitol, and diuretics have not been shown to have any renal sparing effect though dopamine and diuretics (such as furosemide, bumetanide) may play a role in maintaining blood pressure and fluid balance. See below (treatment of acute renal failure) for details.

III. PRERENAL AZOTEMIA

A. Cause and diagnosis. Commonly caused by dehydration (often attributable to excessive diuretic therapy). May be secondary to decreased renal perfusion as with cardiac dysfunction or liver failure. Indicated by signs of decreased renal function with BUN elevated out of proportion to serum creatinine, often greater than 20:1.

B. Treatment.

1. Adequate intravascular volume will prevent progression to oliguric or anuric failure if it is secondary to simply inadequate volume. Unless there is hypoalbuminemia, there is no evidence that albumin is superior to crystalloids in restoring plasma volume.
2. Treat cardiac failure as per CHF in Chapter 2. In those with CHF, consider also prerenal azotemia secondary to excessive diuretic use, ACE inhibitor–induced renal failure, and use of NSAIDs.
3. If prerenal azotemia is secondary to liver failure, outcome is poor unless patient is transplant candidate.

IV. POSTRENAL AZOTEMIA

Usually caused in males by bladder outlet obstruction and is rapidly treatable with a Foley catheter. Other causes include pelvic tumors or surgical injury.

V. GLOMERULONEPHRITIS

A. Causes are legion. Include poststreptococcal glomerulonephritis, hemolytic uremic syndrome, Henoch-Schönlein purpura, collagen vascular diseases, etc.

B. Clinical presentation. Sudden-onset renal failure, hematuria, proteinuria, azotemia, and edema.

C. Diagnosis. See below section on nephrotic syndrome and nephritis.

VI. TREATMENT OF ACUTE RENAL FAILURE

A. Careful monitoring of fluid and electrolyte status. Fluids should be restricted to replacement of losses (urine output, other losses (GI), and approximately 500 ml/day for insensiblc loss). Dietary intake of K^+ and phosphates should be severely restricted. Hyperphosphatemia may be prevented by use of oral calcium carbonate or calcium acetate antacids to absorb dietary phosphates and maintain PO_4 <5.5 mg/dl. Calcium should be monitored, since it will tend to fall if phosphorus rises. Hyperkalemia should be treated as noted in Chapter 5. Fluid overload may require dialysis or diuretics, such as furosemide 20 mg IV or more.

B. Monitor acidosis. Mild to moderate metabolic acidosis should be anticipated and may be well tolerated. Severe acidosis may require oral bicarbonate solutions. These contain significant quantities of sodium.

C. Monitor carefully for signs of infection (a common cause of mortality during acute renal failure).

D. Dialysis is indicated for uremic pericarditis, severe hyperkalemia or other unmanageable electrolyte abnormality, severe acidosis, significant fluid overload, and other uremic symptoms (especially neurologic). Hemodialysis using biocompatible noncellulose membranes has been shown to improve survival.

VII. CHRONIC RENAL FAILURE (CRF)

A. Definition. Clinical syndrome of chronic compromise of renal function, which can be categorized into three major groups:

1. Inadequate renal reserve, characterized by inability to compensate for extreme water or solute loading or deprivation.
2. Renal insufficiency, characterized by elevated BUN and greatly diminished capacity for dealing with water solute fluctuations, but otherwise can maintain homeostasis.
3. Renal failure, characterized by progressive increase in BUN to the point of causing uremia, fluid, and electrolyte imbalance (GFR <6 mg/min/m^2).

B. Causes. Common causes include diabetes, hypertension, glomerulonephritis, polycystic kidney disease, obstructive uropathy, amyloidosis, etc. See section on nephritis and nephrotic syndrome for differential diagnosis (Table 11-2).

Unfortunately deterioration may continue even after initial insult resolves, perhaps because of a change in intrarenal hemodynamics.

C. **Clinical manifestation.** Early manifestations may include only nocturia because of inability to concentrate urine. Fatigue, altered mental status, peripheral neuropathy, anorexia, N&V, pruritus, may indicate uremia. Hypertension is common. Fluid and electrolyte imbalances result in varying signs and symptoms. Loss of erythropoietin and vitamin D function results in anemia and osteodystrophy. Patients may remain asymptomatic until GFR is less than 10% of normal.

D. **Laboratory diagnosis.** Generally reflected in an elevated BUN and creatinine. A 24-hour urine study will show a decreased creatinine clearance. Acidosis is usually present and so too a normochromic-normocytic anemia. Hyperkalemia and hyponatremia are often present.

E. **Preventive methods.** ACE inhibitors (specifically captopril) have been shown to decrease progression to renal failure in both diabetic and nondiabetic patients. Protein restriction may reduce progression of chronic renal disease though the data are conflicting. It seems reasonable to limit patients to 0.6 g/kg/day of protein. Blood pressure control is crucial because hypertension will accelerate renal failure.

F. **Treatment.**

1. ***Sodium and fluid hemostasis.*** Generally not a problem. The kidney maintains ability to regulate sodium until extremely late in course. Use diuretics (such as furosemide) to remove excess free water.
2. ***Potassium.*** May require potassium restriction to 2 g/day late in the course of renal failure. May develop aldosterone resistance (and therefore hyperkalemia) requiring more aggressive therapy such as fludrocortisone and potassium-binding resins. See Chapter 5 for details.
3. ***Acidosis.*** Can be treated with oral sodium bicarbonate (1.2 to 2.4 g/day) if symptomatic (lethargy, fatigue, tachypnea) or if bicarbonate <15 g/day. This will give a sodium load; so be careful in setting of CHF, etc.
4. ***Dietary restrictions.*** Required to maintain appropriate fluid and electrolyte balance. Protein restriction (20 to 25 g/day of balanced amino acid protein) can reduce acidosis and symptoms from elevated BUN. Although the data are inconsistent, protein restriction may slow disease progression.
5. ***Phosphate and calcium ions.*** Phosphate intake should be limited, and hyperphosphatemia should be treated with phosphate binders such as oral calcium acetate or calcium carbonate to prevent the development of renal osteodystrophy. Briefly, elevated phosphate results in lower serum calcium, which leads to elevated parathyroid hormone (see section on hypercalcemia in Chapter 5 for parathyroid evaluation) and resorption of calcium from bone to

TABLE 11-2
Diseases Associated with the Nephrotic Syndrome or Nephritic Urine or Proteinuria

	Approximate incidence	
	Children	Adults
PRIMARY RENAL DISEASE	**90%**	**75%**
Minimal-change disease (MCD)	65	15
Focal glomerulosclerosis (FGS)	10	15
Membranous glomerulonephritis (MGN)	5	30
Membranoproliferative glomerulonephritis (MPGN)	10	7
Others: mesangial proliferative glomerulonephritis, IgA nephropathy, rapidly progressive glomerulonephritis (RPGN)	10	3
SECONDARY DISEASE	**10%**	**25%**

Metabolic	Diabetes mellitus, amyloidosis
Immunogenic	Systemic lupus erythematosus, Henoch-Schönlein purpura, polyarteritis nodosa, Sjögren's syndrome, sarcoidosis, serum sickness, erythema multiforme
Neoplastic	Leukemias, lymphomas, Hodgkin's lymphoma, multiple myeloma, carcinoma (bronchus, breast, colon, stomach, kidney), melanoma
Nephrotoxic and drugs	Gold salts, penicillamine, NSAIDs, lithium carbonate, street heroin
Allergenic	Insect stings, snake venoms, antitoxins, poison ivy, poison oak
Infective	*Bacterial*—postinfective glomerulonephritis, vascular prosthetic nephritis, infective endocarditis, leprosy, syphilis *Viral*—hepatitis B and C, Epstein-Barr, herpes zoster, HIV *Protozoal*—malaria *Helminthic*—schistosomiasis, filariasis
Congenital nephrotic syndrome	Finnish type
Heredofamilial	Alport's syndrome, Fabry's disease
Miscellaneous	Toxemia of pregnancy, malignant hypertension

From Berkow R, editor: *The Merck manual of diagnosis and therapy*, ed 17, Rahway, N.J., 1992, Merck & Co.

maintain normal serum calcium. Avoid magnesium- and aluminum-containing preparations, since these elements tend to cause problems in those with renal failure. Supplements of vitamin D will eventually be needed. Calcitriol 0.25 to 1 µg/day generally a good choice.

6. ***Anemia.*** Generally attributable to decreased erythropoietin production in kidney. Rule out other causes such as slow GI bleed, etc. Give erythropoietin 30 to 50 units/kg SQ 3 × per week (up to 150 U/kg has been used in some studies, and dose should be adjusted to response). Several factors including adequate dialysis and control of renal failure related to hyperparathyroidism will improve the response to erythropoietin.
7. ***Bleeding.*** Can be treated with FFP or cryoprecipitate. Unique to bleeding in uremia is the use of conjugated estrogens for bleeding. A dose of 0.6 mg/kg/day for 5 days has been used.
8. ***Dialysis.*** Hemodialysis and chronic ambulatory peritoneal dialysis. Absolutely indicated for uremic pericarditis, progressive motor impairment, fluid overload not responsive to other interventions or producing CHF, severe acidosis, and hyperkalemia. Early consultation with nephrologist should be considered so that patient can become psychologically adapted to the idea of dialysis and a physician-patient relationship can be developed before the need for dialysis.
9. ***Transplantation.*** An alternative to dialysis. Decision to proceed with dialysis or transplantation requires the assistance of a nephrologist.

PROTEINURIA, NEPHROTIC SYNDROME, AND NEPHRITIC URINE

Nephrotic Urine versus Nephritic Urine

The *nephrotic* urine contains a large amount of protein but does not contain elements indicating active inflammation such as WBCs and red blood cell casts. In contrast, the *nephritic* urine is suggestive of acute renal inflammation and will contain protein, red blood cell casts, blood by dipstick, and white blood cells. The differential diagnosis can be narrowed based on whether a nephritic or nephrotic urine is present.

I. NEPHROTIC SYNDROME

A. General. Nephrotic syndrome is not a particular disease process but rather the renal manifestation of multiple underlying causes. The primary disease may be renal in origin, such as minimal-change disease, or may be a systemic illness with renal manifestations, such as diabetes mellitus with nephropathy. Nephrotic syndrome may be related to glomerulonephritis and other causes of nephritis. Once active renal disease (nephritis) is no longer ongoing (that is, burned out), the patient may end up with nephrotic syndrome and a nephrotic urine.

B. Definition. Nephrotic syndrome manifests as proteinuria of >2 to 3 g/day. Patients with nephrotic syndrome usually also manifest hypoalbuminemia, edema, and hyperlipidemia. Thrombotic events may also occur. Nephrotic syndrome may occur at any age including in children ("nil disease" most common in children).

C. Presentation.
- Anorexia, malaise edema, anasarca, or pleural effusions.
- Focal edema, especially ankles and genitalia.
- May have orthostatic hypotension and can be fluid overloaded or hypovolemic depending on what is intravascular.
- May be hypertensive, especially in those with collagen-vascular disease.
- Thrombotic phenomenon including renal vein thrombosis. Mostly caused by decreased fibrinolytic activity.
- Frothy urine secondary to proteinuria, nocturia at presentation secondary to increased vascular volume at night from fluid mobilization.

D. Laboratory findings.

1. ***Urine.***
   - Pronounced proteinuria (excretion >2 g/day).
   - Urinary protein to creatinine ratio >2.
   - Casts: hyaline, granular, waxy, or epithelial.
   - Urine Na low (<1 mmol/L).
   - K:Na ratio >1.
2. ***Blood.***
   - Hypoalbuminemia.
   - Globulins, adrenocortical hormones, or thyroid hormones may be low.
   - BUN and creatinine are variable depending on progression of renal disease.
   - Aldosterone initially high (aldosterone causes K excretion, Na retention, and hypertension).
   - Lipemia including elevated cholesterol and triglycerides. May have lipiduria.
   - Microcytic anemia from urinary loss of transferrin or poor erythropoietin production.
   - Coagulation disorders may be from loss of factors IX, XII, and thrombolytic factors (urokinase and antithrombin III) in the urine and increased serum levels of factor VIII, fibrinogen, and platelets.

E. Diagnosis. Is focused on determining underlying cause (see Table 11-2). History and associated clinical findings go a long way in making the diagnosis. Family history is very important, since many causes may be familial.

F. Work-up. Overlaps with that of glomerulonephritis. See below.

G. In children. Orthostatic proteinuria, a benign condition, is frequently found in children. In orthostatic proteinuria, protein is found only in the urine after the child has been upright and so a first morning void should be free of protein (if the bladder was emptied just before bedtime). A 24-hour urine analysis can be done with the collection being done in

2 containers–one that collects all of the urine from when the child is lying down overnight and another that collects the urine while the patient is awake and upright. Diagnostic criteria include (1) no or little protein in the first morning void, (2) not greater than a total of 1.5 g of protein in a 24-hour urine, and (3) 80% to 100% of the protein being in the specimen collected while the child is upright (fractionate collection into two 12-hour periods in separate containers). However, many physicians will make the diagnosis with only the absence of protein in the urine on the morning void.

H. **Prognosis and treatment.** Beyond the scope of this manual; treatment is generally complex and suboptimal. The exception is minimal-change disease or "nil disease." Minimal-change disease has the best prognosis, with 90% of children and 50% of adults responding to therapy. In children with a nephrotic urine *and no evidence of nephritis* an empiric trial of prednisone (1 mg/kg/day for 3 months and then tapered off) is indicated, since most will respond. If no response, hypertension, *or any other evidence of active nephritis,* further work-up is indicated. Generally a nephrology consultation should be considered before one embarks on treatment.

Glomerulonephritis and Nephritis

Discussion of specific entities is beyond the scope of this manual. However, diagnostic work-up should proceed as noted below.

Diagnosis and work-up for nephrotic syndrome, nephritis, suspected glomerulonephritis

Use clinical judgment in ordering appropriate tests. This work-up may also be appropriate for those with nephrotic syndrome and proteinuria when looking for an underlying cause. Work-up may include:

- "Minimum." CXR, CBC, screening cancer tests (as appropriate for age [see inside front and back covers] and symptoms), pursue cancer diagnosis in appropriate clinical setting (weight loss, elderly, adenopathy, back pain, etc.), other "routine" chemical analyses.
- Serum and urine protein electrophoresis and immunoelectrophoresis to detect Bence Jones protein and monoclonal gammopathy.
- Check for diabetes mellitus, amyloid, and SLE.
- Check for HBsAg (hepatitis B surface antigen). This causes up to 22% of nephrotic syndrome depending on the population.
- Family history of renal failure or deafness (Alport's nephropathy).
- Sexual history (syphilis, hepatitis B, or HIV).
- Hemoptysis (Wegener's granulomatosis, or Goodpasture syndrome).
- Paresthesias, or neurologic deficits (Fabry's disease).
- ANA or ANCA or both (Wegener's granulomatosis, other vasculitides).
- C3, C4 (low in endocarditis, status post streptococcal glomerulonephritis, lupus, membranoproliferative glomerulonephritis, or cryoglobulinemia).
- ASO and other detection for recent streptococcal infection (status post streptococcal glomerulonephritis).

- Anti–glomerular basement membrane antibodies: positive in Goodpasture syndrome.
- Cryoglobulins.
- Angiotensin-converting enzyme (ACE) or other diagnostic work-up analyte for sarcoid (see p. 150).
- Hepatitis B and C, and HIV serologic tests.
- Biopsy.

URINARY INCONTINENCE

I. GENERAL

Defined as involuntary loss of urine.

II. CAUSES

Causes of transient incontinence include delirium; infection; atrophic vaginitis or urethritis; and drugs including sedatives, hypnotics, diuretics, opiates, calcium-channel blockers, anticholinergics (antidepressants, antihistamines), decongestants, and others. Other less common causes include depression, excess urine production (diabetes, diabetes insipidus), restricted mobility, and stool impaction. Additionally, immobility may contribute to incontinence if patient is unable to get to the bathroom.

III. TYPES OF INCONTINENCE AND THEIR SPECIFIC CAUSES

A. **Urge incontinence.** Involuntary loss of urine corresponding with a sudden urge and desire to void. Associated with involuntary detrusor contractions. Causes include neurologic disorders (such as stroke, multiple sclerosis) and urinary tract infections.

B. **Stress incontinence.** Involuntary loss of urine during coughing, sneezing, laughing, or other increases in intra-abdominal pressure. Most commonly seen in women after middle age (with repeated pregnancies and vaginal deliveries), stress incontinence is often a result of weakness of the pelvic floor and poor support of the vesicourethral sphincteric unit. Another cause is intrinsic urethral sphincter weakness such as that from myelomeningocele, epispadias, prostatectomy, trauma, radiation, or sacral cord lesion.

C. **Overflow incontinence.** Involuntary loss of urine associated with overdistension of the bladder. May have frequent dribbling or be present as urge or stress incontinence. May be attributable to underactive bladder, bladder outlet obstruction (such as tumor, prostatic hypertrophy), drugs (such as diuretics), fecal impaction, diabetic neuropathy, or vitamin B_{12} deficiency.

D. **Functional incontinence.** Immobility, cognitive deficits, paraplegia, or poor bladder compliance.

IV. EVALUATION

Confirm urinary incontinence and identify factors that might contribute:

A. History including medications and provoking factors.
B. Physical including abdominal exam, pelvic exam, rectal exam, sensation in the rectal and perineal area, edema, drugs.
C. Do stress testing. Have patient cough or sneeze.
D. Urinalysis and microscopic examination of urine. Urine culture, if warranted.
E. Check postvoid residual.
F. Follow timing of incontinence. Observe patient urinating and watch for signs of straining, etc.
G. Cystometry with flow rates, etc., may be needed if cause clinically inapparent.

V. TREATMENT

Set goals and scoring system ahead of time. Most patients will respond to behavioral techniques. Most of all require structured nursing personnel input.

A. Bladder training. Need education, scheduled voiding, and rewards. Must inhibit urinating until a set time, and this set amount of time should be progressively increased. Start at 2 to 3 hours and progress upward. 12% may become entirely continent, and 75% may have a 50% reduction in incontinent episodes. Works best in urge incontinence but also may help stress incontinence.
B. Habit training. Prompt them to void when they normally would as in morning, before bed, after meals, etc.
C. Prompted voiding. Especially good in cognitively impaired individuals. Reduced incontinent episodes by 50% or so.
D. Pelvic floor exercises (Kegel exercises). Especially useful in stress incontinence. 16% cure rate and 54% improve.
E. Intermittent catheterization may also be used.
F. Drugs.

1. ***For urge incontinence, bladder spasms, detrusor instability.*** Oxybutynin (Ditropan) 2.5 to 5.0 mg QHS and increase to 10 mg TID if needed. Second-line drugs include propantheline (anticholinergic) and tricyclics antidepressants. Watch for anticholinergic side effects.
2. ***For stress incontinence.*** Phenylpropanolamine 25 to 100 mg in sustained-release form BID or pseudoephedrine 30 to 60 mg up to QID (or long-acting preparation). Helps with sphincter incompetence.
3. ***For men.*** Treating obstructive prostatic symptoms with terazosin or finasteride may be helpful.
4. ***In women.*** Estrogen may be useful for stress and urge incontinence (start with half applicator of estrogen cream every other day and increase to 1 applicator QHS if

needed or used orally as for postmenopausal use). May need surgical repair.

BIBLIOGRAPHY

AHCPR Clinical practice guideline: update guideline for urinary incontinence, Rockville, Md., 1996, Agency for Health Care Policy and Research.

Andersen JT et al: Can finasteride reverse the progress of benign prostatic hyperplasia? A two-year placebo-controlled study, *Urology* 46(5):631, 1995.

Avorn JL et al: Reduction of bacteriuria and pyuria after ingestion of cranberry juice, *JAMA* 271(10):751, 1994.

Benson G: *Priapism,* AUA Update Series, vol XV, lesson 11, Baltimore, 1996, American Urological Association, Inc.

Berkow Z et al, editors: *The Merck manual of diagnosis and therapy,* Rahway, N.J., 1992, Merck & Co.

Cardamakis E et al: Comparative study of systemic interferon alfa-2a plus isotretinoin versus isotretinoin in the treatment of recurrent condyloma acuminatum in men, *Urology,* 45(5):857-869, 1995.

Chen J, Koontz W: *Inflammatory lesions of the kidney,* AUA Update Series, vol XIV, lesson 26, Baltimore, 1996, American Urological Association, Inc.

Cordell WH et al: Indomethacin suppositories versus intravenously titrated morphine for the treatment of ureteral colic, *Ann Emerg Med* 23(2):262, 1994.

Crain EF et al: Urinary tract infections in febrile infants younger than 8 weeks of age, *Pediatrics* 86(3):363, 1990.

Curhan GC et al: A prospective study of dietary calcium and other nutrients and the risk of symptomatic kidney stones, *N Engl J Med* 328(12):833-838, 1993.

Dale DC, Federman DD, editors: *Scientific American medicine,* New York, 1996, Scientific American, Inc.

Driscoll CE et al, editors: *Handbook of family practice,* St. Louis, 1986, Mosby.

Eron LJ et al: Interferon therapy of condylomata acuminata, *N Engl J Med* 315:1059-1064, 1986.

Hannedouche T et al: Randomised controlled trial of enalapril and beta blockers in nondiabetic chronic renal failure, *Br Med J* 309:833, 1994.

Hanno PM, Wein AJ, editors: *A clinical manual of urology,* Norwalk, Conn., 1987, Appleton-Century-Crofts.

Hooton TM et al: Randomized comparative trial and cost analysis of 3-day antimicrobial regimens for treatment of acute cystitis in women, *JAMA* 273(1):41, 1995.

Ifudu O et al: The intensity of hemodialysis and the response to erythropoietin in patients with end-stage renal disease, *N Engl J Med* 334(7):420-425, 1996.

Kapoor DA et al: Use of indomethacin suppositories in the prophylaxis of recurrent ureteral colic, *J Urol* 142:1428, 1989.

Kinkaid T, Menon M: *Renal tubular acidosis,* AUA Update Series, vol XIV, lesson 7, Baltimore, 1995, American Urological Association, Inc.

Krane R et al: *Clinical urology,* Philadelphia, 1994, Lippincott.

Lewis EJ et al: The effect of angiotensin-converting-enzyme inhibition on diabetic nephropathy, *N Engl J Med* 329:1456, 1993.

Linet OI et al: Efficacy and safety of intracavernosal alprostadil in men with erectile dysfunction, *N Engl J Med* 334:873-877, 1996.

Macaluso JN et al: Priapism: review of 34 cases, *Urology* 26(3):233, 1985.

Maschio G et al: Effect of the angiotensin converting enzyme inhibitor benazepril on the progression of chronic renal failure, *N Engl J Med* 334:939-945, 1996.

Macfarlane M: *Urology,* ed 2, Baltimore, 1995, House Officer Series, Williams & Wilkins.

Mcconnell J: Clinical practice guideline N8, *Benign prostatic hyperplasia: diagnosis and treatment,* Feb 1994, U.S. Department of Health and Human Service, Public Health Service, Agency Of Health Care Policy And Research.

Millar LK et al: Outpatient treatment of pyelonephritis in pregnancy: a randomized controlled trial, *Obstet Gynecol* 86(4 Part 1):560-564, 1995.

Nairn SJ et al: Adequacy of follow-up in children diagnosed with urinary tract infections in a pediatric emergency department, *Pediatr Emerg Care* 11(3):156, 1995.

Panzer RJ et al: *Diagnostic strategies for common medical problems,* Philadelphia, 1991, American College of Physicians.

Pedrini MT et al: The effect of dietary protein restriction on the progression of diabetic and non-diabetic renal diseases: a meta-analysis, *Ann Intern Med* 124:627-632, 1996.

Preminger G: *Medical management of urinary calculus disease. Part 1: Pathogenesis and evaluation. Part 2: Classification of metabolic disorders and selective medical management,* AUA Update Series, vol XIV, lesson 5, Baltimore, 1995, American Urological Association, Inc.

Rakel RE, Conn HF, editors: *Textbook of family practice,* ed 3, Philadelphia, 1984, Saunders.

Rao DS et al: Effect of serum parathyroid hormone and bone marrow fibrosis on the response to erythropoietin in uremia, *N Engl J Med* 328(3):171-175, 1993.

Saginur R et al: Single-dose compared with 3-day norfloxacin treatment of uncomplicated urinary tract infection in women, *Arch Intern Med* 152:1233, 1992.

Sanford JP et al: *The Sanford guide to antimicrobial therapy,* Dallas, 1996, Antimicrobial Therapy, Inc.

Schlager TA et al: Explanation for false-positive urine cultures obtained by bag technique, *Arch Pediatr Adolesc Med* 149(2):170, 1995.

Sommer P et al: Analgesic effect and tolerance of voltaren and ketogan in acute renal or ureteric colic, *Br J Urol* 63(1):4, 1989.

Tanagho EA, Mcaninch JW: *Smith's general urology,* ed 14, East Norwalk, Conn., 1995, Appleton & Lange.

Thompson JF et al: Rectal diclofenac compared with pethidine injection in acute renal colic, *Br Med J* 299:1140, 1989.

Tintinalli JE et al: *Emergency medicine: a comprehensive study guide,* New York, 1996, McGraw-Hill.

Turner GM et al: Fever can cause pyuria in children, *Br Med J* 311(7010):924, 1995.

Walsh P et al: *Campbell's urology,* ed 6, Philadelphia, 1992, Saunders.

Watson AJ et al: Treatment of the anemia of chronic renal failure with subcutaneous recombinant human erythropoietin, *Am J Med* 89:432-435, 1990.

Weiss WD: Non-pharmacologic treatment of urinary incontinence, *Am Fam Physician* 44(2):7479-7586, 1991.

Wolfson AB et al: Oral indomethacin for acute renal colic, *Am J Emerg Med* 9(1):16, 1991.

Wrenn K: Emergency intravenous pyelography in the setting of possible renal colic: is it indicated? *Ann Emerg Med* 26(3):304, 1995.

12

Ophthalmology

LAURA BEATY AND ROBERT L. HERTING, JR.

BASIC EXAMINATION

I. PUPIL EXAMINATION

1. Miosis = small pupils; mydriasis = dilated pupil or pupils.
2. ***Assess pupil size, shape, reactivity, and accommodation (pupils should constrict when following finger in nasally).*** Anisocoria refers to pupils of different nerve in right and left eyes. This is normal in a portion of the population, and the patient's baseline pupil size should be established before one looks for a cause. Causes include cranial nerve III palsy (as from diabetes mellitus, multiple sclerosis), uncal herniation (patient comatose, other CNS signs and symptoms), Horner's syndrome (interruption of sympathetic innervation of eye causing miosis, ptosis, ipsilateral decreased sweating; may be secondary to lung cancer, etc.), Adie's syndrome (parasympathetic dysfunction at or distal to the ciliary ganglion from trauma, etc., leading to unilateral dilated pupil), ocular trauma or inflammation, prescription or OTC eye drops, or Argyll-Robertson pupil (pupils may be small, accommodating to near vision but not reacting to light or painful stimuli; seen with neurosyphilis or Lyme disease). Common causes of a weak reaction include the problems just listed plus optic nerve and retinal disease.
3. ***Swinging flashlight test (consensual constriction of a pupil with absent direct response).*** Used to detect relative afferent pupillary defects (that is visual loss at the eye with preserved brain function allowing consensual reflex). May be caused by optic neuritis, ischemic optic neuropathy, chiasmal area tumors, retinal artery or vein occlusion, retinal detachment, or acute angle-closure glaucoma.

II. OCULAR MOTILITY

Check six cardinal positions of gaze, corneal light reflection, and the cover test. Common causes of motility and alignment abnormalities include congenital and childhood-onset strabismus, cranial nerve palsies, orbital trauma, Graves' disease, myasthenia gravis, stroke, or brain tumor.

III. FLUORESCEIN STAINING

Moisten fluorescein paper and gently touch to inner surface of lower lid. Disrupted corneal epithelium will fluoresce under Wood's lamp or cobalt blue slitlamp. However, this may miss up to 21% of defects. A dendritic defect will be highlighted in herpes simplex keratitis.

IV. TOPICAL ANESTHETIC

Can be used to differentiate topical problems such as foreign body and corneal abrasions from deeper problems such as iritis and glaucoma. If pain resolves with topical anesthetic, this finding is suggestive of but does not prove a superficial cause.

V. SOME USEFUL DRUGS FOR:

A. **Mydriasis.** Cyclopentolate: maximal dilatation at 25 to 75 minutes, lasting 6 to 24 hours; homatropine: maximal dilatation is rapid, must be used TID or QID to maintain mydriasis; scopolamine: dilatation at about 1 hour, must be used TID to QID.
B. **Miosis.** Pilocarpine in 0.25%, 0.5%, and 1.0%. Generally needed only every day. See section on acute glaucoma, p. 524, for exception.
C. **Anesthesia.** Tetracaine 1%, proparacaine 0.5%.

THE RED EYE (Table 12-1)

I. CONJUNCTIVITIS

Conjunctival erythema caused by injection and hyperemia of tortuous superficial vessels. May be accompanied by itching, burning, or foreign-body sensation. Often discharge or drainage is present, and crusting of the eyelids may occur while sleeping. Vision is generally not affected. If particularly severe symptoms, consider gonococcal disease. If seen in a neonate, *Chlamydia* may be the culprit. Conjunctivitis may be broken down into:

A. **Viral.** Acute redness, watery discharge with foreign-body sensation. Lasts 1 to 4 days; infectious up to 2 weeks. Antibiotics are not helpful and are not indicated. Boric acid washes, which can be obtained over the counter, often provide excellent symptomatic relief. Patients should throw away eyeliner, etc., which may be infected.
B. **Bacterial.** Acute redness with purulent discharge. *Treatment*: antibiotic ophthalmic preparations (sulfacetamide sodium, erythromycin, or gentamicin drops Q2-4h or ointment Q4-6h). Avoid contact use. Refer if any evidence of corneal ulceration is noted.

TABLE 12-1
The Red Eye

	Conjunctivitis					
	Bacterial	Viral	Allergic	Corneal injury or infection	Iritis	Glaucoma
Vision	NL	NL	NL	↓ or ↓↓	↓	↓↓
Pain	–	–	–	+	+	+++
Photophobia	–	+/–	–	+	++	–
Foreign-body sensation	–	+/–	+/–	+	–	–
Itch	+/–	+/–	++	–	–	–
Tearing	+	++	+	++	+	–
Discharge	Mucopurulent	Mucoid	–	–	–	–
Preauricular adenopathy	–	+	–	–	–	–
Pupils	–	–	–	NL or small	Small	Middilated and fixed
Conjunctival hyperemia	Diffuse	Diffuse	Diffuse	Diffuse and ciliary flush	Ciliary flush	Diffuse and ciliary flush
Cornea	Clear	Sometimes faint punctate staining or infiltrates	Clear	Depends on disorder	Clear or lightly cloudy	Cloudy
Intraocular pressure	NL	NL	NL	NL	↓, NL, or ↑	↑↑

NL, Normal.

C. **Allergic.** Often a history of seasonal allergies. Watery, red, itchy eyes, without purulent drainage. *Treatment*: topical antiallergic agents (levocabastine HCl (an antihistamine), iodoxamide tromethamine (mast cell stabilizer), or ketorolac tromethamine), 1 drop four times daily. Combination decongestant-antihistamine drops may be used as well (such as Naphcon A, 2 drops QID).

II. IRITIS

Photophobia and ciliary injection of straight deep vessels radiating from the limbus. The pupil is small and poorly reactive because of inflammation. Distant vision may be impaired. On slitlamp examination, white precipitates can be visualized on the posterior surface of the cornea, and inflammatory cells in the anterior chamber appear as "dust particles." Topical anesthetic will not relieve pain. Most common is posttraumatic (that is, direct blow or corneal abrasion), but history should include questions about the presence of collagen and autoimmune diseases. Diseases commonly associated with iritis include ankylosing spondylitis, sarcoidosis, juvenile rheumatoid arthritis, lupus, Reiter's syndrome, Wegener's granulomatosis, brucellosis, leptospirosis, and Behçet's syndrome among others. Blocking pupillary sphincter and ciliary body action with a cycloplegic agent (such as 0.25% scopolamine, 2% homatropine, or 1% cyclopentolate) will reduce pain and photophobia. Topical corticosteroids are indicated to suppress inflammation, *but must be used with caution by the family physician.* Patients should be evaluated by an ophthalmologist early in the course.

III. ACUTE CLOSED-ANGLE GLAUCOMA

This is an ocular emergency requiring immediate diagnosis and treatment. Expect greatly decreased visual acuity with peripheral-field losses, orbital pain, headache, middilated fixed pupil, diffuse conjunctival hyperemia, clouded cornea, and tonometry pressures generally greater than 21 mm HG and frequently much higher. *Acute glaucoma may present as abdominal pain and vomiting, and this diagnosis should not be overlooked in those with a GI presentation. An ophthalmologist should be consulted immediately upon making the diagnosis.* Treat with acetazolamide 500 mg PO or IV followed by 250 mg Q4h with or without topical beta-adrenergic antagonists (timolol maleate 0.5% one dose) to decrease aqueous humor production. Constrict pupil with topical pilocarpine 2% one drop every 5 minutes for the first 2 hours. Vitreous humor volume can be decreased with systemic hyperosmotic agents such as mannitol 1 g/kg IV. Sedate the patient, provide adequate analgesia, and refer immediately to an ophthalmologist.

IV. CORNEAL ABRASION

A localized loss of epithelium from the cornea typically caused by foreign bodies, fingernails, or contact lenses.

A. **Symptoms.** Sudden pain and foreign-body sensation in the eye; this is relieved by topical anesthetics. There may be associated injection of the conjunctival vessels, tearing, and light sensitivity.
B. **Diagnosis.** Made by fluorescein staining. Carefully search for any remaining foreign bodies using the slitlamp and everting the lids.
C. **Treatment.** Applying topical antibiotics may reduce the risk of infection. However, aminoglycosides may reduce the rate of reepithelialization. Avoid prescribing topical anesthetics. These decrease healing and may lead to corneal epithelium breakdown. Tetanus status should be ascertained and updated, if needed. Patching "clean" abrasions and those not related to contact lens use is traditional and considered standard of care. However, evidence indicates that patching may be actually associated with a delayed healing time and increased discomfort. Patients should be advised to avoid reading, watching TV, and other "eye-intensive" activities. Short-acting cycloplegic agents (such as 0.25% scopolamine, 2% homatropine, or 1% cyclopentolate) decrease pain by helping to reduce ciliary spasm. Abrasions usually resolve within 48 hours. Close, daily follow-up care is required.
D. *Contact lens-related and "dirty" abrasions (as from dogs, contaminated foreign body) should never be patched and should be treated with an aminoglycoside antibiotic because of increased risk of* Pseudomonas *infection. Patients with contact lens–related ulcers should have an ophthalmologic consultation.*

V. SUBCONJUNCTIVAL HEMORRHAGE

Sharply demarcated area of injection resulting from the rupture of small subconjunctival vessels. Hemorrhages can result from trauma, coughing, vomiting, straining, or viral hemorrhagic conjunctivitis (adenovirus, enterovirus, coxsackievirus). Subconjunctival hemorrhage alone is self-limited and requires no treatment. *The presence of blood in the anterior chamber indicates a hyphema and requires immediate ophthalmologic referral.*

VI. HYPERTHYROIDISM MAY CAUSE CONJUNCTIVAL INJECTION

TRAUMA

I. BLUNT TRAUMA

A. **Orbital wall fracture** should be considered. Signs and symptoms may include diplopia, epistaxis, ecchymosis, crepitus, hypesthesia in the infraorbital nerve distribution, and restricted upward gaze secondary to inferior rectus entrapment. CT scan with axial and coronal cuts is necessary for definitive diagnosis. Visual impairment or globe injury warrants immediate referral.

B. **Hyphema** is the presence of blood in the anterior chamber and is typically easily visualized. Symptoms include pain, photophobia, and blurring of vision. Elevated intraocular pressure is a possible side effect and should be treated like acute angle closure glaucoma. Bed rest with elevation of the head and patching of the affected eye may prevent the frequent complication of rebleeding, but the data are unclear. Immediate ophthalmologic consultation should be obtained to determine need for surgical evacuation.

C. **Periorbital contusions** are treated with ice, head elevation, and reassurance that symptoms will resolve in 2 to 3 weeks.

II. PENETRATING TRAUMA

A. **Corneal laceration, scleral laceration, intraocular foreign body, or globe rupture.** Treatment includes placement of a shield (an inverted paper or Styrofoam cup will do) *without applying pressure to the globe*, initiation of systemic antibiotics to cover both gram-positive and gram-negative organisms (such as vancomycin and gentamicin), tetanus prophylaxis, sedation, analgesia, and urgent referral.

B. **Chemical exposure (especially alkali).** Expect to find lacrimation, blepharospasm, painful red sclera, and photophobia. Direct lavage should be done at the scene for at least 15 minutes with any water or saline solution available. To irrigate in the emergency department, instill a topical anesthetic (Pontocaine, tetracaine and others). Sweep under lids and in conjunctival cul-de-sacs to remove particulate matter. Hang IV solution bags of normal saline connected through IV tubing to an l8-gauge plastic IV catheter or a continuous-flow contact lens. For patients who cannot tolerate saline, balanced salt solution is a good, although expensive, alternative. *Lavage should be continued for at least 20 minutes by the clock.* When adequately lavaged, use fluorescein stain to evaluate for damage or residual abrasions, and use litmus paper to ensure that eye pH is neutral immediately after the lavage is completed and again 10 minutes later. This is especially crucial to document in alkali injuries. Continue to irrigate until the pH is neutral (pH = 7.4 to 7.6). Reapply ophthalmic anesthetic and apply two drops of 0.25% scopolamine, 2% homatropine, or 1% cyclopentolate for cycloplegia into the affected eye or eyes if indicated by severity of injury. This will prevent spasm of the pupil, which can cause pain. Use an antibiotic ointment. Erythromycin is a good choice. Gentamicin and other aminoglycosides inhibit corneal repair. Provide adequate oral analgesia and follow-up within 24 hours. Contact lenses should not be worn for 2 weeks. Refer immediately for any of the following: (1) acid or alkali burn of significance (that is, corneal epithelial damage, any haziness of cornea), or (2) subnormal visual acuity, severe conjunctival swelling. See all others back in 24 hours. Prescribe oral pain medications, since these are often painful injuries.

ORBIT, EYELIDS, AND LACRIMAL APPARATUS

I. ORBITAL CELLULITIS

Infection of tissues posterior to the orbital septum. Rarely seen, it is typically caused by extension of sinusitis or periorbital cellulitis; it is more likely to be seen in children than adults. Common presentation includes dull aching periocular pain, conjunctival injection, fever, symptoms of URI, violaceous swelling, and tenderness of upper and lower lids, impaired vision, and limited ocular movement. CT of orbit and sinuses is necessary for diagnosis and to rule out sinusitis, orbital subperiosteal abscess, or tumor. Treatment includes IV antibiotics to cover penicillinase-resistant bacteria (*Haemophilus influenzae* coverage is necessary in children) and both ophthalmology and otolaryngology personnel should be urgently consulted. Ceftriaxone is a good antibiotic choice.

II. PERIORBITAL CELLULITIS

Infection confined to structures anterior to orbital septum. The possibility of orbital cellulitis must always be considered. Vision is normal, and ocular movements are intact. Adults may be managed as outpatients with pencillinase-resistant antibiotics (such as amoxicillin-clavulanate) and daily examinations. Children should be hospitalized because of a strong association with bacteremia, septicemia, and meningitis.

III. DACRYOCYSTITIS AND DACRYOSTENOSIS

Inflammation of the lacrimal sac, which is usually unilateral and secondary to nasolacrimal duct obstruction.

A. **Congenital.** Generally presents by 3 to 12 weeks and generally resolves by 6 months. It can be treated by BID massaging of the lacrimal duct area. Antibiotics are used if infection develops (see below). Occasionally requires probing to open the duct.
B. **Infectious.** Mucopurulent discharge, excessive tearing, swelling, erythema, and tender swelling of the medial lower lid is seen. Gram stain of the purulent material expressed from punctum should be performed to aid in antibiotic therapy. An antistaphylococcal drug should be used either PO or IV. Daily examinations are necessary because orbital cellulitis is a possible complication. Adults may warrant referral for dacryocystorhinostomy. Surgery may be indicated if abscess develops.

IV. HORDEOLUM

A. **External hordeolum and internal hordeolum (stye).** A hordeolum is an acute infection of the ciliary follicle or accessory glands of the anterior lid margin that is generally caused by staphylococci. An external hordeolum begins at the lid margin, whereas an internal hordeolum begins in a meibomian gland. Exam reveals a painful, tender *focal mounding* of one eyelid that develops over days, often with pustule formation. Treatment includes warm compresses BID to QID as well as systemic antibiotics (an antistaphylococcal drug such as dicloxacillin, erythro-mycin); expect resolution within several days; rarely, if the hordeolum suppurates, incision and drainage is required along with antibiotics (a simple needle may be used). For an internal hordeolum, the lid must be everted to visualize the inflamed area.

B. **Chalazion.** A chalazion (*ch* is pronounced like *k*) is a chronic granulomatous inflammation of a meibomian gland that occurs after the development of an internal hordeolum. The chalazion will continue to grow, and excision or steroid injection is required for cosmetic reasons or when vision is affected.

V. BLEPHARITIS

A. **Anterior blepharitis.** Chronic bilateral inflammation of the skin, cilium follicles, or accessory glands of the eyelids. Recurrent conjunctivitis, burning, stinging, and itching of the eyelids are common complaints. The lid margins are erythematous with dry crusted areas. Treatment involves removing crusts and cleaning the lid margins with baby shampoo several times a day. Antistaphylococcal antibiotic (bacitracin or erythromycin) ointment should be applied to the lid margins twice a day.

B. **Posterior blepharitis.** Chronic bilateral inflammation of the eyelids caused by dysfunction of the meibomian glands. Inflammation and plugging of the meibomian openings occurs. Individuals with rosacea or seborrheic dermatitis of the scalp and face are especially vulnerable to this posterior form. Treatment involves warm compresses, expression of the meibomian gland secretions, and long-term systemic antibiotic therapy (tetracycline 0.5 to 1 g/day in four divided doses or doxycycline 50 to 100 mg once or twice daily.

CORNEA AND LENS

I. CORNEAL ULCERS

The result of an epithelial defect with stromal infiltration. Ulcers of the cornea appear as whitish, infiltrated areas surrounding a corneal epithelial defect. It is usually a complication of conjunctivitis, contact lens use, or corneal abrasion. Fluorescein examination will reveal the lesion. Apply topical gentamicin or tobramycin hourly and obtain immediate ophthalmology consultation.

II. OPTIC PHOTALGIA (FLASH BURNS, "WELDER'S BURNS")

Occurs as a result of exposure to ultraviolet radiation (welders, sun exposure) and generally presents several hours after the insult. Patch both eyes, bed rest, strong oral analgesia, sedation if necessary. If no reduction of symptoms is noted after 24 hours, refer. Topical analgesics produce slow healing and may lead to additional injury.

RETINA

I. RETINAL DETACHMENT

The separation of the neurosensory retinal layer from its underlying pigmented epithelium. Patients will experience some degree of visual loss and may complain of cloudy vision, floaters, flashes of light, or a black curtain across their vision. Risk factors include aging, myopia, eye surgery, inflammation, trauma, a prior retinal detachment, or a family history of retinal detachment. Funduscopic exam reveals a gray or opaque retina instead of the normal pink color. The arterioles and venules may appear dark, and floaters may be visualized. Retinal detachment is an ocular emergency, and prompt surgical intervention is necessary.

II. RETINAL VASCULAR OCCLUSION

May involve either retinal arterial occlusions (resulting from embolism or thrombosis), or venous occlusions (resulting from thrombosis). Either presents as painless monocular vision loss, with arterial occlusion occurring suddenly and venous occlusion causing vision to decrease over hours. The patient may experience transient episodes of blindness before the event.

A. **Retinal arterial occlusion.** On ophthalmoscopic exam, a small occlusion produces a flame-shaped hemorrhage or a cotton-wool spot; a large occlusion produces a pale retina and a "cherry red spot" in the area of the macula. Intermittent digital pressure should be applied to the globe in an attempt to dislodge the embolus. Increasing the P_{CO_2} to dilate the artery can be attempted if one has the patient breathe into a paper bag or inhale carbogen. Urgent consultation should be obtained.

B. **Retinal vein occlusion.** Ophthalmoscopic exam reveals a "blood-and-thunder optic fundus"–massive hemorrhage covering the retinal surface and dilated veins. There is no immediate treatment for retinal vein occlusion, and the deficits are often reversible. Look for a cause including hyperviscosity, hypertension, glaucoma, and diabetes. These patients need to be followed by an ophthalmologist, since many will develop neovascularization of the iris or retina.

OPTIC NERVE AND VISUAL PATHWAY

Strabismus and estropia

Ocular misalignment, affecting 4% of children, causing amblyopia (a vision loss that is uncorrectable by refractive lenses), reduced stereovision, and a deformed appearance. It is described according to the direction of the misalignment: *esotropia* refers to an inturning of the eye; *extropia*, an outward turning of the eye; and *hypertropia*, an upturning of the eye.

It may also be categorized as paralytic or nonparalytic depending on whether the involved eye moves at all. Paralytic strabismus should be suggestive of the possibility of a brainstem lesion. Amblyopia secondary to strabismus is correctable if treatment is begun by 3-4 years of age. Once 6 to 7 years is reached, vision loss is generally permanent.

A. Predominant causes in adulthood include cranial-nerve palsies, ocular myopathies, and myasthenia gravis. Consider MS, diabetes, etc.

B. To determine misalignment, look at flashlight reflection on cornea when the patient looks in all directions. The light should be reflected on the same portion of the cornea bilaterally (that is, light reflects off center of cornea bilaterally when child looks forward). Alternatively, use the cover test. Cover each eye in turn as child looks at an object about 20 feet away. When the eye is covered, the uncovered eye should not move in a normal individual. In those with strabismus, the uncovered eye will move to focus properly on the object being looked at.

C. The four common childhood forms are:

1. ***Strabismus of visual deprivation.*** Often develops when clear vision is interrupted in one or both eyes. The most serious underlying causes are retinoblastoma and optic nerve or chiasmal tumors. *Any strabismus in which there is visual loss at the onset of strabismus must be investigated immediately.*
2. ***Pseudostrabismus.*** Eyes are functioning well, but infant *appears* to have strabismus because of exaggerated nasal skin and lids.
3. ***Esotropia.***
   a. *Infantile esotropia (also known as congenital esotropia) (nonparalytic)– 20%.* An idiopathic form that is present at birth or develops in the first months of life. If it is intermittent, it should resolve by 6 months of age and does not need to be investigated before this age. Generally no systemic findings. If it is constant, it should be investigated immediately, since it is suggestive of a paralytic cause. Treat by patching the normal eye. Permanent visual loss may occur if not treated by 4 years of age.
   b. *Accommodative esotropia–45% to 50%.* Occurs in children who have a hyperopic refractive error and must therefore accommodate to see clearly. Begins as intermittent and then becomes permanent as vision gets worse. As part of this accommodative effort, convergence is triggered, and esotropia may develop. This usually first appears between 6 months to 7 years of age (2 years average) but may appear as early as 2 month of age. Treat with the use of refractive lenses.
   c. *Nonaccommodative esotropia.* Results as a defect of vision in one eye generally as a result of unequal refrac-

tive errors. May also be attributable to cataract formation or corneal scars.

D. Treatment may be surgical for muscle imbalance, use of refractive lenses, or patching the normal eye to allow the affected eye to regain strength and vision.

BIBLIOGRAPHY

Berkow R et al, editors: *The Merck manual of diagnosis and therapy*, ed 17, Rahway, N.J., 1992, Merck & Co.

Chawla HB: *Ophthalmology*, New York, 1993, Churchill Livingstone.

Handler JA, Ghezzi KT: Emergency treatment of the eye, *Emerg Med Clin North Am* 13:521-699, 1995.

Hulbert MFG: Efficacy of eyepad in corneal healing after corneal foreign body removal, *Lancet* 337(8742):643, 1991.

Jampel HD: Questions and answers: patching for corneal abrasions, *JAMA* 274:1504, 1995.

Janda AM: Ocular trauma: triage and treatment, *Postgrad Med* 90:51-60, 1991.

Kirkpatrick JNP et al: No eye pad for corneal abrasion, *Eye* 7:468, 1993.

Klein BR, Sears ML: Consultation with the specialist: eye injury, *Pediatr Rev* 13:127-128, 1992.

Pederson JE: Glaucoma: a primer for primary care physicians, *Postgrad Med* 90:41-48, 1991.

Silverman H et al: Treatment of common eye emergencies, *Am Fam Physician* 45:2279-2287, 1992.

Sklar DP et al: Topical anesthesia of the eye as a diagnostic test, *Ann Emerg Med* 18(11):1209, 1989.

Tintinalli JE et al: *Emergency medicine: a comprehensive study guide*, New York, 1996, McGraw-Hill.

Trobe JD: *The physician's guide to eye care,* San Francisco, 1993, American Academy of Ophthalmology.

Weinstock FJ, Weinstock MB: Common eye disorders: six patients to refer, *Postgrad Med* 99(4):107-117, 1996.

Weinstock FJ, Weinstock MB: Common eye disorders: six patients to treat, pitfalls to avoid, *Postgrad Med* 99(4):107-117, 1996.

13

Dermatology

Robert L. Herting, Jr.

PRURITUS

I. OVERVIEW

Physiologic pruritus is a mild itch sensation caused by trivial stimuli. Moderate to severe itchy sensations, which cause damage and interfere with well-being, are termed "pathologic pruritus." Pruritus is mediated by histamine, prostaglandins, acetylcholine, kinins, and proteases. Common "itch spots" are located in warm areas where sweat is retained, especially the groin, foot, and scalp. Pruritus may occur spontaneously or be precipitated by the presence of chapped, dry skin, retained sweat, or psychologic factors such as anxiety or depression.

II. ETIOLOGY

A. Cutaneous causes.

1. ***Surface causes.***
   a. *Most common irritants.* Fiberglass, wool, foreign bodies, insect bites.
   b. *Infestations.* Scabies, mites, lice (pediculosis).
   c. *Bites.* Mosquitoes.
   d. *Other.* Lichen planus, nodular prurigo, dermatitis herpetiformis, eczema.
2. ***Dermatoses.*** Fungal, bacterial, viral, herpes, miliaria.

B. Systemic causes.

1. ***Drugs.***
   a. *Allergic reactions.* Penicillin, sulfa drugs, etc.
   b. *Vasoactive drugs.* Nicotinic acid, caffeine, alcohol.
   c. *CNS drugs.* Morphine, cocaine, amphetamines, codeine.
2. ***Endocrinopathy.*** Hypothyroidism, hyperthyroidism, diabetes mellitus, diabetes insipidus, hyperparathyroidism secondary to chronic renal failure.
3. ***Hepatic disease.*** Obstructive biliary disease, cholestasis.

4. ***Malignancy.*** Hodgkin's disease, polycythemia rubra vera, leukemia, mycosis fungoides, Sézary syndrome, visceral neoplasia, carcinoid syndrome, multiple myeloma.
5. ***Slowly progressive, chronic renal failure.***
6. ***Infection.*** Trichinosis, onchocerciasis, echinococcosis, focal infection.
7. ***Miscellaneous.*** Gout, iron-deficiency anemia, primary amyloidosis, beriberi.
8. ***Pregnancy.***

C. **Psychogenic causes.** Secondary to psychosis, anxiety, or depression.
1. Delusions of parasitosis.
2. Psychogenic pruritus.
3. Neurotic excoriation.

III. DIAGNOSIS

History should include details about (1) any skin lesions preceding the pruritus; (2) history of weight loss, fatigue, fever, malaise; (3) any recent stress emotionally; and (4) recent medications and travel. Physical examination with emphasis on the skin and its appendages–xerosis, excoriation, lichenification, hydration. Laboratory tests as suggested by the PE, which may include CBC, ESR, fasting glucose, renal or liver function tests, hepatitis panel, thyroid tests, stool for parasites, CXR.

IV. TREATMENT

Treat systemic disorder. Mild pruritus may respond to nonpharmacologic measures (such as avoiding irritants, using cool water compresses, trimming the nails, behavior therapy). Systemic symptomatic treatment includes H_1-blockers such as diphenhydramine or hydroxyzine, H_2-blockers such as cimetidine or ranitidine, tricyclic antidepressants (particularly doxepin HCl and amitriptyline HCl), and as a last resort oral prednisone. Topical symptomatic treatments include moisturizers, emollients, tar compounds, topical corticosteroids, topical anesthetics such as benzocaine or dibucaine, and pramoxine HCl (alone or combined with menthol, petrolatum, or benzyl alcohol). Doxepin 5% cream (Zonalon) was recently introduced for treatment of pruritus. It has a low potential for sensitization and is better tolerated than oral form. It can be used as monotherapy for acute pruritus or as an adjunct to corticosteroids in chronic conditions producing a steroid-sparing effect. Other treatments include localized ultraviolet B phototherapy or intralesional injections of corticosteroid.

SKIN INFECTIONS

I. BACTERIAL INFECTIONS

A. **Impetigo.** Usually caused by group A hemolytic streptococci or coagulase-positive *Staphylococcus aureus.* Appear as redness, thin yellowish crusts, and even bullae, which may be localized or widespread on the skin and develop over days. Itching, pain, and tenderness may occur. Moderately contagious. Treatment is with mupirocin 2% ointment BID or systemic antibiotics (dicloxacillin 500 mg QID × 10 days, cephalexin 500 mg QID × 10 days, or erythromycin 500 mg QID × 10 days), daily bathing with antibacterial soap, and attention to personal hygiene. Need to monitor for the development of poststreptococcal glomerulonephritis.

B. Ecthyma. Considered a deeper extension of impetigo with the same cause, except it may also be caused by *Pseudomonas* organisms. It is characterized by a hemorrhagic crust with erythema or induration that develops over weeks. Treatment includes systemic antibiotics (see 1A above) as well as débridement of the epidermis, which becomes necrotic. Scars may occur after healing.

C. Cellulitis. Usually caused by group A beta-hemolytic streptococci, it is a suppurative inflammation of the dermis and of subcutaneous tissue. Usually follows trauma or underlying dermatosis, and there is moderate local erythema, tenderness, warmth, and tenseness. Area can become indurated, and frequently streaks of lymphangitis can be seen with involvement of the regional lymph nodes. Systemic symptoms are common, and bacteremia and septicemia may follow. Treatment is with systemic antibiotics (if mild, dicloxacillin or cephalexin 500 mg QID × 7 to 10 days or if severe, nafcillin 1.5 g IV Q4h or vancomycin 1.5 g per day initially for a couple of days and then switch to oral form) and the application of local heat, elevation, and immobilization. For necrotizing fasciitis and synergistic gangrene, early wide surgical excision and débridement is necessary in addition to IV antibiotics.

D. Folliculitis (including sycosis barbae [barber's itch], pseudofolliculitis, and hot-tub folliculitis). A common problem with predisposing factors such as maceration, friction, and the use of irritant chemicals. Usually caused by *S. aureus* but occasionally *Klebsiella, Pseudomonas* (hot-tub folliculitis), *Enterobacter* or *Candida albicans* are the causative agents. Appears as a pustule with a central hair (follicle) with or without any surrounding erythema. Scarring may occur with destruction of the hair follicle with severe infections. Tenderness, itching, and pain may occur. Treatment includes avoidance of inciting agents, antiseptic soap washes, and, in severe cases, topical or systemic antibiotics such as dicloxacillin or erythromycin 500 mg QID × 7 to 10 days and mupirocin 2% ointment topically. Complications can include cellulitis, furunculosis, and alopecia.

E. Furuncle (boil). An acute, localized perifollicular abscess of the skin and subcutaneous tissue caused by coagulase-positive

S. aureus resulting in a red, hot, very tender inflammatory nodule that exudes pus from one opening. A carbuncle is an aggregate of connected furuncles and characteristically is painful and has several pustular openings. This can be an acute or chronic problem with lesions commonly on areas of friction such as buttocks, axillae, breasts, and the nape of the neck. Treatment involves systemic antibiotics (see 1D above), local heat, and rest. Incision and drainage is generally required. Prevention is often difficult. Improved personal hygiene, use of antibacterial soaps, frequent hand washing, daily bathing, and change of clothing are important. Elimination of carrier states in the nose and perineum by the use of topical and systemic antibiotics is often possible.

II. VIRAL INFECTIONS

A. Warts (caused by the human papillomaviruses). The lesions are most common on the hands, feet, and face. They are infectious and autoinoculable. Common in children, the elderly, or in patients with immunologic deficiencies or atopic dermatitis. Treatment is with mild destructive chemicals (salicylic and lactic acid preparations), liquid nitrogen therapy, or electrodesiccation. Recurrences are common (25%). Cicatrix caused by treatment may be painful and is often confused with persistence of the wart, especially on the sole of the foot.

B. Herpes simplex viruses types I and II are DNA viruses. The early lesions are multiple, 1 to 2 mm in diameter, yellowish, clear vesicles on an erythematous base. The vesicles can ulcerate and become quite painful. Classic type I herpes occurs around the mouth, and type II occurs on the genitalia, but either type I or type II can occur anywhere on the skin. Diagnosis can be made from the clinical appearance, the serologic reaction in acute and convalescent sera for primary infections. Tzanck smear (Wright's stain of material obtained from the base of the lesion showing multinucleated giant cells), biopsy, or viral culture. A prodrome of pain or discomfort or tingling is often reported a week to 10 days before the lesions are seen. Treatment is symptomatic with cool compresses, analgesics, and topical drying agents (such as Burrow's solution) for the oozing, weeping stages. Acyclovir has only a modest effect on recurrent genital herpes and does not seem to influence subsequent episodes; it is thus not recommended for therapy for recurrent attacks in the immunologically competent host. It may be indicated in persons who experience frequent, severe recurrences with complications. Some clinical infection syndromes are listed below:

1. ***Gingivostomatitis.*** Occurs periorally in children and young adults.

2. ***Keratoconjunctivitis.*** Ophthalmology consultation is warranted. Usually heals without scarring.
3. ***Vulvovaginitis.***
4. ***Herpes gladiatorum.*** Occurs on the head, neck, or shoulder. Common in wrestlers.
5. ***Eczema herpeticum.*** Occurs in those with underlying skin disorders, most commonly in atopic dermatitis. It occurs more frequently in children than in adults. Consists of *disseminated* umbilicated vesicles confined to eczematous skin, which evolve into punched-out erosions that may become confluent.
6. ***Hepatoadrenal necrosis and encephalitis.***
7. ***Herpetic whitlow (herpetic paronychia).*** Occurs on distal portion of fingers.
8. ***Cold sores.***

C. Herpes zoster (shingles). Reactivation of latent virus present in the sensory ganglia. Classic description is that of grouped vesicles on an erythematous base in one dermatome. Thoracic nerve dermatomes are most commonly involved followed by the major branches of the trigeminal nerve. Symptoms are pain, dysesthesia, and pruritus. Healing requires 2 to 3 weeks, and the afflicted persons are infectious until the lesions have crusted over. Persons of any age can be affected, but the disease is more common and more severe in the elderly. Diagnosis is by clinical presentation, though Tzanck smear, biopsy, and viral culture may be performed. Treatment is oral acyclovir, 800 mg 5 times per day, which is effective if treatment is initiated within 2 days of the onset of the rash. Acyclovir is very effective for pain relief. Alternatively, famciclovir 500 mg PO TID for 7 days can be used and may be more effective at preventing postherpetic neuralgia. Capsaicin creams can be used for pain relief after the lesions have healed. Amitriptyline 25 to 150 mg QHS may be useful in the treatment of postherpetic neuralgia. For recurrent herpes zoster, particularly if more than one dermatome is involved, consider a work-up for malignancy or other causes of immunosuppression.

D. Molluscum contagiosum. Caused by a DNA virus. Appear as pearly papules up to 5 mm in diameter having a central dimple. Multiple lesions are usually present. The central core (molluscum body) can be expressed with a blade. The lesions are infectious, and autoinoculation is common. Children are most commonly affected. Spontaneous resolution may occur, but there is often an eczematous reaction before its resolution. Treatment can be limited to simple superficial curettage without anesthesia. The removal of the molluscum body, application of 50% trichloroacetic acid, or liquid nitrogen cryotherapy are equally efficacious.

III. FUNGAL INFECTIONS

A. Candidiasis. Caused by *Candida albicans.* Seen as thrush (infants and immunosuppressed; see Chapters 10 and 16 respectively), diaper dermatitis, perineal infections, and intertriginous dermatitis. Diagnosis is by clinical exam, and microscopic examination of skin scraping in 10% KOH reveals yeast forms and budding hyphae. Treatment of choice miconazole 2% cream BID to affected areas for superficial fungal infections. See Chapter 7 for vaginal candidiasis. Chronic mucocutaneous involvement can be treated with ketoconazole 200 to 600 mg PO daily (alternatives itraconazole or fluconazole). Multifocal invasive disease requires intravenous amphotericin B. Persons who present with recurrent infections should have an investigation of other causes such as diabetes mellitus, hypoparathyroidism, Addison's disease, malignancies, HIV. Use of steroids and antibiotics is also a predisposing factor.

B. Dermatophytoses (tinea). The fungi belonging to the genera *Trichophyton, Microsporum,* and *Epidermophyton* infect the stratum corneum of epidermis, hair. and nails. Commonly referred to by the locus of infection, that is, tinea unguis (nails), tinea pedis (foot, athlete's foot), tinea cruris (perineum, jock itch), tinea corporis (body, ringworm), and tinea capitis (scalp and hair). Lesions can appear as grayish, scaling patches that can be quite pruritic and may lead to autoinoculation or scalp alopecia. Skin scraping in 10% KOH will demonstrate fungal hyphae. Infected hairs when examined under Wood's light will fluoresce a green-yellow color. Treatment is as follows:

1. ***Tinea corporis (body, ringworm), tinea cruris (perineum, jock itch), tinea pedis (foot, athlete's foot).*** Topical tolnaftate (Tinactin) (OTC) or clotrimazole (Lotrimin) TID until clear and then 1 to 2 weeks longer.
2. ***Tinea capitis (scalp and hair).*** Micronized griseofulvin is usually used for up to 4 to 8 weeks. Adjunctive therapy includes selenium sulfide shampoo q2-3 days.
3. ***Tinea unguis, or onychomycosis (nails).*** Griseofulvin 500 mg BID for a period of 4 to 6 months or itraconazole 200 mg BID for 4 months (1 week on; 3 weeks off); latter regimen is very expensive. An alternative is terbinafine 250 mg PO QD for 12 weeks or BID for 1 week of the month for 3 or 4 months.

C. Pityriasis (tinea) versicolor. Appears as slightly pigmented superficial tan scaling plaques of various sizes, primarily on the neck, trunk, and proximal area of the arms. With sun exposure, the infected regions do not tan and appear hypopigmented. Usually caused by *Malassezia furfur (Pityrosporum orbiculare).* Diagnosis is by clinical exam and KOH preparations of skin scraping. Treatment can be with topical miconazole 2% cream twice daily or washing with zinc or selenium shampoos daily for 2 to 3 weeks.

Although not FDA approved, ketoconazole 400 mg in a single dose orally is 97% effective in adults. Have patients exercise to a sweat and not shower for 2 to 4 hours.

IV. PEDICULOSIS

Two species of lice affect humans: *Pediculus humanus (capitis* or *corporis)* and *Phthirus pubis*. Sensitization to louse saliva and antigens results in clinical manifestations.

A. Pediculosis capitis (infestation by head lice). Seen primarily in preschoolers and early elementary school ages but it occurs in all ages and socioeconomic classes (however, low incidence in blacks). Spread by direct contact or on fomites (helmets, combs, etc.). *Diagnosis:* pruritus; erythematous papules usually on occiput, postauricular region, and nape of the neck; lice; and nits (eggs firmly attached to hair shaft ~1 cm from scalp. *Differential diagnosis:* seborrhea, psoriasis, tinea capitis, impetigo.

B. Pediculosis corporis (infestation by body lice). Live in clothing or bedding and not on people. Seen primarily in lower socioeconomic class. The louse bites at night and leaves pruritic vesicles or papules (especially in axillae, groin, and truncal areas). Diagnosis by examination of clothes to find nits or lice.

C. Pediculosis pubis (infestation by pubic lice). Transmitted by intimate contact. *Diagnosis:* pubic or anogenital pruritus, and lice or nits found especially in the pubic hair but also in trunk, beard, eyelashes, or axillae. Often associated with additional STDs.

D. Treatment for all the above by a pediculicide.

1. Treat all sexual partners and household members simultaneously.
2. Wash all bedding, clothes, towels, and hats in hot water and a hot dryer.
3. If eyelashes or eyebrows are infested, avoid a pediculicide in those areas. Instead apply petrolatum 5 times a day until clear. Remove nits with forceps.
4. Pruritus may last for several weeks after successful treatment.
5. ***For head lice or crabs.*** Permethrin (Nix) 1% cream rinse is drug of choice applied to scalp after shampooing, left on for 10 minutes, and then rinsed off. *Alternative:* lindane 1% shampoo (Kwell, Scabene). Wash all linens in hot water. Avoid in infants, since may be neurotoxic.
6. ***For body lice.*** Use pyrethrum with piperonyl butoxide (RID) lotion over the whole body and in bath; wash off after 10 minutes. Re-treat in 7 to 10 days.

V. SCABIES

A. Overview. Caused by mite, *Sarcoptes scabiei,* that burrows in the skin. Most common in children but found in all ages.

Usually transmitted by person-to-person transmission but may be picked up from bedding, clothes, etc.

B. Diagnosis. Characterized by linear burrows (pathognomonic), papules, or nodules with or preceded by intense pruritus, especially at night. Secondary findings include excoriations, crusting, eczematous plaques, and impetigo. In older children and adults, areas of involvement are webs of fingers, axillae, flexures of arms and wrists, belt line, and areas around the umbilicus, nipples, genitals, and lower buttocks. In infants, palms, soles, head, and neck are involved. Confirm with scraping of lesion with scalpel blade placed on slide with mineral oil and look for mites, ova, or fecal pellets.

C. Treatment. Permethrin cream 5% (Elimite) is drug of choice applied head to toe at bedtime and washed off in morning (8 to 14 hours). Alternative is lindane lotion 1% (Kwell) applied to cool, dry skin at bedtime, washed off in morning, and repeated in 1 week. Neither should be used in infants <2 months of age or in pregnant or nursing women; instead use precipitated sulfur (6%) in petroleum applied for three consecutive nights. Family members should be treated even if symptomatic. Bed linens and clothing should be washed in hot water (>120° F) or stored in tightly sealed bags for 1 week. Recently, Meinking et al. reported the use of a single dose of ivermectin 100 mg as effective treatment for scabies, but this is not an approved indication.

ACNE

I. OVERVIEW

Acne commonly begins in adolescence with stimulation of the sebaceous glands by sex hormones, primarily androgens. Can be aggravated by drugs, steroids, stress, cosmetics, comedogenic agents, picking, and squeezing. The role of dietary factors has been exaggerated.

Acne has a predilection for the face, chest, and back. Lesions progress through stages of closed comedones (whiteheads), open comedones (blackheads), pustules, papules, nodules, (cysts), and atrophic and hypertrophic scars. In females with severe acne, consider polycystic ovarian disease, “congenital” adrenal hyperplasia (see Chapter 10), or Cushing’s disease. Consider obtaining plasma-free testosterone levels, dehydroepiandrosterone sulfate levels, or other work-up as appropriate.

II. TYPES OF ACNE AND THEIR TREATMENT

A. Comedones.

1. Appear as whiteheads and blackheads (closed and open comedones respectively).

2. ***Treatment.*** With topical agents and it takes a minimum of 2 weeks to show any improvement. Patient education is important, since attempts to extrude blackheads or pustules may lead to deeper, potentially scarring lesions.
   a. Tretinoin (Retin-A) is the treatment of choice. Begin nightly application of 0.025% cream or 0.01% gel and increase concentration as necessary and as tolerated. Usually requires 3 to 5 months of therapy.
   b. Benzoyl peroxide, available in 2.5%, 5%, and 10% strengths as lotions and gels, should be applied frequently enough (QD to BID) to produce drying and even scaling but without significant irritation.
   c. Can alternate benzoyl peroxide in the morning with topical tretinoin at bedtime.
   d. Despite its popularity, scrubbing the skin roughly is contraindicated.

B. Papulopustular.

1. Have a significant inflammatory component with inflamed papules and pustules.
2. ***Treatment.*** As listed above with the addition of antibiotics. As the inflammation decreases, the antibiotics can be tapered and discontinued.
   a. For less severe cases, use topical erythromycin 2% to 4% solution, gel, or ointment applied BID; clindamycin 1% solution, gel, or lotion; or tetracycline 4% applied BID.
   b. Severe cases require the use of systemic antibiotics. Tetracycline or erythromycin 500 mg to 1 g daily, or minocycline 100 to 200 mg daily, must be taken for at least 6 weeks before efficacy can be ascertained. With improvement, the dose can be tapered gradually. Depending on the patient, maintenance therapy may be continued or therapy may be discontinued. *Do not administer tetracycline to pregnant women or children under 12 years of age.*

C. Nodulocystic.

1. Manifested by comedones, inflammatory papules or pustules, and deep, inflamed nodules and cysts. Can result in scarring. Hypertrophic scars often form on the chest and back.
2. ***Treatment.*** There are two modalities in addition to the regimens previously mentioned.
   a. Injection of enough corticosteroid, triamcinolone 5 mg/ml, to cause the cyst to blanch. Some recommend needle drainage of the cyst first.
   b. Oral isotretinoin (Accutane), 0.5 to 2 mg/kg/day with meals for a 4 to 5 month course, is usually highly effective but expensive. It is absolutely contraindicated in pregnancy; thus a negative pregnancy test must be

obtained within 2 weeks of initiating treatment, and contraception must be used from 1 month before to 1 month after therapy. Careful monitoring of liver function tests and serum lipid levels is required. Monitor for side effects as well (such as dry eyes, chapped lips, epistaxis, pruritus, alopecia, scaling on the palms and soles, inability to wear contacts, and pseudotumor cerebri).

c. Other therapies in consultation with a dermatologist include (1) estrogen (in the form of an oral contraceptive) for girls older than 16 years of age unresponsive to antibiotics and not a candidate for Accutane, (2) low-dose dexamethasone or prednisone for a patient with evidence of androgen excess, or (3) comedo extraction.

III. OTHER ACNEFORM ERUPTIONS

A. Acne in the pediatric population.

1. ***Acne neonatorum.*** Positive family history; occurs in children less than 3 months of age; usually self-limited.
2. ***Acne of infancy.*** Occurs in infants between 3 months and 2 years of age, and there is usually a positive family history; think of comedogenic agents, virilization, and candidiasis.

B. Acne secondary to chemical exposure (acne venenata, chloracne). Acne caused by chemical agents by sufficient contact in sensitive individuals. Good prognosis with avoidance. Example are chlorinated hydrocarbons, insoluble cutting oils (impure paraffin-oil mixtures), and other petroleum products (crude petroleum, heavy coal tar distillates), dioxin.

C. Acne medicamentosa. Induction or aggravation of preexisting acne. Agents include phenobarbital, corticosteroids, isoniazid, iodides and bromides, and vitamins D and B_{12}.

PAPULOSQUAMOUS DISEASES

I. PSORIASIS

A common skin disorder affecting over 1% of the population. It results from excess proliferation of keratinocytes. Primary lesions are erythematous papules and plaques with gray-white, silvery scale. It usually occurs on extensor surfaces (elbows, knees, lumbosacral areas) and frequently only on the scalp (where it is difficult to differentiate from seborrheic dermatitis). Psoriasis does manifest Koebner's phenomenon (lesions may appear at sites of trauma, such as an excoriation, tattoo, burn). Removal of the scale often causes tiny bleeding points (Auspitz's sign). Nails manifest pitting and stippling, and distal and lateral onycholysis is common. Pruritus is a common complaint, and family history is present in two thirds of the cases. Psoriatic arthritis can affect the

DIP and MCP joints, but rheumatoid factor is usually not present. Topical corticosteroids can be helpful, as can keratolytics such as salicylic acid and moisturizers. Calcipotriene (Dovonex) 0.005% applied topically BID is a new topical treatment for mildly to moderately severe psoriasis (but is not used on the face or groin where it may cause irritant dermatitis). The efficacy of calcipotriene is comparable to midpotency topical corticosteroids in efficacy; however, it does not cause skin atrophy or tachyphylaxis. Treatment with topical crude coal tar formulas and daily exposure to ultraviolet radiation may also be used. Careful patient monitoring is recommended, since it can increase serum calcium. Severe forms of psoriasis should be referred to a dermatologist for other forms of treatment including etretinate (Tegison), cyclosporin A (Sandimmune), methotrexate, hydroxyurea, or ultraviolet radiation therapy. Moreover, studies look promising using a new IL-2 fusion protein treatment.

II. NONCONFLUENT PAPULES

A. **Lichen planus.** A pruritic eruption in which violaceous, flat, polygonal papules occur in linear, annular, or confluent groups. Lesions of the mucous membranes appear as whitish, reticulated, lacy plaques of the buccal mucosa, which may be painful (Wickham's striae). Lichen planus exhibits Koebner's phenomenon (lesions may appear at sites of trauma, such as an excoriation, tattoo, burn). Treatment of this chronic, idiopathic, self-limited disease is supportive with topical corticosteroids (anti-inflammatory), systemic antihistamines (antipruritic), and occasionally intralesional corticosteroids (help to flatten large plaques). Short doses of alternate-day prednisone will temporarily suppress active lesions.

B. **Pityriasis rosea.** Characterized by occurrence of a herald patch that is larger than other lesions. It is usually a bright red, round or oval, sharply demarcated plaque (2 to 5 cm) with scaly margins and central clearing. A few days to weeks later a generalized reaction occurs, frequently in a "fir-tree" pattern. Pruritus may be severe. Treatment is not indicated, since the eruption is self-limited (usually clears in 4 to 10 weeks and seldom recurs). Oral antihistamines (Atarax, Vistaril, Benadryl) are used to alleviate the itching, and a mild hydrocortisone cream may soothe the skin. Must differentiate this from secondary syphilis.

VESICULOBULLOUS LESIONS

I. VESICULAR DISEASE.

Dermatitis herpetiformis lesions consist of extremely itchy, tense, grouped herpetiform vesicles usually 3 to 6 mm in diameter and occurring in a distinctive distribution over the elbows, knees, buttocks, upper back, and posterior scalp. Because of excoriation, round crusts are often the only visible sign of the disease. The gold standard for diagnosis is biopsy with direct immunofluorescence of lesional or normal skin showing IgA deposits, usually in a granular pattern at the tips of dermal papillae. About 90% of patients will have evidence of gluten-sensitive enteropathy on small-bowel biopsy. Both skin and bowel disease regress after several months of a gluten-free diet; however, this diet is difficult to maintain. Thus the mainstay of treatment is lifelong dapsone 100 mg PO QD (pruritus and new lesions stop in 24 hours). CBC should be monitored every 1 to 2 weeks for the first 3 months to detect agranulocytosis. Liver function tests should be performed regularly to detect idiosyncratic dapsone-induced hepatitis.

II. BULLOUS DISEASES

A. Bullous pemphigoid. A subepidermal disease with blisters that are tense, round, well defined, and usually occurring on a pink, edematous, inflamed base. Before the bullae form, severely itchy urticarial plaques may be present for several weeks. Flexural areas and the lower legs are the sites of predilection. Diagnosis is confirmed by biopsy of perilesional skin, which reveals many eosinophils and neutrophils in and below the bulla at the dermoepidermal junction. On electron microscopy, the split is seen at the level of the lamina lucida where the bullous pemphigoid antigen is found. Control is usually achieved with a daily dose of 60 to 80 mg of prednisone initially, followed by fairly rapid tapering to 30 to 40 mg and the slower tapering. Dapsone, cyclophosphamide, or azathioprine is often added if there is difficulty tapering the steroid. The disease often remits in 1 to 2 years, and steroids can be stopped. Relapse occurs in only 10%.

B. Pemphigus vulgaris. Lesions begin around or in the mouth, or on the scalp, and can spread to any area. Primary lesions are flaccid, noninflamed bullae, which break easily and leave large denuded areas, which then crust. Nikolsky's sign is positive (lateral pressure results in dramatic extension of blisters). Lesions heal with temporary hyperpigmentation but without scarring. A pemphigus-like eruption has been reported with use of certain medications: penicillamine (Cuprimine, Depen), captopril (Capoten), piroxicam (Feldene), penicillin, rifampin, phenobarbital. Diagnosis is confirmed by biopsy of the skin or oral mucosa adjacent to active blisters; in virtually 100% of pemphigus cases of all types, IgG and component C3 are seen outlining the intracellular spaces of the epidermis. Therapy is with high-dose steroids, which dramatically reduces the mortality, and referral to a dermatologist is indicated. A common approach is to start with 80 mg of prednisone daily and increase the dose by 50% every 7 days until no new blisters form. If the dose nears 200 mg, consider IV pulse therapy with steroids or plasmapheresis.

After control is achieved, an immunosuppressive agent (most commonly azathioprine [Imuran], or cyclophosphamide [Cytoxan, Neosar]) is added to allow steroid tapering.

C. **Erythma multiforme (EM).** A vascular reaction with a wide variety of causes. Herpes simplex infection causes most mild, recurrent cases. More severe, widespread cases may be caused by other infectious agents, especially *Mycoplasma* species and viruses, and by medications, especially penicillins, sulfonamides, anticonvulsants, nonsteroidal anti-inflammatory drugs, and allopurinol. The lesions of EM are often preceded by a prodrome of fever, malaise, myalgias, and upper respiratory symptoms. Early lesions are pink, edematous papules; some of these evolve into characteristic target lesions (flat, dull red macules with central clearing or vesicle formation). The distribution is symmetric with lesions occurring on the palms, soles, extensor extremities, and often on oral mucosa. Mild cases are self-limited over a 7 to 10 day period and may not require treatment. Suppressive doses of antiherpes drug (see Table 11-1) prevent recurrences associated with herpesvirus. For more severe or widespread disease, treatment involves prednisone (see treatment for EM variants below).

D. **Erythma multiforme bullosum variants.**
1. ***Stevens-Johnson syndrome.*** Severe, explosive mucosal erosions, often on more than one mucosal surface, accompanied by high fever and severe constitutional symptoms that are usually associated with extensive bullous erythema multiforme of the skin. It is more often related to infections with herpesviruses or *Mycoplasma* than to a drug allergy. May require ocular steroids to prevent synechia formation. Generally requires dermatology or burn unit care.
2. ***Toxic epidermal necrolysis.*** Almost always drug induced (see drugs listed under EM above). It is manifested by a burning or painful eruption that predominates on the trunk and proximal extremities. Painful edematous erythema of palms and soles often develops. Less often, the initial presentation is of widespread, confluent erythema. Either initial presentation is followed by epidermal necrosis and sloughing of the skin and mucous membranes. 20% to 100% of total body surface area can be affected. The mortalities are ~30%.
3. ***Treatment.*** A short 2- to 3-week course of prednisone, starting at 30 to 40 mg is given. This may abort the process, but it will not restore epidermis that is already necrotic. In full-blown cases of toxic epidermal necrolysis, the patient should be treated in a burn unit, and steroids should be withheld.

III. OTHER DERMATITIDES

A. Allergic contact dermatitis (such as poison ivy, poison oak). A pruritic, inflammatory reaction that progresses from erythema and irritation to a blistering, vesiculobullous exanthem and that is caused by a reaction to a sensitizing chemical (not necessarily a caustic agent) by a delayed cellular (type IV) hypersensitivity mechanism. The reaction requires a prior exposure ranging from a few days to years. May follow a primary irritant dermatitis and may occur because of a medication used to treat it (especially neomycin). The location of the lesion is often suggestive of the diagnosis. The eyelids are very sensitive and may react to substances rubbed on by fingers that remain free of dermatitis. Oleoresins (poison ivy, poison oak, and sumac) and a few chemicals (dinitrochlorobenzene) will sensitize almost everyone. Other common agents are dyes or coloring agents, tanning chemicals, nickel, mercury, soaps, and perfumes. Common drugs include ethylenediamine, thimerosal, bacitracin, and sunscreen lotions. The patch test, in which a dilute solution of the suspected culprit is allowed to react with normal skin, is diagnostic. Treatment is by symptomatic care of less severe lesions with wet to dry soaks of astringent solutions (aluminum acetate topical solution, or Burow's solution) and antipruritics, such as diphenhydramine or hydroxyzine. Acetaminophen or ibuprofen will also help with pruritus. Oral corticosteroids are effective and indicated for the treatment of severe cases with involvement of large areas of the skin, swelling of the face or genitalia, or large areas of bullae.

B. Irritant contact dermatitis. Caused by exposure to caustic agents. Will cause a reaction manifesting as irritation progressing to erythema and inflammation. Treatment is by thorough cleansing of the affected region with cool water and supportive measures ranging from moisturizing lotions and antiseptic creams to systemic steroids and antibiotics, depending on the insult to the skin. Pruritus, which often accompanies the irritation, is treated with topical corticosteroids and antihistamines (diphenhydramine or hydroxyzine). Recurrence is thwarted by avoidance of the particular agent.

C. Seborrheic dermatitis. A common condition, usually first noticed as dandruff. It affects the scalp, the center of the face, the anterior portion of the chest, or the flexural creases of the arms, legs, and groin (that is, areas of the body that have high concentrations of sebaceous glands). Most commonly affects infants (1 to 3 months of age) and adults (30 to 60 years of age). Typically presents as a greasy scale on the scalp, with erythema and scaling of the nasolabial folds and retroauricular skin. Seborrheic dermatitis is said to be associated with deficiencies of riboflavin, biotin, or pyridoxine and various neurologic disorders (parkinsonism, status post CVAs, epilepsy, CNS trauma, facial nerve palsy, and syringomyelia). New-onset severe seborrheic dermatitis may be associated with HIV. Treatment for infants is a mild, nonmedicated shampoo. In adults or refractory infant cases use a shampoo 2 or 3 times a week containing one of the following: salicylic acid (X-Seb T, Sebulex), selenium sulfide (Selsun, Exsel), coal tar (DHS Tar, Neutrogena T-Gel, Polytar), or pyrithione zinc (DHS Zinc, Danex, Sebulon). More severe cases may be treated with medicated shampoos as well as: (1) ketoconazole (Nizoral) 2% twice daily or (2) once or twice daily topical corticosteroid lotions such as hydrocortisone (Hytone) 2.5%, fluocinonide (Lidex) 0.05%, fluocinolone (Synalar) 0.01%, or betamethasone (Valisone) 0.1%. A new therapy is a topical form of gamma-linoleic acid, borage oil, which is effective in infantile seborrheic dermatitis.

D. Xerotic eczema (winter itch, asteatotic eczema). A relatively common dermatitis that occurs in the winter and in the elderly on the legs, arms, and hands and is characterized by dry, cracked, fissured skin and pruritus. Predisposing factors include old age; a genetic tendency for dry skin; too frequent bathing in hot, soapy baths or showers; and dry, nonhumidified heated rooms. Treatment includes (1) avoidance of overbathing with soap, (2) room humidifiers, (3) tepid water baths using bath oils with liberal application of emollients after drying, (4) medium-potency corticosteroids applied BID until eczema clears, and (5) topical alpha-hydroxy acids (such as glycolic acid or lactic acid).

IV. ECZEMA WITH SIGNIFICANT EXCORIATIONS

A. Atopic dermatitis (infantile eczema, neurodermatitis). A genetic predisposition to react with pruritus and inflammation and associated with asthma, hay fever, and urticaria. Elevated levels of IgE have been associated with atopic dermatitis. The features vary with age and commonly begin as infantile eczema, affecting the face, scalp, and upper extremities, often associated with food consumption (cheese, egg white, wheat, legumes, nuts). This usually fades away or may progress in older children to dermatitis of the neck and the upper and lower extremities, especially the popliteal and the antecubital fossae. This too may fade away or persist in localized areas of the hands and face. Vesiculation, oozing, and crusting are common, and lesions are very pruritic, manifesting lichenified, reddened skin caused by excoriation. Again, it may fade away to recur during times of stress. Patients frequently develop irritant dermatitis, and most are particularly sensitive to formaldehyde and nickel. These patients are very susceptible to bacterial and viral infections and can develop severe, widespread pyoderma. Treatment is directed at relieving pruritus, controlling infection, and promoting healing. Vesicular and crusting dermatitis is treated with wet-to-dry dressings of Burow's solution and oral antihistamines to relieve the pruritus. Topical corticosteroids and emollient creams can be used after the lesions are healed. Use of steroids and emollients under occlusion may be helpful (as under gloves or in a PVC body suit at night). A course of antistaphylococcal antibiotics for 2 weeks may be helpful in acute exacerbations. A short course of systemic corticosteroids may also be used. Avoidance is important, and a trial of environmental control, trial elimination of specific foods, and skin testing for food and inhalant allergens might be useful.

B. Stasis dermatitis. Chronic dermatitis of the lower legs in people with chronic venous insufficiency. Associated with mild pruritus, pain (if an ulcer is present), aching discomfort in the limb, swelling of the ankle, and nocturnal cramps. Lesions consist of erythematous scaling plaques with exudation, crusts, and superficial ulcers particularly on the medial aspect of the ankle. Acute treatment of stasis dermatitis is by Burow's wet dressings and cooling pastes, topical corticosteroids, and systemic antibiotics if cellulitis is present. Chronic treatment of stasis dermatitis includes topical corticosteroids, supportive stockings (Jobst, TEDS), compressive bandages, vein surgery; Unna's paste boot (zinc oxide–impregnated gauze) can be placed for 72 hours to promote healing of skin and ulcers. If stasis dermatitis has ulcerated, treatment includes wet-to-dry dressings using normal saline or Dakin's solution; silver sulfadiazine applied between wet-to-dry dressings; elevation of the leg; compressive bandages; supportive stockings; or surgery; or any combination.

C. Dyshidrotic eczema. Deep-seated, pruritic, tapioca-like vesicles on the palms, soles, or sides of the fingers. Dyshidrosis may begin in childhood, but often the initial appearance is found in early adult life. May be an *id* reaction to infection elsewhere. Thereafter, intermittent episodes can be expected up to 60 years of age. When attacks occur frequently, xerosis, desquamation, cracking, and fissuring may occur. Treatment is difficult and requires the use of intermittent high-potency topical steroids or even a burst of systemic steroids. Later in the disease scaling, lichenification, painful fissures, and erosions may be seen. Dietary restriction of certain metals (cobalt, nickel, or chromium) has been suggested to be successful in treatment of two thirds of patients. Treatment of the vesicular stage includes Burow's wet dressings BID with or without "black cat" (10% crude coal tar in equal parts of acetone and flexible collodion) applied once daily. In moderate or severe disease, erythromycin or dicloxacillin 250 mg QID should be started because bacterial infection may be present even without obvious signs (crusts, tenderness, etc.). PUVA is saved for severe refractory disease.

V. OTHER ECZEMATOUS ERUPTIONS

A. Nummular (discoid) eczema. A chronic, pruritic, inflammatory dermatitis occurring in the form of coin-shaped plaques (4 to 5 cm in diameter) composed of grouped small papules and vesicles on an erythematous base with indistinct borders, crusts, and excoriations. Common on lower legs (older men), trunk, hands and fingers (younger females). Especially prevalent during the winter months and in atopic individuals. Treatment includes topical corticosteroids, oral dicloxacillin or erythromycin if infected, crude coal tar pastes, and skin moisturizers.

B. Lichen simplex chronicus. A circumscribed area of lichenification caused by repeated physical trauma (rubbing and scratching). It occurs in both sexes in the anogenital area and in women on the nuchal areas, arms, legs, and ankles. *Treatment*: stop the rubbing and scratching with anti-inflammatory agents (crude coal tar and topical corticosteroids) covered by continuous dry occlusive gauze dressings. Intralesional corticosteroids are effective for small localized areas.

C. Autoeczematization (autosensitization, an *id* reaction). A tendency for severe eczematous disease to spread spontaneously outside of its original distribution pattern. Believed to be secondary to an immune response mounted against antigens located at the original site of involvement (such as bacteria, fungi, keratin, or collagen). Most often seen in connection with stasis dermatitis, diaper dermatitis, external otitis, hand eczema, and foot eczema. Treatment: (1) systemic steroid burst (such as prednisone 60 mg PO QD for 7 days) and (2) treat the original disease.

URTICARIA

I. OVERVIEW

A common disorder that affects 15 % to 20% of the population at some time. Two thirds of cases occur in persons between 20 and 40 years of age. Urticaria is characterized by a transient, pruritic, patchy eruption that consists of lightly erythematous papules or wheals with raised borders and blanched centers involving the superficial skin layers; involvement of the deeper layers or the submucosa is called "angioedema." Lesions vary considerably in size, from 2 mm to over 30 cm, and may be circular or irregularly shaped. The most common site for urticaria is the trunk, though lesions may occur on any part of the body. Urticaria has been divided into two major groups:

A. Acute urticaria. Defined as hives persisting for less than 4 to 6 weeks (usually 2 to 3 days). It occurs with higher incidence in atopic individuals. Commonly identified causes include foods, drugs, and infections, but in over half of the patients there is no known cause (idiopathic).

B. **Angiodema.** Acute attacks tend to be associated with large irregular areas of swelling and may occur with subcutaneous swelling (angioedema) or even with an anaphylactic reaction. Cause is similar to urticaria but may also include hereditary angioedema (p. 550) or, commonly, ACE inhibitors.

C. **Chronic urticaria.** Attacks persist for 6 weeks or more. Patients usually are not atopic. The course is more benign and may involve waxing and waning. Wheals tend to be smaller, with only a few appearing at any given time.

II. TYPES OF URTICARIA

A. **Idiopathic.** Largest category, comprising a third of acute and two thirds of chronic cases of urticaria.

B. **Physical.** Approximately 15% of the cases. Usually an identifiable cause can be found. There are several types:
   1. ***Dermatographism.*** A reaction to firm stroking of the skin that occurs within 1 to 3 minutes and lasts 5 to 10 minutes. It is not true urticaria though it may be severe enough to seek medical help.
   2. ***Cholinergic urticaria.*** Exercise or sweating is the provocative agent. Cause of 10% of reactions, affects young people, and may last 6 to 8 years. Lesions appear as 1 to 2 mm wheals on a confluent erythematous base and are found on the trunk and arms with sparing of the palms, soles, and the axillae.
   3. ***Cold urticaria.*** An uncommon reaction to cold or rewarming after cold exposure (cold winds are an effective stimulus); can be caused by syphilis.
   4. ***Solar urticaria.*** Rare reaction caused by exposure to light. Appears as pruritus and erythema, followed by urticaria. Sudden onset and occurs in any age group.
   5. ***Delayed pressure urticaria.*** Rare reaction caused by sustained pressure.
   6. ***Aquagenic urticaria.*** Rare reaction caused by contact with water.
   7. ***Localized heat urticaria.*** Rare reaction caused by hot water.

C. **Immunologic.** So named when specific reactants (antigen, antibody, sensitized cell) can be identified. Occurs with anaphylaxis and serum sickness and in atopic persons on a seasonal basis when asthma and allergic rhinitis symptoms peak or when exposed to allergic substances including foods (fish, nuts, berries, eggs) or insect stings (bees, wasps, hornets, yellow jackets). Drug-induced urticaria (especially penicillin and sulfonamides) can be immunologic though identification of the reactant can be difficult. Urticaria can also be caused by immune complexes seen in systemic rheumatologic diseases (systemic lupus erythematosus, Sjögren's syndrome, rheumatic fever, juvenile rheumatoid arthritis, necrotizing vasculitis, and polymyositis), cryoglobulinemias, serum sickness, neoplastic disorders, transfusion reactions, and hepatitis, Epstein-Barr virus, and streptococcal infections.

D. Hereditary angioedema. An autosomal dominant disease caused by the functional absence of C1-esterase protein. This enables vascular permeability and is potentially fatal as a result of respiratory compromise caused by recurrent, acute angioedema of the skin and mucosa. Occasionally presents with acute abdominal symptoms mimicking a surgical abdomen. Serum levels of C2 are normal during asymptomatic periods but decreased during an attack. Levels of C4 and CH-50 (a lab study of complement function) are low all the time. Low C1-esterase inhibitor levels are diagnostic. However, there are nonfunctioning alleles of C1-esterase inhibitor, and so some individuals with the disease will have normal levels. A functional assay should be performed if clinically indicated. These patients should be pretreated with fresh frozen plasma before painful procedures or procedures known to induce attacks. Additionally they can be treated with fresh frozen plasma to abort an ongoing attack. C1-esterase inhibitor is currently investigational but should have FDA approval soon. Long-term therapy includes enough danazole to prevent acute attacks (200 mg TID or less).

E. Infections. Urticaria occasionally associated with acute and chronic infections including protozoan, parasitic, bacterial, and viral infections. Sources such as sinusitis, dental abscesses, periodontal disease, gallbladder infection, chronic bronchitis, chronic UTIs, and low-grade fungal (athlete's foot) or yeast (*Candida* vaginitis) infections should be investigated in persons with chronic urticaria.

F. Infestations. Most commonly attributable to scabies, caused by the mite *Sarcoptes scabiei.* See section on scabies for details, p. 538.

G. Urticaria pigmentosa. An uncommon disease with focal dermal infiltration of tissue mast cells; can have infiltrates in other organs as well as with representative organ system disease. It presents as brown patches that form a wheal and flare upon stroking.

H. Miscellaneous.

1. ***Neoplastic disorders.*** Carcinoma (colorectal, lung, ovarian, uterine, liver), choriocarcinoma, Hodgkin's disease, lymphoma, leukemia, or myeloma.
2. ***Endocrinopathy.*** Hypothroidism or hyperthyroidism, hyperparathyroidism, diabetes mellitus, menopause.
3. ***Arthropod assault (insect bite).*** A papular lesion, usually caused by flea or red ant bite.

4. ***Psychogenic.*** A diagnosis of exclusion, but psychogenic and emotional factors are contributory or aggravating in at least a fourth of patients with chronic urticaria.

III. DIAGNOSTIC TESTS FOR UTICARIA

A. Acute urticaria. Laboratory tests generally are not needed.

B. Chronic urticaria. If physical agents have been excluded as a cause, judicious use of the following laboratory, radiographic, and pathologic studies may provide clues to the diagnosis of an occult systemic illness.

1. ***Routine tests.***
   a. *Laboratory.* Complete blood cell count with differential, chemistry profile, erythrocyte sedimentation rate (ESR), T_4, TSH measurements, urinalysis and urine culture, antinuclear antibody.
   b. *Radiographic.* Chest radiograph, sinus films, dental films or Panorex.
2. ***Selective tests.*** Cryoglobulin, hepatitis and syphilis serologic analysis, rheumatoid factor, serum complement, serum IgE, IgM.
3. ***Skin biopsy.*** If the erythrocyte sedimentation rate is elevated, perform to exclude urticarial vasculitis.

IV. TREATMENT OF URTICARIA

A. Treatment of anaphylaxis is described in Chapter 1.

B. Hereditary angioedema does not respond to typical therapy as outlined below. See section on hereditary angioedema for management, p. 550.

C. Eliminate or limit exposure to the causative agent.

D. Treat any underlying disease because it may be a causative factor.

E. Symptomatic care.

1. ***Antihistamines.***
   a. Classic H_1-blockers include chlorpheniramine (Chlor-Trimeton) 4 mg every 4 to 6 hours, Cyproheptadine (Periactin) 4 to 8 mg every 6 hours, diphenhydramine (Benadryl) 25 to 50 mg every 6 to 8 hours, hydroxyzine (Atarax, Vistaril) 25 to 50 mg every 6 to 8 hours, and promethazine (Phenergan) 12.5 to 25 mg every 12 to 24 hours. Hydroxyzine is believed to be one of the most effective agents, but diphenhydramine and chlorpheniramine are less expensive and OTC.
   b. Nonsedating H_1-blockers include terfenadine (Seldane), astemizole (Hismanal), loratadine (Claritin), cetirizine (Zyrtec), and fexofenadine (Allegra). They are equally effective compared to classic agents, are less sedating, and have simpler dosing schedules. Avoid the use of terfenadine or astemizole in patients taking macrolide antibiotics or ketoconazole.

TABLE 13-1
Potency of Topical Corticosteroids*

Group†	%‡	Generic Name§
I	0.05	Betamethasone dipropionate
II	0.01	Amcinonide
	0.05	Fluocinonide
	0.25	Desoximetasone
III	0.5	Triamcinolone acetonide
	0.1	Betamethasone valerate
IV	0.05	Flurandrenolide
	0.025	Fluocinolone acetonide
V	0.1	Betamethasone valerate
VI	0.01	Fluocinolone acetonide
	0.03	Flumethasone pivalate
VII	0.2	Betamethasone valerate
	1-2.5	Hydrocortisone

Adapted from Habif TP; *Clinical dermatology: a color guide to diagnosis and therapy,* ed 3, St. Louis, 1993, Mosby.
*"Rules of nines"; for three-times-daily application, 9 g of cream covers 1% of skin area daily.
†Potencies decrease from group I (strongest) to group VII (weakest).
‡Increasing the concentration increases the potency. At equal concentrations, potency decreases as the viscosity of the substance increases.
§Brand name drugs are available in a variety of strengths and vehicles (such as ointment, solution, cream, lotion).

c. H_2-blockers, such as cimetidine (Tagamet), ranitidine (Zantac), may be considered in patients who do not respond to therapy with H_1-antagonists alone.
d. Beta-agonists such as terbutaline (Brethine, Bricanyl) may be a useful adjunct to antihistamines.
e. Doxepin (Adapin, Sinequan) is a potent H_1-blocker with efficacy comparable to hydroxyzine.

2. Topical application of capsaicin (Zostrix) or local anesthetic can suppress wheal-and-flare reactions in local heat urticaria.
3. Topical or systemic corticosteroids (Table 13-1) should be reserved for patients with refractory symptoms. However, compared to placebo, a short course (40 mg × 5 days of prednisone) is quite effective at symptom control.
4. ***Skin care.*** Patients should be instructed in regular bathing, hydration, and use of emollients.
5. New therapies currently under study in controlled trials include use of nifedipine (Adalat, Procardia), ketotifen (Zaditen), cyclosporin A (Sandimmune), UVB phototherapy, and plasmapheresis. More safety studies are needed before advocating any of these treatments.

BIBLIOGRAPHY

Bart BJ: Annular skin eruptions: not every ring on the skin is ringworm, *Postgrad Med* 96(1):37-50, 1994.

Cohen PR: Genodermatoses with malignant potential, *Am Fam Physician* 46(5):1479-1486, 1992.

Fitzpatrick TB et al: *Color atlas and synopsis of clinical dermatology,* ed 2, New York, 1994, McGraw-Hill.

Forsman KE: Pediculosis and scabies–what to look for in patients who are crawling with clues, *Postgrad Med* 98(6):89-100, 1995.

Gannon T: Dermatologic emergencies: when early recognition can be lifesaving, *Postgrad Med* 96(1):67-82, 1994.

Greaves MW, Weinstein GD: Treatment of psoriasis, *N Engl J Med* 332(9):581-588, 1995.

Healy E, Simpson N: Acne vulgaris, *Br Med J* 308:831-833, 1994.

Janniger CK, Schwartz RA: Seborrheic dermatitis, *Am Fam Physician* 52(1):149-155, 1995.

Kibarian MA, Hruza GJ: Nonmelanoma skin cancer: risks, treatment options, and tips on prevention, *Postgrad Med* 98(6):39-58, 1995.

Kirsner RS: Treatment of psoriasis: role of calcipotriene, *Am Fam Physician* 52(1):237-240, 1995.

Klaus MV, Wieselthier JS: Contact dermatitis, *Am Fam Physician* 48(4):629-632, 1993.

Mahmood T: Urticaria, *Am Fam Physician* 51(4):811-816, 1995.

Millikan LE: Treating pruritus: what's new in safe relief of symptoms? *Postgrad Med* 99(1):173-184, 1996.

Millikan LE, Shrum JP: An update on common skin diseases: acne, psoriasis, contact dermatitis, and warts, *Postgrad Med* 91(6):96-115, 1992.

Olson CL: Blistering disorders: which ones can be deadly? *Postgrad Med* 96(1):53-64, 1994.

Phillips TJ, Dover JS: Recent advances in dermatology, *N Engl J Med* 326(3):167-178, 1992.

Preston DS, Stern RS: Nonmelanoma cancers of the skin, *N Engl J Med* 327(23):1649-1662, 1992.

Shalita AR et al: Topical erythromycin vs. clindamycin therapy for acne: multicenter, double-blind comparison, *Arch Dermatol* 120:351, 1984.

Strauss JS et al: Isotretinoin therapy for acne: results of a multicenter dose-response study, *J Am Acad Dermatol* 10:490, 1984.

Winston MH, Shalita AR: Acne vulgaris: pathogenesis and treatment, *Pediatr Clin North Am* 38:899, 1991.

14

Neurology

ROBERT L. HERTING, JR. AND NORA R. FROHBERG

HEADACHE (HA)

I. HISTORY

Includes nature of headache, family history, psychosocial history, and current medications. Inquire about inciting factors such as smoking, alcohol, vasodilators, or ingestion of tyramine-containing food (such as chocolate or red wine). Oral contraceptive pills and pregnancy can alleviate or intensify headaches. Analgesic overuse can cause "rebound headache."

II. CHARACTERISTICS OF VARIOUS TYPES OF HEADACHES

A. Primary headaches (see Table 14-1).

1. ***Migraine without aura (common migraine).*** Must have at least 5 attacks that meet the following criteria:
   a. Headache attacks last 4 to 72 hours.
   b. Headache has at least 2 of the following:
      - Unilateral location
      - Pulsating quality
      - Moderate or severe intensity (inhibits daily activity)
      - Aggravation by routine physical activity
   c. During the headache, at least 1 of the following:
      - Nausea or vomiting
      - Photophobia and phonophobia
   d. No organic cause found by history, PE, neurologic exam.
2. ***Migraine with aura (classical migraine).*** Must have at least 2 attacks fulfilling the following criteria:
   a. At least 3 of the following are present:
      - One of more fully reversible aura symptoms indicating focal cerebral cortical or brainstem dysfunction.

- At least one aura symptom develops gradually over more than 4 minutes.
- No aura symptom lasts more than 60 minutes (duration proportionally increases if >1 aura symptom present).
- HA follows aura with free interval of less than 60 minutes (may begin before or with the aura). HA usually lasts 4 to 72 hours but may be absent.

b. No organic cause found by history, PE, neurologic exam.

3. ***Tension type.***

a. Headache with at least 2 of the following:
- Pressing or tightening quality
- Mild or moderate intensity
- Bilateral location
- No aggravation by routine physical activity

b. No organic cause found by history, PE, neurologic exam.

c. Tension headache is separated into two subtypes based on frequency:

(1) Episodic
- Headache lasting 30 minutes to 7 days
- No nausea or vomiting with headache
- Photophobia and phonophobia are absent, or one but not the other is present
- At least 10 previous headaches as above, with number of headache days <180/year and <15/month

(2) Chronic
- Headache averages 15 days/month (180 days/year), 6 months
- No vomiting
- No more than 1 of the following: nausea, photophobia, or phonophobia

4. ***Cluster (episodic or chronic).***

a. Severe unilateral orbital, supraorbital, or temporal pain lasting 15 to 180 minutes untreated.

b. Headache is associated with at least 1 of the following on the pain side:
- Conjunctival injection
- Lacrimation
- Nasal congestion
- Forehead and facial sweating
- Rhinorrhea
- Miosis
- Ptosis
- Eyelid edema

c. Frequency of attacks ranges from 1 to 8 daily.

d. At least 5 attacks occur as above.

5. ***Chronic paroxysmal hemicrania.***

TABLE 14-1
Characteristics of Various Types of Primary Headaches

Headache	Quality	Location	Duration	Associated symptoms
Migraine without aura	Throbbing	Unilateral or bilateral	6-48 hours	Nausea, vomiting, photophobia
Migraine with aura	Throbbing	Unilateral	3-12 hours	Visual prodrome, nausea, vomiting, photophobia
Tension type	Dull	Diffuse bilateral	Unremitting	Depression
Cluster (M:F = 5:1)	Boring	Unilateral especially orbital	15-120 minutes	Ipsilateral tearing, Horner's syndrome, nasal stuffiness
Subarachnoid hemorrhage	Throbbing, severe	Variable	Variable	May have focal neurologic symptoms or decreased level of consciousness but may be alert with nonfocal exam
Chronic paroxysmal hemicrania	Severe	Unilateral, orbital, or temporal	2-45 minutes	Conjunctival injection, ptosis lacrimation, rhinorrhea, and relieved with Indocin

a. Severe unilateral orbital, supraorbital, or temporal pain always on the same side, lasting 2 to 45 minutes.
b. Attack frequency >5 a day for more than half the time (periods of lower frequency may occur).
c. Headache is associated with at least 1 of the following on the pain side:
   - Conjunctival injection
   - Lacrimation
   - Nasal congestion
   - Rhinorrhea
   - Eyelid edema
   - Ptosis
d. Absolute effectiveness of indomethacin (150 mg/day or less).
e. At least 50 attacks occur as above.
f. No organic cause found by history, PE, neurologic exam.

B. Secondary headaches.

1. ***Increased intracranial pressure (pseudotumor cerebri).*** Idiopathic, 19 of 100,000 in obese young females. Has been associated with tetracycline use. Often presents with chronic retrobulbar HA exacerbated by eye movements. Also visual changes, diplopia, meningeal signs, and paresthesias. Exam may reveal papilledema and cranial nerve VI palsy. CSF normal except for elevated opening pressure (250 to 450 mm H_2O). *Treatment:* weight loss, serial LPs to remove 20 to 40 ml, diuretics, acetazolamide 500 to 1000 mg QD, prednisone 40 to 60 mg QD, and rarely a shunt.
2. ***Tumor.*** HA most common only complaint, though only 50% of tumors present with HA. 17% have "typical" tumor HA (worse in morning, nausea, vomiting, worse bending over). Usually other neurologic signs or symptoms help localize tumor. Obtain head CT with contrast or MRI for patients with chronic HA presenting with new symptoms or abnormal neurologic signs. *Treatment:* neurosurgical consultation.
3. ***Arteritis (giant cell, temporal).*** Most common symptom is nonspecific headache often with scalp or temporal artery tenderness. Jaw claudication pathognomic. Elderly females at increased risk. Sedimentation rate elevated. Biopsy reveals arteritis. *Treatment:* see Chapter 6.
4. ***Acute effects of substance use.*** Occurs within a discrete period after substance use and disappears with elimination of use.
5. ***Substance withdrawal.*** Occurs after >3 months of high daily dose of substance. Occurs within hours after elimination and relieved by renewed intake. Disappears with withdrawal of substance. This includes caffeine use.

6. ***Meningitis and herpes encephalitis.*** See section on CNS infection, p. 577.
7. ***Drug-rebound headache.*** *Aggravating factors:* ergotamine induced, analgesic abuse (such as >50 g/month ASA or equivalent mild analgesic, >300 mg/month diazepam.) *Treatment:* stop drug.
8. ***Carbon monoxide poisoning.*** See Chapter 1.
9. ***Subarachnoid hemorrhage (SAH).*** Generally have acute onset of worst headache of life. May have nausea, vomiting, mental status changes, or loss of consciousness. Most (59%) have a "warning leak" before severe event and may have antecedent headaches for weeks. Since mortality is 50% for each bleed, if one can pick up the warning leak, one can prevent death and illness.
   a. May have mental status changes and meningeal signs but may not (39% initially free of CNS symptoms or signs).
   b. Only 10% have initially focal exam.
   c. May have fever and leukocytosis from meningeal irritation.
   d. CT scan will find only about 90% of SAH (98% in third-generation scanners). *All those who need a CT also need an LP.* CT should be done on those with severe headache that is different from their usual headache or new onset of headache. In one study, 33% of those with new onset of severe headache *and no CNS signs or symptoms and no other obvious cause of headache* had SAH.
   e. Response to nonnarcotic and narcotic analgesia does not rule out SAH.
   f. Nimodipine reduces the risk of cerebral vasospasm, which may contribute to mortality. Dose is 60 mg Q4h for 21 days.

C. Physical examination. Vitals (BP and temperature), neurologic deficits, papilledema, retinal hemorrhage, cranial bruit, thickened tender temporal arteries, trigger point for fascial pain, ptosis, dilated pupils, and stiff neck.

D. Ancillary tests not necessary if physical exam is negative. Routine CT scanning has low yield except when headaches are severe–an indication that subarachnoid hemorrhage or a neurologic deficit may be present.

1. CT should be done to rule out mass lesion.
2. An LP should be done if CT negative and suspect SAH (CT will miss about 10%).
3. Be sure to rule out meningitis, temporal arteritis by the clinical setting. Obtaining a sedimentation rate in elderly patients with new-onset headaches is prudent.
4. Remember simple causes such as sinusitis, toothache, temporomandibular joint syndrome.

III. TREATMENT FOR MIGRAINE HEADACHE

A. General. Taper off analgesics to prevent rebound HA and start preventive medications. Depression (if identified) needs to be treated.

B. Nonpharmacologic prophylaxis for migraine.

1. ***Dietary changes.***
   a. Avoid monosodium glutamate, nitrates, and alcohol.
   b. Spread out caffeine evenly.
2. ***Lifestyle changes.*** Regular eating, sleeping, and exercise patterns.
3. ***Behavioral therapies.*** Biofeedback, stress management, and self-help groups.

C. Acute therapy (outpatient).

1. Acetaminophen or ASA usually are not effective in severe headaches because of delayed gastric emptying. *The uses of metoclopramide 10 mg PO may enhance the efficacy of oral medication.*
2. ***NSAIDs.*** Such as ibuprofen 400 to 800 mg PO TID or QID or naproxen sodium 550 mg PO BID or TID with food.
3. Fiorinal 1 or 2 tablets Q4-6h up to 4 per day and twice per week. Avoid overuse.
4. ***Abortive therapy for migraines.*** *Ergotamine derivatives contraindicated in peripheral or coronary artery disease. Do not use sumatriptan in those who have had an ergot preparation within the last 24 hours and vice versa.*
   a. Midrin 2 caps PO initially and then 1 capsule Q1h up to 5 in 12 hours.
   b. Sumatriptan (Imitrex) 6 mg SQ; may repeat in 1 hour; maximum 12 mg/24 hours. Contraindicated if concomitant CAD or uncontrolled hypertension. Do not use if patient is given an ergot alkaloid in the last 24 hours. Many (up to 50%) will require rescue medicine because of sumatriptan's 2-hour half-life. Oral sumatriptan available but not so effective.
   c. Cafergot 1 or 2 tablets PO; may repeat up to 4 tabs/attack or 10/week.
   d. Ergotamine 2 mg PO or SL; may repeat in 30 minutes up to 6 mg/24 hours or 10 mg/week.
   e. Prochlorperazine 25 mg PR BID PRN can be used to abort the migraine at home.

D. Acute therapy (emergency room): migraine.

1. Antiemetics may in themselves abort the headache.
   a. Prochlorperazine (Compazine) 10 mg IV or chlorpromazine 25 to 75 mg IV. Chlorpromazine has fallen out of favor because of hypotension, which can be treated with IV NS.
   b. Metoclopramide 5 to 10 mg IV Q8h. Often given with dihydroergotamine (DHE) to prevent DHE-induced nausea. May be combined orally with ASA.

2. NSAIDs (ketorolac [Toradol] 60 mg IM, indomethacin [Indocin] 50 mg PR BID or TID). Not so effective in migraines.
3. Dihydroergotamine (DHE) 0.75 mg IV over a few minutes preceded by prochlorperazine or metoclopramide 10 mg IV. Another 0.5 mg of DHE may be given in 30 minutes. Contraindicated in peripheral or coronary artery disease or those who are >60 years of age or those who have had sumatriptan.
4. Meperidine (Demerol) 50 to 100 mg IM Q3h PRN.
5. Dexamethasone 4 mg IM or a short course of prednisone (40 to 60 mg PO QD), combined with analgesics above, if migraine continues >24 hours.
6. Sumatriptan (Imitrex); see above for dose. Oral sumatriptan also available but less effective.
7. Lidocaine 100 mg IV once for intractable headache. Patient should not drive after treatment. Risk for seizures, arrhythmia, confusion.
8. Transnasal butorphanol 1 mg (1 spray in 1 nostril) repeated if necessary in 60 to 90 minutes.

E. Prophylaxis.

1. Amitriptyline 10 to 200 mg PO QHS. Other tricyclic antidepressants (TCAs) also effective.
2. Propranolol 20 to 60 mg PO BID to QID. Long-acting form can be used. Consider switching to a second beta-blocker if first one fails after adequate trial period (6 to 8 weeks). Contraindicated in asthma, heart failure, and diabetes.
3. Verapamil 40 to 80 mg PO TID (80 to 240 mg/day). Diltiazem and nifedipine are less effective. More beneficial in migraine with aura or cluster headache. Trial should be >2 months. Contraindicated in heart failure and heart block. Constipation is a common side effect.
4. NSAIDs, especially useful for menstrual migraine.
5. Cyproheptadine 2 to 4 mg PO QID. Less effective than methysergide but safe.
6. Methysergide (Sansert) 1 to 2 mg PO QID. Should not use longer than 6 months without a 1-month drug holiday to avoid fibrosis. Contraindicated in peripheral or coronary artery disease.
7. Ergotamine (low dose) 1 mg PO BID, not to exceed 10 mg/week (2 days/week skipped), contraindicated in ischemic diseases.
8. Anticonvulsants.
   a. Carbamazepine 200 to 800 mg PO daily dose divided BID to QID.
   b. Phenytoin 300 to 800 mg PO daily dose divided QD to TID. Efficacy not shown for migraine with aura.
   c. Valproic acid 250 to 1500 mg PO daily dose divided BID to QID titrated up to effective blood levels (50 to 100 mg/L).
9. Fluoxetine 10-30 mg PO QA.M. Other SSRIs are also effective.

IV. TREATMENT FOR SEVERE TENSION HEADACHE

A. Symptomatic treatment.
Simple analgesics, NSAIDs, or TCAs as above.

B. Preventive treatment.
TCAs, beta-blockers, or calcium-channel blockers as above.

V. TREATMENT FOR CLUSTER HEADACHE

A. Acute treatment is by any of the following:

1. Oxygen inhalation through a nonrebreathing mask at a flow rate of 6 to 8 L/min for 15 minutes is 70% effective.
2. Nasal lidocaine 4% solution (15 drops) or 5% ointment (3 swabs) intranasally on ipsilateral side may be abortive.
3. Sumatriptan is especially effective for cluster headache because by definition they last <3 hours. However, this is not an approved usage.
4. Parenteral therapy as above.

B. Prophylactic treatment. Low-dose oral ergotamine, methysergide, prednisone (60 mg QD for 1 week with a rapid tapering off), verapamil (80 to 160 mg TID), lithium carbonate 300 mg BID or TID, with or without valproate 250 to 1500 mg total daily dose divided BID to QID.

DEMENTIA

I. OVERVIEW

A. Prevalence. 3% to 11% in community-dwelling adults >65 years of age and 20% to 50% of individuals >85 years of age. Alzheimer's disease accounts for 60%, and vascular dementia accounts for 5% to 20% of all dementias.

B. (Partially) reversible causes. Medication side effects, infectious disease, dehydration, depression (pseudodementia), schizophrenia, Wernicke-Korsakoff disease, uremia, liver failure, hypothyroidism, hyponatremia, hypercalcemia, hypoglycemia, vitamin B_{12} deficiency, subdural hematoma, stroke, normal-pressure hydrocephalus, neoplastic disease. Partially reversible causes make up 10% to 15% of patients with dementia.

C. Irreversible causes. Alzheimer type of dementia, dementia with Parkinson's disease, multi-infarct dementia, Huntington's chorea, Pick's disease, Creutzfeldt-Jakob disease.

II. DIAGNOSTIC EVALUATION

A. History and physical examination with complete neurologic exam are essential. Babinski's sign, asymmetry of reflexes, and visual-field deficits are suggestive of multi-infarct dementia or focal CNS abnormality rather than Alzheimer type of dementia.

B. Mini–Mental State examination is essential (Box 14-1) Score <21 increases odds of dementia. Dementia can still be present despite a "normal" MMSE score (more likely in younger or well-educated patients).

BOX 14-1
Folstein Mini–Mental State Inventory

Score

( ) 1. What is the year ________, season________, date ________, day ______, month______?

( ) 2. Where are we: state____________, county ____________, town __________, place__________, floor ____________?

( ) 3. Name 3 objects: orange______ airplane ______ tobacco______ (trials) ________

( ) 4. Serial 7's: ______ ______ ______ ______ ______
93 86 79 72 65

or spell "world" backwards ____ ____ ____ ____ ____
d l r o w

( ) 5. Recall 3 objects: orange______ airplane ______ tobacco______

( ) 6. Name a pencil____________, and a watch ____________.

( ) 7. Read and obey____________ ⟶ CLOSE YOUR EYES

( ) 8. Copy design ______________ (below).

9. Write a sentence______________ (below).

10. Repeat the following: "No if, and, or buts"______________

11. Follow a 3-stage command: (a) Take a paper in your right hand.__________

(b) Fold it in half.__________

(c) Put it on the floor. __________

Level of consciousness ________________________ (check)
alert drowsy stupor coma

(One point for each blank. Maximum = 30)

Adapted from Folstein M et al: *J Psychiatr Res* 12:189-198, 1975.

C. Initial lab tests. Should include CBC, ESR, chemistry panel (with electroytes, BUN, creatinine LFTs, calcium, glucose), thyroid function tests.

D. Additional tests. May be obtained if indicated by history, PE, or initial lab tests. These additional tests include UA, vitamin B_{12}, folate, VDRL, HIV, heavy-metal screens (blood and urine), ECG, chest radiograph, head CT, EEG, O_2 saturation, lumber puncture, drug levels, and neuropsychologic testing.

III. DSM-IV DIAGNOSIS OF DEMENTIA

1. The development of multiple cognitive deficits are manifested by both:
   a. Memory impairment (difficulty learning new information or recalling previously learned information).
   b. One (or more) of the following:
      (1) Aphasia (language disturbance).
      (2) Apraxia (difficulty in carrying out motor activities despite intact motor function).
      (3) Agnosia (difficulty recognizing objects despite intact sensory function).
      (4) Disturbance in executive functioning (as in organizing, planning).
2. The cognitive deficits above cause significant impairment in functioning and represent a decline from previous functioning.
3. Symptoms do not occur exclusively during delirium and are not better accounted for by a mental illness.

IV. TYPES OF DEMENTIA (MEETING THE ABOVE DSM-IV CRITERIA)

A. Alzheimer's dementia (AD).

1. Diagnosis of exclusion (other CNS, systemic, or substance-induced conditions that cause dementia symptoms have been ruled out).
2. ***Risk factors.*** Advanced age, family history of Alzheimer's, and presence of apolipoprotein E type 4 allele (apo E-4).
3. ***Course.*** Gradual onset and continuing cognitive decline.
4. ***Treatment.***
   a. Tacrine (Cognex) provides improvement in 20% to 25% of patients with mild to moderate disease at higher doses (120 to 160 mg/day divided QID). LFTs need to be monitored weekly for the first 6 months, and there are multiple side effects.
   b. Donepezil (Aricept) is indicated for the treatment of mild to moderate Alzheimer's dementia. Initial dose is 5 mg PO QHS for 4 to 6 weeks. Then the dose may be increased to 10 mg PO QHS if needed. Easier to use than tacrine because of once-daily dosing and no need for weekly liver function monitoring.

B. Vascular dementia (formerly multi-infarct dementia).

1. Must be evidence of cerebrovascular disease (focal neurologic signs and symptoms or CT or MRI evidence) judged to be the cause of the dementia.
2. ***Risk factors.*** Male, smoking, history of previous strokes or TIAs, HTN, CAD, or atrial fibrillation.
3. ***Course.*** Typically progresses in stepwise deteriorating manner.
4. ***Treatment.*** Reduce modifiable risk factors for stroke. ASA to prevent further strokes. Anticoagulants if an identified

cerebral embolic source and not contraindicated because of risk of falls and intracerebral hemorrhage. Ticlopidine (Ticlid) used in patients unresponsive to ASA or unable to tolerate it.

C. Dementia from other conditions (examples below).

1. ***Normal-pressure hydrocephalus.***
   a. Characterized by triad of gradual onset of dementia, gait disturbance, and urinary incontinence.
   b. CT scan shows enlarged ventricles.
   c. *Treatment.* Surgical ventriculoperitoneal CSF shunting may greatly improve symptoms or even be curative.
2. ***Pick's disease.***
   a. Characterized by changes in personality early in the course, deterioration of social skills, emotional blunting, behavioral disinhibition, and prominent language abnormalities. Later in the course, difficulties with memory, apraxia, and other features of dementia occur.
   b. No specific treatment at this time.

V. OTHER GENERAL MANAGEMENT FOR DEMENTIA

Provide a supportive environment with frequent cues for orientation to the day, date, place, and time. As functioning decreases, nursing home placement may be necessary. Provide the family with supportive therapy and referral to community support groups. For agitation, try behavior modification first, and haloperidol (Haldol) if needed. Avoid benzodiazepines.

DELIRIUM

I. OVERVIEW

A. Prevalence. Affects 10% of all hospitalized patients, 20% of burn patients, 30% of ICU patients, and 30% of hospitalized AIDS patients.

B. Predisposing factors. Extremes of age (young and elderly) and patients with a history of brain damage, dementia, or delirium.

II. DIAGNOSIS BY DSM-IV CRITERIA

A. Disturbance of consciousness with reduced ability to focus, shift, or sustain attention.

B. A change in cognition (such as memory deficit, disorientation) or development of a perceptual disturbance not better accounted for by dementia.

C. Symptoms develop over a short period of time and tend to fluctuate during the day.

III. COMMON CAUSES OF DELIRIUM

A. Organ failure. Renal (uremia), hepatic (hyperammonemia), pulmonary (hypoxia), cardiac (hypotension, low perfusion states).

B. Nutritional. Vitamin B_{12}, folate, and thiamine deficiencies; hypoglycemia.

C. Endocrine. Hypothyroidism, hypercorticism, hypopituitarism, and hyperparathyroidism.

D. Structural-vascular-epileptic. Trauma (burns, postconcussion syndrome, subdural hematoma, fractures (especially of hips), cerebrovascular events (thrombotic, embolic, hemorrhagic), neoplastic (primary and secondary), infectious (encephalitis), epilepsy (postictal, temporal lobe).

E. Infectious. Meningitis, pneumonia, sepsis, pyelonephritis.

F. Drugs. Alcohol and sedative-hypnotics (intoxication and withdrawal); anticonvulsants; antidepressants; antihypertensive drugs, antiparkinsonian drugs, including amantadine and bromocriptine; corticosteroids, digitalis, histamine (H_2)-receptor antagonists, narcotics, and phenothiazines.

G. Electrolyte and acid-base disturbances. Hypernatremia, hyponatremia; hyperkalemia, hypokalemia; hypermagnesemia, hypomagnesemia; hypercalcemia, hypocalcemia; acidosis, alkalosis.

H. Urinary retention or fecal impaction.

IV. DIAGNOSTIC EVALUATION

A. Delirium is considered a medical emergency, and a work-up needs to proceed rapidly to determine the cause.

B. See Table 14-2 to differentiate delirium, dementia, and acute psychosis.

C. History. Ask family or nurse regarding patient's baseline level of function and any recent mental changes or history of mental illness.

D. Physical Examination. Perform a thorough physical and neurologic exam paying attention to signs of the causes listed above. Perform Folstein MMSE (see Box 14-1; score of 24 indicates cognitive disturbance). Another useful test is the Confusion Assessment Method (presence of inattention, acute onset, and fluctuating course plus either disorganized thinking or altered level of consciousness).

E. Laboratory Tests. Basic lab tests include CBC, electrolytes, blood chemistry panel, UA, ECG, oxygen saturation, and CXR. Other labs as indicated by patient's history, PE, and clinical situation: ABG, blood cultures, cardiac isoenzymes, vitamin B_{12}, folate, cortisol, ANA screen, syphilis serologic analysis, TFTs, toxicologic analysis, drug levels, head CT or MRI, lumbar puncture, EEG, or HIV test.

V. MANAGEMENT

A. Treat the underlying medical condition promptly to decrease risk of death (10% to 65%) from the cause of delirium.

B. Minimize any aggravating medications.

C. Optimize nutrition and hydration.

D. Create a supportive environment.

TABLE 14-2
Clinical Features of Delirium Dementia and Acute Functional Psychosis

Clinical feature	Delirium	Dementia	Psychosis
Onset	Sudden	Insidious	Sudden
Course over 24 hours	Fluctuating, with nocturnal exacerbation	Stable	Stable
Consciousness	Reduced	Clear	Clear
Attention	Globally disordered	Normal, except in severe cases	May be disordered
Cognition	Globally disordered	Globally impaired	May be selectively impaired
Hallucinations	Usually visual or visual and auditory	Often absent	Predominantly auditory
Delusions	Fleeting, poorly systematized	Often absent	Sustained, systematized
Orientation	Usually impaired, at least for a time	Often impaired	May be impaired
Psychomotor activity	Increased, reduced, or shifting unpredictably	Often normal	Varies from psychomotor retardation to severe hyper-activity, depending on the type of psychosis
Speech	Often incoherent, slow or rapid	Patient has difficulty finding words, perseveration	Normal, slow, or rapid
Involuntary movements	Often asterixis or coarse tremor	Often absent	Usually absent
Physical illness or drug toxicity	One or both are present	Often absent, especially in senile dementia of the Alzheimer type	Usually absent

1. Family members provide reassurance and familiar items from home to reorient patient.
2. Avoid disturbances of sleep.
3. Place patient near a nursing station for easier monitoring.

E. May treat associated agitation, preferentially with haloperidol (Haldol) initial dose of 0.5 to 2 mg IM or IV. If Haldol not effective, consider adjunctive lorazepam (Ativan) 0.5 to 1.0 mg IM or IV. As last resort, restraints may be necessary for safety.

SEIZURES

I. OVERVIEW

A. Epidemioloy. Annual incidence of approximately 0.5% to 1% of people in thc United States have epileptic seizures. Approximately 2% to 5% of children have febrile seizures with an age range of 3 months to 5 years.

B. Definition. *Epilepsy* refers to recurrent seizures that reflect aberrant electrical activity of cerebral cortical neurons. *Convulsion* applies to a seizure in which motor manifestations predominate. NOTE: A single seizure is not sufficient to warrant a diagnosis of epilepsy.

II. CLASSIFICATION

A. Primary generalized seizures. Bilateral and symmetric without focal onset and usually idiopathic.

1. ***Absence (petit mal).*** Brief (2- to 10-second) lapse of consciousness. Onset 4 to 12 years of age, and decreased frequency of attacks in adolescence. No aura. Manifested by staring, eye blinking, lip smacking. EEG characteristically shows 3 per second spike-and-wave pattern.
2. ***Myoclonic.*** Quick paroxysmal contractions of part of a muscle, whole muscle, or groups of muscles. Can occur as single jerk or intermittently in the same or different places.
3. ***Clonic, tonic, and tonic-clonic (grand mal).*** With or without aura, the patient abruptly loses consciousncss and has a tonic, clonic, or tonic-clonic convulsion, followed by postictal confusion.

B. Partial (focal) seizures.

1. ***Simple.*** Consciousness is not impaired.
2. ***Complex.*** Consciousness is impaired. May have automatic behaviors (such as walking, driving) or repetitive stereotyped behavior.

III. CAUSES.

Seizures result from artificial electrical stimulation of the brain, metabolic disorders, hypoglycemia, physical brain injury including areas of scar, neurosurgery, tumors, withdrawal from drugs, vascular disease, tuberous sclerosis, phenylketonuria, lipid storage diseases, and genetic disorders (benign childhood epilepsy, juvenile myclonic epilepsy). Common causes based on age shown in Table 14-3.

TABLE 14-3
Causes of Epilepsy in Different Age Groups

Age of onset	Probable cause
Adolescence	Idiopathic, trauma
Early adulthood	Idiopathic, trauma, tumor; alcohol or other hypnotic drug withdrawal
Middle age	Trauma, tumor, vascular disease; alcohol or other drug withdrawal
Late life	Vascular disease, tumor, degenerative disease

IV. DIAGNOSIS

A. **History.** Question patient or observers regarding prior seizures, medications, fever, circumstances, precipitating events, history of drug abuse or ingestions, and trauma.

B. **Physical examination.** Assess neurologic (responsiveness, pupils, fundi, fontanelles); cardiovascular (BP, perfusion); pulmonary (cyanosis, irregular breathing). Check for breath odor, rash, signs and symptoms of infection (sepsis, meningitis), signs of trauma, and increased liver size.

C. **Laboratory tests.** Electrolytes, Ca, glucose, BUN, CBC, anticonvulsant levels (if applicable), toxicology screen, sepsis work-up including LP if indication; consider LFTs, Mg, Pb, NH_4^+, CT scan.

D. **EEG.** Supports diagnosis of seizures but not confirmatory. Normal EEG does not rule out seizures. Should be performed 2 weeks after seizure episode. Nasopharyngeal leads add to sensitivity. Gives clues to location of seizure focus.

E. **EEG and videotape monitoring.** Helpful in (1) diagnosis of patients with psychogenic seizures in which there is coexistence of nonepileptic and epileptic events and (2) patients with seizures refractory to medications.

F. **MRI.** Can demonstrate tissue abnormalities and areas of subtle atrophy.

G. **PET and SPECT.** Can confirm an organic cerebral abnormality not seen structurally. Can differentiate between generalized and partial epilepsy or between primary and secondary epilepsy and delineate the dysfunctional region when surgery is considered.

H. **Magnetoencephalography.** Promising new way to localize epileptic focus.

V. FEBRILE SEIZURES AND STATUS EPILEPTICUS

See Chapter 1.

VI. TREATMENT

A. **Principles.** Optimally use single-drug therapy because multiple-drug interactions impair effectiveness and side effects accumulate. Drugs of choice are (1) carbamazepine and phenytoin for partial and generalized seizures and (2) ethosuximide for absence seizures. NOTE: Most antiepileptic drugs decrease the effectiveness of oral contraceptives. This should be discussed with the patient. See Table 14-4.

B. Surgical treatment. Most effective method for patients with intractable partial epilepsy. Consider a patient to be a surgical candidate within 1 year of epilepsy diagnosis if seizures are socially disabling and refractory to maximal dose of standard medication. Moreover, certain epilepsy syndromes (mesial temporal-lobe epilepsy, discrete neocortical lesion, and diffuse hemispheric disturbance) have a poor prognosis with purely medical treatment but respond well to surgical treatment.

VII. OTHER

A. Pseudoseizures. Seizure-like episodes of psychogenic origin. Usually *tightly* related to stress or personal events, such as the immediate triggering of an attack by an argument. Comparison between pseudoseizure and the specific type of epileptic attack mimicked can support the diagnosis; for example, pseudoepileptic "grand mal" patient may report an awareness of surroundings during attacks. NOTE: urinary incontinence, bodily injury, and tongue biting can occur with pseudoseizures but they are uncommon. If an attack occurs in the hospital or office, drawing a prolactin level within 30 minutes and another 2 hours later may clinch the diagnosis. The prolactin may be elevated immediately after a seizure when compared to a "baseline" value drawn at 2 hours. However, a negative test is not helpful. EEG during an attack can also distinguish pseudoseizures from true seizures. CPK may be elevated after seizure as well.

B. Breath-holding spells.
Seen in infants and small children. During crying, the infant holds his breath in expiration, becomes cyanotic, loses consciousness, and has a few convulsive limb movements. Distinguished from seizures because provoked only by crying and because the cyanosis precedes the convulsive movements in breath-holding spells but follows convulsive movements in true seizure. Resolve with maturity (usually by 5 years of age).

PARKINSON'S DISEASE (PD)

I. OVERVIEW

A slowly progressive movement disorder of unknown cause that primarily affects the pigmented, dopamine-containing neurons of the pars compacta of the substantia nigra. Usually appears in late adult life but sometimes as early as the fourth decade. Familial history usually absent.

TABLE 14-4
Common Antiepileptic Drugs for Adults

Generic (trade) Name	Daily dosage (mg)	Principal therapeutic indications	Serum half-life (hours)	Effective levels (mg/L)
Phenobarbital (Luminal)	60-200	Grand mal, absence, simple and complex partial seizures	79 ±12	10-40
Phenytoin (Dilantin)	300-400	Grand mal, simple and complex partial seizures	24 ±12	10-20
Carbamazepine (Tegretol)	600-1200	Grand mal, complex partial seizures	12 ±3	4-10
Valproic acid (Depakene)	1000-3000	Absence, grand mal, complex partial seizures	8 ±2	50-100
Primidone (Mysoline)	750-1500	Grand mal, simple and complex partial seizures	12 ±6	5-15
Ethosuximide (Zarontin)	750-2000	Absence	40 ±6	40-100
Clonazepam (Klonopin)	1.5-20	Absence, myoclonus	18 - 50	NA
		RECENT AGENTS		
Gabapentin (Neurontin)	900-1800	Adjunct therapy in partial seizures if age >12 years	5-7	NA
Lamotrigine (Lamictal)	25-500	Adjunct in partial seizure Unlabeled use: absence, myoclonic, tonic-clonic	24-30	Not known
Vigabatrin	Not known	Not FDA approved yet, expected in 1997	5-7	Not known
Felbamate (Felbatol)	1200-3600	Severe, refractory seizures that outweigh aplastic anemia or liver risk	14-23	NA

Adapted from Adams RA, Victor M: *Principles of neurology,* ed 4, companion handbook, New York, 1991, McGraw-Hill.

II. DIAGNOSIS

Diagnosis is made clinically. Cardinal symptoms are gross resting tremor (often pill-rolling involving mainly the hands and feet), bradykinesia, and muscular rigidity (described as lead pipe and cogwheel). Other features include masked face, decreased blinking, stooped posture, festinating gait (rapid propulsion forward with inability to stop), increased sweating and salivation. Depression and dementia may also be seen. A favorable response to L-dopa is suggestive of Parkinson's disease.

III. DIFFERENTIAL DIAGNOSIS

A. **Essential tremor.** Fine and rapid, intensified with sustained posture (such as holding hands extended), relieved by alcohol, and is usually familial with onset in young adulthood. Head tremor may also be seen. Neurologic exam is otherwise normal without the other features that define Parkinson's disease. Treatments for essential tremor include propranolol 20 to 60 mg PO TID or diazepam 2 to 10 mg PO TID.

B. **Parkinsonism secondary to drugs (such as antipsychotics and metoclopramide) or poisons (such as carbon monoxide, cyanide, manganese).** Usually apparent by history.

C. **Striatonigral degeneration.** Involves the corticospinal tract and extrapyramidal system, producing Babinski's sign (upgoing toes). Does not respond to L-dopa but may partially respond to anticholinergics.

D. **Progressive supranuclear palsy.** Characterized by failure of voluntary vertical conjugate gaze with parkinsonian symptoms. Speech becomes slurred and swallowing difficult.

E. **Shy-Drager syndrome.** Manifested by orthostatic hypotension and other autonomic dysfunction. May be associated with a parkinsonian type of presentation.

IV. TREATMENT

In 1994, a consensus conference was held to determine an algorithm for the management of Parkinson's disease (Fig. 14-1).

A. Medications used in the treatment of Parkinson's disease.

1. ***Selegiline (Eldepryl).*** A selective inhibitor of monoamine oxidase (MAO) subtype B. Promotes symptomatic benefit early in the disease state, and although it may delay disease progression of the disease, by 4 years groups treated with selegiline and L-dopa are equal in disability. Dosed 5 mg PO at breakfast and 5 mg at lunch (if given later in the day, insomnia occurs because of an amphetamine metabolite). No more than 10 mg/day total. Hypertensive crisis may occur with intake of tyramine-containing foods at doses >10 mg/day. Avoid use in combination with TCAs, SSRIs,

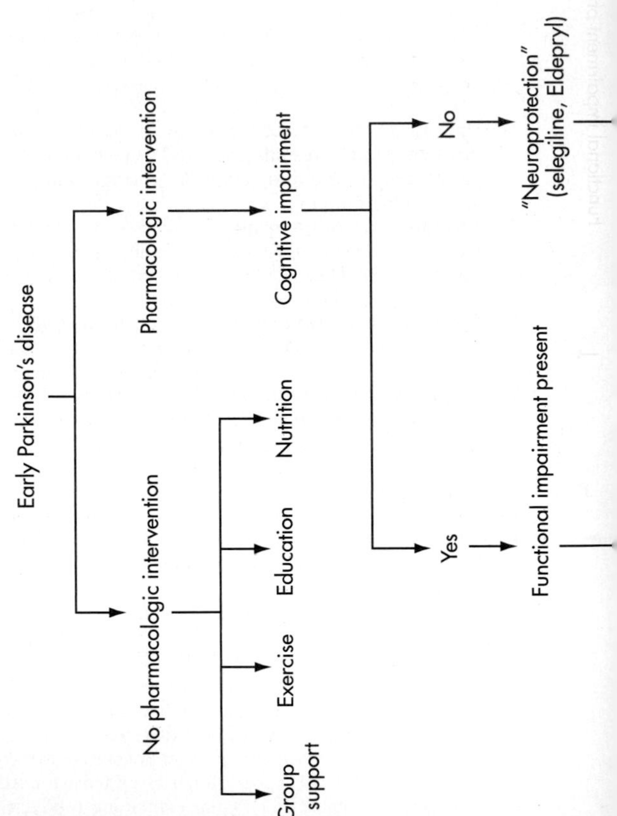
Early Parkinson's disease
No pharmacologic intervention
Pharmacologic intervention
Group support
Exercise
Education
Nutrition
Cognitive impairment
Yes
No
Functional impairment present
"Neuroprotection"
(selegiline, Eldepryl)

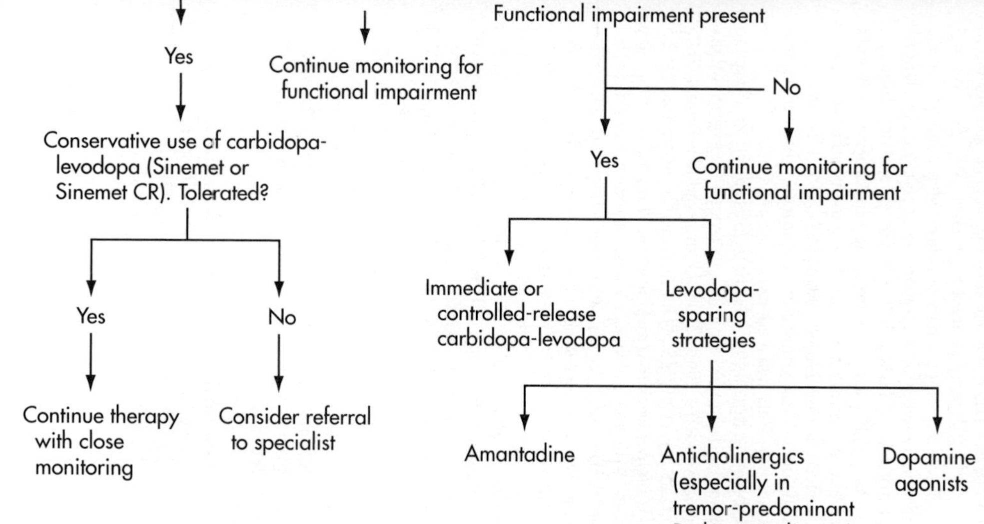

FIG. 14-1 Algorithm for the treatment of early Parkinson's disease. (From Stacy M, Brownlee HJ: *Am Fam Physician* 53(4):1281-1287, 1996.)

or other MAOIs. *Mortality may be up to 60% greater in those treated with selegiline plus L-dopa.*

2. ***Anticholinergics.*** For example, trihexyphenidyl (Artane) 1 to 5 mg PO TID or benztropine mesylate (Cogentin) 0.5 to 4 mg PO BID may be used for tremor. *Side effects:* blurred vision, constipation, urinary retention. Mental status changes and urinary retention limit their use in geriatric population.
3. ***Amantadine.*** Has both anticholinergic and dopaminergic effects; often used as monotherapy in patients with mild akinesia and minimal tremor. Also a useful adjunct in more advanced disease. Dosed 100 mg PO QD to TID. *Side effects:* livedo reticularis, confusion, nightmares, visual hallucinations, and rarely pedal edema.
4. ***Dopamine agonists.*** May be used as adjunct to L-dopa to minimize long-term exposure to L-dopa. Start bromocriptine (Parlodel) 1.25 mg PO QD, or pergolide (Permax) 0.05 to 0.25 mg PO QHS. Then increase bromocriptine by 2.5 mg/day per week to a maximum of 75 mg/day or pergolide by 0.25 mg/day per week to a maximum of 5 mg/day until satisfactory effect is achieved. Side effects include orthostatic hypotension and confusion with visual hallucinations.
5. ***Sinemet.*** For moderate to severe bradykinesia. Initially, immediate-release (Sinemet) or less often controlled release (Sinemet CR) is used. Sinemet 25/100 (carbidopa 25 mg with levodopa 100 mg) PO TID is started with meals to minimize nausea and slowly increased by 1 tablet/day every 3 or 4 days. *Alternatively,* Sinemet CR 25/100 BID is started and slowly increased by ½ tablet/day every 3 or 4 days to target L-dopa dose of 200 to 400 mg/day. When 500 to 800 mg/day of L-dopa is reached, the addition of a dopamine agonist is preferred over further increases in L-dopa. After 5 to 6 years of treatment, only 25% to 50% of patients maintain their initial improvement.

   Side effects of Sinemet

   a. *Peak-dose dyskinesias (similar to tardive dyskinesia).*
      (1) Occur within 20 to 90 minutes after Sinemet or 60 to 150 minutes after Sinemet CR.
      (2) Requires a gradual reduction in dose.
   b. *"Wearing-off" phenomenon.*
      (1) Seen toward the time of next dose.
      (2) Sinemet CR form has less "wearing-off" phenomenon than the immediate-release form has.
      (3) Use regular Sinemet in the morning to obtain rapid control of morning symptoms and Sinemet CR to maintain symptom relief during the day.
      (4) Concomitant use of monamine oxidase (MAO–B) inhibitors and L-dopa may reduce motor fluctuations.

(5) The early combination of L-dopa and a dopamine agonist may reduce the incidence of "wearing-off" fluctuations.
(6) Protein redistribution diets (concentrate protein-rich foods at dinner and use less protein-rich foods at breakfast and lunch) may improve "wearing-off" fluctuations.
(7) Other options include adding amantadine, selegiline, anticholinergics, or apomorphine to reduce "wearing-off."

c. *Nausea and vomiting.* Responds to trimethobenzamide (Tigan) 250 mg TID or add additional carbidopa.
d. Decreased efficacy can be caused by vitamin B_6 high protein diets.

B. Nonpharmacologic therapy for Parkinson's disease. A key component to early Parkinson's disease. See Fig. 14-1.

C. Physical therapy. Often useful in gait training and balance.

D. Surgical treatments such as thalamic stimulation, posteroventral pallidotomy, and fetal tissue transplantation are currently being studied for patients with advanced PD poorly controlled with medications.

V. ASSOCIATED CONDITIONS

A. Dementia. Incidence 15% to 20%. May be related to PD or other dementing illnesses. Aggravated by antiparkinsonian drugs. Should attempt to minimize anticholinergic medications first, followed by dopaminergic medications if tolerated.

B. Depression. Occurs in up to 47% of patients with PD. If sustained, treat with psychotherapy or TCAs (nortriptyline usually tolerated best) or SSRIs. Concurrent use of selegiline and SSRIs or TCAs is discouraged because of adverse interactions. Electroconvulsive therapy is useful for severe depression unresponsive to medications and may provide transient decrease in motor signs of PD.

C. Hallucinations. May be induced by both anticholinergic and dopaminergic antiparkinsonian medications (for example, a 20% incidence with L-dopa). Early symptoms of restlessness or nightmares progress to auditory and visual hallucinations and paranoia. Attempt to minimize medication doses if possible. If symptoms persist, treat with low-potency antipsychotics such as thioridazine, risperidone, or molindone.

BENIGN NOCTURNAL LEG CRAMPS

I. OVERVIEW AND DEFINITION

A. Prevalence. 35% to 95% at some time in all adults, but most common in older adults.

B. Definition. A benign muscle cramp is an involuntary, localized, visible, and usually painful skeletal muscle contraction (calf muscles most commonly). Cramps typically occur at night, are sporadic and random, and usually last only seconds to minutes.

C. Precipitating factors. Muscle fatigue and passive plantar flexion.

II. DIAGNOSIS

A. Causes. May include the following:

1. ***Lower motor neuron disease.*** Amyotrophic lateral sclerosis, polyneuropathies, peripheral nerve injury.
2. Hemodialysis.
3. Heat cramps.
4. ***Altered fluid and electrolyte levels:*** hypoglycemia, severe hyponatremia.
5. ***Certain drugs:*** nifedipine (Procardia), beta-agonists (terbutaline sulfate [Brethine]), clofibrate (Atromid-S), penicillamine (Cuprimine).
6. Alcohol ingestion.
7. ***Contractures:*** McArdle disease (a deficiency in muscle phosphorylase leading to stiffness and decreased exercise tolerance), hyperthyroid myopathy.
8. ***Tetany (often preceded by tingling paresthesias).*** Hypocalcemia, respiratory alkalosis, hypermagnesemia, hypokalemia, hyperkalemia.
9. Dystonias.
10. Claudication.

B. Physical examination. Unrevealing unless a cramp is observed.

III. TREATMENT

A. Acute muscle cramp. Stretching of the affected muscle (as in walking).

B. Mechanical prevention. Advise to stretch calf muscles intermittently throughout the day, use a footboard during sleep, and dangle feet over the edge of bed when lying prone.

C. Pharmacologic prevention.

1. The efficacy of quinine sulfate at low doses (such as 300 mg PO QHS) has been supported by several recent analysis. Its use is controversial since the FDA has banned quinine-based OTC preparations for nocturnal leg cramps. Potentially fatal thrombocytopenia, hypersensitivity reactions, or arrhythmias can occur with quinine use.
2. Other reportedly helpful medications include vitamin E (800 units/day), verapamil (Calan), carbamazepine (Tegretol), diphenhydramine (Benadryl), phenytoin (Dilantin), methocarbamol (Robaxin), and riboflavin; however, no randomized, controlled studies were found in the literature.

RESTLESS LEGS SYNDROME

I. SIGNS AND SYMPTOMS

Unpleasant sensation in the legs (and occasionally arms) that occurs at rest and relieved by movement. Sensations are described as crawling, creeping, aching, jittery, or fidgety in nature. Motor restlessness usually accompanies the paresthesias. Symptoms typically occur at night with associated sleep disturbance. The disorder is intermittent, and long asymptomatic periods can occur. Mild symptoms of restless legs occur in up to 5% of the population. Restless legs syndrome is idiopathic in the majority of patients but may be the presenting sign of iron deficiency, and it is also common in diabetes mellitus, uremia, pregnancy, rheumatoid arthritis, vitamin B_{12} deficiency, and polyneuropathy.

II. DIAGNOSIS

Differential diagnosis includes other conditions that cause nocturnal limb discomfort: burning feet syndrome, muscular cramps, vascular and neurogenic claudication, polyneuropathy, fibromyalgia, meralgia parasthetica, and drug-induced akathisia. History is used to make the diagnosis. Lab tests to rule out other causes include BUN, creatinine, glucose, ferritin, folate, and CBC. Consider needle electromyography and nerve conduction studies if polyneuropathy is suspected. Consider sleep studies to document sleep disturbances and periodic movements of sleep in difficult cases or if sleep apnea is suspected.

III. TREATMENT

A. **General measures.** Limit smoking, alcohol, caffeine. Discontinue aggravating medications.

B. **Treatment of primary condition.** Treat underlying causes: iron deficiency responds to iron supplements; folate is beneficial for those who are folate deficient, especially pregnant women, etc.

C. **Pharmacologic treatment options.**

1. ***Sinemet.*** Levodopa component dosed 50 to 600 mg/day PO (average 100 to 200 mg/day). Be careful, since overmedication with Sinemet can cause symptoms similar to restless legs itself. It may be necessary to titrate the dose carefully.
2. ***Clonazepam*** (Klonopin). 0.5 to 4.0 mg/day PO.
3. ***Carbamazepine*** (Tegretol). 100 to 300 mg/day PO.
4. ***Clonidine*** (Catapres). 0.1 to 0.9 mg/day PO (average 0.1 to 0.3 mg/day).

CNS INFECTION IN THE ADULT

I. CAUSES. *Streptococcus pneumoniae* and *Neisseria meningitidis* are responsible for most adult *bacterial meningitis*. Predisposing factors include sinusitis, otitis media, or mastoiditis. Fever and focal neurologic signs should raise the possibility of brain abscess; a source should be sought (such as lung abscess). *Viral meningitis* is common and is usually caused by enteroviruses, and the course is usually benign. *Herpes simplex virus* is a sporadic cause of encephalitis and requires early institution of therapy. Meningitis may also be caused by unusual bacterial organisms such as *Leptospira* species, *Brucella* species, *Borrelia burgdorferi* and others. Cryptococcal meningitis and tuberculous meningitis should be ruled out whenever suspected. (See Chapter 16 for more information on opportunistic organisms.)

II. CLINICAL PRESENTATION

Fever, headache, nausea, vomiting, malaise, and meningeal signs; neck stiffness and Kernig's sign are characteristic of meningitis. Mental status changes or seizures are suggestive of encephalitis. Important history includes exposure to mosquitoes, ticks or tuberculosis; travel; HIV risk factors; and a prior history of meningitis.

III. DIAGNOSIS

A lumbar puncture should be performed immediately, *unless* there are focal neurologic signs or papilledema, which warrant a head CT first. Marked alterations in consciousness also require head CT or MRI. Do not delay antibiotics if unable to do lumbar puncture immediately. Give antibiotics before sending for CT or MRI scan. A single dose of antibiotics will not change your culture results. Determine opening pressure; send the first tube of cerebrospinal fluid for *protein and glucose,* the second tube for *Gram stain, C&S,* and the third tube for *cell count and differential* (Table 14-5). Acid-fast bacilli stain, India ink preparation, and cryptococcal antigen may be obtained when indicated. Blood glucose is obtained for reference at the same time as LP.

IV. TREATMENT

A. Supportive measures. Give no more fluid than required for maintenance and avoid D_5W especially when brain edema is suspected. Depending on severity of illness, may want to avoid narcotics for pain control because they make assessment of consciousness difficult, may suppress ventilation, and may worsen brain edema caused by CO_2 retention.

B. Empiric therapy.

1. ***Bacterial meningitis in an adult without immunocompromise.*** *Start with a third-generation cephalosporin* (cefotaxime 2 g IV Q4h or ceftriaxone 2 g IV Q12h) *pending culture results and add ampicillin for adults >50 years.* These combinations are not active against *Staphylococcus aureus, Pseudomonas,* or anaerobics, which are extremely rare in uncomplicated adult meningitis. If

TABLE 14-5
Cerebrospinal Fluid Findings in Lumbar Puncture

Condition	Protein (mg/dl)	Fasting sugar (mg/dl)	WBC (number/mm³)
Normal	15-45	45-80	Up to 10 L
Viral meningitis or encephalitis	20-200	Normal	10 to 500 chiefly L; may be P dominant in acute phase
Bacterial meningitis	50-1500	0-45	25 to 10,000 chiefly P; may be L dominant if partially treated
Tuberculous meningitis	45-500	10-45	25 to 1000 chiefly L
Cryptococcal meningitis	<500 in 90%	Moderately decreased in 55%	<800 chiefly L

L, Lymphocyte; *P*, polymorphonuclear leukocyte.

penicillin-resistant *Streptococcus pneumoniae* is prevalent in your institution, initial therapy with vancomycin and rifampin may be indicated. If C&S reveal penicillin-sensitive organism, penicillin G, 2 million units IV Q4h, or ampicillin 3 g IV Q6h for 10 to 14 days will provide effective therapy.

2. ***Viral meningitis.*** If uncertain of diagnosis or bacterial meningitis is suspected, hospitalize and begin antibiotics as above. Otherwise adequate hydration, antiemetics, and analgesics for headache should be sufficient treatment and can be carried out at home with reliable caregivers. Any sign of encephalitis (such as mental changes) warrants admission to watch for acute neurologic deterioration.
3. ***Brain abscess.*** Add metronidazole 500 mg IV Q6h to the regimens noted above for meningitis to cover anaerobes. CT or MRI is diagnostic, but brain abscess can be confused with tumors or cerebrovascular diseases. Neurosurgery or neurology consultation is imperative.
4. ***Herpes encephalitis.*** Treatment with acyclovir 10 mg/kg IV Q8h for 10 days should be started without delay in patient who presents with the abrupt onset of fever, behavioral changes, alteration of consciousness with or without focal neurologic signs, particularly when CSF abnormalities are moderate, a state suggestive of a viral CNS infection. MRI is a sensitive method to detect characteristic temporal lobe abnormalities, but these changes may not be obvious in early stages. Consult a neurologist.

CEREBROVASCULAR DISEASE

I. OVERVIEW

Stroke affects 500,000 people per year. Third leading cause of death in adults. With hemorrhagic stroke, 40% to 84% of patients die within 30 days; with ischemic stroke, 15% to 33% of patients die within 30 days. 80% of strokes are ischemic, and one fourth are caused by cerebral emboli.

II. CLASSIFICATION

A. Infarction.

1. ***Transient ischemic attacks (TIAs).*** Neurologic symptoms or deficits clearing <24 hours.
2. ***Progressing stroke.*** Unstable; progressing neurologic deficits.
3. ***Completed stroke.*** A stable, nonprogressing neurologic deficit.
4. ***Lacunar infarction.*** Caused by hyaline thickening of small penetrating arteries in subcortical brain and com-

monly associated with hypertension. Often asymptomatic but may result in pure motor strokes, pure sensory strokes, clumsy hand–dysarthria syndrome, or ataxic hemiparesis. CT may show small subcortical infarcts, but MRI is more sensitive.

B. **Intracranial hemorrhage.** White color on CT scan. Often evidence of a vascular anomaly (such as an aneurysm or angioma) or hypertension.
   1. ***Intracerebral hemorrhage.*** Hemorrhage in or around brain.
   2. ***Subarachnoid hemorrhage (SAH).*** Accounts for 5% to 10% of strokes.

III. DIAGNOSIS

A. **History and physical.**
   1. ***Intracranial hemorrhage.*** Suggested by coma, vomiting, severe headache, history of warfarin therapy, history of vascular anomaly (aneurysm or angioma), systolic BP >220 mm Hg, or blood glucose ≥170 in nondiabetic.
   2. ***Abrupt onset.*** Suggestive of infarction, but must rule out brain abscess, tumor, or subdural hematoma. Differential diagnosis also includes epilepsy, delirium, intoxication, MS, and conversion reaction.
   3. Suspect subarachnoid hemorrhage if patient has new-onset severe headache that may be followed by nausea and vomiting and loss of consciousness (transient or coma). However, may have only headache and normal exam (see headache, p. 554.
   4. ***Risk factors for embolic stroke.*** Atrial fibrillation, valvular disease especially mitral stenosis and mitral prolapse, CAD, recent MI, ventricular aneurysm, carotid stenosis, peripheral vascular disease, smoking, hyperlipidemia, diabetes, and history of IV drug abuse.
   5. ***Physical examination.*** On PE especially evaluate the level of consciousness, speech, cognitive abilities, visual fields, extraocular muscle function, motor function, and gait. Check for heart murmurs or carotid bruits.

B. **Differential diagnosis.** Seizures and postictal states, delirium intoxications, tumors, syncope, and subdural hematomas. Identify and correct any condition that causes decreased cardiac output (such as arrhythmia, MI, CHF) or hypotension (such as hypovolemia, septic shock).

C. **Diagnostic tests.**
   1. ***Minimal evaluation.*** Neuroimaging study (CT or MRI), ECG, CXR, pulse oximetry or ABG, CBC, PT/PTT, serum glucose, Cr, BUN, and electrolytes. Implications of these tests are interpreted in Box 14-2.
   2. ***Neuroimaging considerations.***

BOX 14-2

Initial Laboratory Work-up in Stroke and Implications of Findings

HEMOGLOBIN AND HEMATOCRIT
Anemia may compromise cerebral oxygenation
Hematocrit greater than 60 percent leads to increased viscosity and decreased perfusion
Anemia can suggest sickle cell or other hemoglobinopathies

WHITE BLOOD CELL COUNT
Increased in leukemia, leading to sludging of capillaries and multiple small infarcts
Increase in infections, including meningitis, which may occasionally mimic a stroke

PLATELETS
A platelet count greater than 1 million leads to hypercoagulability
A platelet count less than 10,000 may increase risk of bleeding
Decreased platelets may imply the following:
- Antiphospholipid syndrome
- Consumptive coagulopathies
- Systemic lupus erythematosus
- Thrombotic thrombocytopenic purpura

PROTHROMBIN TIME AND PARTIAL THROMBOPLASTIN TIME
Screening tests for bleeding disorder

SERUM GLUCOSE
Hypoglycemia or hyperglycemia may mimic stroke
Hyperglycemia may exacerbate cell death

ELECTROLYTES
Abnormalities may be suggestive of systemic illness mimicking or exacerbating stroke

CREATININE AND BLOOD UREA NITROGEN
Abnormalities may indicate dehydration or underlying renal disease

ELECTROCARDIOGRAM
Signs of myocardial ischemia, infarction, or arrhythmia

CHEST RADIOGRAPH
Screens for evidence of cardiac or pulmonary disease mimicking or exacerbating stroke

PULSE OXIMETRY OR ARTERIAL BLOOD GAS
Hypoxia exacerbates cerebral ischemia
Hypercarbia may indicate need for ventilatory support.

Modified from Smucker WD et al: *Am Fam Physician* 52(1):227-234, 1995.

a. Noncontrast CT to rule out intracranial bleed.
b. Contrast CT if suspect abscess, tumor, or granuloma.
c. *MRI.* More sensitive for detecting infarction than CT is especially if lesion in brainstem or posterior fossa. More sensitive for mass lesions than CT is but difficult to obtain emergently.
d. *Comments.* CT will miss approximately 10% of subarachnoid bleeds. When CT scan early in course of presumed ischemic stoke is normal, a repeat scan in 72 hours reliably shows area of infarction. MRI sensitivity offset by fact that it may not accurately differentiate intracerebral hemorrhage from ischemia during acute phase of stroke; thus in most patients CT is preferable to MRI.

3. *Transesophageal echocardiogram* if cardiac embolism suspected. Transthoracic is not sensitive for this indication and should be skipped.
4. *Ultrasonography* to screen for carotid artery stenosis in all patients with ischemic stroke. If posterior cerebral circulation signs and symptoms, may questionably benefit from transcranial Doppler study.
5. *Angiography* is indicated when a patient is a candidate for endarterectomy, or when he or she is young or poses a diagnostic dilemma, such as vasculitis, congenital vascular anomaly.
6. Further testing as indicated by Box 14-3.

IV. TREATMENT

A. General measures.

1. Box 14-4. Approach to lowering blood pressure in acute stroke.
2. Vomiting is common and NG suction may be needed.
3. Avoid IV solutions with large amounts of free water, such as D_5W.
4. Passive range-of-motion exercises are begun 3 or 4 times a day within 24 to 48 hours of complction of thc strokc.
5. New therapies with nimodipine, *N*-methyl-D-aspartate–receptor antagonists, and tissue plasminogen activator (TPA) are currently under further study but look very promising. Their use at this time is still limited to study centers with stroke units and neurosurgeons.

B. Specific measures.

1. ***Cardiogenic embolus.*** Systemic anticoagulation to prevent subsequent emboli. Its timing remains controversial: hemorrhage into an infarct can develop 1 to 7 days after the infarction and may become fatal. Therefore, hold anticoagulation on a large embolic infarct for 1 to 7 days unless thrombus is found in the heart. To anticoagulate,

BOX 14-3

Discretionary Tests in the Assessment of Patients with Acute Stroke

LUMBAR PUNCTURE

Indicated when clinical picture is suggestive of subarachnoid hemorrhage but computerized tomography is negative

Indicated when clinical picture is suggestive of central nervous system infection

ELECTROENCEPHALOGRAM

If clinical picture is suggestive of seizure

TOXICOLOGY SCREENING

Indicated when presentation is unusual or history is suggestive of ingestion

ERYTHROCYTE SEDIMENTATION RATE

Indicated in cases of unexplained stroke

Increased with vasculitis

HEMOGLOBIN ELECTROPHORESIS

Indicated if anemia is present and history is suggestive of racial or genetic predisposition to thrombosis

FIBRINOGEN

Indicated when common stroke risk factors are not present

Increased level causes increased viscosity

Increased as acute-phase reactant in early stroke

IMMUNOELECTROPHORESIS

Indicated when common stroke-risk factors are not present

Increased IgA, IgG or IgM implies autoimmune disease causing thrombosis

Waldenström's acroglobulinemia causes thrombosis

Multiple myeloma causes thrombosis

ANTIPHOSPHOLIPID ANTIBODIES

Indicated when common stroke risk factors are not present

Associated with thrombosis

Modified from Smucker WD et al: *Am Fam Physician* 52(1):227-234, 1995.

use heparin to prolong the PTT. See deep venous thrombosis section, p. 116, for anticoagulation protocols.

2. ***Transient ischemic attacks (TIAs).*** About one third of patients will experience cerebral infarction within 5 years. Start aspirin 325 mg QD, or baby aspirin (81 mg) QD

BOX 14-4

Approach to Lowering the Blood Pressure in Acute Stroke

LOWER BLOOD PRESSURE SLOWLY AND GENTLY

Watch for signs of clinical deterioration in neurologic status

ISCHEMIC STROKE

Lower blood pressure only if repeated measurements are >220 mm Hg systolic or >120 mm Hg diastolic or there is evidence of end-organ failure or aortic dissection

Lower blood pressure from 180 to 185/105 to 110 mm Hg in patients with a history of hypertension

Lower blood pressure from 160 to 170/95 to 100 mm Hg in patients with previously normal blood pressure

INTRACEREBRAL HEMORRHAGE

Lower blood pressure from 180 to 185/105 to 110 mm Hg in patients with a history of hypertension

Lower blood pressure from 160 to 170/95 to 100 mm Hg in patients with previously normal blood pressure

SUBARACHNOID HEMORRHAGE

Lower to prestroke levels

THERAPEUTIC AGENTS

Labetalol (Normodyne, Trandate), 10 mg intravenously over 1 to 2 minutes (may repeat or double dosage every 10 to 20 minutes until blood pressure is controlled or until a maximum dose of 300 mg has been given)

Labetalol, 200 to 300 mg orally every 6 to 8 hours

Enalapril (Vasotec), 1 mg intravenously over 15 to 20 minutes

Captopril (Capoten), 6.25 to 25 mg orally every 8 hours

Nifedipine (Adalat, Procardia), 10 mg orally every 6 hours*

Nimodipine (Nimotop), 60 mg orally every 4 hours†

Modified from Smucker WD et al: *Am Fam Physician* 52(1):227-234,1995.

*Nifedipine should not be given sublingually.

†Nimodipine is recommended in cases of subarachnoid hemorrhage.

in those unable to tolerate the regular dose of aspirin. Ticlopidine 25 mg BID reserved for patients failing aspirin therapy (but monitor for neutropenia or agranulocytosis). Ticlopidine is more effective than ASA, and some authors suggest ticlopidine as primary therapy. However it is more expensive. Carotid endarterectomy is done in symptomatic patients with high-grade carotid stenosis

(70% to 99%). Consider endarterectomy in asymptomatic patients with >60% stenosis but only if complication rate of vascular surgeon is <3% (surgery for asymptomatic lesions is not yet standard of care). If stenosis <60%, use medical therapy and repeat carotid scan in 6 to 12 months.

3. ***Progressing stroke.*** IV heparin still used though studies have not shown any benefit up to now. Obtain head CT without contrast first to rule out hemorrhagic infarction.
4. ***Thrombosis (atherosclerosis) and lacunar infarction.*** Aspirin or ticlopidine as above. Treat risk factors, especially hypertension and diabetes.
5. ***Intracerebral hemorrhage.*** Obtain neurosurgical consultation for possible evacuation in patients with cerebellar hematomas and large superficial cerebral hematomas.
6. ***Subarachnoid hemorrhage.*** Immediate neurosurgical consultation required. Patient advised against straining and is given stool softeners. Phenytoin is given routinely to prevent seizures (15 mg/kg IV at 1 mg/kg/min IV not to exceed 50 mg/min); do not exceed 1 g in adults; mix with NS (50 ml/500 mg in adults).

PERIPHERAL NEUROPATHY

I. CLASSIFICATION

A. Polyneuropathy. Bilaterally symmetric affection of the peripheral nerves, usually involving the legs more than the arms and the distal segments earlier and more severely than the proximal ones, that is, the stocking-and-glove pattern.

B. Mononeuropathy. Involvement of a single nerve.

C. Mononeuropathy multiplex. Random involvement of multiple nerves.

D. Radiculopahty. Involvement of the nerve roots.

E. Demyelination. Commonly affects both proximal and distal segments of the nerve as in Guillain-Barré syndrome.

F. Axonal degeneration. Commonly progresses from distal to proximal segments (that is, dying-back neuropathy).

II. MANIFESTATIONS

Symptoms and signs include pain, paresthesias, sensory loss, weakness, muscle atrophy, reflex loss, anhidrosis, orthostatic hypotension.

III. DIAGNOSIS

A. Full neurologic exam with special attention to muscle weakness, reflex loss, autonomic dysfunction, and sensory deficits (touch, pain, temperature, position, and vibration).

B. Nerve conduction study can confirm neuropathy and differentiate demyelination from axonal degeneration.

C. Electromyography differentiates myogenic from neurogenic causes of weakness and confirms abnormality of neuromuscular junctions.

D. Nerve biopsy is undertaken only when etiologic diagnosis remains in doubt after electrodiagnostic tests have been completed.

IV. DIFFERENTIAL DIAGNOSIS

A. The most commonly acquired neuropathies are those associated with diabetes mellitus, alcoholism, or Guillain-Barré syndrome. Inherited peripheral neuropathies include Charcot-Marie-Tooth disease. Two types of questions must be answered to determine the cause: (1) polyneuropathy or mononeuropathy multiplex? (2) acute, subacute, or chronic?

B. Causes of neuropathy. (Mononeuropathies, plexopathies, and inherited polyneuropathies are not included.)

1. ***Acute ascending motor paralysis with minimal sensory disturbance.***
   - Guillain-Barré syndrome
   - Diphtheritic polyneuropathy
2. ***Subacute sensorimotor disturbance.***
   a. **Polyneuropathy.**
      (1) *Nutritional deficiency:* alcoholism (beriberi), pellagra, vitamin B_{12} deficiency.
      (2) *Poisoning with heavy metals and solvents:* arsenic, lead, mercury, thallium, methyl-*n*-butylketone, *n*-hexane, methyl bromide, organophosphates, acrylamide.
      (3) *Drug intoxications:* isoniazid, ethionamide, hydralazine, nitrofurantoin, disulfiram, vincristine, chloramphenicol, phenytoin, dapsone, etc.
      (4) *Uremic neuropathy.*

   b. **Mononeuropathy multiplex.**
      - Diabetes mellitus
      - Sarcoidosis
      - Polyarteritis nodosa
3. ***Chronic sensorimotor polyneuropathy.***
   - Benign form in the elderly
   - Connective tissue diseases
   - Uremia (occasionally subacute)
   - Beriberi (usually subacute)
   - Carcinoma (paraneoplastic syndrome)
   - Paraproteinemias
   - Hypothyroidism
   - Amyloidosis
   - Diabetes mellitus
   - Leprosy

V. TREATMENT

Removal of the offending agent in toxic neuropathies (such as alcohol) and, where possible, treatment of an associated systemic illness (such as Lyme disease) are important. Physical and occupational therapy may be helpful to prevent contractures and improve function. Vitamin replacement in deficiency states. Steroids and, in some instances, plasma exchanges are useful for relapsing demyelinating polyneuritis. Steroids are useful in polyarteritis. Dysesthetic pain in polyneuropathies is treated with a small QHS dose of a tricyclic antidepressant. Neuralgic pain (stabbing, shooting) is treated with anticonvulsant doses of phenytoin, carbamazepine. Capsaicin cream may also be useful for neuropathy pain. For compression mononeuropathies (such as carpal tunnel "syndrome"), first treat with splints, NSAIDs, or local steroid injections; if failure, then surgical release may be curative.

MULTIPLE SCLEROSIS (MS)

I. OVERVIEW

MS affects young adults and is characterized by multiple areas of demyelination and sclerosis in the CNS. MS affects white matter; peripheral nerves are spared. Cause is unknown. Familial incidence is low. Whites are more susceptible than blacks and Asians. Pregnancy decreases risk of exacerbations, but exacerbations increase immediately post partum. Infection or trauma may precipitate or trigger exacerbations.

II. CLINICAL MANIFESTATIONS

Acute onset of symptoms usually lasting for several weeks but may persist for only a few minutes or hours. A history of fluctuation in the clinical course and signs of neurologic deficits consistent with multiple lesions in the white matter of the CNS is almost pathognomonic of MS. Common symptoms include weakness or numbness of a limb, monocular visual loss, diplopia, vertigo, facial weakness or numbness, sphincter disturbances, ataxia, and nystagmus. A history of symptoms aggravated by a hot bath is sometimes obtained.

III. LABORATORY TESTS.

About 90% of patients have abnormal findings in CSF that include a mild mononuclear pleocytosis, a modest increase in total protein, a greatly increased gamma globulin fraction, a high IgG index, presence of oligoclonal bands, and an increase in myelin basic protein. MRI is as sensitive as CSF exam and is the neuroimaging test of choice with gadolinium enhancement, which can differentiate new lesions from old ones. Pattern-shift visual-evoked responses are abnormal in 80% of patients with definite MS.

IV. DIFFERENTIAL DIAGNOSIS

Behçet's disease, SLE, metastatic tumors, vascular malformation of brainstem, Arnold-Chiari malformation, herniated intervertebral disk, and spinocerebellar degeneration.

V. PROGNOSIS

One study showed that a 25-year mortality was about 26% compared with 14% in the general population. After 25 years two thirds of the survivors were still ambulatory. 60% of those with an initial diagnosis of optic neuritis will develop MS within 40 years.

VI. TREATMENT

Corticosteroids are often used to shorten the duration of acute exacerbations, though their utility has not been shown in controlled studies. Typical regimen is prednisone 60 to 80 mg PO for 10 days with tapering off over 3 weeks. Rapid improvement has been reported in some patients with high-dose IV methylprednisolone (250 to 1000 mg/day for 2 to 7 days) followed by a course of oral prednisone. Optic neuritis is worsened by the use of oral prednisone alone and should be preceded by methylprednisolone (that is, methylprednisolone 1 g/day for 3 days, then prednisone 1 mg/kg/day for 11 days, and then taper off). Additionally, using methylprednisolone may slow progression to MS. In patients with relapsing-remitting MS, treatment with beta-interferon has been shown to reduce the annual exacerbation rate, and further studies of this approach are in progress. Several recent studies have suggested that intensive immunosuppressive therapy with cyclophosphamide or azathioprine may help arrest the course of chronic progressive active multiple sclerosis, but further clinical trials are still in progress. Finally, early studies show that copolymer 1 (a random polymer-simulating myelin basic protein) may benefit patients with the exacerbating-remitting form of MS; further evaluation is pending.

VERTIGO AND DIZZINESS

I. CLASSIFICATION WITH SIGNS AND SYMPTOMS

A. **Vertigo.** A sense that the environment is spinning around or a sensation of feeling impelled forward, backward, or to either side. Others describe "tilting" of their environment or a "back-and-forth" feeling. Acute episodes may be associated with nausea, vomiting, diaphoresis, and ataxia. Vertigo is typically broken down into 2 major types, central and peripheral (see Table 14-6). *Vertigo does not equal presyncope.*

B. **Presyncope.** A feeling of light-headedness or faintness. Often associated with generalized weakness, visual blurring

TABLE 14-6
Comparison of Peripheral and Central Vertigo

Symptom	Peripheral	Central
Occurrence of vertigo	Episodic	May be constant
Vertigo severity	Proportionate to nystagmus	May be disproportionate
Nystagmus axis	Horizontal/rotatory	Horizontal/vertical, oblique, or rotatory and may vary
Nystagmus type	Slow and fast phase	May be irregular or equal phase
Nystagmus latency	About 10 to 20 seconds	None
Nystagmus direction	Single	Direction changing
Nystagmus severity	Varies with vertigo	Independent
Nystagmus duration	Brief	Long
Nystagmus fatigue*	Yes	No
Nystagmus habituation†	Yes	No
Hearing loss, tinnitus	Possible	No
Loss of consciousness	No	Possible
Other neurologic signs/ symptoms	No	Possible

Adapted from Cohen NL: *Med Clin North Am* 75(6):1252-1253, 1991.
*If one holds same position, nystagmus decreases with time.
†Repeating same position change produces decreasing nystagmus.

or blacking out, diaphoresis, SOB, or palpitations. Typically episodic and caused by transient decrease in cerebral perfusion.

C. Disequilibrium. Dizziness is primarily experienced when one is standing or walking. Better when lying or sitting. Crowds and difficult walkways (such as stairs, ramps, and escalators) exacerbate patient's symptoms.

II. VERTIGO SYNDROMES

A. Causes of recurrent episodes of vertigo.

1. ***Benign paroxysmal positional vertigo (BPPV).*** Most common cause of recurrent vertigo. Historical characteristics: change in head position (can be more than one position) brings on vertigo; brief latency to onset of vertigo; fatigability of vertigo with repeated trials; not associated with tinnitus; may be associated with nausea but rarely emesis. Symptoms often reproducible with Hallpike or Barany maneuver (rapidly laying patient

down with hyperextension of the neck over the edge of the bed). Typically idiopathic but may develop after head trauma or viral illness. Typically a waxing and waning course over months to years, but most cases resolve with time. All patients with BPPV should have an audiogram or brainstem auditory evoked responses (BAERs) to screen for tumors. If positive BAER, then MRI or CT should be done; however, if negative, then no further work-up needed. Meclizine (Antivert) is not too useful. Diazepam (Valium) may blunt the sensation; however, it may prolong the illness. Vestibular training is superior to drugs alone and leads to a more rapid resolution of symptoms (4 weeks 75% versus 24%; 8 weeks 62% versus 70%; and 30% in drug plus vestibular training group). BPPV can also be improved with the use of Epley's maneuver, which is an attempt to reposition the presumed otolith into a nonsensitive position in the semicircular canals. However, no controlled trials have been done.

2. ***Positioning vertigo.*** Not a specific syndrome like BPPV but instead a symptom of an underlying peripheral or central vestibular disorder. Lacks the specificity of head position, the latency to onset of vertigo, and the fatigability with repeated trials seen in BPPV.
3. ***Ménière's disease.*** Syndrome with recurrent attacks of vertigo and tinnitus lasting hours to days and associated hearing loss (low frequencies lost first; discrimination is maintained). Generally have feeling of ear fullness that resolves after episodes of vertigo. *Transient vertigo is not Ménière's disease!* May have nausea, vomiting, and ataxia. Onset age 30 to 60 years. All patients should have posterior fossa CT or MRI and bilateral audiometry. 60% resolve spontaneously without treatment. Treatment includes bed rest, IV fluids if unable to maintain hydration, antihistamines, and phenothiazines. Salt restriction and diuretics (such as hydrochlorothiazide or furosemide) may be helpful. Data are poor, but two thirds are reported to respond to either sodium restriction or diuretics. If severe symptoms, surgical ablation may be performed (labyrinthectomy if hearing is lost; vestibular nerve section if hearing is preserved).
4. ***Toxic damage to labyrinth.*** Antibiotics especially aminoglycosides, salicylates, ethanol intoxication, phenytoin toxicity, quinine, benzene, arsenic, etc. Hypothyroidism rare cause.
5. ***Acoustic neuroma.*** Benign tumor arising from cranial nerve VIII. May have tinnitus and hearing loss, *but* discrimination is lost much before hearing loss is complete.

May have associated facial palsy. Auditory brainstem testing is the best test. Nerve stretched by tumor; therefore there is a delay of the signal.

6. ***Migraine.*** Vertigo can arise from migrainous vasospasm of the basilar artery. Other symptoms include scintillating scotoma, homonymous hemianopsia, cortical blindness, diplopia, dysarthria, ataxia, paresthesias. Patients typically young. Migraine HA may occur after vertigo. Treat as for migraine headache.
7. ***Perilymph fistula.*** Vertigo precipitated by change in head position, coughing, sneezing, swallowing, straining, barotrauma, air travel, or loud noises. Often history of head trauma that results in a small tear in the oval or round window. Tends to be better in the morning and worse after being upright for a time because patient has perilymph leak. May be associated tinnitus and hearing loss. *Diagnosis:* pneumatic otoscopy reproduces symptoms. Often heals spontaneously. Surgical correction if ongoing symptoms.
8. ***Temporal lobe epilepsy.*** Vertigo experienced as part of seizure.

B. Causes of a single acute episode of vertigo.

1. ***Acute peripheral vestibulopathy (viral labyrinthitis).*** Acute onset of severe vertigo, vomiting, nausea, and ataxia that lasts hours to days and slowly returns to normal. Hearing loss and tinnitus not typical. Nystagmus with characteristics of peripheral origin. Occurs in all ages. Cause unclear but may be viral (45% cluster around viral infections). Perform audiogram or BAERs for screening. Posterior fossa imaging necessary if screening test abnormal or if >60 years of age with history and risk factors for vascular disease. *Treatment:* bed rest, antihistamines, IV fluids, phenothiazines, diazepam. Some have used steroids (32 mg on day 1, 16 mg BID on days 2 to 4, taper to 4 mg on day 8) with success.
2. ***Vertebrobasilar vascular disease.*** Sudden vertigo less severe than other syndromes. Nausea, vomiting, ataxia may be seen. Hearing loss and tinnitus not seen. Nystagmus with characteristics of central disorder. Often history of risk factors for cerebrovascular disease (CVD). If headache or stiff neck, obtain head CT immediately to rule out cerebellar hemorrhage. Any patient at risk for CVD should have posterior fossa imaging (MRI preferred; CT if MRI unavailable). Consider neurology consultation for further work-up.
3. ***Multiple sclerosis.*** Vertigo less severe than in peripheral disorders. Nausea, vomiting, and ataxia may be seen.

Hearing loss rare. Usually associated with other neurologic symptoms of demyelination in CNS. Work-up includes brain MRI, evoked potentials, and LP (showing oligoclonal bands). *Treatment:* ACTH or corticosteroids for demyelination and phenothiazines or antihistamines for vertigo.

4. ***Head trauma.*** Dizziness usually attributable to postconcussion syndrome (that is, disequilibrium dizziness). Less common: BPPV, perilymph fistula, or basilar skull fracture. Work-up includes skull radiographs, head CT with bone windows, and ENT evaluation.

III. PRESYNCOPE AND SYNCOPE

See Chapter 2.

IV. DISEQUILIBRIUM

A. Processes that disturb equilibrium.

1. ***Abnormalities of sensory input.*** Diseases that decrease or distort vision, degenerative disease of the vestibular system, neoplasms (such as acoustic neuroma), toxins (such as aminoglycosides), peripheral neuropathies, and hearing loss. Especially common in the elderly, especially with falls at night because they have peripheral sensory loss and are unable to compensate with vision in low light.
2. ***Abnormalities of central integration.*** Dementia, metabolic encephalopathy, and sedative medications.
3. ***Abnormalities of motor response.*** Disturbance in pyramidal, extrapyramidal (such as Parkinson's disease), or cerebellar function (such as alcohol-related, degenerative, or neoplastic disease).

B. Diagnostic evaluation of disequilibrium. Review medications. Ask about visual problems, hearing loss, sensory loss, paresthesias, and if history of vertigo. Check for hyporeflexia or hyperreflexia, positive Romberg's sign, signs of Parkinson's disease. If hearing loss, obtain audiometry or BAER. If unilateral abnormality, perform posterior fossa imaging. If no identifiable cause, consider imaging study, ENG (to rule out cerebellopontine angle tumors), and neurologic consultation.

C. Therapy for disequilibrium. Discontinue aggravating medications. Correct metabolic derangements. If visual symptoms present, refer to ophthalmologist. If bilateral hearing abnormality on audiometry or BAER, refer to ENT. Treat peripheral neuropathy or Parkinson's disease as discussed earlier. Patients may benefit from use of a light cane, a soft cervical collar, vestibular exercises, or low-dose CNS stimulants (such as ephedrine or methylphenidate).

APPENDIX: DERMATOMAL SENSORY PATTERNS

(Figs. 14-A and 14-B)

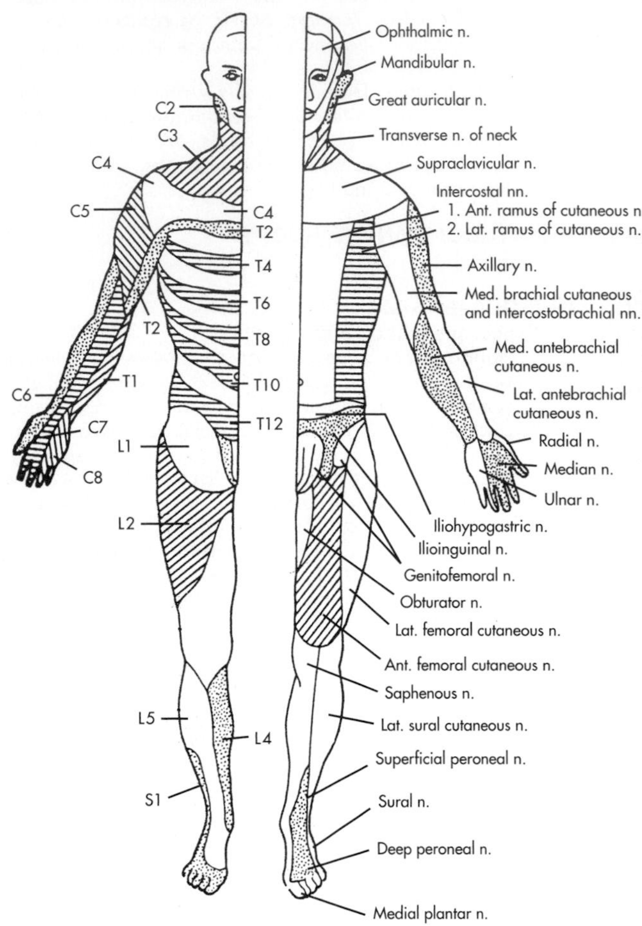

FIG. 14-A Anterior view of dermatomes *(left)* and cutaneous areas supplied by individual peripheral nerves *(right)*. (Modified from Carpenter MB, Sutin J: *Human neuroanatomy,* Baltimore, 1983, Williams & Wilkins, and from Isselbacher KJ et al, editors: *Harrison's principles of internal medicine,* ed 13, New York, 1994, McGraw-Hill.)

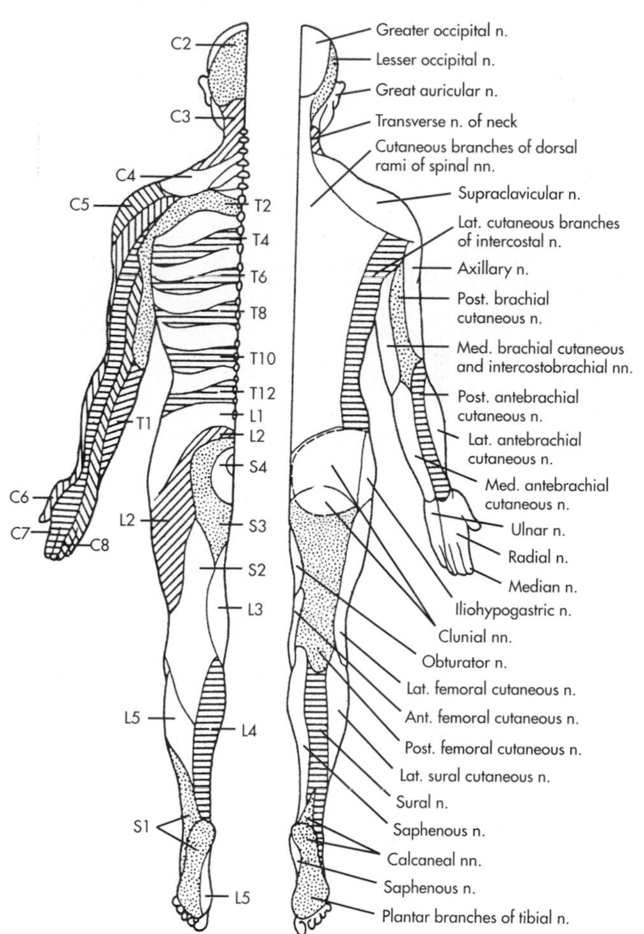

FIG. 14-B Posterior view of dermatomes *(left)* and cutaneous areas supplied by individual peripheral nerves *(right)*. (Modified from Carpenter MB, Sutin J: *Human neuroanatomy,* Baltimore, 1983, Williams & Wilkins, and from Isselbacher KJ et al, editors: *Harrison's principles of internal medicine,* ed 13, New York, 1994, McGraw-Hill.)

BIBLIOGRAPHY

Adams HP Jr et al: Guidelines for the management of patients with acute ischemic stroke: a statement for healthcare professionals from a special writing group of the Stroke Council, *Stroke* 25:1901-1913, 1994.

American Psychiatric Association: *Diagnostic and statistical manual of mental disorders,* ed 4, Washington, D.C., 1994, American Psychiatric Association.

Ariyasu L et al: The beneficial effect of methylprednisolone in acute vestibular vertigo, *Arch Otolaryngol Head Neck Surg* 116(6):700, 1990.

Arnold SE, Kumar A: Reversible dementias, *Med Clin North Am* 77(1):215-213, 1993.

Avorn J et al: Increased incidence of levodopa therapy following metoclopramide use, *JAMA* 274(22):1780, 1995.

Baumel B: Migraine: a pharmacologic review with newer options and delivery modalities, *Neurology* 44(suppl 3):S13-S17, 1994.

Beck RW et al: The effect of corticosteroids for acute optic neuritis on the subsequent development of multiple sclerosis, *N Engl J Med* 329(24):1764-1769, 1993.

Benbadis SR et al: Value of tongue biting in the diagnosis of seizures, *Arch Intern Med* 155(2):2346, 1995.

Bernat JL, Vincent FM: *Neurology: problems in primary care,* ed 2, Los Angeles, 1993, Practice Management Information Corp.

Brodie MJ, Dichter MA: Antiepileptic drugs, *N Engl J Med* 334(3):168-175, 1996.

Bross MH, Tatum NO: Delirium in the elderly patient, *Am Fam Physician* 50(6):1325-1332, 1994.

Cascino GD: Epilepsy: contemporary perspectives in evaluation and treatment, *Mayo Clin Proc* 69:1199-1211, 1994.

Cohen NL: The dizzy patient: update on vestibular disorders, *Med Clin North Am* 75(6):1251-1261, 1991.

Comerota AJ et al: Is transcranial Doppler a worthwhile addition to screening tests for cerebrovascular disease? *J Vasc Surg* 21(1):90-95, 1995.

Corey-Bloom J et al: Diagnosis and evaluation of dementia, *Neurology* 45:211-218, 1995.

Cummings JL: Dementia: the failing brain, *Lancet* 345:1481-1484, 1995.

Engel J Jr: Surgery for seizures, *N Engl J Med* 334(10):647-652, 1996.

Epley JM: The canalith repositioning procedure: for treatment of benign paroxysmal positional vertigo, *Otolaryngol Head Neck Surg* 107(3):399-404, 1992.

Fleming KC et al: Dementia: diagnosis and evaluation, *Mayo Clin Proc* 70:1093-1107, 1995.

Folstein MF et al: "Mini–mental state": a practical method for grading the cognitive state of patients for the clinician, *J Psychiatr Res* 12:189-198, 1975.

Fontanarosa PB: Recognition of subarachnoid hemorrhage, *Ann Emerg Med* 18(11):1199, 1989.

Forsyth PA et al: Headaches in patients with brain tumors: a study of 111 patients, *Neurology* 43(9):1678, 1993.

Fujino A et al: Vestibular training for benign paroxysmal positional vertigo: its efficacy in comparison with antivertigo drugs, *Arch Otolaryngol Head Neck Surg* 120(5):497-504, 1994.

Green JD Jr et al: Longitudinal follow-up of patients with Ménière's disease, *Otolaryngol Head Neck Surg* 104(6):783-788, 1991.

Headache Classification Committee of the International Headache Society: Classification and diagnostic criteria for headache disorders, cranial neuralgias, and facial pain, *Cephalalgia* 8(suppl 7):1-96, 1988.

Hoffert MJ: Treatment of migraine: a new era, *Am Fam Physician* 49(3):633-638, 1994.

Inaba-Roland KE, Maricle RA: Assessing delirium in the acute care setting, *Heart Lung* 21(1):48-55, 1992.

Inouye SK et al: Clarifying confusion: the confusion assessment method: a new method for detection of delirium, *Ann Intern Med* 113:941-948, 1990.

Jones EB et al: Safety and efficacy of rectal prochlorperazine for the treatment of migraine in the emergency department, *Ann Emerg Med* 24:237-241, 1994.

Kaplan HI, Sadock BJ: *Pocket handbook of clinical psychiatry,* ed 2, Baltimore, 1996, Williams & Wilkins.

Koller WC, Silver DE, Liberman A, editors: An algorithm for the management of Parkinson's disease, *Neurology* 44(12:suppl 10):S1-S52, 1994.

Leclerc KM, Landry FJ: Benign nocturnal leg cramps: current controversies over use of quinine, *Postgrad Med* 99(2):177-184, 1996.

Lee KJ: Essential otolaryngology, a board preparation and concise reference, New York, 1991, Medical Examination Publishing Co.

Lees AJ on behalf of the Parkinson's Disease Research Group of the United Kingdom: Comparison of therapeutic effects and mortality data of levodopa combined with selegiline in patients with early, mild Parkinson's disease, *Br Med J* 311:1602-1607, 1995.

Lempert T et al: Benign positional vertigo: recognition and treatment, *Br Med J* 311:489-491, 1995.

Lledo A et al: Acute headache of recent onset and subarachnoid hemorrhage: a prospective study, *Headache* 34(3):172, 1994.

Man-Son-Hing M, Wells, G: Meta-analysis of efficacy of quinine for treatment of nocturnal leg cramps in elderly people, *Br Med J* 310(6971):13-17, 1995.

Mizuno Y et al: Various aspects of motor fluctuations and their management in Parkinson's disease, *Neurology* 44(suppl 6):S29-S34, 1994.

O'Keefe ST: Restless legs syndrome: a review, *Arch Intern Med* 156:243-248, 1996.

Perkins AT, Ondo W: When to worry about headache: head pain as a clue to intracranial disease, *Postgrad Med* 98(2):197-208, 1995.

Petruk KC et al: Nimodipine treatment in poor-grade aneurysm patients: results of a multicenter double-blind placebo-controlled trial, *J Neurosurg* 68:505, 1988.

Rodriguez M et al: Optic neuritis: a population-based study in Olmsted County, Minnesota, *Neurology* 45:244-250, 1995.

Ruckenstein MJ: A practical approach to dizziness, *Postgrad Med* 97(3):70-81, 1995.

Santilli JD et al: Prevention of stroke caused by carotid bifurcation stenosis, *Am Fam Physician* 53(2):549-556, 1996.

Seymour JJ et al: Response of headaches to nonnarcotic analgesics resulting in missed intracranial hemorrhage, *Am J Emerg Med* 13(1):43, 1995.

Silberstein SD: Tension-type and chronic daily headache, *Neurology* 43:1644-1649, 1993.

Silverstein PM: Moderate Parkinson's disease–strategies for maximizing treatment, *Postgrad Med* 99(1):52-68, 1996.

Slivka A et al: Clinical and angiographic features of thunderclap headache, *Headache* 35(1):1, 1995.

Smucker WD et al: Systematic approach to diagnosis and initial management of stroke, *Am Fam Physician* 52(1):225-234, 1995.

Snyder H et al: Signs and symptoms of patients with brain tumors presenting to the emergency department, *J Emerg Med* 11(3):253, 1993.

Sweeney PJ: Parkinson's disease: managing symptoms and preserving function, *Geriatrics* 50(9):24-31, 1995.

Troost BT, Patton JM: Exercise therapy for positional vertigo, *Neurology* 42:1441-1444, 1992.

van der Wee N et al: Detection of subarachnoid haemorrhage on early CT: is lumbar puncture still needed after a negative scan? *J Neurol Neurosurg Psychiatry* 58(3): 357, 1995.

Walling A: Cluster headache, *Am Fam Physician* 47(6):1457-1463, 1993.

Weiner HL, Levitt LP: *Neurology for the house officer,* ed 4, Baltimore, 1989, Williams & Wilkins.

Weiner WJ, Goetz CG, editors: *Neurology for the non-neurologist,* ed 3, Philadelphia, 1994, Lippincott.

15

Psychiatry

NORA R. FROHBERG AND ROBERT L. HERTING, JR.

MOOD DISORDERS

I. MAJOR DEPRESSIVE DISORDER (MDD)

A. Overview. Lifetime risk 7% to 12% for men, 20% to 25% for women. *Risk factors:* female (especially post partum), history of depressive illness in first-degree relatives, prior episodes of major depression, prior suicide attempts, age <40 years, medical comorbidity, decreased social support, stressful life events, and current substance or alcohol abuse.

B. Tip-offs for depression in a primary care setting. May include fatigue, somatic complaints (such as headache, backache, chest pain, dyspepsia, and limb pain), anxiety symptoms, depressed mood, or insomnia.

C. Symptoms can be divided into:

1. ***Emotional.*** Dysphoria, irritability, anhedonia, withdrawal.
2. ***Cognitive.*** Self-criticism, sense of worthlessness or guilt, hopelessness, poor concentration, memory impairment, delusions or hallucinations.
3. ***Vegetative.*** Fatigue, decreased energy, insomnia, hypersomnia, anorexia, psychomotor retardation or agitation, impaired libido.

D. Diagnosis. DSM-IV criteria for a major depressive episode include at least five of the following symptoms present for at least 2 weeks that represent a change from previous level of functioning:

- Depressed mood (most of day, almost daily). NOTE: In children and adolescents there may be an irritable mood.
- Diminished interest or pleasure in all or most activities
- Significant weight loss or gain, or decrease or increase in appetite nearly every day
- Insomnia or hypersomnia
- Psychomotor retardation or agitation (observable by others)
- Fatigue or decreased level of energy

- Feelings of worthlessness or inappropriate guilt
- Poor concentration or indecisiveness
- Recurrent thoughts of death or suicidal ideation

NOTE: At least one of the above symptoms must be either (1) depressed mood or (2) loss of interest or pleasure.

E. To be defined as a major depressive episode, the symptoms (1) must cause clinically significant distress or impairment in functioning and (2) must not be attributable to the effects of substance use, general medical condition, or bereavement.

F. Evaluation.

1. ***History.*** May use Beck Inventory (Box 15-1), or Geriatric Depression Scale (Box 15-2) to screen for high-risk patients. If depressive symptoms are present, determine:
   a. Time course and severity.
   b. Any prior episodes and level of recovery.
   c. Any history of manic or hypomanic episodes.
   d. If other major psychiatric disorders are present.
   e. Any suicidal ideation, plan, or intent.
2. ***Examination.*** Evaluate for possible related medical conditions: anemia, hypothyroidism, chronic infection, substance abuse, or medication side effects (oral contraceptives, antihypertensives, etc.).
3. ***Lab tests.*** Screen for medical causes of depression (if suspected by history or physical examination). Lab tests may include complete blood count with differential, electrolytes, renal and liver functions, thyroid studies, etc.

G. Treatment

1. ***Hospitalization.*** Indicated if serious suicidal ideation is present (with a plan and access to the means), patient is dangerous to self or others, there is a complicating medical condition, or there is a lack of support system at home.
2. ***Medication.*** Most antidepressants believed to be equally effective in equivalent therapeutic doses. Expect a 2- to 6-week latent period before the full effect is seen at therapeutic doses. To prevent relapse, continue medication for at least 4 to 9 months after patient becomes asymptomatic. For recurrent depression, consider chronic prophylactic therapy.
   a. *Tricyclic antidepressants (TCAs).* A rational method for selecting a TCA is to narrow the choice to a dimethylated TCA (such as imipramine) and a monomethylated TCA (such as nortriptyline). Choose between them based on patient's sedation requirements and ability to tolerate orthostatic hypotension, weight gain, and anticholinergic adverse effects

Text continued on p. 604

BOX 15-1

Beck Inventory for the Screening of Depression

Beck Inventory

Name: **Date:**

On this questionnaire are groups of statements. Please read each group of statements carefully. Then pick out the one statement in each group that best describes the way you have been feeling the PAST WEEK INCLUDING TODAY. Circle the number beside the statement you picked. If several statements in the group seem to apply equally well, circle each one. Be sure to read all the statements in each group before making your choice.

1.
0 I do not feel sad.
1 I feel sad.
2 I am sad all the time and can't snap out of it.
3 I am so sad or unhappy that I can't stand it.

2.
0 I am not particularly discouraged about the future.
1 I feel discouraged about the future.
2 I feel I have nothing to look forward to.
3 I feel that the future is hopeless and that things cannot improve.

3.
0 I do not feel like a failure.
1 I feel I have failed more than the average person.
2 As I look back on my life, all I can see is a lot of failures.
3 I feel I am a complete failure as a person.

4.
0 I get as much satisfaction out of things as I used to.
1 I don't enjoy things the way I used to.
2 I don't get real satisfaction out of anything anymore.
3 I am dissatisfied and bored with everything.

5.
0 I don't feel particularly guilty.
1 I feel guilty a good part of the time.
2 I feel quite guilty most of the time.
3 I feel guilty all of the time.

6.
0 I don't feel I am being punished.
1 I feel I may be punished.
2 I expect to be punished.
3 I feel I am being punished.

7.

0 I don't feel disappointed in myself.
1 I am disappointed in myself.
2 I am disgusted with myself.
3 I hate myself.

8.

0 I have not lost interest in other people.
1 I am less interested in other people than I used to be.
2 I have lost most of my interest in other people.
3 I have lost all of my interest in other people.

9.

0 I make decisions about as well as I ever could.
1 I put off making decisions more than I used to.
2 I have greater difficulty in making decisions than before.
3 I can't make decisions at all anymore.

10.

0 I don't feel I look worse than I used to.
1 I am worried that I am looking old or unattractive.
2 I feel that there are permanent changes in my appearance that make me look unattractive.
3 I believe that I look ugly.

11.

0 I can work about as well as before.
1 It takes an extra effort to get started to do something.
2 I have to push myself very hard to do anything.
3 I can't do any work at all.

12.

0 I can sleep as well as usual.
1 I get tired more easily than I used to.
2 I get tired from doing almost anything.
3 I am too tired to do anything.

13.

0 I don't get tired more than usual.
1 I get tired more easily than I used to.
2 I get tired from doing almost anything.
3 I am too tired to do anything.

14.

0 My appetite is no worse than usual.
1 My appetite is not as good as it used to be.
2 My appetite is much worse now.
3 I have no appetite at all anymore.

15.

0 I don't feel I am any worse than anybody else.
1 I am critical of myself for my weaknesses or mistakes.
2 I blame myself all the time for my faults.
3 I blame myself for everything bad that happens.

Continued

BOX 15-1
Beck Inventory for the Screening of Depression—cont'd

16.
0 I don't have any thoughts of killing myself.
1 I have thoughts of killing myself but would not carry them out.
2 I would like to kill myself.
3 I would kill myself if I had the chance.

17.
0 I am no more worried about my health than usual.
1 I am worried about physical problems such as aches and pains or upset stomach or constipation.
2 I am very worried about physical problems, and it is hard to think of much else.
3 I am so worried about my physical problems that I cannot think of anything else.

18.
0 I don't cry any more that usual.
1 I cry more now than I used to.
2 I cry all the time now.
3 I used to be able to cry, but now I can't cry even though I want to.

19.
0 I have not noticed any recent change in my interest in sex.
1 I am less interested in sex than I used to be.
2 I am much less interested in sex now.
3 I have lose interest in sex completely.

20.
0 I am no more irritated now than I ever am.
1 I get annoyed or irritated more easily than I used to.
2 I feel irritated all the time now.
3 I don't get irritated at all by the things that used to irritate me.

21.
0 I haven't lost much weight, if any lately.
1 I have lost more than 5 pounds.
2 I have lost more than 10 pounds.
3 I have lost more than 15 pounds.
(I am purposely trying to lose weight by eating less. Yes___ No___)

Scoring:
0-9 normal
10-15 mild depressive symptoms
16-19 mild-moderate depressive symptoms
20-29 moderate-severe depressive symptoms
30 severe depressive symptoms

BOX 15-2
Geriatric Depression Scale

This may be administered in oral or written format. If written, the answer sheet must have printed Yes/No after each question. The subject is instructed to circle the better response. If given orally, the question may need to be repeated to get a response of "yes" or "no." The GDS seems to work well with other age groups.

1. Are you basically satisfied with your life? N*
2. Have you dropped many of your activities and interests? Y
3. Do you feel that your life is empty? Y
4. Do you often get bored? Y
5. Are you hopeful about the future? N
6. Are you bothered by thoughts that you just cannot get out of your head? Y
7. Are you in good spirits most of the time? N
8. Are you afraid that something bad is going to happen to you? Y
9. Do you feel happy most of the time? N
10. Do you often feel helpless? Y
11. Do you often get restless and fidgety? Y
12. Do you prefer to stay home at night, rather than go out and do new things? Y
13. Do you frequently worry about the future? Y
14. Do you feel that you have more problems with memory than most? Y
15. Do you think it is wonderful to be alive now? N
16. Do you often feel downhearted and blue? Y
17. Do you feel pretty worthless the way you are now? Y
18. Do you worry a lot about the past? Y
19. Do you find life very exciting? N
20. Is it hard for you to get started on new projects? Y
21. Do you feel full of energy? N
22. Do you feel that your situation is hopeless? Y
23. Do you think that most people are better off than you are? Y
24. Do you frequently get upset over little things? Y
25. Do you frequently feel like crying? Y
26. Do you have trouble concentrating? Y
27. Do you enjoy getting up in the morning? N
28. Do you prefer to avoid social gatherings? Y
29. Is it easy for you to make decisions? N
30. Is your mind as clear as it used to be? N

*__Scoring__: count 1 point for each depressive answer shown after each question. 0 to 10 = normal; 11 to 20 = mild depression; 21 to 30 = moderate or severe depression.

(see Table 15-1). TCAs are usually given QHS to take advantage of sedating effects. All TCAs may cause slowing of cardiac conduction. May be fatal in overdoses around 2000 mg or more in adults. A therapeutic trial usually is considered >100 mg/day of amitriptyline or its equivalent for at least 3 weeks. *NOTE: Nortriptyline (Pamelor) has a "therapeutic window" plasma level of 50 to 150 ng/ml for optimal efficacy. It has the lowest risk for orthostatic hypotension of all TCAs making it a safe choice in the geriatric patient.*

b. *Second-generation antidepressants*
   (1) *Selective serotonin reuptake inhibitors (SSRIs).* Much safer in overdose than TCAs. Expensive in contrast to generic TCAs. Initial dose often an effective dose. May need to start at lower doses in the elderly of others sensitive to side effects. Side effects vary and may include nausea, anorexia, insomnia or mild sedation, sweating, headache, tremor, *sexual dysfunction,* and nervousness. Fluoxetine may have a slower onset of action than other SSRIs. Safety in patients with cardiovascular disease not well studied. Fluvoxamine is contraindicated with astemizole and terfenadine. All SSRIs contraindicated with MAOIs. If switching from a SSRI to a MAOI, need a drug-free period of 14 days for paroxetine, sertraline or fluvoxamine or 5 weeks for fluoxetine.
   (2) *Bupropion (Wellbutrin).* Safer in overdose than TCAs. Safer choice in patients with history of cardiac disease. Very low incidence of sexual dysfunction compared to SSRIs, TCAs, and MAOIs. TID schedule and 150 mg maximum single dose to minimize the risk of seizures (0.4%). Contraindicated in patients with seizure disorder, bulimia, or anorexia nervosa.
   (3) *Venlafaxine (Effexor).* Monitor for blood pressure elevation.
   (4) *Trazodone (Desyrel).* Patients with cardiac disease should be closely monitored. Used as monotherapy or adjunct to certain antidepressants for sedation at bedtime. Risk of priapism 1:6000.
   (5) *Nefazodone (Serzone).* A newer treatment option for patients experiencing either poor response or intolerable side effects from other antidepressants. Contraindicated with astemizole and terfenadine.
   (6) *Mirtazapine (Remeron).* A newer option for patients with a poor response or an inability to tolerate other antidepressants.

Relative Comparison of Antidepressants

Drug	Dosage range (mg/day)*	Dosage schedule	Orthostatic hypotension	Anticholinergic†	Sedation	Weight gain
TRICYCLIC ANTIDEPRESSANTS						
Amitriptyline (Elavil)	50-300	QHS	++++	+++++	+++++	+++
Desipramine (Norpramin)	50-300	QHS	++	+	+	+
Imipramine (Tofranil)	50-300	QHS	+++	++++	+++	++
Nortriptyline (Pamelor)	30-100	QHS	++	+++	++	+
SEROTONIN-SPECIFIC REUPTAKE INHIBITORS (SSRIs)						
Fluoxetine (Prozac)	1-100	QAM	Minimal to neutral with regard to sedative, anticholinergic, and orthostatic hypotensive side effects; may cause mild weight loss in some individuals			
Paroxetine (Paxil)	10-50	QAM or QHS				
Sertraline (Zoloft)	12.5-200	QAM or QHS				
SEROTONIN-NONSELECTIVE REUPTAKE INHIBITORS						
Venlafaxine (Effexor)	25-375	QD-TID	0	+/−	+/−	0
DOPAMINE ACTIVE						
Bupropion (Wellbutrin)	150-450	BID-TID	0	+	+	—
OTHER						
Trazodone (Desyrel)	50-400	QHS-TID	+++	++	+++++	+
Nefazodone (Serzone)	300-600	BID	+/−	+/−	+	0
Mirtazapine (Remeron)	15-60	QHS	+/−	+/−	++	++

Adapted from Bernstein JG: *Handbook of drug therapy in psychiatry,* ed 3, St. Louis, 1995, Mosby.
*Doses should be lowered in the elderly.
†Blurred vision, constipation, dry mouth, urinary retention.

c. *Monoamine oxidase inhibitors (MAOIs).* Sometimes used in depression refractory to the other treatments. Consider consulting psychiatrist before starting because of the serious adverse effect potential.

3. ***Psychotherapy.*** Supportive therapy is always part of depression treatment. Other types of psychotherapy may be helpful in mild to moderate depression, alone or with medication.
4. ***Electroconvulsive therapy.*** ECT is the most effective, rapid method of treating severe major depressive disorder (MDD). Indicated for patients with poor response to medications, poor tolerance of usual antidepressants, severe vegetative symptoms, or psychotic features. The decision to administer ECT should be made by a psychiatrist.

II. BIPOLAR AFFECTIVE DISORDER (BPAD)

A. Overview.

1. ***Lifetime prevalence ~1%.*** Affects males and females equally. Age of onset usually late teens to mid-30s.
2. ***Bipolar I disorder.*** Characterized by *one or more manic episodes, or mixed (manic and depressive) episodes.* Individuals affected often have a history of one or more episodes of depression. More than 90% of individuals with a manic episode have future episodes of depression or mania.

B. DSM-IV criteria for manic episode.

1. A distinct period of abnormally and persistently elevated, expansive, or irritable mood lasting at least 1 week (or any duration if hospitalized). During this period, the patient must exhibit at least three of the following (four if mood is only irritable):
   - Grandiosity
   - Decreased need for sleep
   - Pressured speech or unusually talkative
   - Racing thoughts or flight of ideas
   - Distractibility
   - Psychomotor agitation or increased goal-directed activity (social, work, school, or sexual)
   - Excessive involvement in pleasurable activities with a high potential for painful consequences (such as unrestrained buying sprees, sexual indiscretions).
2. Symptoms are not better accounted for by another general medical, mental, or substance abuse disorder.
3. Symptoms cause pronounced impairment of functioning, require hospitalization, or are associated with psychotic features.

C. Evaluation.

1. ***History.*** Interviews with family or friends are essential. Often a family history of affective disorders and alcoholism

is present in first-degree relatives. If patient is >40 years of age and has first manic episode, look for medical causes.

2. ***Examination.*** Evaluate for medical cause, such as drug abuse or intoxication.
3. ***Laboratory tests.*** Tests are needed before starting lithium carbonate, carbamazepine, or valproate (see below under specific medications). They should also be performed to rule out certain causes of secondary mania, such as megaloblastic anemia, hyperglycemia and hypoglycemia, hyperthyroidism and hypothyroidism, systemic lupus erythematosus, syphilis, HIV, and liver disease induced by alcohol or other substances.

D. Treatment. *Hospitalization is usually indicated for* full manic syndromes, since the patient's well-being is at risk because of impaired judgment. This includes a risk of death from exhaustion. Consider ECT in medication nonresponders and pregnant women.

E. Medications.

1. ***Antipsychotics (such as haloperidol).*** Often required initially for sedation, control of behavior, or psychotic symptoms. Benzodiazepines may be a useful adjunct for sedation.
2. ***Antimanic drugs (mood stabilizers).***
   a. *Lithium carbonate.* Best studied and usually the drug of choice for mania with response rates of 80%. Up to 3 weeks generally needed at therapeutic blood levels before clinical effects noted. Also beneficial for prophylaxis of depressive episodes associated with bipolar illness.
      (1) Dose is 600 to 2400 mg/day. Give with food and initially in divided doses to minimize GI side effects. Then change to a single dose QHS (if ≤1800 mg/day) or BID (if ≤3000 mg/day) to minimize potential tremor and polyuria.
      (2) Monitor serum trough levels (12 hours after last dose) at least twice weekly initially and then Q2-3 months for maintenance. In acute mania, 0.9 to 1.4 mEq/L levels needed. Maintenance levels range from 0.4 to 0.8 mEq/L (with elderly requiring the higher range).
      (3) Side effects. Polyuria and polydipsia, muscle weakness, tremor, GI upset or diarrhea, and hypothyroidism.
      (4) Toxicity may occur at serum levels just over the therapeutic range. Mild toxicity symptoms are exacerbations of side effects listed above. More severe toxicity includes primarily neurologic manifestations (lethargy, confusion, coma, seizures, ataxia, dysarthria, nystagmus) and nephropathy.

Overdose not responsive to charcoal but may respond to polystyrene resins and dialysis.

(5) Lab monitoring. Baseline tests before starting lithium include BUN and creatinine, pregnancy test, thyroid function tests (TFTs) (lithium may induce hypothyroidism), ECG for patient >40 years of age and consider a CBC. During the first 6 months of lithium treatment, monitor BUN and Cr every 2 to 3 months and TFTs 1 or 2 times. Subsequently check creatinine (Q6-12 months) and thyroid functions (every year) while patient is receiving maintenance lithium treatment.

(6) Warnings. Avoid use in pregnancy (especially first trimester) unless benefits outweigh risks. Dehydration and sodium-restricted diets may increase lithium levels and risk for toxicity.

(7) Drug interactions. Any medication that can decrease renal clearance (such as NSAIDs); sodium-depleting diuretics should be used with caution.

b. *Carbamazepine (Tegretol).* Second-line treatment to lithium for treatment of mania. Dosage 600 to 2000 mg/day for acute mania. Onset of action 1 to 2 weeks; therapeutic trial 3 weeks. No established therapeutic blood levels for treatment of mania. Monitor for leukopenia and liver dysfunction. Avoid use in pregnancy unless benefits outweigh risks.

c. *Valproic acid (Depakene, Depakote).* Third-line treatment for mania behind lithium and carbamazepine. However, it is the preferred choice in rapid cycling and mixed mania. Usual starting dose is 15 mg/kg/day in 2 or more divided doses. Therapeutic blood level not established for mania. Increase dose until therapeutic response or adverse effects occur. Obtain baseline hematologic and hepatic tests. Instruct patients about potential symptoms of leukopenia and liver disease. Depakote may be less likely to produce GI side effects than Depakene. Avoid use in pregnancy unless benefits outweigh risks.

d. *Verapamil (Calan).* Fourth-line treatment for mania until its efficacy compared to other treatments is determined. Antimanic dosages range from 160 to 480 mg/day.

ANXIETY DISORDERS

I. OVERVIEW

A. Definition of anxiety. Unpleasant and unwarranted feelings of apprehension, sometimes accompanied by physiological symptoms.

B. Types of anxiety disorders.

1. Generalized anxiety disorder
2. Panic disorder

3. Agoraphobia
4. Social or simple phobias
5. Obsessive compulsive disorder
6. Posttraumatic stress disorder

C. Differential diagnosis of anxiety disorders.

1. ***Psychiatric.***
    a. Anxious depression
    b. Drug abuse or withdrawal (alcohol, benzodiazepines)
    c. Stimulant use (caffeine, amphetamines)
    d. Some personality disorders
2. ***Medical.***
    a. Cardiovascular (such as mitral valve prolapse, angina, cardiac arrhythmias, CHF, HTN, MI).
    b. Respiratory (such as asthma, COPD, hyperventilation, hypoxia, PE).
    c. Endocrine (such as hypoglycemia, hyperthyroidism, menopause, pheochromocytoma, Cushing's syndrome).
    d. Neurologic (such as delirium, multiple sclerosis, partial complex seizures, postconcussion syndrome, vestibular dysfunction).
    e. Drugs (such as theophylline, bronchodilators, steroids, calcium-channel blockers, neuroleptics, anticholinergics).
    f. Gastroesophageal reflux.

II. GENERALIZED ANXIETY DISORDER (GAD)

A. Overview. Probably the most common anxiety disorder in primary care with lifetime prevalence of 5%. Gradual onset with peak onset in the teen years. High risk for other comorbid psychiatric disorders

B. DSM-IV diagnosis.

1. Excessive anxiety and worry on most days for at least 6 months, about a number of issues.
2. Difficulty controlling the worry.
3. The anxiety and worry are associated with at least 3 of the following 6 symptoms for the past 6 months:
    - Restlessness or feeling on edge
    - Irritability
    - Being easily fatigued
    - Difficulty concentrating
    - Muscle tension
    - Sleep disturbance
4. Focus of the anxiety and worry does not relate to another major emotional disorder (for example, worry is *not* about having a panic attack as in panic disorder).
5. Anxiety causes significant distress or impairment in functioning.
6. The symptoms are not attributable to substance use or a medical condition and are not present only during the course of a mood, psychotic, or developmental disorder.

C. Treatment.

1. ***Therapy.***
   a. *Psychotherapy.* Most patients with mild symptoms can be treated with supportive counseling and education without need for medication.
   b. *Other therapies.* Relaxation training and cognitive therapy.
2. ***General measures.*** Regular exercise and avoidance of caffeine and alcohol.
3. ***Medications.***
   a. *TCAs.* Imipramine 25 to 150 mg/day. Does not become effective for 2 to 3 weeks. Most beneficial in patients with comorbid depression or sleep disturbance.
   b. *Antihistamines.* Hydroxyzine (Atarax, Vistaril) 50 to 100 mg QID may be used PRN, as an adjunct to other medications, or as an alternative therapy for patients with addiction potential.
   c. *Benzodiazepines.* Usually of short-term use with no long-term efficacy proved. Use lowest dose that alleviates anxiety. Longer half-life drugs may be easier to taper. May cause rebound anxiety with taper or withdrawal. *Examples:* alprazolam (Xanax) 0.25 to 0.5 mg PO TID initial dose; rarely need to exceed 4 mg/day. Diazepam (Valium) 2 to 10 mg PO BID to QID. Lorazepam (Ativan) 1 mg PO BID or TID initially; rarely need to exceed 10 mg/day. Use lower doses than above in the elderly.
   d. *Buspirone.* May be less effective than other agents. Start 5 mg PO TID and increase to typical dose of 20 to 30 mg/day. Takes 2 weeks to be effective. Nonsedating. Little abuse potential.
   e. *SSRIs.* Clinically appear helpful but not well studied yet. Use in doses similar to those for panic disorder (see below). In select patients may add a benzodiazepine for first several weeks of treatment, since it has a quicker onset of action and avoids potential initial side effect of increased anxiety with SSRIs.
   f. *Beta-blockers.* Propranolol (Inderal) may help physical symptoms (not FDA approved) but has no effect on psychic component of anxiety.

III. PANIC DISORDER

A. Overview. Estimated lifetime prevalence is greater than 3%.

B. DSM-IV diagnosis. Recurrent unexplained panic attacks (discrete periods of intense fear).

1. At least one of the attacks has been followed by 1 month (or more) of one (or more) of the following:
   a. Concern about having future attacks

b. Worry about consequences of the attack
c. Change in behavior related to the attacks

2. Panic attacks are not substance induced, related to a general medical condition, or better accounted for by another mental disorder.
3. During the attack at least 4 of the following symptoms develop quickly and peak within 10 minutes:
   - Palpitations or tachycardia
   - Trembling or shaking
   - Feelings of choking
   - Nausea or abdominal discomfort
   - Feeling dizzy, unsteady, or faint
   - Fear of losing control or going crazy
   - Derealization (feelings of unreality) or depersonalization (being detached from oneself)
   - Sweating
   - Feelings of dyspnea
   - Chest pain or discomfort
   - Fear of dying
   - Paresthesias
   - Flushing or chilling

C. Treatment.

1. ***Medications.***
   a. *SSRIs* are the drugs of choice (currently only Paxil is FDA approved for this indication). *Recommended dosage ranges:* Paxil (paroxetine) 10 to 50 mg/day, Luvox (fluvoxamine) 25 to 300 mg/day, and Prozac (fluoxetine) 5 to 60 mg/day. Start at lowest dose and may increase after first week as tolerated (such as Prozac 10 mg PO QOD for week 1, 10 mg QD for week 2, and then 20 mg QD for week 3). Monitor for initial paradoxical anxiety secondary to drug side effect, which usually resolves with time.
   b. *Tricyclic antidepressants.* For example, start imipramine at 10 to 25 mg QHS and increase by 10 to 25 mg every 3 or 4 days until effective, side effects predominate, or initial target dose of 150 to 200 mg QHS is reached. If no response after 4 to 6 weeks at target dose, may increase to maximum dose of 300 to 400 mg QHS as tolerated. Clinical experience has shown that serotonergic TCAs are more effective than noradrenergic TCAs.
   c. *Benzodiazepines* have a quicker onset of action than other drugs; may use as a short-term adjunct to SSRIs if initial paradoxical anxiety arises. They may be used long term if patients fail treatment or are unable to tolerate SSRIs or TCAs.
   d. *MAOIs* are reserved for patients who do not respond to SSRIs or TCAs because of serious adverse drug reactions. Before starting, consider consulting a psychiatrist.

e. *Propanolol* is not a first-line agent for panic disorder but is very effective for physical symptoms of panic attacks associated with performance anxiety.
f. *Buspirone (Buspar)* has demonstrated *little* efficacy in patients with panic disorders.

2. ***Psychotherapy.***
a. Supportive therapy is always included.
b. Addition of cognitive therapy may be beneficial.

IV. AGORAPHOBIA

A. Overview. Age of onset most often in 20s and 30s. More common in women. Often occurs with panic disorders.

B. DSM-IV diagnosis criteria require:

1. Fear of being in place or situations from which escape might be difficult or embarrassing in the event of suddenly developing a panic attack or panic-like symptoms.
2. The situations are avoided, or else endured with considerable anxiety about having panic-attacks symptoms, or require a companion.
3. Anxiety and avoidance are not better accounted for by another mental disorder.

C. Treatment.

1. ***Agoraphobia with panic attacks.*** Choices include SSRIs, TCAs, benzodiazepines, or MAOIs. See section on panic disorder above. Medications in combination with behavioral therapy most beneficial.
2. ***Agoraphobia alone.*** Systematic desensitization with exposure to real-life feared situations is the treatment of choice. Consult a psychologist.

V. SPECIFIC AND SOCIAL PHOBIAS

A. Overview. Social phobia has a lifetime prevalence of 13% with onset most common in the midteens. Specific phobias are more common in females, and impairment is usually minimal.

B. DSM-IV criteria.

1. Persistent fear of humiliation or embarrassment in certain social situations (social phobia) or irrational fear of other circumscribed stimuli (specific phobia).
2. Exposure to the particular stimulus provokes anxiety, which may include a situationally bound panic attack.
3. The person usually realizes that the fear is excessive.
4. The fear results in avoidance of the stimulus that interferes with patient's social environment or produces significant distress.
5. The fear or avoidance is not attributable to substance use, a general medical condition, or another mental disorder.

C. Treatment.

1. Systematic desensitization and exposure (for specific phobias) and cognitive behavioral therapy (for social phobias).
2. Beta-blockers may be effective in treating performance-anxiety symptoms.
3. Drugs used in generalized social phobias include SSRIs (doses higher than those used in depression) *or* an MAOI (such as phenelzine).

VI. OBSESSIVE-COMPULSIVE DISORDER (OCD)

A. Overview. Lifetime prevalence of 2.5%. Onset usually in adolescence or early adulthood.

B. DSM-IV diagnosis. Obsessions or compulsions that significantly interfere with daily functioning because of distress or time consumption.

1. ***Obsessions.*** Recurrent, persistent thoughts that are experienced as intrusive and inappropriate. The person recognizes the thoughts as a product of his or her own mind and attempts to ignore or suppress them.
2. ***Compulsions.*** Repetitive, purposeful behaviors performed in response to an obsession or according to certain rules. These are designed to neutralize or prevent discomfort. In general, recognized by the patient as unreasonable.

C. Treatment. Generally not curative but can obtain significant improvement.

1. Behavior therapy uses the technique of exposure and response prevention to limit the amount of dysfunction resulting from the obsessions or compulsions.
2. ***Medications.***
   a. *Clomipramine (Anafranil).* Start with 25 mg, and titrate up to 100 to 250 mg daily. Give in divided doses with meals to minimize GI side effects, or at bedtime to minimize sedation.
   b. *SSRIs* Have better side effect profiles than clomipramine does. Start at low dose and titrate to doses higher than those used for depression (such as fluoxetine (Prozac) start 20 mg daily; usual daily dose 40 to 80 mg). If a therapeutic trial with one SSRI fails, another one may be efficacious.
3. ***Cingulotomy.*** A last resort for severe treatment-resistant patients. May benefit up to 80% of patients receiving the surgery, but results may be inconsistent.

VII. POSTTRAUMATIC STRESS DISORDER (PTSD)

A. Overview. Lifetime prevalence 1% to 14%. PTSD can occur at any age. Symptoms usually begin within 3 months after the inciting trauma.

B. DSM-IV diagnosis criteria. PTSD occurs in individuals who experienced an extraordinarily distressing event (combat, sexual abuse or rape, natural disasters) involving self or others. In addition, the person's response includes intense fear or helplessness.

1. Characterized by persistent reexperiences of the event in at least one of the following ways:
    - Intrusive, recurrent recollections of the event
    - Recurrent distressing dreams of the event
    - Sudden sense of reliving the experience (flashbacks, hallucinations)
    - Intense distress with exposure to symbols or representations of the event (such as anniversaries)
2. Results in avoidant behavior of stimuli associated with the trauma or decreased responsiveness to the external world (psychic numbing).
3. Associated with 2 or more symptoms of increased arousal (insomnia, irritability, anger, poor, concentration, hypervigilance, or exaggerated startle).
4. The disturbance lasts more than 1 month and causes significant distress or functional impairment.

C. Treatment.

1. Supportive therapy that is appropriate for grief reaction.
2. Group therapy may be helpful.
3. Individuals may benefit from medical treatment (such as treating depressive or anxiety symptoms).

SUBSTANCE-USE DISORDERS

I. OVERVIEW (Tables 15-2 to 15-4)

A. Epidemiology. Marijuana is the most commonly used illicit drug with 10 million current users. Cocaine is used by 2 million Americans. Substance use rates are highest in ages 18 to 25 years. Substance use is involved in 50% of all highway deaths and over 50% of domestic violence.

B. Substance-dependence DSM-IV criteria. Maladaptive pattern of substance use leading to significant impairment or distress with at least 3 of the following occurring within a 12-month period:

1. Tolerance (increased amount of substance required to produce desired effect).
2. Withdrawal syndrome, or using a substance to relieve withdrawal symptoms.
3. Substance taken in larger amounts or over longer periods than intended.
4. Persistent desire or unsuccessful attempts to cut down use.
5. Significant amount of time spent in obtaining, consuming, or recovering from the substance.
6. Important social or occupational activities reduced because of substance use.

TABLE 15-2
Drugs of Abuse

Opioids	Hallucinogens	Depressants	Stimulants	Cannabinoids
Heroin	Phencyclidine (PCP)	Alcohol	Cocaine	Marijuana
Hydromorphone	Lysergic acid diethylamide (LSD)	Benzodiazepines	Amphetamines	Hashish
Oxycodone	Mescaline	Barbiturates		
Methadone	Psilocybin	Methaqualone		
Meperidine	MDMA (3,4-methylenedioxy-methamphetamine, "ectasy")	Meprobamate		
		Glutethimide		
		Ethchlorvynol		

Adapted from Hyman SE, Tesar GE: *Manual of psychiatric emergencies*, ed 3, Boston, 1994, Little, Brown & Co.

TABLE 15-3
Intoxication and Overdose

Signs or symptoms	Opioids	Depressants	Stimulants	Hallucinogens	Phencyclidine (PCP)
Anxiety	–	+	+	+	+
Arrhythmia	–	–	+	–	–
Coma	+	+	–	+	+
Delirium	+	+	–	+	+
Diaphoresis	–	–	+	+	+
Euphoria	+	+	+	+	+
Hallucinations	–	–	+	+	+
Hypertension	+	–	+	+	+
Hypotension	+	–	–	–	–
Hyperthermia	–	–	+	+	+
Nausea and vomiting	+	–	+	+	+
Nystagmus	–	+	–	–	+
Pupils, dilated	–	–	+	+	–
Pupils, pinpoint	+	–	–	–	–
Reflexes increased	–	–	+	+	+
Respiratory depression	+	+	+	–	+/–
Seizures	–	–	+	–	+
Tachycardia	–	–	+	+	+
Tremor	–	–	+	+	+
Violent or bizarre behavior	–	+	+	+	+

Compiled from Hyman SE, Tesar GE: *Manual of psychiatric emergencies,* ed 3, Boston, 1994, Little, Brown & Co.

TABLE 15-4
Withdrawal

Signs or symptoms	Opioids	Depressants	Stimulants
Anxiety	+	+	−
Depression	−	+	+
Fatigue	−	−	+
Hallucinations	−	+	+
Hypertension	+	+	−
Hypotension (orthostatic)	−	+	−
Insomnia	+	+	−
Nausea and vomiting	+	+	−
Pupils, dilated	+	−	−
Reflexes, hyperactive	−	+	−
Seizures	−	+	−
Tachycardia	+	+	−

Compiled from Hyman SE, Tesar GE: *Manual of psychiatric emergencies*, ed 3, Boston, 1994, Little, Brown & Co.

7. Persistent use despite knowledge of social, psychologic, or physical problems caused by its use.

C. Substance-abuse DSM-IV criteria.

1. Maladaptive pattern of use leading to a significant impairment or distress with at least one of the following within a 12-month period:
   a. Recurrent substance use resulting in a failure to fulfill major role obligations at work, school, or home.
   b. Recurrent use in situations where use is physically hazardous (driving while intoxicated).
   c. Recurrent substance abuse–related legal problems.
   d. Continued use despite knowledge of having a persistent/recurring social or interpersonal problem that is caused or worsened by the substance use.
2. Symptoms have never met criteria for substance dependence for this class of substance.

II. ALCOHOL

A. Prevalence. Lifetime prevalence of alcohol abuse or dependence at 15% to 20% in males. Males outnumber females 4:1.

B. Suspect alcohol abuse if any of the following complaints are present:

- Chronic anxiety or tension
- Legal or marital problems
- Headaches or blackouts
- Frequent falls or minor injuries
- Vague GI problems

- Chronic depression
- Insomnia
- Seizures

C. Complications.

- Gastritis or peptic ulcer disease
- Hypertension
- Liver disease (cirrhosis, ascites)
- Depression
- Myopathy
- Nutritional deficiencies
- Pancreatitis
- Insomnia
- Impotence
- Cardiomyopathy

D. Alcohol-withdrawal syndromes.

1. ***Uncomplicated alcohol withdrawal.*** Begins 12 to 18 hours after cessation of drinking. Peaks between 24 to 48 hours. Untreated, shakes subside within 7 days. Characterized by tremors, nausea, vomiting, tachycardia, and hypertension.
2. ***Alcohol seizures.*** Occur 7 to 38 hours after cessation, and peak at 24 to 48 hours.
3. ***Alcohol-induced psychotic disorder, with hallucinations.*** Onset within 48 hours of cessation and may last 1 week or more. Characterized by unpleasant auditory hallucinations without evidence of delirium.
4. ***Alcohol-withdrawal delirium (delirium tremens, DTs).*** May begin 2 or 3 days after cessation and peak in 4 or 5 days. Typically lasts 3 days but can persist for weeks. Symptoms include mild fever, autonomic hyperarousal, and delirium. Important to monitor closely in the hospital as risk for mortality if untreated.

E. Evaluation.

1. ***Screening with CAGE questions.*** One positive answer to any of the following questions may be significant:
   - Have you ever felt you should *cut down* on your drinking?
   - Have people *annoyed* you by criticizing your drinking?
   - Have you ever felt bad or *guilty* about your drinking?
   - Have you ever had a drink first thing in the morning to steady your nerves or get rid of a hangover (*eye-opener*)?
2. ***Physical exam.*** Early findings may include hepatomegaly, tremor, or mild peripheral neuropathy. In later stages, sequelae such as pneumonia, hypertension, Wernicke's syndrome (ophthalmoplegia, ataxia, and confusion), Korsakoff's syndrome (amnesia, disorientation, impairment of recent memory, and confabulation), gynecomastia, and spider angiomas may occur.
3. ***Laboratory tests.*** Blood alcohol level, CBC, liver enzymes, PT/PTT, general screen. Consider other tests: hep-

atitis B and C, RPR, vitamin B_{12}, folate, Mg, amylase, UA, urine drug screen, stool guaiac, CRX, TB skin test, and HIV based on risk factors and clinical situation.

F. Management.

1. ***Psychotherapy.*** Includes cognitive behavioral therapy that stresses goal setting, self-monitoring, identifying antecedents to drinking, learning alternative coping skills, and social skills training. Total abstinence and relapse prevention are the goals.
2. ***Alcoholics Anonymous.*** Encouraged patient to attend AA meetings.
3. ***Detoxification.*** May be required if tolerance or withdrawal present.
   a. *Vitamins*
      (1) To prevent Wernicke-Korsakoff syndrome give thiamine 50 to 100 mg IV or IM immediately and then 100 mg PO QD.
      (2) Folate 1 mg PO daily.
      (3) Multivitamin daily.
   b. *Benzodiazepines* should be used to decrease withdrawal symptoms in medically unstable patients and as prophylaxis in patients with history of DTs. In medically stable patients, benzodiazepine treatment is necessary only if 3 of 7 signs or symptoms of withdrawal occur: temperature >38.3° C, pulse >110 bpm, SBP >160 mm Hg, DBP >100 mm Hg, nausea, vomiting, or tremors. Chlordiazepoxide (Librium) or diazepam (Valium) taper may be used, such as chlordiazepoxide 50 mg PO Q4h × 24 hours, then 50 mg Q6h × 24 hours, then 25 mg Q4h × 24 hours, and then 25 mg Q6h × 24 hours. Hold dose if any of the following occur: nystagmus, sedation, ataxia, slurred speech, or the patient is asleep. An alternative regimen involves treating the patient with a benzodiazepine *only when the patient has symptoms* as opposed to scheduled doses with a tapering off (such as 25 to 50 mg PO Q4h PRN symptoms). This may reduce total dose of benzodiazepines needed.
   c. *Beta-blockers* are sometimes used with benzodiazepines to reduce autonomic nervous system hyperactivity.
   d. *Haloperidol* PO or IM for patients with alcohol-induced psychotic disorder and agitation associated with DTs.
   e. *For DTs,* supplement benzodiazepine as necessary for agitation. Seclusion and restraints as necessary. Adequate hydration and nutrition.
4. ***Disulfiram (Antabuse).*** Controlled trials have not demonstrated benefits over placebo in achieving total abstinence or delaying relapse. May benefit some individuals who remain employed, socially stable, and motivated. Advise patient to

avoid all forms of alcohol (24 hours before starting disulfiram to 14 days after last dose) to prevent toxic and potentially fatal reaction. Dosage range 125 to 500 mg PO QHS.

5. ***Naltrexone (Revia).*** FDA approved for alcohol dependence to decrease risk for relapse. No disulfiram-like reactions as a result of ethanol ingestion. Average dose is 50 mg PO QD for 12 weeks. Revia proved superior to placebo in measures of drinking including abstention rates (51% versus 23%), number of drinking days, and relapse (31% versus 60%).

ACUTE PSYCHOSIS

I. DEFINITION

Significant impairment of sense of reality (incoherence, looseness of associations, delusions, hallucinations, catatonic or disorganized behavior) that results in impairment of ability to communicate, emotional turmoil, and impaired cognitive abilities

II. DIFFERENTIAL DIAGNOSIS

A. **Substance-induced (intoxication or withdrawal).** For example, hallucinogens, amphetamines, cocaine, alcohol withdrawal, anticholinergic drugs, corticosteroids, and L-dopa.

B. **Acute exacerbation or initial episode of chronic psychotic disorder (schizophrenia).**

C. **Major affective syndrome,** anxiety disorder, or personality disorder (cluster A).

D. **Secondary to general medical condition.** For example, temporal lobe epilepsy, CNS tumors, stroke, trauma, endocrine or metabolic disorders, infections autoimmune disorders, vitamin deficiency, and toxins. Suspect psychosis caused by a medical condition if:

1. Delirium is present (clouding of the sensorium)
2. No personal or family history of psychotic disorder
3. Age over 35 years
4. Rapid development of psychosis in a previously functioning individual

III. LABORATORY TESTS

May include CBC, UA, liver enzymes, electrolytes, BUN, Cr, TFTs, VDRL, and HIV. Also urine drug screen and occasionally heavy-metal screen. Also perform head CT or MRI in selected patients.

IV. TREATMENT

A. **General.** Antipsychotics initially used to control behavior, including rapid tranquilization. Long-term treatment will depend on the cause. Further history may need to be obtained from family or friends to evaluate baseline functioning. Hospitalization may be indicated for patient safety.

B. Rapid tranquilization. Used to treat violent, assaultive, or extremely agitated patients. It is very useful in the emergency department as well as for inpatients. It is effective for treatment of symptoms regardless of the cause of the aggression that is, it works for schizophrenia, mania, dementia, delirium, etc.).

C. Medications used is rapid tranquilization. *Patients who have been tranquilized must have vital signs closely monitored.*

1. ***Typical antipsychotics.*** Use Q30-60 min IM until behavior subsides or limited by side effects (Table 15-5). Side effects may dictate antipsychotic chosen. NOTE: Side effects are similar within potency groups. Haloperidol produces less hypotension than other preparations do and is relatively safe in large doses. See Table 15-6 for details. May use Haldol in IV form for more rapid effect. Use PRN Benadryl (25 to 50 mg PO/IM/IV up to TID or QID) or Cogentin (1 to 2 mg PO/IM/IV up to BID or TID) for treatment of extrapyramidal symptoms (such as parkinsonism, dystonic reactions [torticollis, facial grimacing, or oculogyric crisis], or akathisia [restlessness, pacing]).
2. ***Benzodiazepines.*** Drug of choice for alcohol or benzodiazepine withdrawal (see previous alcohol abuse section). May be used as an adjunct to antipsychotics for sedative effect, such as lorazepam (Ativan) 2 to 4 mg IM Q30 min to 2 hours up to 120 mg/24 hours, offering more rapid and complete IM absorption than other benzodiazepines. Watch for respiratory depression.
3. ***Droperidol (Inapsine).*** Used for the short-term symptomatic treatment of acute violence or agitation, especially

TABLE 15-5

Recommended Antipsychotic Dose for Rapid Tranquilization

Drug	IM (mg)	Oral concentrate (mg)
HIGH POTENCY		
Haloperidol (Haldol)	5	10
Fluphenazine (Prolixin)	5	10
Thiothixene (Navane)	10	20
Trifluoperazine (Stelazine)	10	20
LOW POTENCY		
Chlorpromazine (Thorazine)	50	100
Thioridazine (Mellaril)	NA	100
OTHER		
Droperidol (Inapsine)	2.5-10	NA

NA, Not applicable.

in young, healthy patients. *Produces much more rapid sedation than Haldol.* Usual dosage 2.5 to 10 mg IM or IV (dose should be individualized, based on weight, age, and clinical situation). Increased risk of hypotension, sedation, and cardiovascular effects (ECG changes, dysrhythmias in doses >25 mg) make it second-line drug to Haldol. Do not use in those with underlying cardiac disease.

SCHIZOPHRENIA AND OTHER PSYCHOTIC DISORDERS

I. SCHIZOPHRENIA

A. Prevalence. The most common psychotic disorder, affecting 1% of the world population, and having a strong familial tendency. Between one third and one half of homeless Americans have schizophrenia.

B. DSM-IV criteria.

1. ***Characteristic symptoms.*** Two (or more) of the following, each present for a significant time during a 1-month period (or less if treated successfully):
   - Delusions
   - Hallucinations
   - Disorganized or catatonic behavior
   - Disorganized speech
   - Negative symptoms (such as, affective flattening, alogia [poverty of speech or thought content], or avolition [inability to initiate and persist in goal-directed activities])
2. ***Social or occupational dysfunction.*** Significant impairment in work, relationships, or self-care since onset of illness.
3. Continuous signs of the disturbance persist for at least six months.
4. ***Exclusions.*** Symptoms not attributable to a mood disorder or to the effects of a general medical condition or psychoactive substance.

C. Subtypes

1. ***Paranoid.*** Preoccupation with one or more delusions or frequent auditory hallucinations. *No* incoherence, loosening of associations, catatonic or disorganized behavior. Best prognosis.
2. ***Disorganized.*** Characterized by disorganized speech or behavior and flat or inappropriate affect. No catatonic features. Worst prognosis.
3. ***Catatonic.*** At least two of the following: immobility/stupor, negativism/mutism, bizarre posturing, purposeless excitement, or echolalia/echopraxia. Must differentiate from catatonia found in affective disorders and physical illnesses.
4. ***Undifferentiated.*** Does not fit criteria for the categories above.
5. ***Residual.*** Absence of prominent psychotic symptoms but continuing evidence of the disturbance in attenuated form.

D. Differential diagnosis. Any condition that can produce acute psychosis (see section above on acute psychosis).

E. Treatment.

1. ***First psychotic episode.*** Typical antipsychotic chosen based on side effects the patient will tolerate best (see examples in Table 15-5). Need 6 to 8 weeks at a therapeutic dose for adequate trial. If no response, consider switching to another typical antipsychotic class. If two typical antipsychotic trials fail, consider atypical antipsychotics (usually risperidone first, then olanzapine, and then clozapine). Prophylactic treatment is recommended for at least 6 months to 1 year. The above is usually done in consultation with a psychiatrist.
2. ***Relapsing psychosis.*** Requires long-term treatment with antipsychotics (Table 15-6). Minimize dose to prevent long-term complications of antipsychotics (tardive dyskinesia).

TABLE 15-6

Antipsychotic Doses and Side Effects for Chronic Use

Drug	Relative potency (milligram equivalents)	Dose (mg)/ day)	Anticholin-ergic*	EPS†	Sedation	Orthostatic hypoten-sion
TYPICAL ANTIPSYCHOTICS						
Chlorprom-azine (Thorazine)	100	100-2000	++++	++	+++++	+++++
Thioridazine (Mellaril)	100	100-600	+++++	+	++++	+++++
Trifluo-perazine (Stelazine)	5	5-60	++	++++	+	++
Thiothixene (Navane)	5	5-60	++	++++	++	++
Fluphenazine (Prolixin)	4	5-30	++	+++++	++	++
Haloperidol (Haldol)	4	2-100	+	+++++	++	+
ATYPICAL ANTIPSYCHOTICS						
Risperidone (Risperdal)	1	1-6	+/−	+	+	++
Clozapine (Clozaril)‡	50	25-900	+++++	+/−	+++++	+++++
Olanzapine (Zyprexa)	2	5-20	+/−	+/−	++	+

Adapted from Bernstein JG: *Handbook of drug therapy in psychiatry,* ed 3, St. Louis, 1995, Mosby.

*Dry mouth, constipation, blurred vision, urinary retention.

†Extrapyramidal side effects (dystonia, parkinsonism, akathisia, tardive dyskinesia).

‡Requires weekly WBC count because of risk of agranulocytosis.

3. ***Supportive psychotherapy.*** Individual or family counseling may be a helpful adjunct to reduce risk for relapse.
4. ***Community programs.*** Beneficial in providing support, social skills training, and vocational rehabilitation.

II. SPECIAL ANTIPSYCHOTIC ADVERSE REACTIONS

A. Neuroleptic malignant syndrome. May occur at any point during the course of treatment. Includes symptoms of autonomic instability, altered mental status, which may progress to hypothermia, stupor, and muscle hypertonicity. Death may occur. See section on neuroleptic malignant syndrome in Chapter 1 for treatment.

B. Tardive dyskinesia. Involuntary movements of the tongue, face, mouth, or jaw associated with long-term administration of antipsychotics. Elderly females at highest risk. May be irreversible.

EATING DISORDERS

I. ANOREXIA NERVOSA (AN)

A. Overview. Onset is usually in adolescence and affects females 10:1 over males. Prevalence in young women is up to 1%. Some will also have episodes of binge eating or purging. Anorexia is a life-threatening disorder, with mortality over 10%.

B. Diagnosis.

1. Early signs may include withdrawal from family and friends, increased sensitivity to criticism, sudden increased interest in physical activity, anxiety or depressive symptoms.
2. ***DSM-IV criteria.***
   a. Refusal to maintain body weight over a minimal normal weight for age and height (such as weight less than 85% of expected).
   b. Intense fear of becoming fat even though underweight.
   c. Disturbed body image or denial of seriousness of current low body weight.
   d. Absence of 3 consecutive menstrual periods.

C. Laboratory tests. No single lab test helps with the diagnosis; however, a battery of tests should be performed to rule out medical complications of starvation. CBC, general screen (to include electrolytes, glucose, calcium, phosphate, BUN, and Cr), Mg, liver and thyroid function tests, amylase, carotene, UA, ECG. Other useful tests include CK with isoenzymes if an ipecac abuser; or bone densitometry if amenorrheic for >6 months.

D. Potential medical complications.
Dry skin, hypothermia, bradycardia, hypotension, dependent edema, anemia, lanugo, infertility, osteoporosis, cardiac failure, and death (most commonly results from starvation, suicide, or electrolyte imbalances).

E. Treatment.

1. Indications for hospitalization may include any of the following:
   a. Patient's weight ≤70% of ideal body weight.
   b. Persistent suicidal ideation.
   c. Need for withdrawal from laxatives, diet pills, or diuretics.
   d. Failure of outpatient treatment.
3. ***Outpatient.***
   a. Treat the medical complications of starvation.
   b. Nutritional counseling to establish a balanced diet, an expected rate of weight gain (up to 2 lbs. per week), and a final goal weight.
   c. Use behavioral techniques to reward weight gain.
   d. Individual and group cognitive therapy to alter anorexic attitudes, enhance autonomy, and improve self-esteem.
   e. Family therapy may also be useful.
   f. Treat any associated mood disorder.

II. BULIMIA NERVOSA (BN)

A. Overview. Onset is usually in late adolescence or early adulthood and is more prevalent in females than in males. As many as 17% of college-aged women engage in bulimic behaviors. Bulimics tend to be of normal weight to slightly overweight. Associated dysphoria or depression is common. 30% to 80% of bulimics have a history of anorexia nervosa.

B. DSM-IV criteria.

1. Recurrent episodes of binge eating characterized by:
   a. Eating large amounts of food in a discrete period of time.
   b. Lack if control over eating behavior.
2. Regular inappropriate compensatory behavior to prevent weight gain (such as use of self-inducing vomiting, laxatives, diuretics, fasting, or excessive exercise).
3. Binge episodes and compensatory behaviors both occur on average twice a week for at least 3 months.
4. Persistent overconcern with body shape and weight.

C. Laboratory tests. No single lab test helps with the diagnosis; however, to check for complications, several tests should be performed: general screen (to include electrolytes, glucose, calcium, phosphate, BUN, and Cr), Mg, and amylase.

D. Potential medical complications. Erosion of dental enamel, dental caries, parotitis, menstrual irregularity, laxative dependence, electrolyte disturbances, gastric rupture, cardiac arrhythmias, and chronic pancreatitis.

E. Treatment. Should include medical stabilization, routine monitoring of serum K^+ and Mg^{++}, education about medical complications, supportive and cognitive behavioral therapy and nutritional counseling. Prozac 20 to 60 mg PO QA.M. May lessen the number of binge episodes and associated dysphoria (not yet FDA approved). Treat comorbid depression if present. Hospitalization in a minority of patients (admission criteria similar to those of anorexia nervosa except for weight loss).

BIBLIOGRAPHY:

American Psychiatric Association: *Diagnostic and statistical manual of mental disorders,* ed 4, Washington, D.C., 1994, American Psychiatric Association.

American Psychiatric Association: *Diagnostic and statistical manual of mental disorders,* ed 4, *Primary Care Version,* ed 1, Washington, D.C., 1995, American Psychiatric Association.

American Psychiatric Association: Practice guidance for the treatment of patients with bipolar disorder, *Am J Psychiatry Suppl* 151(12):1-36, 1994.

American Psychiatric Association: Practice guideline for the treatment of patients with substance use disorders: alcohol, cocaine, and opioids, *Am J Psychiatry Suppl* 152(11): 5-80, 1995.

Andreasen NC, Black DW: *Introductory textbook of psychiatry,* Washington, D.C., 1991, American Psychiatric Press, pp 293-308.

Andreasen NC: Symptoms, signs, and diagnosis of schizophrenia, *Lancet* 346:477-481, 1995.

Beumont PJV et al: Treatment of anorexia nervosa, *Lancet* 341:1635-1640, 1993.

Blumenreich PE, Lippmann SB: Phobias: how to help patients overcome irrational fears, *Postgrad Med* 96(1):125-134, 1994.

Boyer W: Serotonin uptake inhibitors are superior to imipramine and alprazolam in alleviating panic attacks: a meta-analysis, *Int Clin Psychopharmacol* 10(1):45-49, 1995.

Carpenter, WT Jr, Buchanan RW: Medical progress–schizophrenia, *N Engl J Med* 330(10):681-690, 1994.

Depression Guideline Panel: *Depression in primary care,* Vol 1, *Detection and diagnosis,* Clinical Practice Guideline, no. 5, AHCPR Pub No. 93-0550, Rockville, Md., April 1993, U.S. Department of Health and Human Services, Public Health Service, Agency for Health Care Policy and Research.

Goldman HH, editor: *Review of general psychiatry,* ed 4, East Norwalk, Conn., 1995, Appleton & Lange.

Guze B et al: *The psychiatric drug handbook,* ed 2, St. Louis, 1995, Mosby.

Haller E: Eating disorders–a review and update, *West J Med* 157(6):658-662, 1992.

Kane JM, McGlashen TH: Treatment of schizophrenia, *Lancet* 346:820-825, 1995.

Kaplan HI, Sadock BJ: *Pocket handbook of clinical psychiatry,* ed 2, Baltimore, 1996, Williams & Wilkins.

Kaplan HI et al: *Synopsis of psychiatry,* ed 7, Baltimore, 1994, Williams & Wilkins.

Noyes R, Hoehn-Saric R: *Anxiety disorders,* New York, 1996, Cambridge University Press.

Nymberg JH, Van Noppen B: Obsessive-compulsive disorder: a concealed diagnosis, *Am Fam Physician* 49(5):1129-1137, 1994.

Perry P et al: Clinical Psychopharmacology Seminar, 1994-1995, University of Iowa.

Perry P et al: *Psychotropic drug handbook,* ed 7, Washington D.C., 1996, American Psychiatric Press.

Thase ME: Do we really need all these antidepressants? Weighing the options, *J Practical Psychiatry and Behavioral Health* 3(1):3-17, 1997.

Weiden PJ: Olanzapine: a new "atypical" antipsychotic, *J Practical Psychiatry and Behavioral Health* 3(1):49-53, 1997.

16

AIDS

Melissa J. Gamponia and Mark A. Graber

AIDS (ACQUIRED IMMUNODEFICIENCY SYNDROME)

The treatment of AIDS and related illnesses is a rapidly changing field. Although the recommendations below were current at the time of writing, changes in the treatment regimens may have occurred since then.

I. AIDS is a spectrum of disease manifestations, ranging from asymptomatic to life-threatening conditions characterized by severe immunodeficiency, opportunistic infections, and cancers occurring in individuals not receiving immunosuppressive drugs and with no other immunosuppressive disease. It is caused by the HIV-1 and HIV-2 viruses. These retroviruses cause a progressive loss of helper T cells (also known as T4 lymphocytes, or CD4+ lymphocytes) leading to a progressive loss in immune competence and subsequent opportunistic infections. See diagnosis of AIDS on p. 633 for the list of AIDS-defining conditions.

II. HIGH-RISK BEHAVIORS AND MODES OF TRANSMISSION

The HIV virus is transmitted by the exchange of infected body fluids including blood and semen. High-risk behaviors include:

A. Unprotected sexual intercourse with multiple partners, a high-risk partner (commercial sex worker, IV drug user), or an infected partner.

B. IV drug use, or exchanging sexual intercourse for drugs.

C. Persons receiving blood products before 1985.

1. Although infected transfusions are almost 100% effective in transmitting HIV, seroconversion after a "routine" exposure to infected blood in health care workers (such as a splash or a needle stick) occurs in only 4 per 1000. The risk of transmission is increased if the needle stick is deep or directly enters a vein or a large volume of blood is involved. **A recent analysis of data by the CDC indicates that postexposure transmission may be decreased by 79% if AZT prophylaxis is used after an exposure to known infected**

material! Prophylaxis should be started ASAP and preferably within 1 hour of exposure. See Table 16-1 for CDC recommendations.

2. HIV transmission through hemodialysis has not been reported in the United States, though it has been documented in other countries.
3. Transmission has occurred in women who were artificially inseminated.

D. Perinatal and vertical transmission.

1. Whether in utero, intra partum, or by breast-feeding, there is a perinatal transmission rate of 15% to 30%. Risk factors include advanced maternal disease status, low maternal CD4+ cell count, infant exposure to maternal blood, prolonged duration of ruptured membranes, maternal vitamin A deficiency, and an increased quantity of HIV in maternal blood at delivery (as with acute infection). Breast-feeding is not recommended for HIV-seropositive mothers in the United States. See below for details of perinatal diagnosis of HIV.
2. There is no evidence implicating an insect vector in the transmission of AIDS. Likewise, living with an HIV-infected person or even sharing the same toothbrush is not considered high-risk behavior for contracting the AIDS virus.

III. AIDS BY ORGAN SYSTEM

Use this list to help identify a particular illness in a patient with AIDS who has symptoms referable to a particular organ system.

A. Pulmonary disease. *Pneumocystis carinii* pneumonia, bacterial pneumonia, mycobacterial disease, fungal disease (histoplasmosis, coccidioidomycosis, cryptococcosis, aspergillosis), viral diseases (including CMV, varicella zoster, influenza), Kaposi's sarcoma, AIDS-related non-Hodgkin's lymphoma, lymphoid interstitial pneumonitis.

B. Gastrointestinal disease.

1. ***Esophageal diseases.*** Including candidal esophagitis, CMV and HSV esophagitis, rarely Kaposi's sarcoma and AIDS-related non-Hodgkin's lymphoma.
2. ***Intestinal disease.***
   a. Bacteria. *Salmonella, Shigella,* and *Campylobacter* organisms; *Mycobacterium avium-intracellulare* complex.
   b. Parasites. *Cryptosporidium, Isospora, Entamoeba, Giardia* organisms.
   c. Viruses. CMV, herpes simplex, HIV enteropathy.
   d. Tumor including AIDS-KS and AIDS-NHL, anogenital carcinoma, condylomata acuminata.

C. Hepatobiliary and pancreatic diseases.

1. Any AIDS-related infection or neoplasm.
2. Drugs including DDI, DDC, sulfonamide antibiotics, pentamadine-induced pancreatitis, DDI-induced pancreatitis.

TABLE 16-1

Provisional Public Health Service Recommendations for Chemoprophylaxis after Occupational Exposure to HIV, by Type of Exposure and Source Material—1996

Type of exposure	Source material*	Antiretroviral prophylaxis†	Antiretroviral regimen§
Percutaneous	Blood‖		
	Highest risk	Recommend	ZDV plus 3TC plus IDV
	Increased risk	Recommend	ZDV plus 3TC, ± IDV¶
	No increased risk	Offer	ZDV plus 3TC
	Fluid containing visible blood, other potentially infectious fluid,# or tissue	Offer	ZDV plus 3TC
	Other body fluid (e.g., urine)	Not offer	
Mucous membrane	Blood	Offer	ZDV plus 3TC, ± IDV¶
	Fluid containing visible blood, other potentially infectious fluid,# or tissue	Offer	ZDV, ±3TC
	Other body fluid (e.g., urine)	Not offer	

Continued.

TABLE 16-1

Provisional Public Health Service Recommendations for Chemoprophylaxis after Occupational Exposure to HIV, by Type of Exposure and Source Material—1996—cont'd

Type of exposure	Source material*	Antiretroviral prophylaxis†	Antiretroviral regimen§
Skin, increased risk**	Blood	Offer	ZDV plus 3TC, ±IDV¶
	Fluid containing visible blood, other potentially infectious fluid,# or tissue	Offer	ZDV, ±3TC
	Other body fluid (e.g., urine)	Not offer	

*Any exposure to concentrated HIV (e.g., in a research laboratory or production facility) is treated as percutaneous exposure to blood with highest risk.

†*Recommend*—Postexposure prophylaxis (PEP) should be recommended to the exposed worker with counseling. *Offer*—PEP should be offered to the exposed worker with counseling. *Not offer*—PEP should not be offered because these are not occupational exposures to HIV.

§*Regimens:* zidovudine (ZDV), 200 mg three times a day; lamivudine (3TC), 150 mg two times a day; indinavir (IDV), 800 mg three times a day (if IDV is not available, saquinavir may be used, 600 mg three times a day). Prophylaxis is given for 4 weeks. For full prescribing information, see package inserts.

‖*Highest risk*—BOTH larger volume of blood (e.g., deep injury with large-diameter hollow needle previously in source patient's vein or artery, especially involving an injection of source-patient's blood) AND blood containing a high titer of HIV (e.g., source with acute retroviral illness or end-stage AIDS; viral load measurement may be considered, but its use in relation to PEP has not been evaluated). *Increased risk*—EITHER exposure to larger volume of blood OR blood with a high titer of HIV. *No increased risk*—NEITHER exposure to larger volume of blood NOR blood with a high titer of HIV (e.g., solid suture needle injury from source patient with asymptomatic HIV infection).

¶Possible toxicity of additional drug may not be warranted.

#Includes semen; vaginal secretions; cerebrospinal, synovial, pleural, peritoneal, pericardial, and amniotic fluids.

**For skin, risk is increased for exposures involving a high titer of HIV, prolonged contact, an extensive area, or an area in which skin integrity is visibly compromised. For skin exposures without increased risk, the risk for drug toxicity outweighs the benefit of PEP.

3. *Mycobacterium avium-intracellulare* complex.
4. AIDS cholangiopathy.
   a. Severe RUQ abdominal pain.
   b. Spiking fevers.
   c. Elevated alkaline phosphatase levels.
   d. Pathologically sclerosing cholangitis and papillary stenosis.
   e. Can use ERCP to diagnose.

D. Ophthalmologic disease.

1. ***Cornea.*** Ulcerative keratitis, dry eye, herpes simplex keratitis, herpes zoster ophthalmicus, Microsporida order.
2. ***Retina and choroid.*** Microvasulopathy (cotton-wool spots, retinal hemorrhages), cytomegalovirus retinitis, acute retinal necrosis, progressive outer retinal necrosis, syphilis, toxoplasmosis, *Pneumocystis* choroidopathy, cryptococcosis, mycobacterial infection, intraocular lymphoma, candidiasis, histoplasmosis.
3. ***Drug-associated ocular toxicity.*** Didanosine-associated ocular toxicity, rifabutin-associated uveitis.
4. ***Neuro-ophthalmic.*** Disk edema (papilledema), optic neuropathy, cranial nerve palsies.
5. ***Orbital disorder.*** Orbital lymphoma, orbital infection.

E. Neurologic disease.

1. ***Primary viral (HIV) syndromes.*** HIV encephalopathy, atypical aseptic meningitis, spinal vacuolar myelopathy.
2. ***Opportunistic viral illnesses.*** Cytomegalovirus, herpes simplex virus (types 1 and 2), varicella-zoster virus, papovavirus (progressive multifocal leukoencephalopathy), adenovirus (type 2)
3. ***Nonviral infections.*** *Toxoplasma gondii, Cryptococcus neoformans, Candida albicans, Aspergillus fumigatus, Coccidioides immitis,* mucormycosis (caused by *Mucor, Absidia,* and *Rhizopus* species). *Acremonium alabamensis, Histoplasma capsulatum, Mycobacterium tuberculosis, Mycobacterium avium-intracellulare, Listeria monocytogenes, Nocardia asteroides.*
4. ***Neoplasms.*** Primary CNS lymphoma, metastatic systemic lymphoma, metastatic Kaposi's sarcoma.
5. ***Cerebrovascular complications.*** Infarction, hemorrhage, vasculitis.
6. ***Complications of systemic AIDS therapy.***
7. ***Peripheral neuropathic syndromes.***
   a. Distal symmetric peripheral neuropathy.
   b. Inflammatory demyelinating polyradiculoneuropathy.
   c. Mononeuropathy multiplex.
   d. Progressive polyradiculopathy.

F. Gynecologic diseases.

1. ***Sexually transmitted diseases.*** There is a three- to five fold increased risk of HIV transmission with both ulcerative and nonulcerative STDs.

a. *Neisseria gonorrhoeae, Chlamydia,* and *Trichomonas.* Few data.
b. PID. Recurrent PID is more common in HIV-seropositive women and such women are more likely to require surgical intervention than women with PID in the general population.
c. Genital ulcerative infections. HSV is more severe and frequent, and has atypical recurrences with progressive immunosuppression. Syphilis also has atypical presentations, abnormally high titers, and more persistent primary lesions with increased risk of treatment failure for secondary disease. Chancroid may present atypically and have increased risk for treatment failure.

2. ***HPV, CIN, and cervical cancer.***
   a. Increased diagnosis of HPV with progressive immunosuppression.
   b. Increased proportion of abnormal Pap smears.
      (1) If a Pap smear obtained during initial evaluation is normal, a follow-up Pap smear should be obtained in 6 months to rule out false-negative results. With a normal follow-up Pap smear, HIV-infected women should be advised to have a Pap smear annually. If an HIV-infected woman has a history of abnormal Pap smears, follow-up should be more frequent at every 6 months.
      (2) If either the initial or follow-up Pap smear reveals severe inflammation with reactive squamous cellular changes, the next follow-up Pap smear should be obtained in 3 months, and management should be guided by the cause of the inflammation. Monitoring with annual Pap smears is advised for HIV-infected women with Pap smears showing only atypical cells of undetermined significance.
      (3) Management for HIV-infected women with Pap smears showing low-grade squamous intraepithelial lesions (SIL) is controversial. Some experts would obtain a follow-up Pap smear at 3 months and then refer the patient for colposcopy if the lesion persisted. Other experts elect to monitor Pap smears at frequent intervals (3 to 6 months), whereas still other health care providers refer all HIV-infected patients with low-grade SIL for colposcopy.
      (4) With a Pap smear result showing a high-grade SIL or squamous cell carcinoma, the woman should be referred for colposcopy and biopsy (if indicated).
      (5) Colposcopy is not indicated for HIV-infected women with normal Pap smears.

c. CIN tends to be more severe and multifocal and may involve the vagina, vulva, perianal area. Rapid progression occurs; recurrence rates are higher and lesions tend to be more refractory to treatment as the patient becomes more immunocompromised.

3. ***Amenorrhea and menstrual disorders.*** Associated with weight loss and wasting. Often secondary to anemia, which may be a direct result of HIV, marrow infection, malignancy, or drug treatment and prophylaxis regimens.

IV. HOW TO DIAGNOSE HIV INFECTION

A. The criteria for HIV infection in persons ≥13 years of age.

1. Reactive screening test for HIV antibody (ELISA: false positive <1%, false negative <3%) with specific antibody identified by the use of supplemental tests (Western blot, immunofluorescence assay). With an intermediate result, may want to retest at a later date if high clinical suspicion or pursue dCD4+ (helper T-cell) counts, or make a clinical diagnosis.
2. Direct identification of virus in host tissues by virus isolation.
3. HIV antigen detection of p24 antigen by standard assay or immune complex–dissociated assay.
4. Demonstration of HIV viral RNA in the blood.
5. A positive result on any other highly specific licensed test for HIV.
   a. The FDA has approved an oral HIV test (Orasure manufactured by Epitope, Inc., Beaverton, Oreg.) that detects HIV antibody using a specially treated cotton swab that obtains a sample of saliva when the swab is placed between the patient's lower gum and the cheek.
   b. An HIV dipstick test is being used in China, Thailand, Indonesia, Argentina, India, Cameroon, and Zimbabwe (using serum or plasma samples).

B. The CDC 1993 revised classification system for HIV infection and AIDS surveillance case definition is based on three ranges of CD4+ T-lymphocyte counts and three clinical categories and is represented by a matrix of nine mutually exclusive categories.

1. Category A includes (1) asymptomatic HIV infection, 2) persistent generalized lymphadenopathy, and (3) acute (primary) HIV infection with accompanying illness or history of acute HIV infection (without the occurrence of conditions in B or C).
2. Category B conditions take precedence over those in category A and must meet the following criteria: (1) are attributed to HIV infection, (2) are indicative of a defect in cell-mediated immunity, or (3) are considered by physicians

to have a clinical course or to require management that is complicated by HIV infection. These conditions are not included in category C (the AIDS surveillance case definition). Examples are bacillary angiomatosis, oropharyngeal candidiasis (thrush), vulvovaginal candidiasis (persistent, frequent, or poorly responsive to therapy), cervical dysplasia (moderate to severe or cervical carcinoma in situ, constitutional symptoms (fever of ≥38.5° C or diarrhea lasting >1 month), oral hairy leukoplakia, herpes zoster (shingles, involving 2 or more distinct episodes or more than 1 dermatome), idiopathic thrombocytopenic purpura, listeriosis, PID (especially if complicated by a tubo-ovarian abscess), or peripheral neuropathy.

3. Conditions included in the 1993 CDC AIDS surveillance case definition or category C. HIV-positive patients with any of these clinical manifestations are defined as having AIDS: candidiasis (esophageal, bronchial, tracheal, or pulmonary), invasive cervical cancer, coccidioidomycosis (disseminated or extrapulmonary), cryptosporidiosis (chronic intestinal >1 month in duration), cytomegalovirus retinitis (with loss of vision), cytomegalovirus disease (other than liver, spleen, or nodes), HIV-related encephalopathy, herpes simplex (chronic ulcers >1 month in duration, or bronchitis, pneumonitis, or esophagitis), histoplasmosis (disseminated or extrapulmonary), isosporiasis (chronic intestinal >1 month in duration), Kaposi's sarcoma, Burkitt's lymphoma, immunoblastic lymphoma, primary CNS lymphoma. *Mycobacterium avium-intracellulare* complex or *M. kansasii* (disseminated or extrapulmonary), *M. tuberculosis* (any site), other *Mycobacterium* species (disseminated or extrapulmonary), *Pneumocystis carinii* pneumonia, recurrent pneumonia, progressive multifocal leukoencephalopathy, recurrent *Salmonella* septicemia, toxoplasmosis of brain, HIV wasting syndrome.

C. Seroconversion to HIV positive usually occurs within 9 to 12 weeks of exposure to the HIV virus, but patients may remain seronegative for up to 36 months so that sequential testing may be required. For high-risk individuals, the CDC recommends testing every 6 months.

D. The diagnosis in the neonatal period is more complicated because, although transmission rates for the virus from mother to child are 15% to 30%, a high percentage of the children born to HIV-positive mothers will test positive using the Western blot and ELISA tests because of the passive transmission of maternal antibody transplacentally. This antibody will be present for up to 18 months.

1. ***For a child <18 months of age who is known to be HIV seropositive or born to an HIV-infected mother,*** the diagnosis is confirmed with positive results on 2 separate determinations with one or more of the following tests:

a. Culture, very good but expensive. 48% sensitive at birth and 75% sensitive at 3 months.
b. PCR or other technique for demonstrating viral RNA in the blood. This is highly sensitive and specific, is reasonably priced, and requires a small sample of whole blood. Accuracy is 84% at birth and 98% to 100% at 1 month of age.
c. Can check for the p24 antigen (a major core protein of the HIV virus). However, this is only 18% sensitive at birth.
d. Or meets criteria for acquired immunodeficiency syndrome diagnosis based on the 1987 AIDS surveillance case definition (see section on AIDS in the Pediatric Patient, p. 652).

2. ***For a child ≥18 months of age born to an HIV-infected mother or any child infected by blood, blood products, or other known modes of transmission,*** the diagnosis of HIV is confirmed under the following conditions:
   a. HIV-antibody positive by repeatedly reactive enzyme immunoassay (EIA) and confirmatory test (Western blot or immunofluorescence assay (IFA).
   b. Or meets any of the criteria listed above (IV D1).
3. ***A child is given the diagnosis of perinatally acquired HIV if:***
   a. The child does not meet the above criteria but is HIV seropositive by EIA and confirmatory test (Western blot or IFA) and is <18 months of age at the time of the test.
   b. And has unknown antibody status at birth but was born to a mother known to be infected with HIV.
4. ***If the child is born to an HIV-infected mother, the child is diagnosed as a seroconverter if:***
   a. There is documentation of negative HIV-antibody testing (≥2 negative EIA tests performed at 6 to 18 months of age and 1 negative EIA test after 18 months of age)
   b. And there is no other laboratory evidence of infection (has not had 2 positive viral detection tests, if performed)
   c. And has not had an AIDS-defining condition.

E. While obtaining informed consent to test for the HIV virus, it is important to discuss with the patient the implications of a positive test including insurance and work or school ramifications. Despite federal antidiscrimination legislation enacted in 1990, many HIV-infected persons still face substantial public intolerance. Anonymous testing and confidentiality in diagnosis and treatment are therefore useful for HIV-infected individuals to remain active in their communities and in the work force. Posttest counseling is also recommended to include information on high-risk behaviors and retesting for seronegative individuals, behaviors to prevent transmission, strategies for health protection with an immunocompromised system, and the necessity of contact tracing for HIV-seropositive individuals.

V. THE INITIAL EVALUATION OF THE HIV-POSITIVE PATIENT

Initial laboratory data should include (1) HepB core antibody, (2) HepB surface antigen, (3) CD4+ count and viral RNA load, (4) CBC with differential, platelet count, (5) VDRL + FTA if VDRL positive, (6) PPD (some authors consider >3 mm positive in HIV patients), (7) mumps and *Candida* skin tests (documents anergy, control for PPD), (8) liver and renal function studies, electrolytes, (9) UA, (10) GC culture–genital, rectal, and oral and *Chlamydia* testing, (11) stool for ova and parasites × 3, (12) stool for culture, (13), toxoplasmosis and cytomegalovirus titers, (14) CXR, (15) G6PD if indicated, and (16) Pap smear and wet mount in women.

VI. NATURAL HISTORY WITH VARIABLE COURSE

A. The acute phase occurs soon after exposure and may present as an influenza or a mononucleosis-like illness with fever, sweats, fatigue, adenopathy, diarrhea, arthralgias, headache, and occasionally thrombocytopenia (HIV infection may present with epistaxis). There may also be an acute drop in the CD4+ lymphocyte count with an occasional opportunistic infection.

B. The incubation period may be up to 10 years long. Therefore HIV is a chronic disease with a better prognosis than diseases such as congestive heart failure.

1. Antigenic stimulation (intercurrent infections, parasites, etc.) of CD4+ cells hastens viral replication and cell death.
2. There is some evidence that repeated exposure to the HIV virus shortens the time to the development of AIDS. Therefore it is important to practice safe sex even if one's partner is also HIV positive.

C. Asymptomatic phase is characterized by a decline in the CD4+ count with persistent lymphadenopathy but active viral replication.

D. AIDS-related complex (ARC) comprises lymphadenopathy, fever, and malaise in the absence of opportunistic infections.

1. Biopsy specimens of lymph nodes show a nonspecific hyperplasia. The regression of lymphadenopathy may herald a worsening of the disease. The cells necessary to support a hyperplasia may no longer be available.

VII. MANAGEMENT OF HIV INFECTION

A. Immunize. Give Pneumovax and tetanus and influenza vaccines.

1. Should fully immunize including hepatitis B if not already immune *but do not give live, attenuated vaccines to these patients.* The following vaccines are live: BCG, measles, MMR, MR,

mumps, OPV (oral poliovirus), rubella, oral typhoid, varicella, and yellow fever.

B. Ongoing evaulation should include:

1. A follow-up at 2 to 4 weeks to discuss questions, lifestyle changes, and support systems and to deal with emotional issues and suicidal ideation (rates of suicide are increased in HIV-positive patients).
2. Therapy based on CD4+ counts, clinical manifestations, and viral RNA counts. Draw CD4+ counts at the same time each visit, since there is a diurnal variation.
   a. If CD4+ count **>600**, check every 6 months with a brief history, CBC, CD4+ count.
   b. If CD4+ count **>500 but <600**, check every 3 months with a brief history, CBC, CD4+ count.
   c. If CD4+ count **<500 or** if patient develops opportunistic infections regardless of CD4+ count, start antiviral drugs.
   d. If CD4+ count **<200**, patient is susceptible to opportunistic infections and prophylaxis should be begun (see below).
3. ***Viral RNA.***
   a. Should be assessed in all HIV-positive patients using same assay and type of collection tube, since assays vary widely.
   b. Check initially and then at 2 to 4 weeks to examine trend.
   c. Check every 3 to 4 months or more frequently if need to consider changes in therapy.
   d. Check viral RNA 3 to 4 weeks after any change in therapy to see if there is an adequate response (decrease in viral RNA by 0.5 log or greater).
      - If RNA count decreases but then returns to within 0.5 log of the pretreatment value, treatment should be considered a failure.

C. Initiate antiviral therapy if:

1. ***Symptomatic HIV disease (AIDS) regardless of CD4+ count:*** Start combination therapy as noted below.
2. ***Asymptomatic individuals with CD4+ >500:*** If have >30,000 copies/ml of viral RNA or if CD4+ cells decreasing at >10 cells/month. Many would start if viral RNA >5,000 to 10,000 copies/ml.
3. ***Asymptomatic individuals with CD4+ counts <500/µl:*** Start combination therapy in all patients. Some experts would defer treatment in those individuals with stable CD4+ counts between 350 to 500/µl and low levels of viral RNA (<5000 copies/ml) but decision to withhold should be done in consultation with an infectious disease specialist.
4. ***For initial therapy:*** AZT + DDI, AZT + DDC, AZT + 3TC, DT4 + DDI, AZT + indinavir, DDI, AZT + 3TC +

indinavir or ritonavir. *AZT monotherapy is not indicated for initial therapy.*

D. Nucleoside analog dosing.

1. *Nucleoside analogs* inhibit reverse transcriptase, an enzyme used by the HIV to replicate. The ACTG 175 and Delta trials have shown combination therapy to be more effective than AZT alone. The ACTG 175 Trial studied patients with CD4+ counts of 200 to 500/µl. It showed that DDI alone, AZT + DDI, or AZT + DDC were more likely than AZT alone to prevent a ≥50% decrease in CD4+ cells and development of AIDS-defining conditions. The Delta Trial showed that either AZT + DDL or AZT + DDC decreased the mortality by 38% compared to AZT alone. The rationale supporting combination therapy is based on viral resistance: when 2 nucleoside analogs are administered, virions that had previously developed resistance to AZT are believed to revert to AZT sensitivity as they develop resistance to the other nucleoside analog.
2. *AZT (zidovudine, ZDU, Retrovir)* 100 mg every 4 hours while awake *or* 200 mg PO Q8h has been shown to be just as effective. Side effects include granulocytopenia, myopathy (get CPK increase), nausea, anemia, headache, paresthesias. Check CBC Q2 weeks until stable.
3. *DDI (dideoxyinosine, didanosine, ddI, Videx)* if >75 kg, give 300 mg PO Q12h; if 50 to 75 kg, give 200 mg Q12h; if 35 to 49 kg, give 125 mg Q12h. Must take on an empty stomach for absorption. Side effects include pancreatitis (27%), peripheral neuropathy (42%), and abdominal pain (6%).
4. *DDC (zalcitabine, dideoxycytidine, ddC, HIVID)* 0.75 mg PO TID. Side effects include mouth ulcers (66%), peripheral neuropathy (50%), granulocytopenia, and thrombocytopenia.
5. *D4T (stavudine, Zerit)* 15 to 40 mg (15, 20, 30, 40 mg tablets) PO Q12h. Side effects include peripheral neuropathy (18%), aminotransferase elevations, anemia, macrocytosis, and psychologic disturbances (insominia, anxiety, panic attacks).
6. *3TC (lamivudine)* 150 to 300 mg BID. Side effects include headache, fatigue, insomnia, peripheral neuropathy, muscle aches, rash, and aphthous ulcers.
7. Resistance may develop to one drug or another, and so if the patient deteriorates clinically with decreasing CD4+ counts, consider changing drug combinations. Also, try to minimize adverse effects by using combinations that do not compound side effects.

E. Protease inhibitors.

1. *Protease inhibitors* act to prevent the cleavage of viral polyproteins into functional proteins. Clinical trials evalu-

ating the effectiveness of protease inhibitors in combination with nucleoside analogs are ongoing. In a multicenter placebo-controlled clinical trial involving 1110 patients with CD4+ counts <100/µl and >9 months of prior anti-HIV treatment, only 13% of 543 patients receiving ritonavir died or developed a new AIDS-related condition in contrast to 27% of 547 patients receiving a placebo. In this study, the mortality was halved at 8.4% compared to 4.8%. Trials using saquinavir and indinavir have been similarly encouraging. *Protease inhibitors cannot be used as single-agent therapy because of the rapid induction of resistant HIV strains.*

2. *Saquinavir mesylate (Invirase)* 600 mg PO TID (take after a full meal). Side effects include headache, confusion, nausea, fever, abdominal pain.
3. *Indinavir (Crixivan)* 800 mg PO TID (take after a full meal). Side effects include nausea, vomiting, diarrhea, hyperbilirubinemia, aminotransferase elevations, rash, dry skin, nephrolithiasis, insomnia.
4. *Ritonavir (Norvir)* 600 mg PO BID (take after a full meal). Side effects include nausea, vomiting, diarrhea, aminotransferase elevations, hypercholesterolemia, hypertriglyceridemia, paresthesias.

VIII. INFECTIONS IN AIDS PATIENTS

Remember, AIDS patients get the usual organisms too and have an increased incidence of *Haemophilas influenzae, Streptococcus pneumoniae, Salmonella* sepsis, etc. Do not forget the common organisms. Always pursue a definitive diagnosis and treat broadly in life-threatening conditions until you have isolated an organism. AIDS patients may not mount a white blood cell count response and may not run a fever with infections. Maintain a high clinical suspicion.

IX. INFECTION PROPHYLAXIS IN THE HIV-POSITIVE PATIENT

The following are prophylaxis doses. If chronic suppression is required, this is discussed under the treatment of each disease respectively.

A. Prophylaxis by CD4+ count and other indications. (See specific indications under each entity.)

1. *CD4+ count of <200: Pneumocystis.*
2. *CD4+ count of <100: Toxoplasma.*
3. *CD4+ count of <75:* MAC.
4. *CD4+ count of <50:* CMV, *Cryptococcus, Coccidioides immitis.*
5. *Prophylaxis* indicated for multiple recurrences regardless of CD4+ count: candidiasis, herpes simplex, CMV.

B. *Pneumocystis* prophylaxis.

1. ***Indications.*** For all AIDS patients with CD4+ count <200 and all patients with prior *Pneumocystis* disease

(get 60% recurrence in first year without prophylaxis). Also indicated for patients with an unexplained fever for ≥2 weeks or oropharyngeal candidiasis.

2. ***Protocols.***
   a. TMP-SMX 1 DS PO QD or 1 SS PO QD or 1 DS PO 3 days a week or
   b. Dapsone 50 mg PO BID or 100 mg PO QD (cannot use in patients with G6PD deficiency) or
   c. Dapsone 50 mg PO QD + pyrimethamine 50 mg PO every week + leucovorin 25 mg PO every week or
   d. Aerosolized pentamadine 300 mg every month by nebulizer.
      (1) Least desirable because of cost, side effects of bronchospasm and cough.
      (2) High failure rate with occurrence of extrapulmonary disease.
      (3) Must assure patient is TB negative before giving aerosols.
   e. Clindamycin 450 to 600 mg PO BID or TID + primaquine 15 mg PO QD or
   f. Atovaquone 750 mg PO BD with or without pyrimethamine 25 to 75 mg PO every week or
   g. Pyrimethamine + sulfadoxine 500 mg PO Q2 weeks.

C. *Candida* prophylaxis.

1. ***Indications.*** Prophylaxis or suppression after active disease.
2. ***Protocol.*** Fluconazole 100 to 200 mg PO QD or ketoconazole 200 mg PO QD.

D. *Cytomegalovirus* prophylaxis.

1. ***Indications.*** CD4+ <50 and CMV antibody positive or history of CMV disease.
2. ***Protocol.*** Ganciclovir 1 g PO TID or 5 to 6 mg/kg IV 5 to 7 days/week or foscarnet 90 to 120 mg/kg IV QD.

E. *Toxoplasma* prophylaxis.

1. ***Indications.*** CD4+ counts <100 and IgG *Toxoplasma* antibody positive.
2. ***Protocol.*** TMP/SMX 1 DS PO QD. Alternatively, may use dapsone 50 mg PO QD + pyrimethamine 75 mg PO every week + leucovorin 25 mg PO every week or clindamycin + pyrimethamine or atovaquone + pyrimethamine.

F. *Cryptococcus* prophylaxis.

1. ***Indications.*** CD4+ <50
2. ***Protocol.*** Fluconazole 200 mg PO QD or itraconazole 200 mg PO QD.

G. *Coccidiodes immitis* prophylaxis.

1. ***Indications.*** CD4+ counts <50
2. ***Protocol.*** Fluconazole 200 mg PO QD or itraconazole 200 mg PO QD

H. *Mycobacterium avium-intracellulare* prophylaxis.

1. ***Indications.*** CD4+ count <75
2. Clarithromycin 500 mg PO BID or azithromycin 500 mg PO QD + one or more of the following: ethambutol 15 mg/kg PO QD or clofazimine 100 mg PO QD or rifabutin 150 mg PO BID or ciprofloxacin 500 to 750 mg PO BID. Do not use this regimen in those with active TB.

OPPORTUNISTIC INFECTIONS IN THE HIV-POSITIVE PATIENT

A. *Pneumocystis carinii.*

1. ***Diagnosis.***
   a. Presenting infection in 50% of those with AIDS.
   b. Clinically have subacute, nonproductive cough, tachypnea, and hypoxia (cardinal signs). May have clear lungs or only wheezes.
   c. An interstitial pneumonitis pattern is common on radiograph, but the patient may have a normal radiograph. Occasionally, cavitary lesions are seen.
   d. Diagnose in sputum especially by immunofluorescent techniques. The patient may require bronchoscopy and biopsy if the diagnosis is suspected, but the sputum is normal.
2. **Management of *Pneumocystis.***
   a. If not acutely ill with Po_2 >60 mm Hg.
      (1) Trimethoprim/sulfamethoxazole (TMP/SMX) 10 to 15 mg/kg PO BID-TID based on the TMP component for 21 days. Frequently get rash and fever in AIDS patients taking TMP/SMX; can continue drug if not severe.
      (2) Alternatives for mild or moderate disease.
         - TMP + dapsone 100 mg PO QD or pyrimethamine 50 to 75 PO QD.
         - Atovaquone 750 mg PO BID-TID + pyrimethamine.
         - Clindamycin 600 mg PO or IV TID + primaquine 30 mg base PO QD for 21 days.
   b. If unable to take PO or acutely ill or Po_2 <60 mm Hg, take TMP/SMX 20 mg/kg or TMP IV Q6H × 21 days.
   c. Should start prednisone 40 mg PO BID × 5 days and then 40 mg QD × 5 days, followed by 20 mg PO QD × 11 days, and then taper off to zero. This reduces the rate of respiratory failure and mortality though it increases the rate of herpes zoster. Important to get definitive diagnosis if going to use steroids because prednisone may worsen TB.

   d. May get clinical and radiographic worsening during the first 3 to 5 days of therapy but usually get improvement within 7 to 10 days.
   e. Alternative therapy includes pentamadine 4 mg/kg/day IV or isethionate for 21 days or trimetrexate 45 mg/m^2 IV QD + leucovorin 20 mg/m^2 IV or PO Q6h + dapsone 100 mg PO QD.

B. Mucosal candidiasis/esophagitis.

1. Presents with oral curd like lesions or dysphagia, odynophagia.
2. May have esophageal disease without oral disease.
3. ***Therapy.***
   a. Orally may use nystatin (100,000 units/ml swish and swallow 5 ml or 500,000 U tablets PO Q6h) or clotrimazole (troches 10 mg 5 × day or vaginal suppositories 100 mg QD or BID) dissolved in mouth, or fluconazole 100 to 200 mg PO QD for 2 weeks or ketoconazole 400 mg PO QD, followed by 200 mg PO QD or BID × 7 days or amphotericin B mouthwash 0.1 mg/ml, swish and swallow 5 ml QID.
   b. For esophageal candidiasis:
      (1) Fluconazole 200 to 400 mg PO or IV daily for 14 to 28 days or ketoconazole 200 mg PO BID or itraconazole 200 mg PO QD.
      (2) If no response in 1 week, change to amphotericin B 0.3 to 0.4 mg/kg IV QD.

C. Cytomegalovirus (CMV).

1. ***Retinitis.*** Presents with visual changes, decreased vision, floaters, flashes of light, blind spots, and blurred vision. Diagnosed by funduscopic exam. Fluffy white infiltrates associated with central pallor, surrounding retinal hemorrhage, and perivascular sheathing are seen. Can cause retinal hemorrhage.
2. ***Pneumonitis.*** Must add IgG to therapy.
3. ***Treatment.*** Median survival is longer with foscarnet. However, both ganciclovir and foscarnet are fairly toxic. (Ganciclovir is associated with myelosuppression and foscarnet is associated with nephrotoxicity and hypocalcemia.)
   a. Ganciclovir 5 mg/kg IV over 1 hour Q12h for 14 days (induction) followed by 5 mg/kg/day. May be given with granulocyte-macrophage colony-stimulating factor.
   b. Foscarnet 60 mg/kg IV over 2 hours Q8h for 14 to 21 days (induction) followed by 90 to 120 mg/kg/day in 1 dose IV daily.
   c. Must continue lifelong suppression for CMV retinitis. For prophylaxis, CD4+ <50 and CMV antibody positive, ganciclovir 1 g PO TID or 5 to 6 mg/kg IV 5 to 7 days/week or foscarnet 90 to 120 mg/kg IV QD.

d. Sustained-release ganciclovir as disk implants in the vitreous cavity (lasting 6 to 8 months) appears promising but is investigational for now.
e. Studies are currently being done to determine if combination treatment is cost effective.
f. Side effects may be lessened with intravitreal injections.
g. *Other drugs under investigation.* Cidofovir (Vistide, an acyclic nucleoside analog) 5 mg/kg IV with probenecid every week for 2 weeks and then Q2 weeks and Isis 2922 (phosphorothioate oligonucleotide, a CMV-neutralizing antibody).
h. Efficacy not established in CMV hepatitis.

D. Toxoplasmosis.

1. Most common cause of CNS mass lesion in AIDS. 47% of patients with AIDS develop CNS toxoplasmosis.
2. Presents with frequent headache, lateralizing signs, altered mentation, fever, and seizures.
3. CT shows enhancing lesions, usually bilateral.
4. ***Treatment.***
   a. Pyrimethamine 200 mg loading dose and then 50 to 75 mg QD *and* sulfadiazine 1 to 1.5 PO Q6h + leucovorin 10 to 25 mg/day. Use this regimen for 4 to 6 weeks. Alternatively, may use clindamycin 600 to 900 mg PO or IV Q6h + pyrimethamine 100 to 200 mg load and then 50 to 75 mg/day or atovaquone with or without pyrimethamine or macrolides (clarithromycin or azithromycin) with or without pyrimethamine or immunomodulators (interferon-γ, interleukin-2, or interleukin-12) or doxycycline 100 mg PO TID or QID or minocycline 200 mg PO BID or dapsone 100 mg PO QD or TMP/SMX as for acute PCP.
   b. Must use chronic suppression for life, which is done by sulfadiazine 1 to 1.5 g PO Q6h + pyrimethamine 25 to 75 mg PO QD + leucovorin 10 to 25 mg PO QD to QID. Alternatively may use clindamycin 300 to 450 mg PO Q6-8h + pyrimethamine 25 to 75 mg PO QD + leucovorin 10 to 25 mg PO QD to QID.

E. Herpes zoster (varicella zoster).

1. Presents with grouped vesicles over one or more dermatomes.
2. ***Treatment.*** Acyclovir 800 mg PO 5 × a day or 10 mg/kg IV Q8h for 7 to 10 days.
   a. Resistance may develop and so if the patient has been treated previously with acyclovir, may have to use foscarnet 40 mg/kg IV Q8h for 14 to 26 days, or famciclovir 500 mg PO TID or valacyclovir HCl 500 mg PO BID for 5 days.
   b. Must begin antiviral therapy within 72 hours of the development of lesions in order to be effective.

3. The HZ vaccine should be avoided because it is a live vaccine.

F. **Cryptococcal meningitis.**
   1. Presents with headache, fever, delirium, nausea, and vomiting. Only 20% have meningismus and photophobia. Rarely patients present with seizures.
   2. Only 21% have CSF WBC counts >20 WBC/mm^3.
   3. Diagnose with India ink or CSF cryptococcal antigen.
   4. Do head CT before LP because of high incidence of mass lesions in AIDS patients to avoid transtentorial herniation.
   5. ***Treatment.***
      a. Amphotericin B 0.7 to 1 mg/kg/day IV with or without flucytosine 25 mg/kg PO Q6h for 2 to 4 weeks. Follow with fluconazole 400 mg PO QD or itraconazole 200 mg PO BID for 10 weeks.
      b. Must continue suppression with fluconazole 200 to 400 mg QD or itraconazole 200 mg PO QD indefinitely.

G. **Bacterial infections (only in selected patients).** For neutropenia, start granulocyte colony-stimulating factor 5 to 10 µg/kg SQ QD for 2 to 4 weeks; or granulocyte-macrophage colony-stimulating factor 250 µg/m^2 IV over 2 hours QD for 2 to 4 weeks.

I. AIDS-ASSOCIATED DIARRHEA

A. **General.** 30% to 50% of AIDS patients in the United States have diarrhea at some point during their illness. Since the causes of diarrhea in these patients are protean, empiric therapy is almost never indicated. It is important to try to identify the organism. A general approach includes stool for (1) culture and sensitivity (need to culture for *Salmonella* species, which is 100 × more common than in "normal" population, *Shigella flexneri,* and *Campylobacter jejuni*); (2) ova and parasites × 3 and *Giardia* antigen; (3) *Clostridium difficile* toxin; (4) acid-fast stains and in advanced disease chromotrope-based stains × 2 (see below for details). It may be necessary to proceed to colonoscopy (culture and biopsy for CMV, *Mycobacterium,* adenovirus, and herpes simplex) or esophagogastroduodenoscopy (culture for CMV and *Mycobacterium*). General supportive measures are also indicated including fluids and antimotility drugs *unless* the patient has fecal leukocytes or abdominal pain.

B. **Dietary and drinking water precautions.**
   1. Avoid raw meat (eggs, sushi, etc.). Cook meat thoroughly. Do not use cracked eggs. Thaw frozen meat in the refrigerator or microwave, not at room temperature.
   2. Wash fruits and vegetables thoroughly.
   3. Use only pasteurized milk.

4. Keep hot foods hot (cooked at 165° to 212° F and held at 140° to 165° F). Keep cold foods cold (refrigerate at 35° to 40° F). Do not allow foods to stand at a temperature between 45° and 140° F for more than 2 hours.
5. Refrigerate perishable foods immediately upon return from the store. Store foods that have been opened in airtight containers or a moisture- and vapor-proof wrap. Do not crowd or overpack food in the refrigerator. Avoid moldy or spoiled foods. Do not eat foods after the recommended date on the label.
6. Always wash hands before handling food. Use different cutting boards for raw and cooked foods.
7. Listeriosis is a rare disease; however, it may be contracted by eating hot dogs and cold cuts from delicatessen counters. These foods should be reheated before consumption.
8. Avoid drinking water from lakes or rivers because of the risk of cryptosporidiosis and giardiasis. Even accidental ingestion while swimming carries a risk.

C. Specific causes of AIDS-associated diarrhea.

1. ***Cryptosporidium.***
   a. Transmitted by fecal-oral route.
   b. Presents with chronic voluminous diarrhea and abdominal pain, anorexia, nausea, and malabsorption.
   c. Diagnosis made by biopsy of colon or small bowel or by acid-fast stain of the stool.
   d. Treatment octreotide 50 µg SQ Q8h × 48 hours and then increased by 100 to 200 µg Q1-2 weeks to maximum dose of 500 µg Q8h. Alternatively, can give paromomycin 750 mg PO TID.
      - Treatment outcome for *Cryptosporidium* is not good with only a 42% response rate.
2. ***Giardia lamblia.***
   a. Transmitted by water and fecal-oral route.
   b. Diagnosed by duodenal biopsy (90% yield) or stool for O & P with a 50% yield. Can also use immunofluorescent technique, which has higher yields, or a new test that detects antigen in the stool.
   c. Treatment is metronidazole 250 mg PO TID for 5 days *or* quinacrine 100 mg PO TID after meals for 5 days (see Chapter 4 for further information).
3. ***Isospora.***
   a. Constitutes 1% to 3% of AIDS diarrhea in the United States (higher elsewhere).
   b. Symptoms are similar to those of *Cryptosporidium,* but the patient gets an associated eosinophilia.
   c. Diagnosed by acid-fast stain of stool.
   d. Treatment is by TMP/SMX DS 1 PO QID for 21 days. Maintain on TMP/SMX DS 1 PO QOD.

4. ***Microsporida order: Enterocytozoon bieneusi, Septata intestinalis.***
   a. Diagnose by duodenal biopsy and electron microscopy *or* stain formalin fixed stool with chromotrope-based technique and use light microscopy.
   b. No standard treatment. However, albendazole 400 mg PO BID for 1 month has been used with a good response in 50% to 100% of treated patients.
5. ***CMV.***
   a. Culture biopsy of colon.
   b. No good treatment for CMV diarrhea but can try ganciclovir of foscarnet (see protocol above).
   c. May cause necrosis and perforation.
6. ***Histoplasma capsulatum.***
7. ***Mycobacterium avium-intracellulare*** (MAC). Diarrhea is usually associated with disseminated disease. See section below on mycobacterial disease.
8. AIDS-associated enteropathy. Comprising villous atrophy, malabsorption, and lactase deficiency in the absence of an identifiable pathogen after extensive work-up. Antiretroviral drugs may improve symptoms.
9. ***Bacterial disease.***
   a. Diagnosed by culture.
   b. Treatment is by ciprofloxacin 500 mg PO BID; however, should base on culture sensitivities when known.
10. ***HSV proctitis.***
   a. May have proctitis, esophagitis, or genital and perianal lesions.
   b. Presents with tenesmus, constipation, dysphagia, and anorectal pain.
   c. Treatment is acyclovir 200 mg 5 × per day. Alternatively, valacyclovir HCl 500 mg BID × 5 days.
   d. Can suppress with acyclovir 200 mg TID if there is recurrence.
11. ***Suppression.*** Suppression indicated for *Salmonella, Shigella,* HSV, and *Candida if* there is recurrent disease frequently. Must suppress CMV; see protocol above.

II. TUBERCULOSIS IN HIV INFECTION

A. Because *Mycobacterium tuberculolsis* is more virulent than *Pneumocystis* species, will often present at an earlier stage of HIV infection than *Pneumocystis* will.

B. Of those with TB, extrapulmonary disease develops in 70% of those patients with preexisting AIDS and 45% of those with HIV infection.

C. Incidence is inversely associated with baseline CD4+ count and is directly associated with CDC clinical class. Among those who have disease, it is most likely reactivation rather than from a recent exposure.

D. Clinical presentation. Persistent cough >2 weeks, dyspnea, hemoptysis, fever, night sweats, and significant weight loss >10% of body weight.

E. Diagnosis.

1. ***Positive PPD.*** Must do controls for *Candida* and mumps.
   a. 5 mm result is considered a positive test in those with HIV infection. Some authors use 2 to 3 mm as a positive test result.
   b. Must do at least 3 sputums for AFB.
2. Can diagnose by CXR with perihilar adenopathy and cavitary lesions. May have effusions. Miliary TB may mimic *Pneumocystis* on CXR.

F. Treatment.

1. Treat prophylactically in all patients with positive PPD regardless of age, since 8% will develop active disease every year. Treat prophylactically for 12 months.
2. Treat active disease as per the protocol recommended in your area. Pockets of drug-resistant TB make blanket recommendations unwise at this time.

G. Precautions. Do not use nebulized pentamidine in those with TB because of the possibility of transmission of the disease to others.

III. *MYCOBACTERIUM AVIUM-INTRACELLULARE* (MAC/MAI)

A. May present as diarrhea, fever, night sweats, and generalized wasting.

B. Can generally culture from blood or stool.

C. Treatment regimens include clarithromycin 500 to 1000 mg PO BID or azithromycin 500 mg PO QD plus clofazimine 100 mg PO BID or rifampin 600 mg PO QD. Another, more accepted regimen includes ciprofloxacin 750 mg PO BID + ethambutol 15 mg/kg PO QD + rifampin 600 mg PO QD + amikacin 7.5 mg/kg IV QD.

AIDS-ASSOCIATED WEIGHT LOSS AND WASTING

A. Weight loss and malnutrition are major problems in the AIDS patient for several reasons, including increased metabolic demand, loss of appetite, eating difficulties from oral and esophageal disease, as well as diarrhea and malabsorption.

B. Marijuana is widely used by patients with AIDS to improve their appetite, and anecdotal evidence indicates that it may be effective. However, no controlled study has been done up to now.

C. The use of megestrol acetate 800 mg/day has been associated with a significant weight gain and improved feeling of well-being in patients with AIDS-associated wasting. Megestrol may be associated with adrenal suppression and should not be discontinued abruptly.

NEUROPSYCHIATRIC DISEASE

I. GENERAL

About 60% of individuals with AIDS have some neuropsychiatric manifestations of the illness. This may be because macrophages and monocytes carry the HIV into the CNS. The virus may also gain direct access because many CNS components are CD4+. It is critical to ascertain that neurologic manifestations are not attributable to infectious causes or CNS lymphoma before attributing symptoms to the direct effects of the AIDS virus. Remember that individuals with AIDS or HIV infection are undergoing a major stress. Psychologic support of these patients is critical to the successful management of their illness. Drug therapies are helpful, but social and psychologic support is also very important to their overall care.

II. TERMINOLOGY

Subacute encephalitis (AIDS encephalopathy, AIDS dementia complex).

- **A.** Defined by progressive dementia, psychomotor retardation, focal motor abnormalities, behavioral changes, and short-term memory deficits.
- **B.** May manifest headache with problems of coordination, apathy, and affective blunting. Later manifestations include inappropriate behavior, emotional lability, seizures, aphasia, and psychotic manifestations.
- **C.** Advanced cases develop global cognitive deterioration, incontinence, sensory loss, and visual disturbances.
- **D.** 75% of AIDS patients manifest these symptoms, but 90% show pathologic changes on autopsy.

III. TESTING

- **A.** Useful tests include the Symbol Digit Modalities Test and Parts A & B of the Trail Making Test, which test psychomotor function. A newly developed screening instrument has also been developed, the HIV Dementia Scale, which is a reliable and quantitative scale superior to the Minimental Status Exam and the Grooved Pegboard in identifying HIV dementia.
- **B.** Double-dose contrast-enhanced CT alone cannot provide a definitive diagnosis. The most common abnormality reported on CT scans of these patients is cerebral atrophy. Radiographically MRI is best at demonstrating degeneration. The most common white matter lesions are diffuse over a wide area, typically in the centrum semiovale and periventricular white matter. Less commonly, there is localized involvement with patchy or punctate lesions.
- **C.** In atypical aseptic meningitis, there is an increase in the ICP and in the CSF mononuclear pleocytosis, multinucleated giant cells, protein content, and oligoclonal bands.
- **D.** EEG is not particularly helpful.

IV. DIFFERENTIAL DIAGNOSIS OF NEUROPSYCHIATRIC DISORDERS IN HIV DISEASE ONCE ONE HAS EXCLUDED INFECTIOUS AND OTHER MEDICAL CAUSES

A. Most common are affective disorders.

B. Dementia.

1. Responds to some degree to antiretroviral agents.
2. Some promising results with methylphenidate and dextroamphetamines. Using methylphenidate, start with a 5 mg trial dose and follow with 2.5 to 5 mg PO BID. Increase by 5 mg QOD split into 2 doses. Give last dose before 3 PM.
   a. Do not use in those with florid psychosis.
   b. Document changes with tests noted above.

C. Agitation secondary to delirium may be treated by lorazepam 0.5 mg IV slow push.

D. Psychotic symptoms may be treated with haloperidol starting at 0.5 to 1 mg PO QID.

E. Depression can be treated with standard antidepressants. Patients may be sensitive to anticholinergic side effects late in illness.

F. AIDS patients can get a manic syndrome related to the use of ganciclovir, zidovudine, and fluoxetine, which may respond to lithium. Treat agitation as above.

G. Anxiety can be treated with standard drugs. See Chapter 15.

DERMATOLOGIC MANIFESTATIONS OF AIDS

I. CUTANEOUS INFECTIONS

A. Viral. Herpesviruses produce disseminated, extensive, or chronic herpetic ulcers. Treat with acyclovir 200 to 400 mg PO 5 × a day or 5 mg/kg IV Q8h × 7 to 14 days if severe. Maintenance dose acyclovir 200 to 400 mg PO BID or TID.

B. Fungal.

1. ***Dermatophytosis (tinea) by fungi of the genera Trichophyton, Microsporum, and Epidermophyton.*** For treatment, see Chapter 13.
2. ***Yeasts and mucosal candidiasis.*** Treat with systemic antifungals (see section on candidiasis).
3. ***Histoplasmosis.*** Rare.
4. ***Cryptococcosis.*** Rare.

C. Bacterial.

1. ***Bacterial folliculitis.*** For treatment, see Chapter 13.
2. ***Impetigo.*** For treatment, see Chapter 13.
3. ***Syphilis.***
   a. Penicillin is recommended for treatment in all HIV-infected patients in all stages of syphilis. Skin testing is advised to confirm allergy though the utility in immunocompromised patients is questionable. For HIV-infected

patients who are penicillin allergic, the CDC recommends desensitization and then treatment with PCN.

b. For primary and secondary syphilis among HIV-infected individuals, the treatment is benzathine penicillin G 2.4 million units IM as one dose. However, these patients may have CSF abnormalities of unknown prognostic significance, and therefore some experts elect to obtain an LP before treatment and modify therapy accordingly. If have positive CSF pleocytosis **or** positive CSF VDRL test, treat for neurosyphilis. May also have elevated CSF total protein.

c. For latent syphilis among HIV-infected individuals, the treatment is benzathine penicillin G 7.2 million units as 3 weekly doses of 2.4 million units each. Again, some experts advise obtaining CSF examination before treatment to adjust therapy accordingly.

d. For treatment failure, evaluation of CSF is indicated. If the CSF is normal, the penicillin dose is the same as that for latent syphilis. Follow-up study for treatment failure includes clinical and serologic evaluation at 1 month and then 2, 3, 6, 9, and 12 months after treatment.

4. ***Mycobacteriosis.*** Treatment involves systemic antibiotics; see previous section on *Mycobacterium.*

5. ***Bacillary angiomatosis.*** Treat with erythromycin 250 to 500 mg PO QID until lesions resolve or doxycycline 100 mg PO BID.

II. CUTANEOUS NEOPLASMS

A. Kaposi's sarcoma. A herpes virus was recently shown to be the etiologic factor. Clinically appear as purplish macules, papules, plaques, nodules, tumors. Histopathologic analysis reveals immunostain to type IV collagen. Therapy includes observation, cryotherapy, laser surgery, excisional surgery, or radiation therapy until lesions and symptoms are resolved or controlled. Additional modalities include intralesional vinblastine (0.2 mg/ml every 2 weeks) or systemic chemotherapy (vinblastine + vincristine, or with combination doxorubicin, bleomycin, and vincristine, or paclitaxel as well as systemic interferon).

B. Lymphoma cutis. Skin is rarely involved, usually B cell in origin.

C. Possible increased incidence of melanoma, basal cell carcinoma, and squamous cell carcinoma

D. Oral hairy leukoplakia. Well-demarcated verrucous plaque with an irregular, corrugated, or hairy surface, most commonly on the lateral or inferior surface of the tongue, or on the buccal and soft palatal mucosa.

III. INFLAMMATORY DERMATITIDES

A. Seborrheic dermatitis, psoriasis, eczematous dermatitis, and folliculitis. See Chapter 13 for treatment options. However, avoid the use of methotrexate in those with HIV.

B. Pruritus, prurigo, eosinophilic folliculitis.

1. Extremely common and extremely debilitating with 3 to 5 mm edematous, follicular papules, and pustules.
2. Treatment is often unsatisfactory. Antihistamines, potent topical fluorinated corticosteroids (such as clobetasol propionate BID), phototherapy with natural sunlight or UVB radiation.

C. Cutaneous eruption of HIV. Presents as erythematous macules soon after infection.

AIDS IN PREGNANCY

I. In a randomized, multicenter, double-blind, placebo-controlled clinical trial (ACTG 076) of HIV-seropositive pregnant women with a CD4+ count >200, AZT was given during pregnancy, intra partum, and to the newborn for 6 weeks after birth. This significantly decreased the vertical HIV transmission rate from 25% to 8% (a 67% reduction). These women had no antiviral therapy before pregnancy and no clinical indication for AZT. Follow-up testing at 6 months also showed no significant difference in CD4+ counts.

A. To start AZT begin with a dose of 100 mg 5 × PO QD at 14 to 34 weeks of gestation and continue throughout the remainder of the pregnancy. The side effects of AZT when given during the first trimester are unknown. In the ACTG 076 trial, the rates of congenital anomalies were equal in the treatment and control groups, an indication that AZT may not be teratogenic.

B. IV AZT during labor should be given as 2 mg/kg over 1 hour and then followed by a continuous infusion of 1 mg/kg/hour until delivery.

II. HIV-seropositive women have a higher miscarriage rate. In a prospective study, 124 HIV-seropositive women were followed over a 4-year period. 14 (11%) had spontaneous abortions with half of the miscarried fetuses testing positive (by culture) for HIV. HIV-seropositive women should be counseled about their options regarding pregnancy. Information about contraception, prenatal care, and abortion services should be provided.

III. Procedures that increase the likelihood of direct fetal exposure to maternal blood should be minimized during the antepartum and intrapartum periods. Examples include amniocentesis, fetal scalp electrode placement, and fetal scalp pH measurements. Although more data are needed, C-sections may actually reduce the incidence of perinatal infection and are done only as indicated.

IV. Prophylaxis of opportunistic infections during pregnancy HIV in pregnancy presents a special dilemma in which the health care provider must carefully weight the risks and benefits. Unfortunately, there are very few data in this area of medicine. Listed below are generally accepted guidelines.

1. Try to limit drug exposures during the first trimester, the most critical period for organogenesis.
2. PCP prophylaxis is important with CD4+ <200. Although animal studies have shown TMP-SMZ to be associated with cleft palate, retrospective human studies have shown no increased risk of congenital malformations. Aerosolized pentamidine and dapsone are believed to be safe during pregnancy; however, pyrimethamine should be used with caution.
3. Preventive therapy should be instituted in pregnant women who have a positive tuberculin skin test or who are exposed to persons with infectious tuberculosis. Treatment with isoniazid should be deferred until after the first trimester and, when started, should be given with pyridoxine 25 to 50 mg PO BID secondary to the risk of peripheral neuropathy. Experience with rifampin and rifabutin is limited.

AIDS IN THE PEDIATRIC PATIENT

Perinatal transmission accounts for >85% of HIV infection in United States children. For infants who are born to HIV-seropositive mothers, AZT should be given for the first 6 weeks of life beginning 8 to 12 hours after birth. The AZT syrup is 2 mg/kg PO Q6h. Anemia (Hb <8 g/dl) should be corrected before the initiation of AZT treatment. There are several case reports of infants being "cured" of the HIV with prompt perinatal AZT treatment. Additionally, all infants born to an HIV-positive mother should have PCP prophylaxis started at 4 to 6 weeks and continued until 12 months of age unless the child is proved to be HIV negative.

BIBLIOGRAPHY

AMA Advisory Group on HIV Early Intervention: *HIV early intervention physician guidelines,* ed 2, Chicago, 1994, American Medical Association.

Barnes PF, Block AP: Tuberculosis in patients with human immunodeficiency virus infection, *N Engl J Med* 324(23):1644-1650, 1991.

Bender BS: Outpatient management of patients infected with human immunodeficiency virus, *J Fam Practitioner* 34(4):313-329, 1992.

Berger JR: How to distinguish HIV dementia from progressive multifocal leukoencephalopathy, *HIV Newsline* 1(1):11-13, Feb 1995.

Blanche S et al: Relation of the course of HIV infection in children to the severity of the disease in their mothers at delivery, *N Engl J Med* 330(5):308-812, 1994.

Blanshard C et al: Electron microscopic changes in *Enterocytozoon bieneusi* following treatment with albendazole, *J Clin Pathol* 46(10):898-902, 1993.

Bryson YJ et al: Clearance of HIV infection in a perinatally infected infant, *N Engl J Med* 332(13):833-838, 1995.

Blendon RJ, Donelan K, Knox RA: Public opinion and AIDS: lessons for the second decade, *JAMA* 267(7):981-986, 1992.

Burgard M et al: The use of viral culture and p24 antigen testing to diagnose human immunodeficiency virus infection in neonates, The HIV Infection in Newborns French Collaborative Study Group, *N Engl J Med* 327(17):1192-1197, 1992.

Centers for Disease Control and Prevention: 1993 revised classification system for HIV infection and expanded surveillance case definition for AIDS among adolescents and adults, *MMWR* 41(No RR-17):1-19, 1992.

Centers for Disease Control and Prevention: Classification system for human immunodeficiency virus infection in children under 13 years of age, *MMWR* 36:225-235, 1987.

Centers for Disease Control and Prevention: USPHS/IDSA guidelines for the prevention of opportunistic infections in persons infected with human immunodeficiency virus: introduction, clinical infectious diseases 21(suppl 1):S1-S43, 1995.

Centers for Disease Control and Prevention: USPHS/IDSA guidelines for the prevention of opportunistic infections in persons infected with human immunodeficiency virus: a summary, *MMWR* 44(No RR-8):1-34, 1995.

Centers for Disease Control and Prevention: 1994 Revised classification system for human immunodeficiency virus infection in children less than 13 years of age; official authorized agenda: human immunodeficiency virus infection codes and official guidelines for coding and reporting ICD-9-CM, *MMWR* 43(No RR-12):1-9, 1994.

Committee on Infectious Diseases: *1994 Red book: report of the Committee on Infectious Diseases,* pp. 254-270, Elk Grove Village, Ill., 1994, American Academy of Pediatrics.

Connor EM et al: Reduction of maternal-infant transmission of human immunodeficiency virus type 1 with zidovudine treatment, Pediatric AIDS Clinical Trials Group Protocol 076 Study Group, *N Engl J Med* 331(18):1173-1180, 1994.

Dale DC, Federman DD, editors: *Scientific American Medicine,* New York, 1996, Scientific American, Inc.

Dickover, RE et al: Identification of levels of maternal HIV-1 RNA associated with risk of perinatal transmission: effect of maternal zidovudine treatment on viral load, *JAMA* 275(8):599-610, 1996.

Dore GJ et al: Disseminated microsporidiosis due to *Septata intestinalis* in nine patients infected with the human immunodeficiency virus: response to therapy with albendazole, *Clin Infect Dis* 21(1):70-76, 1995.

Fitzpatrick TB et al: *Color atlas and synposis of clinical dermatology,* New York, 1994, McGraw-Hill, pp 376, 415-441.

Gilmer WS, Busch KA: Neuropsychiatric aspects of AIDS and psychopharmacology management, *Psychiatr Med* 9(2):313-329, 1991.

Goldschmidt RH, Dong BJ: current report–HIV: treatment of AIDS and HIV-related conditions–1996, *J Am Board Fam Pract* 9(2):125-147, 1996.

Kafity AA, Thomas FB: AIDS-associated diarrhea, *The AIDS Reader,* pp 160-171, Sept-Oct 1991.

Leinung MC et al: Induction of adrenal suppression by megestrol acetate in patients with AIDS, *Ann Intern Med* 122(11):843-845, 1995.

Levy RM, Bredesen DE, Rosenblum ML: Neurologic complications of HIV infection, *Am Fam Physician* 41(2):517-536, 1990.

Medical News and Perspectives: New anti-HIV drugs and treatment strategies buoy AIDS researchers, *JAMA* 275(8):579-580, 1996.

MMWR 44(50):933, 1995.

Power C et al: HIV Dementia Scale: a rapid screening test, *J Acquir Immune Defic Syndr and Hum Retrovirology* 8(3):273-279, 1995.

Sanford JP: *Guide to antimicrobial therapy,* Dallas, 1996, Antimicrobial Therapy, Inc.

Siena Consenus Workshop: Early diagnosis of HIV infection in infants, *J Acquir Immune Defic Syndr* 5:1169-1178, 1992.

Small P et al: Treatment of tuberculosis in patients with advanced human immunodeficiency virus infection, *N Engl J Med* 324(5):289-294, 1991.

Smith PD et al: Gastrointestinal infections in AIDS, *Ann Intern Med* 116(1):63-76, 1992.

Talan DA, Kennedy CA: The management of HIV-related illness in the emergency department, *Ann Emerg Med* 20:1355-1365, 1991.

Volberding PA: *Management of HIV infection treatment team workshop handbook,* Research Triangle Park, N.C., 1991, Burroughs-Wellcome.

Von Roenn JH et al: Megestrol acetate in patients with AIDS-related cachexia, *Ann Intern Med* 121(6):393-399, 1994.

Weber R et al: Improved light-microscopical detection of microsporidia spores in stool and duodenal aspirates, *N Engl J Med* 326(3):161-165, 1992.

Whitcup SM: Ocular manifestations of AIDS, *JAMA* 275(2):142-150, 1996.

17

Office and Hospital Procedures

Melissa J. Gamponia and Robert L. Herting, Jr.

TYMPANOMETRY

I. INDICATIONS

Useful in detecting fluid in the middle ear, negative middle ear pressure, tympanic membrane perforation, ossicular chain disruption, or the patency of ventilation tubes.

II. PROCEDURES

A. Examine the ear canal and remove any occluding cerumen or exudate. Inspect tympanic membrane. Select the appropriate tip for the tympanometer.

B. Grasp the helix and straighten the ear canal. Position the probe. When the probe is positioned properly, the automatic recording device will be triggered.

C. Leave the probe in position until the tympanometer signals the conclusion of the test. Repeat in the contralateral ear. See Fig. 17-1 for interpretation.

ARTHROCENTESIS

I. INDICATIONS

- Analysis of joint fluid.
- Therapeutic (relief of pain by drainage of tense effusion or instillation of medication).

II. CONTRAINDICATIONS

- Infection of nearby skin or soft tissue.

III. TECHNIQUE

A. General principles of technique.

1. Careful identification of landmarks.

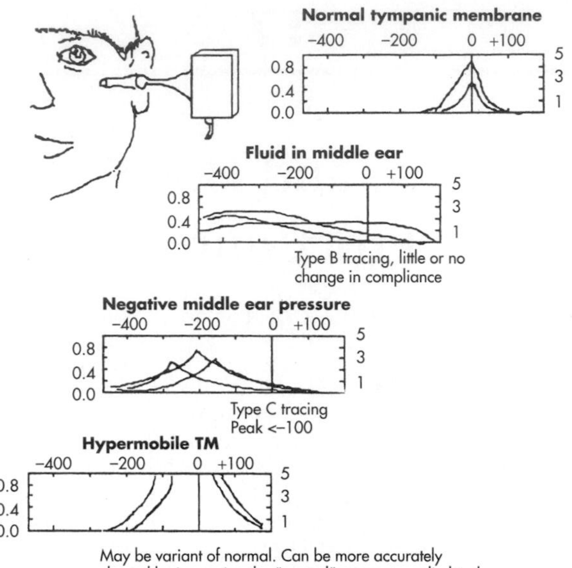

FIG. 17-1 Tympanometry.

2. Preparation of skin with povidone-iodine complex and alcohol.
3. Local anesthesia of overlying soft tissues with 1% lidocaine.
4. Advancement of needle with constant negative pressure.

B. Shoulder (Fig. 17-2).

1. Patient should be in a sitting position with arm in lap (this positions the shoulder in mild internal rotation and adduction). Identify insertion site inferior and slightly lateral to tip of coracoid.
2. Prepare site as above.
3. Direct needle dorsally, laterally, and slightly superiorly into joint space.

C. Wrist (Fig. 17-3).

1. The wrist should be positioned prone with about 20 degrees of flexion. Identify insertion site by marking the distal ends of the ulna and radius. The insertion site is ulnar to the extensor pollicis longus tendon.
2. Prepare the site as above.
3. Direct needle perpendicular to the skin.

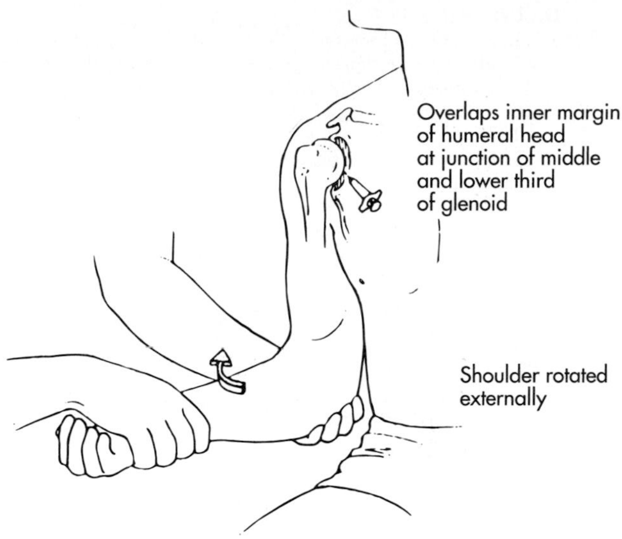

FIG. 17-2 Shoulder joint access (anesthetics or aspirates).

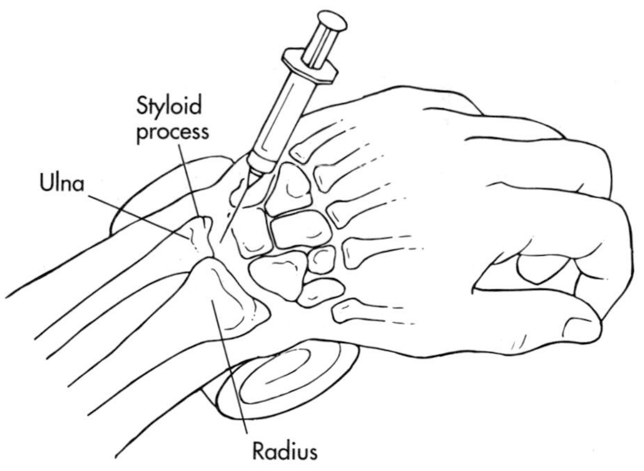

FIG. 17-3 Wrist joint access.

D. Elbow (Fig. 17-4).

1. Position patient with elbow at 90 degrees, palm prone. Identify insertion site on the lateral aspect of the elbow in the shallow depression immediately anterior and inferior to the lateral epicondyle of the humerus.
2. Prepare the skin as above.
3. Direct the needle perpendicularly to the skin.

E. Knee (Fig. 17-5).

1. Patient should be supine with quadriceps muscle relaxed (patella should be freely movable). Identify the insertion site immediately beneath the lateral or medial edge of the patella.
2. Prepare the skin as above.
3. Direct the needle parallel to the plane of the underside of the patella.

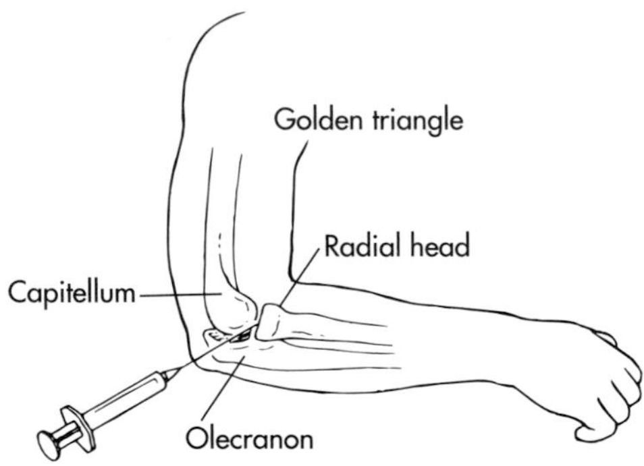

FIG. 17-4 Elbow joint access.

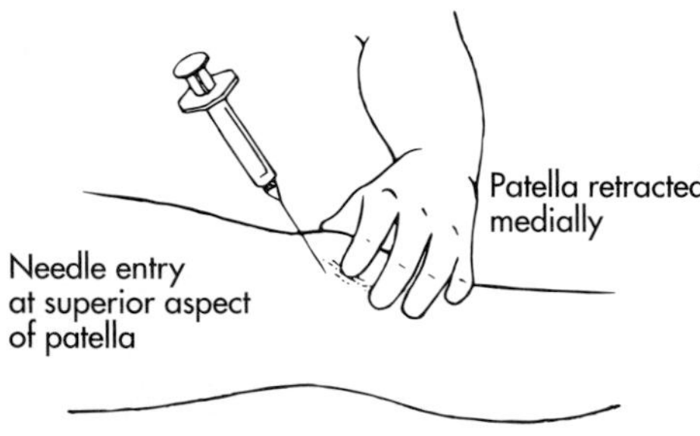

FIG. 17-5 Knee joint access.

IV. INTRA-ARTICULAR STEROIDS

A. Large joints such as the knee or shoulder may be injected with the equivalent of 80 mg of methylprednisolone acetate in 1 to 2 ml of 1% lidocaine.

B. Smaller joints such as the wrist, elbow, or ankle may be injected with 20 to 40 mg of methylprednisolone acetate in 0.5 to 1 ml of 1% lidocaine.

CHEST TUBE PLACEMENT

I. INDICATIONS

- Pneumothorax.
- Hemothorax.
- Drainage of pleural effusion.

II. CONTRAINDICATIONS

There are no contraindications to chest tube placement in patients symptomatic from the above-listed indications. However, care should be used in patients with a potential for serious bleeding.

III. MATERIALS NEEDED

- Iodine and alcohol swabs for preparing skin.
- Sterile drapes and gloves.
- No. 11 scalpel blade and handle.
- Mayo clamp.
- Kelly clamp.
- Silk suture (size 0).
- Needle holder.
- Petrolatum-impregnated gauze.
- Sterile gauze.
- Tape.
- Suction apparatus.
- Chest tube (size 32 to 40 French depending on clinical setting).
- 1% lidocaine with epinephrine, 10 ml syringe, 25- and 22-gauge needles.

IV. TECHNIQUE (Fig. 17-6)

A. Position patient with affected side up. Identify the insertion site, which is generally at the anterior axillary line just behind the lateral edge of the pectoralis major at the level of the nipple. Prep and drape the insertion site. Generously anesthetize the insertion site along the insertion tract to the pleura. Appropriate position can be checked by aspiration through the needle used for instilling the local anesthetic.

B. The skin should be incised directly over the body of the rib, with the incision length being 1½ times the diameter of the chest tube to be used. The Kelly or Mayo clamp is then used to bluntly dissect superiorly over the superior margin of the next higher rib. The Mayo clamp is then pushed through the

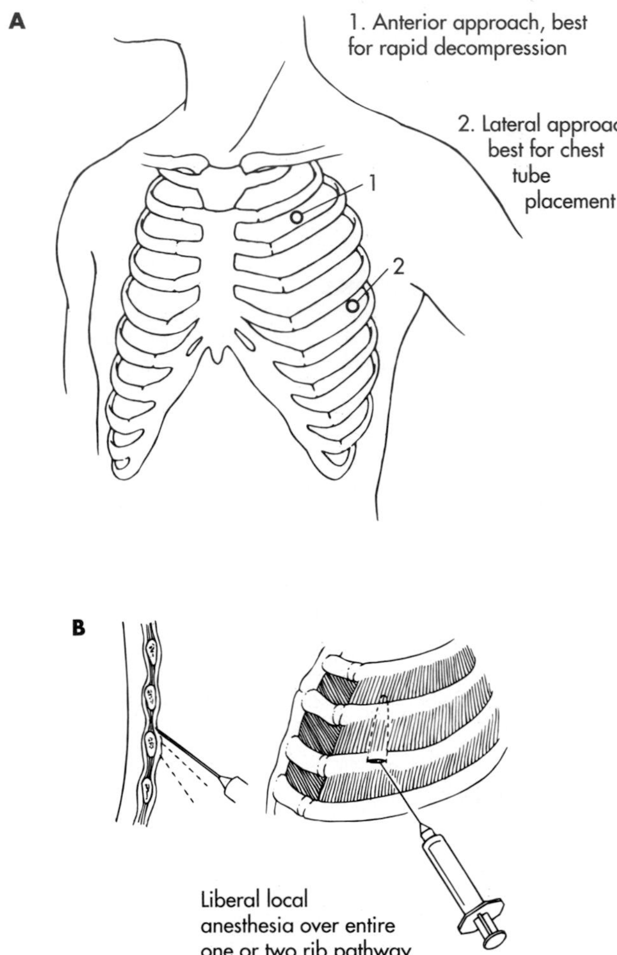

FIG. 17-6 A-D, Chest tube placement.

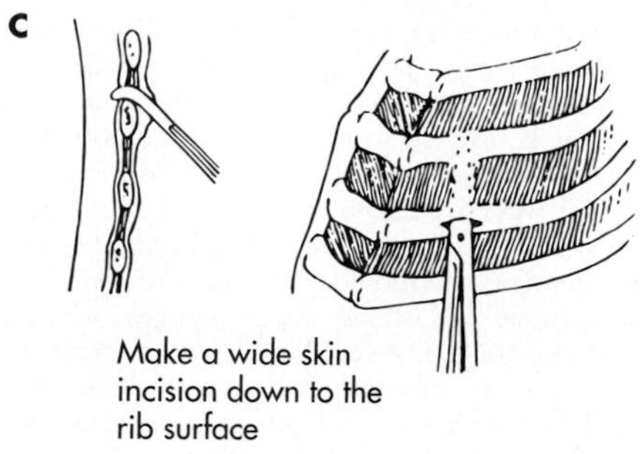

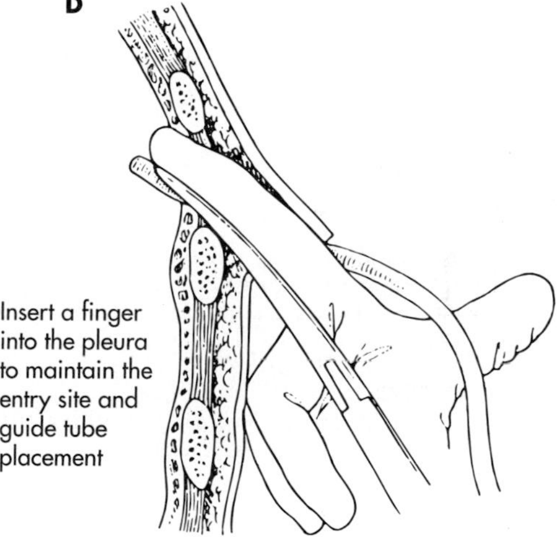

FIG. 17-6, cont'd. For legend see opposite page.

parietal pleura with tips closed and with slow steady pressure. Once the pleura has been penetrated, the clamps are opened wide to enlarge the insertion tract and remove. Operator's index finger can also be inserted along the tract to further enlarge the opening if needed.

C. The chest tube is grasped near the end to be inserted with the Mayo clamp (jaws of the clamp parallel to the length of the tube) and advanced into the pleural space. Once the tube is inserted so that all drainage ports are inside the thoracic cavity, the tube is connected to suction and sutured in place with silk suture by closure of the skin edges of the incision around the tube and tying the suture ends up around the tube. The area should be dressed with petrolatum-impregnated gauze and sterile gauze sponges. Chest radiograph should be obtained to confirm proper placement.

D. Removal is accomplished by having the patient inhale fully, hold his or her breath, and pulling the tube out swiftly. Cover with antibiotic-impregnated gauze.

V. COMPLICATIONS

- Hemorrhage at the site of insertion.
- Infection.
- Hematoma.
- Lung laceration.
- Laceration of intra-abdominal organs if tube is inadvertently inserted into the abdominal cavity.

INTRAOSSEOUS INFUSION

Intraosseous infusion can provide a very rapid and dependable route of vascular access in children 3 years of age or less (where vascular access is likely to be difficult in settings where it is most urgent). Almost any infusate can be instilled at a rapid rate through an intraosseous line, including blood and blood products, Plasmanate, glucose, crystalloids, pressor agents including epinephrine, dopamine and dobutamine, and atropine.

I. INDICATIONS

- Emergency fluid infusion, especially in setting of circulatory collapse where rapid IV access is essential.
- Difficult IV access.
- Burn or other injury preventing access to the venous system at other sites.

II. CONTRAINDICATIONS

- Overlying cellulitis.
- Bony lesion at site.
- Osteomyelitis.

III. MATERIALS

- Material for preparing the area (alcohol and iodine prep solutions).

- 1% lidocaine if local anesthesia is appropriate.
- 3 ml syringe with 25-gauge needle for infiltration of local anesthetic.
- Sterile gloves and drape.
- IV infusion set.
- 18- or 20-gauge short spinal needle or bone marrow needle.

IV. TECHNIQUE (Fig. 17-7)

A. Identify landmarks and prepare the insertion site with iodine or alcohol solution. Sites for insertion:

1. Proximal tibia 2 to 5 cm below the tibial tuberosity in the midline in children.
2. Distal tibia in the midline 2 to 5 cm above medial malleolus in adults.

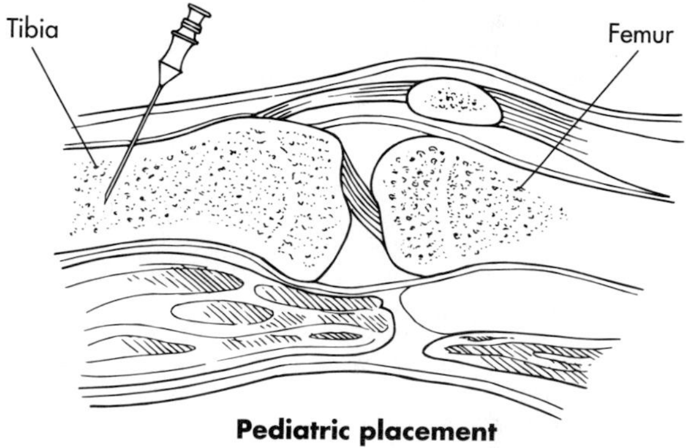

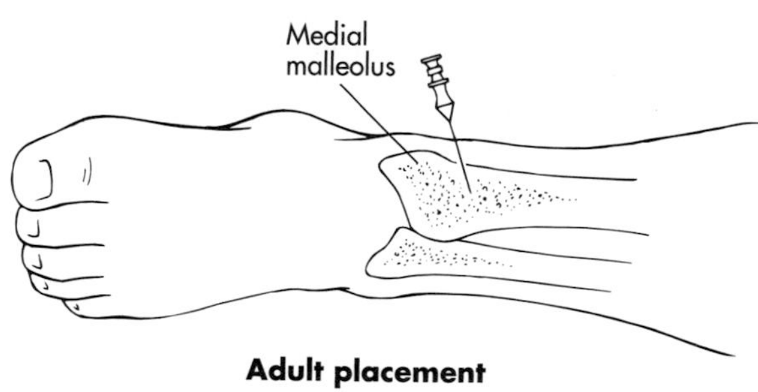

FIG. 17-7 Intraosseous infusion.

B. Infiltrate the overlying skin to the periosteum if the patient is sensitive to pain.
C. For insertion into the proximal end of the tibia, the spinal needle is directed inferiorly at a 45-degree angle from the perpendicular. If the insertion site is the distal tibia, the needle should be angled 45 degrees superiorly. In both instances the goal is to angle away from the region of the growth plate or joint, or both.
D. Advance needle (with stylet in place) through skin, subcutaneous tissue, and cortex of bone into the marrow space using a rotary motion.
E. Remove stylet and confirm placement by aspirating back marrow. Try infusing 5 ml of saline with a syringe.
F. Detach syringe and connect IV tubing to begin infusion. Secure in position with tape.

V. COMPLICATIONS

- Local abscess or cellulitis.
- Osteomyelitis.
- Injury to growth plate has not been identified as a complication that occurs with any significant frequency.

REGIONAL BLOCKS

A. **Prep skin and draw up anesthetic.** Always raise skin wheal before advancing the needle, and always inject slowly and aspirate to avoid intravascular administration.
B. **Digital blocks.** For complete finger anesthesia and for reductions or repair of lacerations (Fig. 17-8).
   1. Raise skin wheal using 1% lidocaine without epinephrine at base of digit at the level of the interphalangeal skin creases.
   2. Angle 5/8-inch 25-gauge needle 45 degrees from finger in the horizontal and vertical planes and advance until the bone is reached.
   3. While butting the needle tip against the bone of the proximal end of the phalanx and aspirating for blood and injecting local anesthetic periodically, "walk" the needle through the same puncture site over the dorsal and volar aspects of the phalanx to leave a complete "half-ring' of anesthetized tissues on both sides of the digit. Use no more than 3 to 5 ml through either puncture site and set the syringe aside for further use if needed. Gently massage the zone of anesthesia to ensure that an adequate block occurs after 5 to 10 minutes. If distal pinprick sensation is still present by 10 minutes, you may repeat the procedure through the same puncture sites using another 1 ml of lidocaine on either side.
C. **Supraorbital nerve block.** Anesthesia for upper eyelid to scalp line from midline to lambdoid suture. (Fig. 17-9).
   1. With the patient looking directly ahead, palpate the supraorbital notch above the midline pupil in the middle to lower part of the eyebrow.

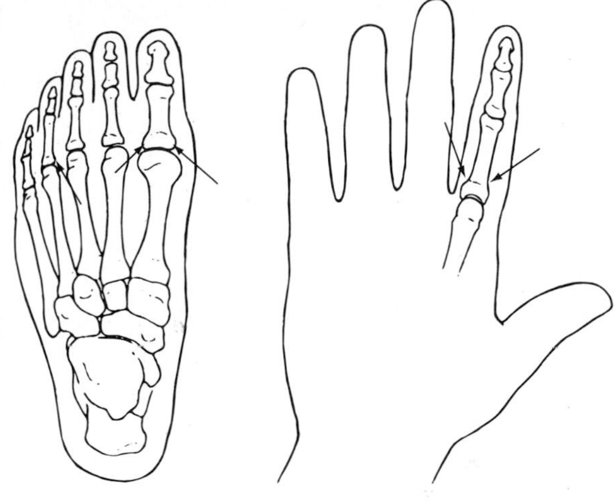

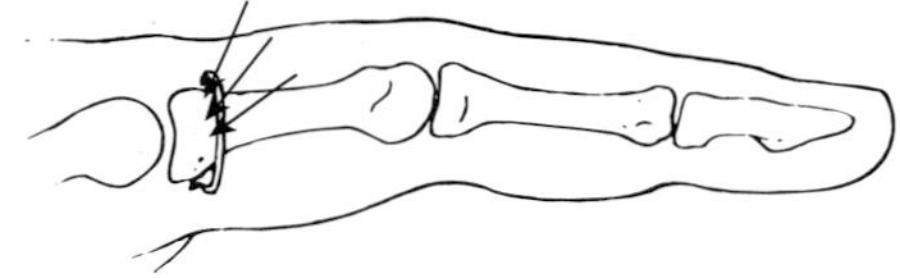

FIG. 17-8 Digital nerve block techniques.

2. Advance needle superiorly until paresthesias are noted. Apply pressure to the upper lid and inject 2 ml of 1% lidocaine without epinephrine.

D. Infraorbital nerve block. Anesthesia of the upper lip, nose, lower portion of the eyelid, and maxillary portion of the face.

1. Palpate infraorbital foramen immediately below midline of pupil. Raise skin wheal at this site.
2. Advance the needle until paresthesias are elicited, and inject 2 ml of 1% lidocaine without epinephrine while applying pressure above the infraorbital rim.

E. Mental nerve block. Anesthesia of the chin and lower lip.

1. Identify the mental foramen, which is palpable subcutaneously halfway between the upper and lower border of the mandible. A line drawn connecting the supraorbital and infraorbital foramina and the corner of the mouth would

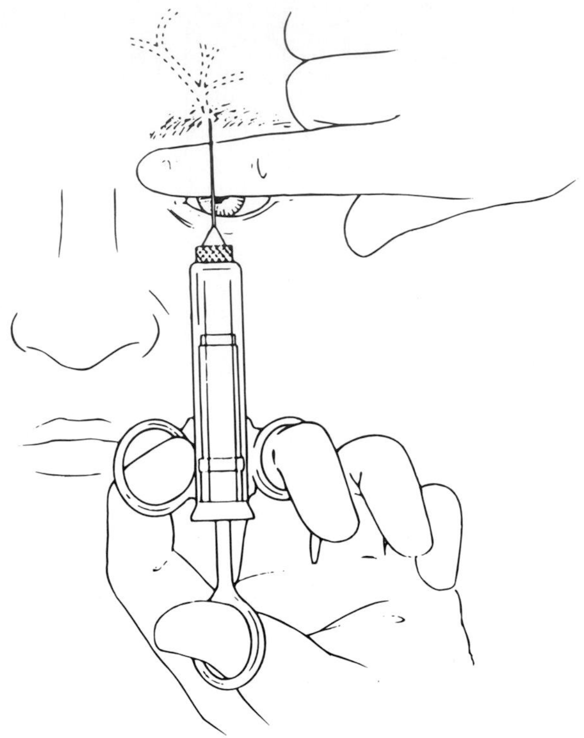

FIG. 17-9 Supraorbital nerve block.

pass through the mental foramen. Prep the skin with povidone-iodine complex. Raise a skin wheal at the injection site.

2. Advance the 25-gauge needle to but not into the foramen, and inject 3 ml of 1% lidocaine without epinephrine.

F. Intercostal nerve block. Relieve chest wall pain caused by rib fractures (Fig. 17-10).

1. Have patient sit, leaning forward onto a Mayo tray. Identify affected rib and the angle formed by the rib and paraspinous muscle. Raise skin wheal at this angle, over the inferior border of the rib.
2. Advance the needle to just under the inferior border of the rib, aspirate, and inject 5 ml of 1% lidocaine with

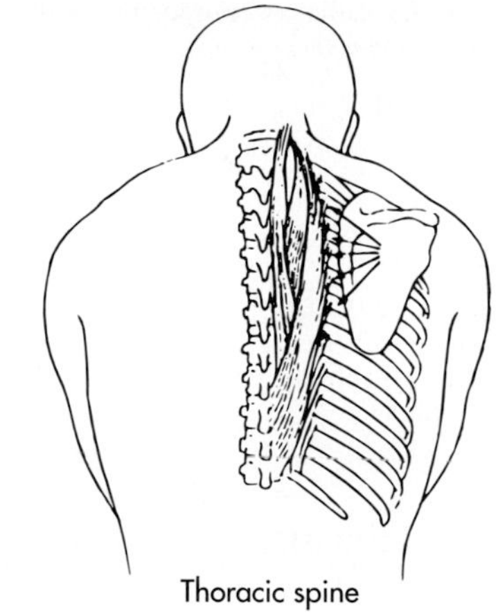

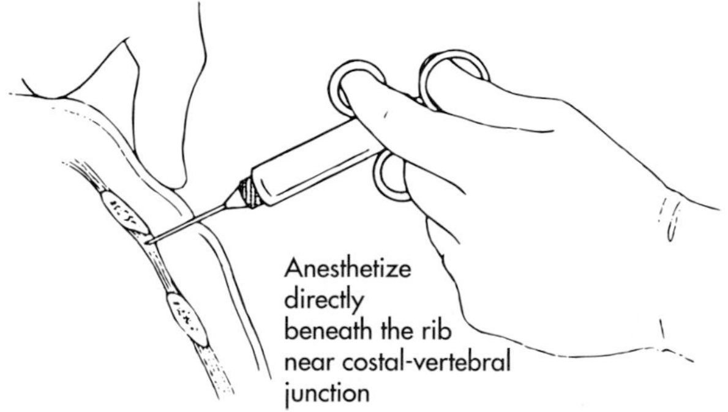

FIG. 17-10 Intercostal nerve block.

epinephrine. Bupivacaine HCl (Marcaine) may also be used for prolonged effect.

CENTRAL VENOUS LINES

I. INDICATIONS

- CVP monitoring.
- Medication administration.
- Parenteral nutrition.
- Poor peripheral access.

- Conduit for Swan-Ganz catheters, temporary cardiac pacemakers, hemodialysis catheters.

II. CONTRAINDICATIONS

- Bleeding diathesis.
- Overlying skin infection.

III. MATERIALS

- Sterile gloves and drapes.
- Povidone-iodine and alcohol swabs.
- 16-gauge central venous catheter kit.
- 1% lidocaine without epinephrine.
- Pressure monitor–optional.
- Heparinized saline.
- Sterile gauze.

IV. SELDINGER TECHNIQUE (USING INFRACLAVICULAR APPROACH TO THE SUBCLAVIAN VEIN)

(Fig. 17-11). For other approaches or access sites see ACLS manual.

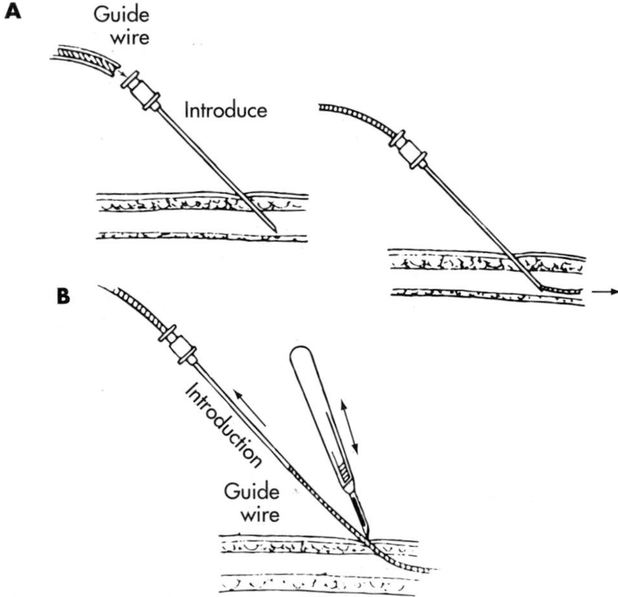

FIG. 17-11 A-D, Seldinger catheter-over-wire technique.

A. Position patient supine in slight Trendelenburg position. Identify insertion site. Prep, drape, and anesthetize the desired access site.

B. The introducer needle is inserted at the junction of the medial and central thirds of the clavicle and "walked" around and under the clavicle toward the sternal notch while aspirating back with the syringe held parallel to the chest wall. Free blood flow indicates vessel entry. If bright red, pulsating blood return is encountered, withdraw and redirect the needle.

C. Advance the needle another 2 to 3 mm and then remove the syringe. Quickly place finger over hub to avoid air embolism. A free flow of blood confirms placement.

D. The flexible guide wire is inserted through the needle and into the vein. Do not advance the wire into the right atrium. Remove the needle over the guide wire, making sure the guide wire is securely held throughout removal of the needle. Make a skin incision next to the wire to allow passage of the catheter.

E. Slide the vein dilator onto the wire and advance it through the skin and into the vein. Be sure not to advance the guide wire.

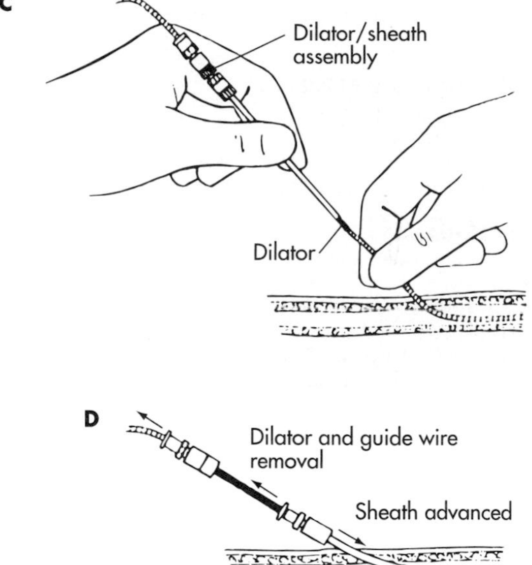

FIG. 17-11, cont'd. For legend see opposite page.

Remove vein dilator and slide the venous catheter over the wire and into the vein. Be sure to maintain guide wire in position.

F. Remove guide wire and attach IV tubing to catheter. Suture catheter into position and dress site with sterile gauze and antibiotic ointment.,

G. Obtain chest radiograph to check line placement and to rule out pneumothorax.

V. COMPLICATIONS

- Infection.
- Catheter tip embolus or thrombotic embolus.
- Bleeding.
- Hematoma formation.
- Arterial cannulation.
- Pneumothorax.
- Hemothorax.
- Chylothorax.
- Air embolism.
- Arrhythmias.

THORACENTESIS

I. INDICATIONS

Evaluation of a pulmonary effusion or relieve respiratory distress caused by large effusion.

II. CONTRAINDICATIONS

- Severe coagulopathies.
- Small stable effusions.
- Patients who are unable to cooperate.
- Patients responding to medical therapy.

III. MATERIALS

- Povidone-iodine solution and swabs.
- Gauze.
- Alcohol pads.
- Sterile drape and gloves.
- 5/8-inch, 25-gauge needle and 1% lidocaine.
- 2-inch, 22-gauge needle.
- 3-way stopcock gauge.
- 5 ml syringe.
- 50 ml syringe.
- 3 specimen tubes with stoppers.
- Adhesive tape.
- Optional: vacuum bottle, to attach to 15-gauge needle clamp.

IV. TECHNIQUE

A. Determine puncture site by CXR and percussion. Have patient sit leaning forward. put on sterile gloves. Prep and drape area.

B. Choose entry site below air-fluid interface and at the upper edge of the rib. Raise skin wheal with 25-gauge needle and carry anesthesia down through the chest wall. Use 2-inch, 22-gauge needle to anesthetize the pleural surface. Pop the needle into the pleural space and confirm location with aspiration of fluid.

C. Remove needle and attach it to the 3-way stopcock and 50 ml syringe. Reinsert and withdraw enough fluid to fill the specimen tubes.

D. To remove a large volume of fluid, fill 50 ml syringe and turn the stopcock to permit emptying. Repeat if necessary. If you will be emptying up to 1 liter of fluid, attach a vacuum bottle by rubber tubing to a 15-gauge needle clamp tubing, and insert needle in clamp and allow vacuum to aspirate the fluid.

E. When finished aspirating, withdraw needle and apply pressure over site for a few minutes and dress with pressure dressing. Observe for dyspnea. Send fluid for white blood cell count and differential, protein, glucose, LDH, culture, Gram stain, specific gravity, cytologic analysis, AFB, fungal cultures. Obtain posttap CXR.

V. INTERPRETATION

See the section on pleural effusion, Chapter 3.

VI. COMPLICATIONS

- Pneumothorax.
- Hematoma.
- Hemothorax.
- Infection.

NASAL FOREIGN-BODY REMOVAL

I. INDICATIONS

Common in young children and mentally retarded adults. Suspect nasal foreign body with sudden-onset respiratory distress, nasal flaring, unilateral mucopurulent discharge, foul smell.

II. CONTRAINDICATIONS

Few contraindications exist. ABCs take precedence over any procedures.

III. MATERIALS

None.

IV. TECHNIQUE

A. Reassure and calm the patient and instruct the caregiver or parent to give the patient a breath "mouth to mouth" while occluding the unobstructed naris.

B. Place the child supine in Trendelenburg position. Then place the child's head in a "sniffing position" with his or her mouth open widely.

C. The parent may obtain full cooperation by telling the child that he or she is going to give the child a big kiss. Then the parent delivers a breath with a tight seal. Subsequently the obstructing object is dislodged, often onto the cheek of the caregiver.

D. Reattempts may be required with minor adjustments. Alternatively, an Ambu-Bag may be used to deliver a "breath." A drop of local vasoconstrictor may also be used before the procedure to minimize mucosal edema.

V. COMPLICATIONS

Recommend ENT referral for objects that are sharp or not dislodged with this technique. Other techniques, using a Foley catheter or Fogarty biliary balloon catheter, positive-pressure ventilation or high-frequency ventilation, or bronchoscopic removal are not discussed here.

BIBLIOGRAPHY

Backlin SA: Positive pressure technique for nasal foreign body removal in children, *Ann Emerg Med* 25(4):544-555, 1995.

Driscoll CE et al, editors: *Handbook of family practice,* St. Louis, 1986, Mosby.

Driscoll CE, Rakel RE, editors: *Procedures for your practice,* Oradell, N. J., 1988, Medical Economics, Co.

Mills J et al, editors: *Current emergency diagnosis and treatment,* ed 2, Los Altos, Calif., 1985, Lange Medical Publishers.

Pfenninger JL, Fowler GC: *Procedures for primary care physicians,* St. Louis, 1994, Mosby.

Roberts JR, Hedges JR: *Clinical procedures in emergency medicine,* Philadelphia, 1985, Saunders.

Weiner HL, Levitt LP: *Neurology for the house officer,* ed 4, Baltimore, 1989, Williams & Wilkins.

18

Infectious Disease

ELIZABETH VALDES

GRAM STAIN

A. Protocol for performing Gram stain.

1. Spread specimen thinly on slide.
2. Heat-fix the slide and allow it to cool.
3. Flood slide with crystal violet for 10 to 30 seconds.
4. Rinse with tap water and shake off excess.
5. Flood slide with iodine for 20 to 60 seconds (2 × longer than with crystal violet)
6. Rinse with tap water and shake off excess.
7. Flood slide with decolorizer (acetone-alcohol) for 10 seconds and rinse immediately.
   - Repeat until blue dye no longer runs off slide.
8. Rinse with tap water and shake off excess.
9. Flood slide with counterstain (safranin) for 30 seconds.
10. Rinse with tap water and gently blot dry with paper towels or air dry.

B. Interpretation of Gram-stain results (Table 18-1).

SEPSIS

A. Definition.

1. ***Septicemia.*** Acute invasion of bloodstream by microorganisms producing fever, chills, tachycardia, tachypnea, and altered mentation.
2. ***Sepsis and septic shock.*** Characterized by the presence of two or more of these: (1) temperature above 38° C or less than 36° C, (2) heart rate >120 or $Pa{CO_2}$ <32 torrs, (3) WBC >12,000/mm^3 or <4000 or >10% bands. Septic shock includes a BP <90 mm or drop of 40 mm Hg from baseline value in absence of other causes. May also have organ dysfunction, hypoperfusion, hypotension, lactic acidosis.

TABLE 18-1
Microbiologic Characteristics of Bacteria Based on Gram Staining

Organism		Microbiologic characteristic		
GRAM-POSITIVE BACTERIA		**CATALASE**	**MISCELLANEOUS**	**AEROBIC?**
Cocci				
	Streptococcus	Negative		Yes
	Enterococcus	Negative		Yes
	Aerococcus	Negative		Yes
	Lactococcus	Negative		Yes
	Staphylococcus aureus	Positive	Coagulase positive	Yes
	Staphylococcus epidermidis	Positive	Coagulase negative	Yes
	Micrococcus	Positive	Coagulase negative	Yes
	Peptostreptococcus			Anaerobic
Bacilli				
	Bacillus		Spore forming	Yes
	Nocardia		Branching	Yes
	Actinomyces	Negative		Yes
	Lactobacillus	Negative		Yes
	Corynebacterium	Positive		Yes
	Listeria	Positive		Yes
	Clostridium		Spore-forming	Anaerobic
	Actinomyces		Non–spore forming	Anaerobic
	Propionibacterium		Non–spore forming	Anaerobic
	Eubacterium		Non–spore forming	Anaerobic

		OXIDASE	MISCELLANEOUS	AEROBIC?
Bacilli				
	Haemophilus		No growth on sheep blood agar	Yes
	Campylobacter		No growth on sheep blood agar	Yes
	Legionella		No growth on sheep blood agar	Yes
	Enterobacter, including: *Escherichia coli, Salmonella, Shigella, Klebsiella, Serratia, Proteus, Yersinia*	Negative	Ferments glucose	Yes
	Actinobacillus	Negative	Ferments glucose	Yes
	Gardnerella	Negative	Ferments glucose	Yes
	Acinetobacter	Negative	No glucose fermentation	Yes
	Pseudomonas	Negative	No glucose fermentation	Yes
	Vibrio	Positive	Ferments glucose	Yes
	Pasteurella	Positive	Ferments glucose	Yes
	Brucella	Positive	No glucose fermentation	Yes
	Campylobacter	Positive	No glucose fermentation	Yes
	Helicobacter pylori	Positive	Urease producing	Yes
	Bordetella	Positive	No glucose fermentation	Yes
	Pseudomonas	Positive	No glucose fermentation	Yes
	Bacteroides fragilis		Bile resistant	Anaerobic
	Bacteroides ureolyticus		No bile resistance	Anaerobic
	Fusobacterium		No bile resistance	Anaerobic
Cocci				
	Neisseria	Positive	No glucose fermentation	Yes
	Moraxella			Yes

Continued.

TABLE 18-1
Microbiologic Characteristics of Bacteria Based on Gram Staining—cont'd

Organism		Microbiologic characteristic		
GRAM-NEGATIVE BACTERIA		**OXIDASE**	**MISCELLANEOUS**	**AEROBIC?**
Acid-fast				
	Mycobacterium tuberculosis	Positive		Yes
	Mycobacterium marinum	Positive		Yes
	Cryptosporidium			
Weakly acid-fast				
	Nocardia			

B. Causes (percentage of cases).

1. ***Gram-negative bacteria (60% to 70%).***
   a. *Escherichia coli*
   b. *Klebsiella* with *Enterobacter*
   c. *Proteus*
   d. *Pseudomonas*
   e. *Serratia*
   f. *Neisseria meningitidis*
2. ***Gram-positive bacteria (20% to 40%).***
   a. Staphylococci
   b. Streptococci, especially pneumococci
3. Opportunistic fungi (2% to 3%).
4. Rarely, mycobacteria, viruses, protozooans.

C. Epidemiology.

1. 2/3 are in already hospitalized patients (other underlying illnesses and procedures).
2. Higher risk of gram-negative septicemia (mortality 25%).
   a. Neonates and elderly with urinary dysfunction (*very* high risk).
   b. *Underlying diseases:* diabetes, cirrhosis, alcoholism, cancer.
   c. Iatrogenic immunosuppression (such as cytotoxic drugs).
   d. TPN.
   e. Urinary, biliary, or GI infections.
3. Higher risk of gram-positive septicemia.
   a. Community acquired.
   b. Indwelling IV catheters.
4. Higher risk of fungal septicemia.
   a. Immunosuppressed.
   b. Postoperative patient with IV catheter and prolonged antibiotics.

D. Clinical manifestations.

1. Sudden onset and severe, being easily recognized: fever, chills, tachycardia, tachypnea, hypotension, mental status changes.
2. More gradual onset or presentations at the extremes of age can be subtle.
   a. May be hypothermic (T <36.5° C).
   b. Hyperventilation with respiratory alkalosis.
   c. *Rash:* pustules or vesicles may contain organism (bacterium or fungus).
      (1) Petechiae are suggestive of meningococcus.
      (2) Ecthyma gangrenosum (necrotizing or bullous lesions) are suggestive of *Pseudomonas.*
   d. Nausea, vomiting, diarrhea, ileus may obscure diagnosis of sepsis.

E. Work-up.

1. ***CBC.***
   a. Leukocytosis with left shift or leukopenia.

b. Toxic granulations, Döhle bodies, or intracytoplasmic vacuolization in PMNs.
c. Thrombocytopenia (suggestive of onset of DIC).
d. RBC morphology normal unless DIC; then may have microangiopathic hemolytic anemia.

2. ***Blood cultures.***
3. ***Culture all possible sources of infection.*** Sputum, urine, skin lesions, CSF, lines.
4. ***Urinalysis.*** Mild proteinuria early, may develop ATN secondary to shock. UTI can be cause of sepsis, especially in the elderly.
5. ***Electrolytes and glucose.***
   a. Hypoglycemia is rare; diabetics become hyperglycemic.
   b. Low bicarbonate with anion gap suggestive of metabolic acidosis caused by lactic acidemia from hypoperfusion.
6. ***Liver function tests.***
   a. Mild hyperbilirubinemia, elevated transaminases.
   b. Hypoalbuminemia progresses with malnutrition.
7. ***CXR.***
8. Lumbar puncture as indicated.
9. Abdominal radiographs if abdomen is possible source: perforation, ischemic bowel, cholecystitis, diverticulitis, etc.

F. Differential diagnosis. Other causes of shock including myocardial infarction, pulmonary embolus, drug overdose (especially salicylates), occult hemorrhage, cardiac tamponade, rupture of aortic aneurysm, aortic dissection, toxic shock syndrome.

G. Treatment. See Table 18-2 for empiric antibiotics in sepsis.

1. ***ABCs first (especially for those in shock).***
   a. Keep oxygen saturation >95%.
   b. IV fluid boluses, starting with normal saline or lactated Ringer's.
      (1) *Adults.* 1 to 1.5 liters in first 1 to 2 hours; likely will need more (generally about 5 liters behind on presentation).
      (2) *Children.* 20 ml/kg over 2 to 5 minutes (neonates over 20 minutes) repeated twice in first hour if needed to maintain good perfusion. Good evidence that a total of 60 ml/kg in first hour enhances survival.
      (3) Transfuse as needed.
      (4) Try to keep urine output between 30 and 60 ml/hour in adults and 0.5 to 1.5 ml/kg/hour in pediatric patients.
   c. Consider dopamine (5 to 10 μg/kg/min) or dobutamine (2 to 20 μg/kg/min). If these unsuccessful, consider norepinephrine infusion at 2 to 12 μg/min.
   d. Lanoxin may be helpful in septic shock but only small, uncontrolled case series have been done. (See Chapter 2 for details on digitalization.)

TABLE 18-2
Empiric Antibiotics in Sepsis

Likely source of sepsis	Likely organisms	Antibiotics
Urosepsis	Gram-negative rods, enterococci	Ampicillin and gentamicin Vancomycin and gentamicin Third-generation cephalosporin with or without gentamicin
Intra-abdominal infection	Polymicrobial, anaerobes	Ampicillin, gentamicin, and metronidazole Ticarcillin and gentamicin Third-generation cephalosporin and metronidazole
Nosocomial pneumonia	Resistant gram-negative rods	Amnioglycoside (gentamicin or tobramycin with an antipseudomonal (ticarcillin, piperacillin, ceftazidime)
Cellulitis	Streptococci or staphylococci	First-generation cephalosporin (such as cefazolin or oxacillin)
Intravenous catheter	*Staphylococcus aureus*, *S. epidermidis* or gram-negative rods	Vancomycin and gentamicin
Unknown or unclear	Broad-spectrum	Vancomycin, gentamicin, and metronidazole Cefotaxime and gentamicin

e. Naloxone may be helpful: 0.03 mg/kg bolus and 0.25 mg/kg/hour drip. Temporizing only and not without risk.
f. *Steroids have no use in septic shock and may be harmful unless patient has adrenal insufficiency or needs stress doses of steroids secondary to prior steroid use.*
g. Monoclonal antibodies against gram-negative endotoxin are available but are expensive and the lack of good selection criteria for candidates limits the usefulness of these agents at this time. No survival advantage has been demonstrated with the use of these agents or with anti–tumor necrosis factor antibodies.

2. ***Antibiotics.*** Start ASAP, preferably after cultures are obtained. Try to tailor antibiotics to likely source until culture results are known.

FEVER OF UNKNOWN ORIGIN

A. Definition.

1. ***Classic.*** Fever (temperature >38.2^0 C) without identifiable source after 3 days of hospital investigation or 3 outpatient visits.
2. ***Nosocomial.*** Fever in patients who had no fever on admission but persists without identifiable source after 3 days of hospital investigation.
3. ***Neutropenic.*** As with nosocomial origin, in a patient with <500 PMNs (needs empiric therapy).
4. ***HIV-associated.*** Fever for more than 3 days of hospital investigation or 4 weeks outpatient in a patient with confirmed HIV infection.

B. Causes.

1. ***Infection.***
   a. Abscess, TB, fungi, viral syndrome, endocarditis.
   b. As duration of fever increases, likelihood of infectious cause decreases.
2. ***Malignancy.*** Lymphoma, leukemia most common.
3. Autoimmune.
4. Collagen-vascular diseases.
5. Inflammatory bowel disease.
6. ***Miscellaneous.*** Drug fever, erythema multiforme, granulomatous hepatitis, regional enteritis, pulmonary embolism, sarcoidosis, familial Mediterranean fever, Fabry's disease, hypertriglyceridemia, alcoholic hepatitis, factitious, Behçet's syndrome, heavy-metal intoxication.
7. Many remain undiagnosed.

C. Work-up.

1. ***Observe temperature pattern: QAM and QPM.***
   a. Exaggerated circadian rhythm.
   b. Malaria, babesiosis, and cyclic neutropenia have patterns, occasionally Hodgkin's disease.

c. Factitious will have no circadian rhythm.

2. ***History.***
   a. Myalgias, malaise, rigors, sweating, weight loss.
   b. Medications, travel, exposure to chemicals or animals, occupation.
   c. Transient skin rashes can be seen with autoimmune infectious or collagen-vascular causes.
   d. Hematuria suggestive of renal carcinoma.
3. ***Physical exam.*** Daily exam of skin, eyes, nails, lymph nodes, heart, abdomen.
4. ***Laboratory tests.***
   a. CBC.
   b. UA.
   c. Cultures.
      (1) Multiple blood cultures (up to 6; otherwise may miss endocarditis or osteomyelitis) (polymicrobial suggestive of factitious).
      (2) Multiple urine cultures despite lack of classic UTI symptoms, especially in children and elderly.
      (3) Consider multiple cultures of sputum, CSF, stool, bone marrow.
      (4) Culture any tissues removed during biopsy (such as liver, lymph nodes).
   d. Direct examination of blood, CSF, stool.
   e. Consider freezing serum for possible titer testing of an agent later isolated.
   f. Acute-phase reactants are nonspecific and seldom helpful (such as ESR, CRP, fibrinogen, haptoglobin, ceruloplasmin, low iron or zinc, cytokines).
5. ***Noninvasive procedures.***
   a. "Routine":
      (1) CXR (repeat periodically).
      (2) Evaluation or inflammatory bowel disease.
   b. Most sensitive imaging study to evaluate:
      (1) *Brain and spine:* MRI
      (2) *Thorax:* CT
      (3) *Heart:* tranesophageal echocardiography
      (4) *Abdomen:* CT
      (5) *Kidneys, pancreas:* CT and ultrasonography
      (6) *Biliary tract:* Ultrasonography, radionuclide scan, ERCP
      (7) *Pelvis:* CT and ultrasonography
      (8) *Focal infection:* ^{111}In-labeled immunoglobulin G scintigraphy
      (9) *Bone:* radionuclide scan, MRI

B. Treatment of patients with FUO (that is, work-up is negative).

1. Acetaminophen or aspirin in maximum doses.
2. If fever persists, try ibuprofen or indomethacin.
3. Thorough reevaluation periodically (up to Q4-6 months).

IMMUNOSUPPRESSED HOST

Those who are immunosuppressed (taking steroids over long term, neutropenia, diabetes, elderly and very young) must be treated aggressively and may not manifest the usual signs or symptoms of sepsis. Specifically they may not mount a fever or white blood cell response. Localizing symptoms may be absent, and the patient may not have the ability to manifest adenopathy. Urinary tract infections may be present even in the absence of pyuria (especially in neutropenic patient). In addition to usual sites, consider sinuses, candidal sepsis, etc., to be source of fever.

- A. **Chronic corticosteroids.** Those taking steroids over long term will require stress doses of steroids (such as 60 mg of prednisone PO QD). Look hard for illness in the ill-appearing patient even in the absence of fever or localizing symptoms. Treat any infection aggressively because patients who are immunosuppressed secondary to steroids can get ill rapidly.
- B. **Diabetics.** Diabetics are a greater risk of listeriosis, osteomyelitis, infection in a prosthetic joint, etc. Because of neuropathy, the diabetic patient may present with a relatively advanced infection.
- C. **Neutropenia and neutropenic fever.** Need to start empiric antibiotics quickly if work-up does not reveal a specific source. Traditionally an aminoglycoside (such as gentamicin) has been paired with either a cephalosporin or an antipseudomonal penicillin (such as ticarcillin, piperacillin). The most cost effective may be ceftriaxone + gentamicin; piperacillin + gentamicin is another commonly used combination. Another option is treatment with a single agent such as imipenem or ceftazidime for those with a granulocyte count of $>100/mm^3$. Can add aminoglycoside to these as well for the sicker patient. Although not yet standard of care, the use of granulocyte colony–stimulating factor (G-CSF) and granulocyte-macrophage colony–stimulating factor (GM-CSF) have shown promise in reducing length of stay and length of neutropenia. It is not known if this will translate into better survival rates.
- D. **Elderly.** Confusion or change in mental status is characteristic of infection in the elderly. The presentation may be otherwise nonspecific, perhaps even lacking a fever and localizing signs and symptoms. Sepsis should be strongly suspected in any elderly person with vomiting, mental status changes, or an elevated WBC and band count. Hospital admission and a septic work-up should be strongly considered for the geriatric patient with these symptoms.
- E. **Infants and neonates.** See Chapter 10.

ZOONOSES NOT COVERED ELSEWHERE

- A. **Lyme disease.** This diagnosis should be entertained in those patients who present with a flu-like illness during the spring or summer if the patient has a known risk factor (such as camping, other outdoor activities).

1. ***Epidemiology.***
   a. Worldwide distribution, 3 foci in the United States.
      - Northeast: Massachusetts to Maryland
      - Upper Midwest, especially Wisconsin and Minnesota
      - Coastal California and Oregon

   b. Onset of illness is usually May to November, peaking in June and July.
2. ***Pathogenesis.***
   a. *Cause. Borrelia burgdorferi*, a spirochete.
   b. *Transmission.* Bite from deer tick, *Ixodes*, during spring nymph stage.
   c. An infected tick that is attached <24 hours unlikely to transmit infection but >72 hours causes almost 100% transmission. *However, even in endemic areas, the risk of transmission from any tick bite is only 1% to 5%.*
3. ***Clinical characteristics.***
   a. Early manifestations.
      (1) Erythema migrans: red macules enlarge centrifugally to >5 cm.
         - Central clearing in <40% if rash <2 weeks of age; >70% if rash >3 weeks.
         - *Onset.* 3 to 32 days after tick bite.
         - *Differential.* Cellulitis, hypersensitivity reaction to arthropod bites, plant dermatitis, tinea, granuloma annulare.
         - About 50% develop multiple annular lesions.

      (2) Myalgia, arthralgia, fatigue.
      (3) Headache, neck pain, stiffness.
         - Fever, chills, sore throat.
         - *Borrelia* lymphocytoma: red, firm nodule on ear pinna in children, on nipple and areola in adults.

   b. Late manifestations.
      (1) Neurologic involvement in 15%.
         - Usually weeks to months after erythema migrans.
         - Meningitis, encephalitis, chorea.
         - Bilateral facial nerve palsy or any cranial nerve palsy.
         - Radiculoneuritis, mononeuritis multiplex.
         - Diffuse peripheral sensorimotor neuropathy.

      (2) Cardiac involvement in 8%.
         - Fluctuating AV block (can be first, second, or third degree).
         - Myopericarditis with ST-segment changes, arrhythmias.
         - Syncope, presyncope or palpitations.
         - Valvular involvement rare.

      (3) Arthritis in 60%.
         - Onset can be weeks to years after tick bite.
         - Varies from migratory musculoskeletal pain to overt inflammatory arthritis.

- Asymmetric oligoarticular intermittent pain and swelling, usually of large joints, such as knee.
- 10% of those with arthritis develop chronic form with pannus formation resembling rheumatoid arthritis.

c. Later manifestations years after tick bite.
   (1) Acrodermatitis chronica atrophicans.
   (2) Demyelinating encephalopathy.
   (3) Mild axonal polyneuropathy.
   (4) Transverse myelitis.
   (5) Memory impairment, mood changes, chronic fatigue.

4. ***Diagnosis.***
   a. Best if based on clinical and epidemiologic evidence.
   b. Best currently available lab test is immunofluorescent antibody (IFA) or ELISA confirmed by Western blot.
   c. IFA or ELISA test for antibody levels.
      (1) False-negative results. First 3 to 4 weeks of illness, history of antibiotics, variable assay sensitivities.
      (2) False-positive results. *Treponema pallidum,* oral treponemes, *Escherichia coli,* juvenile rheumatoid arthritis, SLE, mononucleosis, bacterial endocarditis.
5. ***Differential diagnosis.***
   a. Erythema multiforme.
   b. Systemic lupus erythematosus.
   c. Prodromal phase or hepatitis B.
   d. Erythema marginatum.
   e. Aseptic meningitis.
   f. Infectious mononucleosis.
   g. Lymphoproliferative disorder.
   h. *Rheumatologic manifestations:* rheumatic fever, reactive arthritis, juvenile rheumatoid arthritis.
   i. *Neurologic manifestations:* Bell's palsy, multiple sclerosis, Guillain-Barré syndrome, brain tumor.
6. ***Treatment.***
   a. Early disease.
      (1) Doxycycline 100 mg PO BID × 10 to 21 days, or
      (2) Amoxicillin 500 mg TID (if <9 years of age, 40 to 50 mg/kg/day) × 10 to 21 days, or
      (3) Erythromycin 500 mg/QID (if <9 years of age, 30 to 40 mg/kg/day) × 10 to 21 days.
      (4) Azithromycin and cefuroxime axetil are more expensive alternatives.
      (5) Jarisch-Herxheimer–like reaction seen in 15%.
      (6) Constitutional symptoms may continue for extended periods despite adequate treatment.
   b. Late disease.
      (1) Bell's palsy alone (even bilateral) may be treated the same as early disease.

(2) Lyme meningitis, serious carditis, or persistent arthritis.
- Ceftriaxone 1 g IV BID (children 75 to 100 mg/kg/day), or
- Penicillin G, 20 to 24 million U/day (children 300,000 U/kg/day) IV divided Q4h × 10 days.

7. ***Prevention.***
   a. *Protective clothing:* long sleeves & pants, tucked into socks.
   b. Insect repellent.
   c. Check for ticks BID when in endemic areas.
   d. Remove attached ticks by grasping near skin with tweezers and pulling straight up.
   e. Prophylaxis after a tick bite may be reasonable in areas where there is >3.5% chance of disease occurrence after a tick bite. However, all those with tick bites should not have prophylaxis.

B. Ehrlichiosis.

1. ***Epidemiology.***
   a. Onset April to September, peaking in June and July; two thirds are rural residents.
   b. Human monocytic ehrlichiosis (HME) more common southeast and south-central United States (Oklahoma, Georgia, Arkansas).
   c. Human granulocytic ehrlichiosis (HGE) more common in Minnesota, Wisconsin, New York, Maryland.
2. ***Pathogenesis.***
   a. HME caused by *Ehrlichia chaffeensis.*
   b. HGE caused by *Ehrlichia equi.*
   c. Transmitted by deer ticks or dog ticks.
3. ***Clinical characteristics.***
   a. Fever, diaphoresis, myalgias, arthralgias, malaise, headache, nausea, vomiting.
   b. Leukopenia, anemia, thrombocytopenia, mild elevations of AST, ALT, LDH.
   c. 15% with severe complications: renal failure, DIC, pulmonary hemorrhage, interstitial pneumonitis, BOOP, seizures, coma.
4. ***Diagnosis.***
   a. Usually clinical, since therapy should be started before lab results are obtained.
   b. May see morulae in circulating peripheral WBCs.
   c. Can be confirmed by serum antibody or PCR testing, with fourfold rise in titer.
5. ***Treatment.*** Doxycycline 100 mg BID for adults (3 mg/kg/day divided BID for children) until 3 days after defervescence (minimum 5 to 7 days). Rifampin works in vitro, but clinical trials have not been done up to now.
6. ***Prevention.***

a. When outdoors in tick-infested areas wear light-colored clothing, use insect repellent, and check thoroughly for ticks afterwards.
b. Antibiotic prophylaxis is not recommended after a tick bite.

C. Babesiosis.

1. ***Epidemiology.***
   a. Most cases from Nantucket Island but also common on Cape cod.
   b. Also New England, Wisconsin, California.
   c. Transmission by *Ixodes dammini,* same vector as for Lyme disease.
   d. Mice and moles are rodent reservoirs.
2. ***Causes.***
   a. *Babesia microti* and *B. divergens.*
   b. Intraerythrocytic protozoan parasite.
3. ***Clinical features.***
   a. Malaria-like illness.
   b. Fever, chills, drenching sweats, lethargy, malaise, myalgias, arthralgias, darkened or red urine.
   c. May have been splenectomized or may have splenomegaly.
   d. *Laboratory findings.* Elevated liver enzymes, leukopenia, hemolytic anemia, hemoglobinuria.
4. ***Diagnosis.*** Can find the intracellular organisms with Giemsa stain.
   a. Multiple parasites per RBC, with pronounced pleomorphism.
   b. Often 4% to 7% RBCs infected (rarely up to 40%).
   c. Serologic is characteristics may also be diagnostic (ELISA, IFA).
   d. PCR appears most specific.
5. ***Treatment.***
   a. Generally self-limited except in the splenectomized.
   b. Clindamycin 12 to 2400 mg/day IV divided TID or QID plus oral quinine 650 mg Q6-8h × 7 to 10 days. (*Children:* clindamycin 20 mg/kg/day, quinine 25 mg/kg/day).
   c. May consider pentamidine.

D. Rocky Mountain spotted fever.

1. ***Tick-borne febrile illness caused by Rickettsia rickettsii.***
   a. Intracellular pathogen.
   b. Primary vector is dog tick: ticks and rodents are natural reservoir.
   c. Tick has to be attached for hours for transmission to occur; disease can be transmitted when one crushes tick during removal.
2. ***Epidemiology.***
   a. All states except Maine and Alaska.

   b. Peak incidence between April and October 1.
   c. Most cases are in children 5 to 9 years.
3. ***Physical findings.***
   a. Incubation 2 to 7 days.
   b. Sudden-onset fever with spiking pattern.
   c. Headache may progress to obtundation (aseptic meningitis-like characteristics with CSF pleocytosis).
   d. Confusion, nausea, rigors, myalgias, weakness.
   e. Rash starting on extremities, spreading to trunk.
      (1) Generally appears as erythematous macules on wrist and ankle within 24 hours, becomes petechial by day 4 if not treated.
      (2) 4% to 10% have no rash, and in others it may be evanescent.
   f. May have acute abdomen from abdominal musculature involvement.
   g. May have splenomegaly, hepatomegaly.
   h. Frequent nausea, vomiting, diarrhea, abdominal pain.
   i. Rarely pulmonary edema.
   j. Myocardial vasculitis with nonspecific ST/T changes.
4. ***Laboratory tests.***
   a. Slightly decreased WBCs, thrombocytopenia (may develop DIC), anemia, elevated aminotransferases.
   b. Serologic testing should be used to confirm the diagnosis.
   c. Weil-Felix reaction positive in only RMSF.
   d. Diagnostic titers not elevated until 10 to 14 days.
   e. PCR is in the works to diagnose rickettsial disease.
5. ***Treatment:***
   a. *In adults*: doxycycline 100 mg PO BID or tetracycline 500 mg PO QID.
   b. *In children:* doxycycline 2.2 mg/kg PO BID for 1 day, and then 2.2 mg/kg QD.
   c. Chloramphenicol 50 to 75 mg/kg/day divided QID is another alternative.
   d. Treat both for 5 to 7 days or until afebrile for 2 to 5 days.

TUBERCULOSIS

A. TB screening is recommended for:

1. *Those with high-risk conditions:* HIV positive, intravenous drug abuser, unexplained weight loss, chronic renal failure, DM, prolonged corticosteroids, leukemia, lymphoma, silicosis, CXR consistent with TB.
2. Close contact with those having known or suspected TB.
3. Immigrants from Latin America, SE Asia, Pacific Islands, Africa.
4. Residents and employees of high-risk institutions (correctional facilities, nursing homes, mental institutions, shelters).

5. Health-care workers serving high-risk clients.
6. Medically underserved, low-income populations.
7. Infants, children, and adolescents exposed to high-risk adults.

B. Screening methods.

1. ***Protein purified derivative (PPD).*** Use 5 tuberculin units of PPD in 0.1 ml injected intradermally; read in 48 to 72 hours. In the elderly, a second dose repeated 1 week later may uncover otherwise-unsuspected disease.
   a. False-positive results. Nontuberculotic mycobacteria; BCG-induced reactivity decreases with time, frequently gone after 1 year.
   b. False-negative results. Impaired immunity (controls also negative).
2. ***CXR.***

C. Interpretation of PPD. The PPD should be interpreted in the same way in those who have had BCG and those who have not. A positive reaction of >10 mm in those who have had BCG should be considered as a positive reaction!

1. Measure induration (elevated, firm area, not erythema).
2. 5 to 10 mm induration is considered positive among:
   a. Recent close contact of patients with active TB.
   b. HIV-positive or high-risk patient with unknown HIV status.
   c. Chest radiograph consistent with healed TB.
3. 10 mm or greater: 90% of reactors are infected with TB. 10 mm or greater induration is considered positive among:
   a. IV drug abusers known to be HIV seronegative.
   b. Medical conditions with increased risk: DM, high-dose steroids, immunosuppressive therapy, chronic renal failure, lymphoma, leukemia, other cancer, weight loss >10% below ideal, silicosis, gastrectomy, jejunoileal bypass.
   c. Residents and employees of prisons, jails, nursing homes, residential mental health facilities, shelters.
   d. Foreign-born and arrived from countries with high incidence of TB within last 5 years.
   e. Medically underserved, low-income populations.
   f. <4 years of age.
   g. Any child or adolescent exposed to high-risk adult.
4. >15 mm induration. Essentially 100% with 15 mm induration are infected with Mycobacterium tuberculosis. 15 mm is positive in anyone who does not meet above criteria.

B. Prevention.

1. ***Isolation.***
   a. *Indication.* Any patient known or suspected to have TB.
   b. Should be single-patient room with negative-pressure ventilation.
   c. Persons entering the room should wear appropriate respiratory protection.

2. ***Indications for preventive therapy after a positive PPD.***
   a. Prophylaxis for all those <35 years of age.
   b. No age limit for prophylaxis of reactors in the following groups:
      - PPD conversion from negative to positive within 2 years (3% risk of active disease in first year; must have baseline negative PPD within last 2 years).
      - All HIV-positive reactors (risk of active disease 10% per year).
      - Household contacts of those with active TB.
      - Those with past TB who have not had adequate treatment.
      - Positive reactor with underlying illness such as DM, high-dose steroids, immunosuppressive therapy, chronic renal failure, lymphoma, leukemia, other cancer weight loss >10% below ideal, silicosis, gastrectomy, jejunoileal bypass, IV drug abuse, malnutrition.
      - Those who have evidence on radiography of nonprogressive TB disease.
   c. Must always weigh risk of INH-hepatitis against benefits.
3. ***Preventive therapy.***
   a. *Adults:* isoniazid (INH) 300 mg PO QD × 6 to 12 months (12 if HIV positive). Add pyridoxine 10 to 50 mg PO per day to prevent development of peripheral neuropathy.
   b. *Children:* INH 10 mg/kg/day PO QD × 9 months (up to 300 mg/day total).
   c. If multidrug-resistant TB is likely (Korea, New York, SE Asia, New Jersey), consider multidrug preventive therapy. Check with your local health department about resistance in your area.

C. Therapy for active pulmonary TB (non–drug resistant).
1. Multiple regimens available, best to contact your local TB experts.
2. INH, rifampin, pyrazinamide, and ethambutol or streptomycin QD for 8 weeks and then INH and rifampin once susceptibility is demonstrated.
3. Treat for at least 9 months if HIV positive.

D. Therapy for active multidrug-resistant TB.
1. Many are now using 5 to 7 drugs, continuing at least 3 of them for 12 to 24 months total.
2. Empirically INH, rifampin, ethambutol, pyrazinamide, aminoglycoside, ciprofloxacin, and either cycloserine, ethionamide, or aminosalicylic acid.

BIBLIOGRAPHY

ACCP/SCCM Consensus Conference Committee for American College of Chest Physicians/Society of Critical Care Medicine Consensus Conference: Definitions for sepsis and organ failure and guidelines for the use of innovative therapies in sepsis, *Crit Care Med* 20(6):864, 1992.

American Thoracic Society and CDC Recommendations, *Am J Respir Crit Care Med* 49:1359-1374, 1994.
Barnes PF, Barrows SA: Tuberculosis in the 1990s, *Ann Intern Med* 119(5):400-410, 1993.
Baron EJ et al, editors: *Bailey and Scott's diagnostic microbiology,* ed 9, St. Louis, 1993, Mosby.
Bates JH et al: Microbial etiology of acute pneumonia in hospitalized patients, *Chest* 101(4):1005 1992.
Campos JM: Detection of bloodstream infections in children, *Eur J Clin Microbiol Infect Dis* 8:815, 1989.
Centers for Disease Control and Prevention: Screening for tuberculosis and tuberculosis infection in high-risk populations: recommendations of the Advisory Council for the Elimination of Tuberculosis, *MMWR* 44(RR-11):19-34, 1995.
Centers for Disease Control and Prevention: Guidelines for preventing the transmission of *Mycobacterium tuberculosis* in health-care facilities, 1994, *MMWR* 43(RR-13):27-68, 1994.
Centers for Disease Control and Prevention: Human granulocytic ehrlichiosis–New York, 1995, *MMWR* (44)32:593-595, 1995.
Chapnick EK et al: Technique for drawing blood for cultures: is changing needles truly necessary? *South Med J* 84(10):1197, 1991.
Dumler JS, Bakken JS: Ehrlichial diseases of humans: emerging tick-borne infections, *Clin Infect Dis* 20:1102-1110, 1995.
Fontanarosa PB et al: Difficulty in predicting bacteremia in elderly emergency patients, *Ann Emerg Med* 21(7):842, 1992.
Friedland JS, Warrell DA: The Jarsich-Herxheimer reaction in leptospirosis: possible pathogenesis and review, *Rev Infect Dis* 13:207-210, 1991.
Gelfand JA, Wolff SM: Fever of unknown origin. In Mandell G et al, editors: *Principles and practices of infectious diseases,* New York, 1995, Churchill Livingstone.
Harkess JR: Ehrlichiosis, *Infect Dis Clin North Am* 5(1):37-51, 1991.
Jantausch BA: Lyme disease, Rocky Mountain spotted fever, ehrlichiosis: emerging and established challenges for the clinician, *Ann Allergy* 73:4-11, 1994.
Kalmanti M et al: Effect of granulocyte colony–stimulating factor on chemotherapy induced neutropenia in children with cancer, *Pediatr Hematol Oncol* 11(2):147-155, 1994.
Kirkland KB et al: Therapeutic delay and mortality in cases of Rocky Mountain spotted fever, *Clin Infect Dis* 20(5):1118, 1995.
Lefering R et al: Steroid controversy in sepsis and septic shock: a meta-analysis, *Crit Care Med* 23(7):1294, 1995.
Magid D et al: Prevention of Lyme disease after tick bites: a cost-effectiveness analysis *N Engl J Med* 327(8):534, 1992.
Magnarelli LA: Current status of laboratory diagnosis of Lyme disease, *Am J Med* 98(4A):10S-12S, 1995.
Mandell GL, Bennett JE, Colin R: *Mandell, Douglas, and Bennett's principles and practice of infectious disease CD-ROM,* ed 4, New York, 1996, Churchill Livingston.
Mayordomo JI et al: Improving treatment of chemotherapy-induced neutropenic fever by administration of colony-stimulating factors, *J Nat Cancer Inst* 87(11):803-808, 1995.
Mermel LA et al: Detection of bacteremia in adults: consequences of culturing an inadequate volume of blood, *Ann Intern Med* 119(4):270, 1993.
Minocha A et al: Gram's stain and culture of sputum in the routine management of pulmonary infection, *South Med J* 86(11):1225, 1993.
Morris AJ et al: Rationale for selective use of anaerobic blood cultures, *J Clin Microbiol* 31(8):2110, 1993.
Nadelman RB, Wormser GP: Erythema migrans and early Lyme disease, *Am J Med* 98(4A):15S-23S, 1995.

National Committee for Clinical Laboratory Standards: *Procedures for the collection of diagnostic blood specimens by venipuncture,* ed 3: *approved standard,* Villanova, Pa., 1991, NCCLS.

Plorde JJ: Babesiosis. In Wilson JD et al, editors: *Harrison's principles of internal medicine,* ed 12, New York, 1991, McGraw-Hill.

Pruthi RK et al: Human babesiosis, *Mayo Clin Proc* 70:853-862, 1995.

Rahn DW, Malawista SE: Lyme disease, *West J Med* 154:706-714, 1991.

Reese RE, Betts RF: *A practical approach to infectious disease,* Boston, 1996, Little, Brown, & Co.

Rolston KVI et al: A comparison of imipenem to ceftazidime with or without amikacin as empiric therapy in febrile neutropenic patients, *Arch Intern Med* 152(2):283, 1992.

Sanders JW et al: Ceftazidime monotherapy for empiric treatment of febrile neutropenic patients: a metanalysis, *J Infect Dis* 164:907, 1991.

Sanford JP: *A guide to antimicrobial therapy,* Dallas, 1996, Antimicrobial Therapy, Inc.

Sanford JP: Leptospirosis. In Wilson JE et al, editors: *Harrison's principles of internal medicine,* ed 12, New York, 1991, McGraw-Hill.

Sexton DJ et al: Rocky Mountain "spotless" and "almost spotless" fever: a wolf in sheep's clothing, *Clin Infect Dis* 15(3):439, 1992.

Smart D et al: Effect of needle changing and intravenous cannula collection on blood culture contamination rates, *Ann Emerg Med* 22(7):1164, 1993.

Villanova PA, Root RK, Jacobs R: Septicemia and septic shock. In Wilson JD et al, editors: *Harrison's principles of internal medicine,* ed 12, New York, 1991, McGraw-Hill.

Vlessis AA et al: New concepts in the pathophysiology of oxygen metabolism during sepsis, *Br J Surg* 82:870-876, 1995.

Wasserman M et al: Utility of fever, white blood cells, and differential count in predicting bacterial infections in the elderly, *J Am Geriatr Soc* 37(6):537, 1989.

Weissman AF et al: The role of scintigraphy in the evaluation of fever of unknown origin, *Am Fam Physician* 50(8):1717-1727, 1994.

19

Otolaryngology

MARK A. GRABER AND LAURA BEATY

BASIC EXAMINATION

I. ACUTE HEARING LOSS

A. General. Hearing loss may develop over days or acutely. It may be either conductive in nature (ossicle disruption from trauma, tympanic-membrane perforation from cotton-tipped applicator or from noise, etc., cerumen in the canal, otitis media, barotrauma, etc.) or sensorineural (CVA, infectious, tumor, Ménière's disease, herpes zoster oticus (may see vesicles), syphilis, collagen-vascular disease, ototoxic drug exposure, etc). An isolated vascular event causing unilateral hearing loss is not uncommon in young adults.

B. Presentation. Decrease in auditory acuity. May document using audiologic testing or by Rinne and Weber tests (see above).

C. Approach. Treat cause if found. If no obvious cause is found and serious illness has been ruled out by a complete history and physical (especially neurologic exam), patient may be discharged with a follow-up appointment with ENT for further, specialized evaluation.

II. TRAUMA

A. Auricular trauma.

1. **Auricular hematoma** is a subperichondrial collection of blood typically caused by blunt trauma to the pinna. The hematoma separates the perichondrium from the cartilage predisposing the cartilage to avascular necrosis, infection, and "cauliflower-ear" deformity. *The hematoma must be evacuated by needle or an incision.* A compressive dressing is then placed to prevent re-collection of the hematoma. The ear should be examined daily for signs of infection or recurrence of the hematoma.
2. **Lacerations** involving cartilage should be thoroughly cleaned, sutured, covered with antibiotic ointment, and reevaluated daily for signs of infection or hematoma collection.

B. Nasal trauma.

1. ***Septal hematoma.*** Diagnosis requires a high index of suspicion, direct inspection of the septum after any nasal trauma, and recognition. The main symptom is progressive posttraumatic nasal obstruction. The nostril may be obstructed by a large, soft, red, or bluish mass. Its appearance can be confused with a polyp, a deviated septum, or enlarged turbinates. Septal hematomas can be easily missed unless the entire septum is observed visually and palpated with a blunt instrument.
   a. *Evacuation of the hematoma* within 48 hours is necessary to avoid avascular necrosis of the cartilage, abscess formation, or saddle deformity of the nose.
   b. Any finding of a boggy, fluctuant septum that is tender out of proportion to other findings warrants treatment.
   c. *Treatment of septal hematoma.*
      (1) Vasoconstrict and anesthetize the nasal mucosa with topical phenylephrine-tetracaine or cocaine.
      (2) Make a long vertical incision through the mucosa overlying the hematoma.
      (3) Use suction or normal-saline lavage to clean out all clots and place a sterile rubber band drain above the exposed cartilage.
      (4) Pack with a Merocel "rocket" or with petrolatum (Vaseline) gauze as described in the epistaxis section.
      (5) Place the patient on broad-spectrum antibiotic therapy. Reexamine, reaspirate, and repack daily while instructing the patient to avoid activities (nose-blowing, nasal sneezing) that increase nasal and sinus pressures.
      (6) If no recurrence of hematoma is seen, remove the drain and repack the nasal passage for final removal 24 hours later. Antibiotics may be stopped when the packing is discontinued.
      (7) Bilateral hematomas are handled in a similar manner, but ensure that the incisions are staggered over the septum so that no cartilage is underperfused on both sides.

1. ***Nasal fracture.*** Palpate dorsum of nose for deformity, instability, crepitus, and tenderness after any blunt injury causing bleeding from the nose. Diagnosis is confirmed by radiographs. However, treatment is based on presence of deformity when swelling is resolved, and so deferring radiographs until swelling is resolved is acceptable; this should be discussed with the patient. *Initial bleeding should be controlled and septal hematoma ruled out.* Early reduction is possible if the injury is acute and swelling insignificant.

Closed reduction should occur within 3 to 7 days for children and 5 to 10 days for adults.

EAR

I. OTITIS EXTERNA

A. Examination.

1. Expect to find canal maceration, erythema, edema, perhaps fungal colonization, ulceration, and pain with manipulation of the pinna.
2. The canal can be anesthetized with 4 drops of ophthalmic tetracaine for 5 minutes. Lidocaine aerosol 10% and lidocaine 4% topical suspension have also been shown to be very effective at providing local analgesia, whereas lidocaine 5% solution has not.
3. Clean debris from the canal. Depending on severity of disease, insert a wick (cotton or Merocel sponge packs) into the canal and then moisten the wick with 4 to 5 drops of either polymyxin B–neomycin otic suspension (Cortisporin otic suspension and others) or a drying, acidic agent (Vosol and others) every four hours for 2 or 3 days for nonfungal infections.
4. If cotton-like fibers of otomycosis are seen (especially in warm, moist climates), add topical clotrimazole 1% solution. Frequent removal of debris from the ear is crucial; the wick will help. Alternatives include amphotericin B (Fungizone), nystatin (Mycostatin), acetic acid (otic Domeboro), or gentian violet (2% in 95% alcohol).
5. Change the wick or wicks daily in all cases.

B. Malignant otitis externa. A progressive, necrotizing *Pseudomonas* infection typically occurring in elderly diabetic patients. The infection extends to involve the parotid gland, cartilage, bone, nerves, and blood vessels. Potential complications include osteomyelitis of the temporal bone, facial nerve paralysis, meningitis, and brain abscess. Prolonged IV antibiotics with an aminoglycoside and third-generation cephalosporin may result in complete resolution. CT scan is necessary to evaluate bony involvement. Hyperbaric oxygen and surgical débridement may be necessary for more advanced cases.

II. OTITIS MEDIA

A. General. Otalgia, fever, irritability, previous or coexisting URI, ear rubbing, and feeding problems are common presenting symptoms. However, any of the above symptoms, including ear pain and fever, may be absent. Many episodes are viral in origin. The most common bacterial pathogens are *Pneumococcus, Haemophilus influenzae,* and *Moraxella catarrhalis.*

B. Diagnosis. Diagnosis involves adequate observation of the tympanic membrane (TM), which may require cerumen removal. Hyperemia of the TM is an early sign of otitis media, but "red ear" alone does not establish the diagnosis. Other findings include bulging of the TM, indistinct landmarks, diminished light reflex, and limited mobility on pneumatic insufflation. Mastoiditis, meningitis, and abscess are possible complications. Of most concern, however, is impairment of hearing associated with middle ear effusion. Tympanometry may be used to establish the presence of fluid in the middle ear.

C. Treatment. Treatment with antibiotics is standard of care in the United States though this is not the case in many other developed countries. 81% of cases of OM will resolve spontaneously. It is necessary to treat 7 patients to effect the outcome in 1 patient. It is difficult if not impossible to demonstrate the superiority of one antibiotic over another. Start with low-cost agents and those that are well tolerated. If no response in 48 to 72 hours, consider changing antibiotic.

1. ***The most cost-effective agents.***
   a. Amoxicillin 40 mg/kg/day divided TID (125 mg/5 ml or 250 mg/5 ml suspensions) for 10 days [$14].
   b. Trimethoprim-sulfamethoxazole oral suspension 1 ml/kg/day divided BID (8 mg/kg trimethoprim and 40 mg/kg sulfamethoxazole per day) for 10 days [$25]. Avoid in children less than 2 months of age.
   c. Erythromycin-sulfisoxazole dosed as 50 mg of erythromycin per kilogram per day divided QID (suspension is 200 mg of erythromycin per 5 ml) for 10 days [$47].
2. ***The "second-line" drugs, which are more expensive.***
   a. Cefaclor 40 mg/kg/day divided BID for 10 days (suspensions dosed 125 mg/5 ml, 250 mg/5 ml) [$68].
   b. Amoxicillin-clavulanate dosed as 40 mg amoxicillin/kg/day divided TID for 10 days [$66].
   c. Cefixime 8 mg/kg single daily dose or divided BID (100 mg/5 ml suspension) for 10 days [$71].
   d. Clarithromycin 500 mg PO BID or 7.5 mg/kg PO BID for children.
3. Recently, ceftriaxone 50 mg/kg IM has been shown to be almost as effective as a traditional 10-day course of antibiotics. However, it is expensive and, because of emerging resistant bacteria, should be reserved for cases in which compliance is questionable.
4. If there is evidence of TM rupture (purulent drainage from canal), add Cortisporin otic *suspension* QID. The solution is acidic and tends to sting when administered.
5. Although traditional, a follow-up exam is not necessary in the asymptomatic patient who is older than a range of 15 months to 2 years of age. If, however, the patient is still symptomatic or the parent does not believe the otitis is resolved, follow-up exam can be done at 2 weeks.

6. In adults, complete resolution of symptoms such as ear fullness may take 6 weeks.
7. Decongestants play no role in the resolution of acute otitis media though they may be needed for associated conditions.
8. Pain control with topical solutions (such as Auralgan) or systemic agents such as acetaminophen, ibuprofen, or acetaminophen with codeine or hydrocodone may be required from patient comfort.

III. FOR RECURRENT ACUTE OTITIS MEDIA

Antibiotic prophylaxis (such as a single dose of amoxicillin or TMP/SMX at bedtime) should be considered for recurrent disease. Avoiding exposure to cigarette smoke may be helpful. Referral for discussion of tympanostomy tube placement should be considered if there is chronic bilateral effusions of more than 3 months in duration, unilateral effusion of more than 3 months in duration, language-development delay, hearing loss of >20 dB, or failure of antibiotic prophylaxis.

IV. FACIAL NERVE PARALYSIS

A. Bell's palsy is the most frequent diagnosis but is a diagnosis of exclusion.

1. Symptoms include preceding retroauricular headache, numbness of middle and lower areas or the face, otalgia, hyperacusis, decreased tearing, altered taste, and facial weakness with equal weakness in all branches of the seventh cranial nerve.
2. Onset is rapid, often occurring overnight.
3. Bell's palsy (a peripheral seventh cranial nerve lesion) can be differentiated from a central seventh nerve lesion by exam. In Bell's palsy, the motor fibers of all three branches are involved including the ophthalmic branch (forehead weakness). In a central seventh nerve lesion, the forehead is partially spared.
4. ***Differential and possible causes.*** Lyme disease, *Mycoplasma,* sarcoid, vasculitis, diabetes, rickettsial disease, intracranial pathologic condition. Herpes zoster oticus (Ramsay Hunt syndrome) will present with vesicular eruptions. There is some evidence that herpes simplex virus may be an inciting factor in at least some cases of Bell's palsy. History of facial twitching, slow progression, hearing loss, or additional cranial nerve involvement is suggestive of tumor and should be evaluated with CT. An intracranial pathologic condition (tumor, meningitis, CVA, multiple sclerosis) should be ruled out by history, physical exam, and testing as indicated.
5. ***Treatment.***
   a. If patient is unable to close eye, tape or patch the eye with lubricating ointment (such as Lacri-Lube) to prevent corneal drying and injury.

b. Although steroids continue to be used, their use is controversial, and there is no good evidence that they change the course of the illness. If you choose to use steroids, a reasonable course is 60 mg PO QD for 5 days with a tapering off over 7 to 10 days. It will certainly be of no benefit if started over 72 hours after onset of symptoms. Over 85% will resolve without treatment within 3 weeks. Many others will improve up to 6 months out.
c. Those with a dense paralysis or with evidence of complete muscle denervation by EMG have a worse prognosis. An EMG can be checked during the second week of disease if there is no evidence of improvement.
d. There is not proved benefit in the use of acyclovir.

6. Influenza-like symptoms and erythema chronicum migrans should be suggestive of Lyme disease. See Chapter 18 for further information.

NOSE

I. RHINITIS

A. General. Rhinitis is a hyperfunction of the nose resulting in rhinorrhea and nasal obstruction. Examination of a smear of nasal mucus stained with Wright stain can often make the diagnosis:

1. The presence of eosinophils is suggestive of an allergic rhinitis or, in the absence of other allergic symptoms, a nonallergic eosinophilic rhinitis.
2. The presence of many PMNs is suggestive of an infectious cause.
3. If cells are not present, it indicates vasomotor rhinitis.

B. Allergic rhinitis. Often has a seasonal component or specific inciting agents such as animals or dust. Exam often reveals excessive tearing, pale mucous membranes, and allergic facies (long face, dark color beneath eyes, arched palate). Antihistamines may be helpful. Chlorpheniramine is the most cost effective. Other options include the nonsedating antihistamines such as cetirizine (Zyrtec) and loratadine. Nasal steroids such as aqueous beclomethasone or flunisolide can be helpful just as cromolyn (Nasalcrom) can. Ipratropium nasal spray (0.03%) has recently been approved for use in allergic rhinitis.

C. Vasomotor rhinitis. Characterized by nasal mucosal swelling and rhinorrhea secondary to nospecific, nonallergic causes such as recumbency, cold, and humidity. Oral decongestants, topical decongestants (such as Afrin), as well as nasal steroids and ipratropium nasal spray (0.06%) may be helpful.

D. Nonspecific eosinophilic rhinitis. May respond to the same measures as vasomotor rhinitis, especially by topical steroids.

II. ACUTE SINUSITIS

A. General. Sinusitis can occur in any age group and will frequently involve the maxillary and ethmoid sinuses in children. Although the information below applies to all age groups, often a CT scan or MRI is needed to evaluate radiographically the sinuses in children under 3 years of age. However, abnormal CT findings occur in many asymptomatic children and show a high false-positive rate. Children are also prone to mucopurulent rhinitis. The major causative organisms include *Pneumococcus, Haemophilus influenzae,* and *Moraxella catarrhalis. Staphylococcus* and anaerobes may also be involved in those with chronic and recurrent disease.

B. Clinically. A history of a recent URI, facial "fullness," purulent nasal drainage, dental pain (especially with maxillary infection), and failure of over-the-counter preparations to resolve the symptoms are all predictive of sinusitis. Other clinical findings may include fever, facial headache with pain worsened with bending over, failure of the sinus to be transilluminated (indicating a fluid-filled sinus).

C. Positive history and clinical findings are sufficient to treat. Although many cases of sinusitis will resolve spontaneously, antibiotics do shorten the time course and provide symptomatic relief.

D. Treatment. Topical decongestants (oxymetazoline [Afrin] two inhalations each nostril BID for 3 days or phenylephrine nasal spray 2 sprays Q4h), with rinsing of the nose several times a day with saline solution, use of topical steroid spray (beclomethasone nasal, two inhalations each nostril BID for 3 to 6 weeks), oral decongestants, increased clear liquid intake with occasional shower or sauna steamy air inhalation and gentle mucus expectoration for the entire treatment course, and finally antibiotics. Traditionally, a 10 to 14 day course has been prescribed for initial episodes though a 3-day course of TMP/SMX given with a topical decongestant (oxymetazoline [Afrin] or phenylephrine) has recently been found to be effective in many with an acute uncomplicated sinusitis. Those who fail a 3-day course can be treated with a 10 to 14-day course. For recurrent disease, 4 to 6 weeks of antibiotics may be needed.

1. ***"First line" regimen (by far the most cost effective). Remember to check for drug allergy history.***
   - Amoxicillin 500 mg PO TID
   - Trimethoprim-sulfamethoxazole DS PO BID
2. ***"Second line" if initial protocol fails to reduce symptoms.***
   - Amoxicillin-clavulanate 500 mg PO TID
   - Cefuroxime axetil 500 mg PO BID
   - Cefixime 400 mg PO QD
   - Clarithromycin 500 mg PO BID
   - Clindamycin 300 mg PO TID

3. If a "second-line" regimen is deemed necessary to treat a *refractory acute sinusitis,* sinus radiographs or CT scan should be done to rule out neoplasm, smooth-walled retention cysts, abscesses, etc. Frequently, it is necessary to treat refractory sinusitis for 4 to 6 weeks with antibiotics. Refer for possible surgical intervention if pathologic condition is discovered or sinusitis becomes recurrent or refractory to treatment.

III. EPISTAXIS

A. Causes. Nose picking, external trauma, dry nasal mucosa with vascular fragility, foreign bodies, blood dyscrasias, neoplasms, infections, vitamin deficiencies, toxic metal exposures, septal deformities, telangiectasias, angiofibromas, and aneurysm ruptures.

B. Determining the source of bleeding is often the most difficult part of the examination.

C. The posterior area of the nose is supplied by the ethmoid arteries (from the superior internal carotids) and the sphenopalatine arteries (from the external carotids); bleeding from these vessels is often difficult to control.

D. Kiesselbach's arterial plexus supplies the more easily controlled anterior nasal mucosa.

E. If the bleeding has been prolonged, check the patient's Hb and HCT. A PT/INR, PTT, and platelet count may also be indicated depending on the clinical situation.

F. Gather a nasal speculum, a "hands-free" head mirror or lamp, suction with a Frazier suction tip, cocaine or tetracaine-epinephrine solution spray applicator, an electrocautery pencil, silver nitrate sticks, nasal packing (Merocel sponge "nasal rocket" packs, Vaseline gauze), and bayonet forceps to examine and treat a comfortable sitting or supine patient.

1. If bleeding is easily seen and is coming from the septum, direct pressure to the site after generously spraying of the area with the vasoconstrictor analgesic solution may be sufficient (pinch nose for 10 to 15 minutes).
2. If this doesn't work, try silver nitrate for small bleeders or electrocautery for the larger vessels on a well-anesthetized septum. Although there is no clear advantage to electrocautery, it may be effective in a patient who fails chemical cautery.
3. If this is ineffective, or if the bleeding is from under the turbinates, insert the dry Merocel pack entirely into the nostril (using a lubricant such as K-Y Jelly) and moisten it with phenylephrine or saline until it has completely formed to the convoluted nasal passage, leaving it in as necessary for bleeding control for at least 48 hours. Alternatively, pack with Vaseline gauze soaked with phenylephrine.

4. *Patients with COPD could suffer hypoxic distress because the nasopulmonary reflex produces a drop in the Po_2 by 15 mm Hg in most people who have their noses packed!*

G. Prescribe to all patients requiring nasal packing broad-spectrum antibiotics while they are packed; TMP/SMX, amoxicillin-clavulanate, clarithromycin, or cefadroxil are good choices.

H. Examine the uvula. If it's still dripping blood, hemostasis is inadequate and posterior packing may be required. Temporizing measures include the use of one of several commercially available posterior nasal packs or the use of a Foley catheter inserted into the posterior nasal area and inflated. Anyone requiring posterior packing should also have an anterior pack placed. Obtain an otolaryngologic consultation and hospitalize any patient with a posterior nose bleed for observation or vascular intervention.

I. *Consult with an otolaryngologist if posterior packing is required, if nose requires repacking several times during a single ED visit, or for any patients develop signs or symptoms of an infection.*

TONGUE AND MOUTH

I. APHTHOUS ULCERS, "CANKER SORES"

Aphthous ulcers are recurrent painful lesions of nonkeratinized mucosa that vary in size and may appear as solitary lesions or in clusters (herpetiform ulcerations). The typical appearance involves an erythematous periphery with a white or yellow depressed center. Healing within 10 to 14 days is the rule.

A. Causes. Viral (coxsackievirus, herpesvirus), systemic illness (Crohn's disease, lupus, Behçet's disease, erythema multiforme), toothpaste (sodium lauryl sulfate), stress, and smoking. Dental trauma, vitamin $B_{12,}$ folate, and iron deficiency have also been implicated in some cases.

B. Treatment. Symptomatic relief can be obtained by the use of diphenhydramine elixir as a mouth rinse that is then expectorated. Alternatively, viscous lidocaine 2% can be used in the adult. This may suppress the gag reflex, however, and may result in systemic toxicity in children. The application of a topical steroid (triamcinalone as 0.1% in Orabase) or steroid mouth rinse (betamethasone syrup) may accelerate recovery. Herpetiform ulcerations may respond to tetracycline syrup, which is used as a mouth rinse and then swallowed. A burst of oral prednisone may be required in some cases. The use of multiple other drugs including cyclosporin A, colchicine, thalidomide, and dapsone attest to the stubborn nature of these lesions. A mixture of nystatin 12,500 units, diphenhydramine 1.25 mg, and hydrocortisone 0.25 mg/ml has been used as a "shotgun" solution. Some also include tetracycline syrup in the mixture.

C. Prevention. Using a toothpaste free of sodium lauryl sulfate or changing toothpastes has been shown to be helpful in some cases. Topical use of steroids mouth rinses may decrease recurrence. Recently, pentoxifylline has been used to prevent recurrent aphthous ulcers in an open label trial. However, blinded studies are lacking.

D. Herpes simplex virus infrequently causes recurrent intraoral herpes. The lesions occur as a cluster of vesicles that rupture leaving superficial ulcerations that remain for 3 to 10 days. Keratinized tissues, attached gingiva, and the hard palate are often involved, and such features distinguish herpes from aphthous ulcers. Treatment with acyclovir may decrease healing time.

II. XEROSTOMIA (DRY MOUTH)

A. Causes. Sjögren's syndrome, anticholinergics, radiation changes, dehydration, surgical changes, infection (as by CMV), mouth breathing.

B. Treatment. Artificial saliva, mouth washes, hard candy, pilocarpine tablets 5 mg PO TID, pilocarpine solution 15 gtt 1% in 4 oz of water and swish and spit. This can also be swallowed and will provide 5 mg of pilocarpine.

THROAT

I. PHARYNGITIS AND TONSILLITIS

A. General. Acute tonsillitis and pharyngitis present with sore throat, pain radiating to the ears and dysphagia. Fever is more commonly associated with group A beta-hemolytic streptococci (*Streptococcus pyogenes*). The proportion of pharyngitis and tonsillitis that is cause by group A streptococci is related to the patient's age. In children 6 to 15 years of age, approximately 50% of the pharyngitis that presents for care is caused by streptococci. Other causes include *Mycoplasma,* Epstein-Barr virus, adenovirus, *Influenzavirus, Arcanobacterium hemolyticum,* gonococcal pharyngitis, and others. Noninfectious causes include mouth breathing secondary to nasal obstruction (as with a URI). Viral thyroiditis may present as a "sore throat" as may carotidynia, an ill-defined entity characterized by tenderness over the carotid artery, painful swallowing, and pain radiating to the ears. Carotidynia will respond to NSAIDs; antibiotic treatment is not indicated. Consider adult epiglottis in the febrile adult with severe sore throat, with trouble in swallowing and anterior neck tenderness. Also consider peritonsillar abscess. See Table 19-1.

B. The central question in pharyngitis is deciding which patients require antibiotics and doing so in a cost-effective manner. The treatment and approach to pharyngitis is mired in controversy.

TABLE 19-1
Partial Differential Diagnosis of "Sore Throat" with Some Distinguishing Features

Cause	Oral examination	Skin examination	Systemic symptoms	Adenopathy	Age group
Streptococcal pharyngitis	Beefy red pharynx, palatal petechiae	Sandpaper-like rash with scarlet fever only	Fever, absent URI symptoms	Tender anterior cervical adenopathy	Children
Mononucleosis-like illnesses (EBV, CMV)	Injected pharynx, exudate	Rash in response to amoxicillin	Fatigue, fever	Postcervical adenopathy, axillary adenopathy, perhaps splenomegaly	Young adults
Arcanobacterium hemolyticus	Injected pharynx with exudate	May have morbilliform rash			Young adults
Viral pharyngitis	Mild injection, pain out of proportion to exam	No rash	URI symptoms may be present	Rare	All
Adenovirus	Exudative pharyngitis	No rash	Conjunctivitis, cough, bronchitis		Primarily children but also adults
Carotidynia	Throat exam normal	No rash	None	Tender over carotid, no adenopathy	Adults

1. ***Adults.*** A reasonable approach in adults is to treat all patients with fever, systemic symptoms, and tonsillar exudate with antibiotics because they are likely to have streptococcal pharyngitis. Patients exhibiting little or no evidence suggestive of bacterial pharyngitis (those with concurrent URI symptoms, obvious cause such as mouth breathing, little or no visual evidence of pharyngitis, absent adenopathy) may be reassured and treated symptomatically with lozenges or addressing the underlying problem (humidity, nasal congestion, etc.). Streptococcal cultures or quick streptococcal tests can be reserved for those patients in whom the diagnosis is not clear. Testing for mononucleosis can be reserved for those with appropriate adenopathy (see Table 19-1) and those who do not respond to conservative treatment.
2. ***Children.*** Most authors recommend a quick streptococcal test followed by a pharyngeal culture for group A beta-hemolytic streptococci if the quick streptococcal test is negative. This recommendation is based on the increased incidence of streptococcal pharyngitis and sequelae in pediatric patients as well as the frequently limited reliability of the physical examination in this age group. Many clinicians advocate empiric therapy with antibiotics and systemic analgesia while awaiting culture results. Rapid streptococcal tests demonstrate a sensitivity of approximately 80%. The newer tests have a concordance of 91% to 95% with those of a culture.

C. Treatment.

1. Currently, there are no isolates of group A beta-hemolytic streptococci that are penicillin resistant in the United States.
2. Isolates resistant to erythromycin have been found primarily in Japan. Only 3.5% of isolates in the United States are erythromycin resistant. However, these are becoming *less* prevalent with time.
3. Some resistance to treatment may be noted if the patient is simultaneously colonized with *H. influenzae* that is beta-lactamase producing.
4. Therefore the first drug or drugs of choice are penicillin (that is, Pen-VeeK 500 mg PO BID or TID or Penicillin G Benzathine 1.2 million U IM in adults, 600,000 U IM in children) and erythromycin 250 to 500 mg PO Q6h for 10 days. If these fail, a first-generation cephalosporin (such as cephalexin 250 mg PO QID or 500 mg PO BID) may be used.
5. Children may return to school after 24 hours of therapy.

D. Indications for tonsillectomy. History of peritonsillar abscess, history of airway obstruction (sleep apnea) secondary to tonsil hypertrophy; some would suggest 4 or 5 episodes of streptococcal pharyngitis in a 1-year period or "chronic sore throat" with adenopathy for 6 months that is unresponsive to treatment.

E. **Scarlet fever.** Scarlet fever is a self-limited systemic manifestation of streptococcal pharyngitis. Symptoms include "strawberry tongue" (a red tongue with red or whitish papillae), a fine "sandpaper" rash that appears as a diffuse erythema beginning and concentrating in the skin folds (especially axillary) but spares the palms and soles. Frequently, there is circumoral pallor. There may occur a fine desquamation that begins on the fingers and toes. The differential diagnosis includes Kawasaki's disease.

F. **For recurrent disease**, attempt to identify carrier in family with throat and nasal cultures. Treat any identified carriers. Consider IM treatment to rule out noncompliance as a reason for treatment failure.

II. PERITONSILLAR ABSCESS (QUINSY)

A. **General.** A localized area of abscess that is typically unilateral and occurs in patients with tonsillitis.

B. **Cause.** Depending on the series, the most common organism is *Streptococcus* followed by anaerobes.

C. **Clinically.** Symptoms include severe throat pain with radiation to the ear, drooling from inability to swallow saliva, trismus, and fever. Almost pathognomonic of a peritonsillar abscess is a muffled, "hot potato," voice. On exam there is unilateral swelling of the palate and anterior pillar with displacement of the tonsil downward and medially and movement of the uvula away from the involved side.

D. **Treatment.** IV or IM penicillin and tonsillectomy. Several series have documented good results using oral antibiotics and needle drainage, which may need to be done many times. The major concern is the possibility of airway obstruction though this is a very rare event. ENT consultation is recommended.

III. MONONUCLEOSIS

A. Classically, the term "mononucleosis" has referred to the syndrome caused by the Epstein-Barr virus, which is characterized by pharyngitis with exudate, diffuse lymphadenopathy (including splenomegaly in 50%), malaise, fever, and fatigue. So-called heterophil negative mononucleosis may be caused by other organisms including CMV or *Toxoplasma* or by acute HIV infection or leptospirosis. Mononucleosis is most common in young adults, and most of the adult population has had clinically inapparent EBV disease. If patients with mononucleosis are treated with amoxicillin, they will almost uniformly develop a morbilliform rash.

B. Diagnosis. Diagnosis is by CBC revealing the typical lymphocytosis with atypical lymphocytes. A positive heterophil antibody (monospot test) may or may not be present in the early stages of the disease (only 60% by 2 weeks) but will eventually become positive in 90% of young adults. The heterophil test rarely becomes positive in those <5 years of age. If there is any doubt, an EBV antibody titer can be performed. Liver enzymes are almost uniformly elevated.

C. Complications. CNS problems including encephalitis and aseptic meningitis, hematologic complications including hemolytic anemia and splenic rupture, as well as airway obstruction secondary to paratracheal lymphadenopathy.

D. Treatment. Symptomatic, and the illness generally resolves within 2 weeks. However, prednisone has been shown to reduce the length of the illness. A steroid burst of 30 to 60 mg of prednisone PO per day for 3 days or 4 mg of methylprednisolone PO TID for a week may be used but is generally reserved for treating the complications of mononucleosis, including respiratory obstruction, myocarditis-pericarditis, aseptic meningitis, and hemolysis-thrombocytopenia. Contact sports or activities producing other forms of trauma should be avoided because of the risk of splenic rupture.

IV. HOARSENESS

A. Hoarseness. An abnormality of vocal cord vibratory function that results from injury, mucosal tear, or edema.

B. Causes. Infectious laryngitis is the most likely cause; however, history should elicit information regarding smoking and alcohol (risk factors for laryngeal cancer), voice abuse (risk factors for singers' nodules), and trauma. Hypothyroidism may cause a gradual and progressive hoarseness that will resolve with treatment. Gastroesophageal reflux disease and tumor should also be considered. Other causitive entities include neurologic disease (stroke, Eaton-Lambert syndrome, Myasthenia gravis), lung malignancy, and other pulmonary processes (Wegener's granulomatosis, sarcoid), especially with hilar involvement, inhalation injury (smoke etc.).

C. Hydration and voice rest are the primary therapy of suspected infectious laryngitis. Address the underlying cause. If symptoms persist without an obvious cause, referral for complete ENT evaluation is indicated.

TEMPOROMANDIBULAR JOINT

I. TEMPOROMANDIBULAR JOINT DISORDERS

A. General. TMJ disorders include arthritis of the joint, anterior cartilage (meniscus) displacement, and pain in the muscles of mastication (myofascial pain dysfunction).

B. Symptoms. May include ear pain, pain on chewing or opening the mouth wide with pain radiating to the ear, limited jaw mobility, clicking or crepitance, and tenderness on palpation of the joint.

C. Treatment. Avoiding clenching and grinding the teeth, eating a soft diet, moist heat, massage, and NSAIDs. Some patients may benefit from the use of muscles relaxants, bite appliances worn at night, or physical therapy. Referral to otolaryngology, oral surgery, or TMJ centers should be considered for refractory pain.

BIBLIOGRAPHY

Austin JR et al: Idiopathic facial nerve paralysis: a randomized double blind controlled study of placebo versus prednisone, *Laryngoscope* 103(12):1326, 1993.

Barloon TJ et al: Diagnostic imaging in the evaluation of dysphagia, *Am Fam Physician* 53:535-546, 1996.

Bluestone CD et al: Appropriateness of tympanostomy tubes setting the record straight, *Arch Otolaryngol Head Neck Surg* 120:1051-1053, 1994.

Cantor RM: Otitis externa and otitis media: a new look at old problems, *Emerg Med Clin North Am* 13:2, 1995.

Claessen JQPJ: A review of clinical trials regarding treatment of acute otitis media, *Clin Otolaryngol* 17(3):251, 1992.

Coonan KM et al: In vitro susceptibility of recent North American group A streptococcal isolates to eleven oral antibiotics, *Pediatr Infect Dis J* 13(7):630, 1994.

Cummings CW et al: *Otolaryngology–head and neck surgery,* ed 3, St. Louis, 1993, Mosby; ed 5, 1995; CD-ROM, 1996.

Danielides VG et al: Value of the facial nerve latency test in the prognosis of childhood Bell's palsy, *Childs Nerv Syst* 8(3):126-128, 1992.

Del Mar C: Managing sore throat: a literature review. Do antibiotics confer benefit? *Med J Aust* 156(9):644, 1992.

Dippel DWJ et al: Management of children with acute pharyngitis: a decision analysis, *J Fam Pract* 34(2):149, 1992.

El-Daher NT et al: Immediate vs. delayed treatment of group A beta-hemolytic streptococcal pharyngitis with penicillin, *Pediatr Infect Dis* 10(2):126, 1991.

Green SM et al: Single-dose intramuscular ceftriaxone for acute otitis media in children, *Pediatrics* 91(1):23, 1993.

Hathaway TJ et al: Acute otitis media: Who needs posttreatment follow-up? *Pediatrics* 94(2):143, 1994.

Heikkinen T et al: Signs and symptoms predicting acute otitis media, *Arch Pediatr Adolesc Med* 149(1):26, 1995.

Herlofson BB, Barkvoll P: Sodium lauryl sulfate and recurrent aphthous ulcers: a preliminary study, *Acta Odontolog Scand* 52(5):257-259, 1994.

Honda H, Takahashi A: Virus-associated demyelination in the pathogenesis of Bell's palsy, *Internal Med* 31(11):1250-1256, 1992.

Kennedy DW, editor: Sinus disease: guide to first line management, Deerfield Beach, Fla., 1994, Health Communications, Inc.

Lee KJ: Essential otolaryngology: head and neck surgery, East Norwalk, Conn., 1995, Appleton & Lange.

Logan M et al: The utility of nasal bone radiographs in nasal trauma, *Clin Radiol* 49(3): 192, 1994.

Maharaj D et al: Management of peritonsillar abscess, *J Laryngol Otol* 105(9): 743, 1991.

Marchant CD et al: Measuring the comparative efficacy of antibacterial agents for acute otitis media: the "Polyanna phenomenon," *J Pediatr* 120(1):72, 1992.

Maximum Access to Diagnosis and Therapy, Electronic Library of Medicine, Boston, 1996, Little, Brown & Co.

Møller A, Grøntved A: Topical anesthesia of the normal tympanic membrane: a controlled clinical trial of different suspensions of lidocaine, *ORL J Otorhinolaryngol Relat Spec* 52(3):168, 1990.

Niemela M et al: Lack of specific symptomatology in children with acute otitis media, *Pediatr Infect Dis J* 13(9):765, 1994.

Reese R et al: *A practical approach to infectious disease,* Boston, 1991, Little, Brown & Co.

Roddey OF et al: Comparison of an optical immunoassay technique with two culture methods for the detection of group A streptococci in a pediatric office, *J Pediatr* 126(6):931, 1995.

Rosenfeld RM: What to expect from medical treatment of otitis media, *Pediatr Infect Dis J* 14(9):731, 1995.

Schaefer SD: The treatment of acute external laryngeal injuries, *Arch Otolaryngol Head Neck Surg* 117:35-39, 1991.

Shafshak TS et al: The possible contributing factors for the success of steroid therapy in Bell's palsy: a clinical and electrophysiological study, *Laryngol Otol* 108(11):940-943, 1994.

Sharp JF et al: Routine X-rays in nasal trauma: the influence of audit on clinical practice, *J R Soc Med* 87(3):153, 1994.

Snellman LW et al: Duration of positive throat cultures for group A streptococci after initiation of antibiotic therapy, *Pediatrics* 91(6):1166, 1993.

Tintinalli JE et al: Emergency medicine: a comprehensive study guide, New York, 1996, McGraw-Hill.

Toner JG et al: Comparison of electro and chemical cautery in the treatment of anterior epistaxis, *J Laryngol Otol* 104(8):617, 1990.

Vincent SD et al: Clinical, historic, and therapeutic features of aphthous stomatitis, *Oral Surg Oral Med Oral Pathol* 74(1):79, 1992.

Wahba-Yahav AV: Pentoxifylline in intractable recurrent aphthous stomatitis: an open trial, *J Am Acad Dermatol* 33(4):680-682, 1995.

Wald ER: Sinusitis, *Pediatr Rev* 14:345-351, 1993.

Wegner DL et al: Insensitivity of rapid antigen detection methods and single blood agar plate culture for diagnosing streptococcal pharyngitis, *JAMA* 267(5):695, 1992.

Williams JW et al: Randomized controlled trial of 3 vs. 10 days of trimethoprim-sulfamethoxazole for acute maxillary sinusitis, *JAMA* 273(13):1015, 1995.

Williams JW et al: Clinical evaluation for sinusitis: making the diagnosis by history and physical examination, *Ann Intern Med* 117(9):705, 1992.

Williams JW et al: Does this patient have sinusitis: diagnosing acute sinusitis by history and physical examination, *JAMA* 270(10):1242, 1993.

20

Drug Doses of Commonly Prescribed Medications

MARK A. GRABER AND MICHAEL KELLY

Generally, drug dosages (Table 20-1) are for those without underlying renal or hepatic failure. This is intended as a quick reference. Please be familiar with indications, side effects, etc. before using this reference.

Space has been provided so that you may add additional medications therein.

BIBLIOGRAPHY

Physician's GenRX, electronic edition, St. Louis, 1966, Mosby.
AskRX plus (based on USP DI, vol I), San Bruno, Calif., 1996, Hearst Corporation.
Rudolph AM: *Rudolph's pediatrics,* ed 19, East Norwalk, Conn., 1991, Appleton & Lange.
Sanford JP: *A guide to antimicrobial therapy,* Dallas, 1996, Antimicrobial Therapy, Inc.

TABLE 20-1
Commonly prescribed medications

Drug	Pediatric dose	Adult dose	Maximum dose	Important side effects	Indications and notes
Acetaminophen (See codeine for acetaminophen + codeine)	10-15 mg/kg Q6h	650-1000 mg Q6h	1000 mg per dose, 4 g/day	Liver toxicity	Pain, fever
Acyclovir	Same as adult for these indications	Immunosuppressed (skin and mucosal): HSV 1 and HSV 2 5 mg/kg IV over 1 hour Q8h (total: 15 mg/kg/day) for 7 days For herpes encephalitis: 10 mg/kg over 1 hour Q8h for 10 days See Chapter 11 for oral dose for suppression, treatment of genital herpes, dermatology for zoster dose			

Continued

TABLE 20-1
Commonly prescribed medications—cont'd

Drug	Pediatric dose	Adult dose	Maximum dose	Important side effects	Indications and notes
Albuterol (oral)	Preparation is 2 mg/5 ml (0.4 mg/ml) Dose: 0.1 mg/kg TID with initial dose not to exceed 2 mg (5 ml) TID By MDI: 2-8 puffs by spacer Q1-2h PRN	6-12 years: 2 mg PO Q6h Over 12 years: 2-4 mg PO Q6h or extended-release tablets 4-8 mg Q12h By MDI: 2-8 puffs by spacer Q1-2h PRN	16 mg BID	Tremor, tachycardia, anxiety	Inhaled form preferable
Albuterol, inhaled	Nebulized 2.5 mg in 5 ml nebulized as needed	Nebulized: 2.5 mg in 5 ml NS nebulized as needed	Judged by response	Same as above	Very safe and nontoxic
Allopurinol	<6 years: 150 mg/day 6-10 years: 300 mg/day Evaluate response at 48 hours and increase as needed	Mild gout: 200-300 mg/day Severe gout: 400-600 mg/day	800 mg/day	Rash, liver toxicity, precipitation of gout attacks, aplastic anemia, and other hematologic abnormalities	Start 100 mg/day and increase weekly to effect
Alprazolam	Not recommended	For anxiety: 0.25-0.5 mg TID For panic disorder: 0.5 to 2.0 mg TID	10 mg/day	Somnolence, addiction	

Amantadine	Preparation: 50 mg/5ml For influenza A: 1-9 years: 4.4-8.8 mg/kg/day not to exceed 150 mg/day 9-12 years: 200 mg in 1 or 2 doses	For influenza prophylaxis and treatment: 200 mg/day given in 1 or 2 doses Parkinson's disease: 100 mg BID	400 mg/day	Nausea, dizziness, light-headed-ness, depression, ataxia, etc.	
Amikacin	Premature: 10 mg/kg loading dose and then 7.5 mg/kg Q18-24h Neonatal: 10 mg/kg load-ing and then 7.5 mg/kg Q12h Older children: same as adult dose	Load with 10 mg/kg and then 15 mg/kg/24 hours divided Q8-12h	1.5 g/day	Adjust for renal failure Side effects in-clude renal failure, deafness	Loading dose not changed for renal fail-ure Therapeutic level generally 25-30 μg/ml with trough of 5-8 μg/ml
Amitriptyline	Adolescent: 25-50 mg PO QHS or divided; may need more as tolerated.	25-200 mg PO at bedtime or divided TID Start low (25-75 mg QHS) and increase as needed	300 mg (hospita-lized patients)	Sedation, anticho-linergic side ef-fects, prolong-ed QT interval	Be careful in the elderly; may cause falls, mental sta-tus changes, constipation

Continued

TABLE 20-1
Commonly prescribed medications—cont'd

Drug	Pediatric dose	Adult dose	Maximum dose	Important side effects	Indications and notes
Amlodipine	Not indicated	2.5-10 mg PO QD	10 mg	Start low in elderly Usually requires 10 mg to have results in angina	Generally have neutral effect on cardiac output
Amoxicillin	20-40 mg/kg/day in 3 divided doses For children >20 kg use adult dose	250-500 mg PO TID	3 g as single dose for gonorrhea but not recommended	Diarrhea (especially in children) Rash when given in presence of mononucleosis Anaphylaxis	125 to 250 mg/ 5 ml. Available as chewable tablet
Amoxicillin/ clavulanate	Same as amoxicillin	Same as amoxicillin			Two 250 mg tablets do not equal one 500 mg tablet because of the clavulanate component

Ampicillin	50-100 mg/kg PO divided Q6h IV for sepsis, meningitis, etc.: 50 mg/kg/IV Q6h	PO: 250-500 mg Q6h 8-12 g/day divided Q4h			125 and 250 mg/5 ml available
Aspirin	Antipyretic: 10-15 mg/kg Q6h (use only in those >16 years old) Avoid in those with chickenpox or influenza-like symptoms	Pain: 650 mg PO Q6h Antiplatelet: 81-325 mg PO per day			Several timed-release products are available for BID dosing in rheumatoid arthritis (Easprin, ZORprin)
Atenolol	Not established	Hypertension: 50-100 mg PO QD 1-2 weeks to effect Angina: 50-200 mg PO QD IV for MI: 5 mg over 5 minutes and repeat in 10 minutes	HTN: 100 mg Angina: 200 mg		
Azithromycin	Not well studied For those 2-15 years: 10 mg/kg at day 1 and then 5 mg/kg on days 2 to 5 Use adult doses for those >16 years	Most indications: 500 mg day 1 and then 250 mg PO on days 2 to 5 *Chlamydia trachomatis:* 1 g PO once For gonorrhea: 2 g			

Continued

TABLE 20-1
Commonly prescribed medications—cont'd

Drug	Pediatric dose	Adult dose	Maximum dose	Important side effects	Indications and notes
Aztreonam	Neonate: 30 mg/kg/dose Up to 7 days old: 30 mg/kg Q12h 1-4 weeks old: 30 mg/kg Q8h >4 weeks old: 30 mg/kg IV Q6-8h Older children: 90-120 mg/kg 24 hours given divided Q6-8h	Moderately severe infections: 1-2 g IV Q8-12h Severe infections: 2 g IV Q6-8h			
Beclomethasone	6-12 years: For asthma: 1-2 puffs QID with 4 puffs BID as an option and up to 10 puffs/day	For asthma: 2 puffs QID or 4 puffs BID or more if needed (up to 20 puffs/day)		Little systemic effect, oral candidiasis	May not have maximal effect for 1-2 weeks
Benzonatate	>10 years of age give adult dose	100 mg TID-QID	600 mg		

Benztropine	>3 years of age must individualize Not recommended under 3 years of age	1-4 mg PO or IM BID or 1-2 mg TID	6 mg		
Bethanechol	0.6 mg/kg PO divided TID-QID 0.2 mg/kg IM divided TID-QID	5-50 mg PO TID-QID or 2.5-10 mg IM TID-QID	200 mg/day		Start low and increase as needed For IM (adult) give 2.5 mg and repeat Q10 min until have desired effect
Bumetanide	>6 months: 0.015-0.1 mg/kg/dose given QD <6 months: not established	0.5-2 mg PO or IV QD May need higher doses if no response	Start low Maximum dose depends on effect	Hypokalemia, hypotension	0.5 mg to about 20 mg of furosemide
Captopril	Newborn: 0.01 mg/kg BID-TID; adjust as needed Children: 0.3 mg/kg Q8-24h; adjust up as needed	6.25-100 mg PO BID-TID	450 mg/day adults	Dry cough and angioedema Hyperkalemia Aspirin may be helpful for cough (325 mg QAM)	Start low for those sodium and fluid depleted.

Continued

TABLE 20-1
Commonly prescribed medications—cont'd

Drug	Pediatric dose	Adult dose	Maximum dose	Important side effects	Indications and notes
Carbamazepine	Up to 6 years: 10-20 mg/kg divided BID-TID and increase weekly by 100 mg/day; generally need 250-300 day mg/day and rarely 400 mg/day 6-12 years: 50 mg QID or 100 mg BID and increase weekly by 100 mg/day Generally need 400-800 mg/day; don't exceed 1000 mg	100 mg PO QID and then increase weekly by 200 mg/day until therapeutic	12-15 years: 1000 mg >15 years: 1200 mg (occasionally 1600 mg)	CNS toxicity including confusion, lethargy, nausea, lightheadedness Marrow suppression rare but serious	Maintenance in adults generally 800-1200 mg/day Blood levels of 4-10 mg/L
Cefaclor	20-40 mg/kg divided Q8h not to exceed 1 g/day	250-500 mg PO Q8h	1500 mg/day adults		In vitro some *Haemophilus influenzae* are resistant

Cefadroxil	30 mg/kg PO divided into 2 doses	1-2 g/day in single or 2 doses	2 g		Available as 125, 250, and 500 mg/5 ml suspension
Cefamandole	50-100 mg/kg/day divided Q4-8h May need up to 150 mg/kg/day in serious infections not to exceed 12 g/day	500 mg to 1 g IV Q4-8h but may use up to 2 g IV Q4h for serious, life-threatening infections	12 g/day		Lower doses (50 mg/kg for children; 500 mg IV Q6-8h for adults) appropriate for uncomplicated UTI
Cefazolin	25-100 mg/kg IV divided Q6-8h; rarely 150 mg/kg/day has been used Not recommended in neonates though has been used at 40 mg/kg/day divided Q6-8h	500-1.5 g IV Q6h In life-threatening infections, 12 g/day has been used	12 g/day but generally not >9 g/day		

Continued

TABLE 20-1
Commonly prescribed medications—cont'd

Drug	Pediatric dose	Adult dose	Maximum dose	Important side effects	Indications and notes
Cefixime	8 mg/kg/day in single dose or divided BID	400 mg PO QD or 200 mg PO BID			Available as suspension with 100 mg/5 ml NOTE: Studies of treatment of otitis media were done with suspension only, which achieves higher blood levels. Manufacturer recommends using suspension only when treating otitis media.

Cefotaxime	0-1 week: 50 mg/kg IV Q12h 1-4 weeks: 50 mg/kg IV Q8h 1 month to 12 years: 50-180 mg/kg divided Q4-6h; If >50 kg, use adult dose	1-2g IV Q6-12h, but up to 2g Q4h has been used for severe, life-threatening infections			
Cefoxitin	80-160 mg/kg divided Q4-6h Not recommended <3 months	1-2 g IV Q6-8h			
Ceftazidime	0-4 weeks: 30 mg/kg IV Q12h 1 month to 12 years: 30-50 mg/kg per dose Q8h; maximum 6 g/day though higher doses have been used in meningitis and cystic fibrosis	1g IV Q8-12h but may use up to 2 g IV Q8h for serious, life-threatening infections			
Ceftizoxime	50 mg/kg IV up to 200 mg/kg day divided TID-QID	500 mg to 1 g IV Q8-12h (UTI Q12h; others Q8h) For severe infections: 1-4 g IV Q8-12h PID: 2 g IV Q8h	12 g/day		

Continued

TABLE 20-1
Commonly prescribed medications—cont'd

Drug	Pediatric dose	Adult dose	Maximum dose	Important side effects	Indications and notes
Ceftriaxone	50-100 mg/kg Q24h Meningitis dose: 100 mg/kg Soft tissues: 50-75 mg/kg	1-2 g IV Q24h	4 g in adults		May cause cholestasis
Cephalexin	6.25-25 mg/kg PO Q6h Skin, streptococcal pharyngitis: 12.5-50 mg/kg BID	250-500 mg PO Q6H For cystitis, streptococcal pharyngitis, and skin infections: 500 mg PO BID	4 g in adults		Available as pediatric drops 100 mg/ml, 125 and 250 mg/5 ml preparations
Chlorpromazine	Children >6 months for behavior disturbance: Oral: 0.25 mg/lb Q4-6h PRN Rectal: 0.5 mg/lb Q6-8h IM: 0.25 mg/lb Q6-8h PRN	For acute psychosis: 25 mg IM followed by another 25-50 mg IM in 1 hour if needed; increase dose gradually to maximum dose of 400 mg IM Q6h to control symptoms Oral: 10-25 mg BID-TID, increase as needed	1 g/day though doses of up to 1 g/day and 2 g/day have been used	Hypotension, dystonic reactions, sedation	

Cimetidine	20-40 mg/kg PO divided QID Intravenous: 5-10 mg/kg IV Q6h	Ulcer treatment: 400 mg PO BID or 800 mg QHS Prophylaxis: 300 mg PO BID or 400-800 mg QHS IV: 300 mg Q6h	2.4 g/day (higher doses have been used)	Many drug interactions including theophylline, tricyclics, warfarin, anticonvulsants, cyclosporin A, etc.	Can give IV as continuous infusion (900 mg over 24 hours)
Ciprofloxacin	Not indicated in children unless no other option 10-20 mg PO or IV BID but generally not indicated in children!	Oral: 250-750 mg BID IV: 200-400 mg BID			Almost no indication for IV use Can use oral ofloxacin and get good blood levels
Cisapride	Gastroparesis: 0.15-0.3 mg/kg TID-QID before meals	Reflux: 10 mg BID or 20 mg QHS but up to 20 mg bid Gastroparesis: 10-20 mg 15 minutes AC and HS		May interact with terfenadine, clarithromycin, antifungals, others to cause torsades	Available 1 mg/ml (Canada only)
Clarithromycin	7.5 mg/kg PO Q12h	250 or 500 mg PO Q12h	Maximum in child: 500 mg Maximum in adult: 1000 mg		Available in 125 and 250 mg/5 ml

Continued

TABLE 20-1
Commonly prescribed medications—cont'd

Drug	Pediatric dose	Adult dose	Maximum dose	Important side effects	Indications and notes
Clindamycin	PO: 8-16 mg/kg/day given divided TID-QID but up to 20 mg/kg/day IV: neonates: 15-20 mg/kg/day divided TID to QID Children >1 month: 20-40 mg/day TID-QID	PO: 150-300 mg Q6h but up to 450 mg Q6h IV:600-1200 mg/day divided TID-QID More serious infections: 1200-2700 mg/day but 4800 mg has been used			May cause pseudomembranous colitis *(Clostridium difficile* colitis)
Clonidine	For >16 years of age use adult dose; no pediatric indication	0.1 mg PO BID; increase by 0.1 mg/day; most need 0.2-0.6 mg/day	Up to 2.4 mg/day (rarely needed)	May have rebound effect if stopped abruptly	Can cause drowsiness
Codeine	<1 year: dose not established but 0.5 mg/kg Q4-6h has been used >1 year: 0.5-1.0 mg/kg Q4-6h	15-60 mg PO Q4-6h (or 1 or 2 acetaminophen tablets [Tylenol #3])	360 mg/24h		Acetaminophen elixir: 120 mg of acetaminophen and 12 mg of codeine per 5 ml

Colchicine	For familial Mediterranean fever: <5 years: 0.5 mg PO QD >5 years: 0.5 mg PO BID	Acute gout: IV: 2 mg followed by 0.5 mg IV Q6h up to 4 mg in 24 hours. Do not use IV form in those already receiving oral colchicine. Also, after 4 mg IV dose, give no further colchicine for 7days. PO: Acute gout 1-1.2 mg Q2h until pain resolves or have GI symptoms or 6 mg total. Chronic gout: 0.5-0.6 mg PO QD-TID	4 mg IV 6 mg PO		Fab antibody fragments available for acute overdose (not FDA approved)
Desipramine	Not indicated in young children: In adolescents: 25-100 mg PO either divided or in one dose	100-300 mg PO in divided doses or in one dose HS	300 mg/day	Drowsiness, dry mouth, constipation, prolonged QT interval	Start low and increase as tolerated
Dexamethasone	For croup: 0.6 mg/kg IM once up to 5 mg Neonatal: 0.3 mg/kg/24h Pediatric: 0.05-0.5 mg/kg/24h See specific indication in text for doses	0.75-10 mg Q6-24h Generally higher doses for cerebral edema			

Continued

TABLE 20-1
Commonly prescribed medications—cont'd

Drug	Pediatric dose	Adult dose	Maximum dose	Important side effects	Indications and notes
Dextro-methorphan	Neonatal: not indicated 1-4 mg/kg/24h divided Q6h	Adult: 15-60 mg Q6h	Children: 45 mg/dose Adult: 60 mg/dose	Similar to narcotics if overdose	
Diazepam	Neonatal: IV/IM 0.1-0.2 mg/kg/dose for 5 mg maximum PO: 0.2-0.5 mg/kg/dose Children: 0.1-0.5 mg/kg repeat twice for seizures	PO: Anxiety, muscle spasm: 2-10 mg TID-QID. Vertigo: 2 mg TID-QID IV: sedation: 2-10 mg or more Seizure: 10 mg IV repeated as needed		Sedation, respiratory depression, addiction	Lorazepam preferred for seizures Reverse with flumazenil
Dicloxacillin	Not for neonates PO: 12.5-25.0 mg/kg/24h divided Q6h	250-500 mg PO Q6h	2000 mg		
Digoxin	Loading: Preterm: IV 0.015-0.025 mg/kg/24h Term: IV 0.02-0.03 mg/kg/24h	See chapter 2 for loading schedule Average daily dose is 0.125-0.25 mg PO		Check levels and maintain within normal limits (check your lab's normal).	Indicated for CHF not caused by diastolic dysfunction

	Maintenance: 1/4 of digitalizing dose civided Q12h Loading: 2 week to 2 years: 0.03 mg/kg PO or IV >2 years: 0.02 mg/kg/24h Maintenance: 1/5 of IV loading dose divided Q12h For all loading: give 1/2 in first dose and other 1/4 at 6 and 12 hours			Side effects include arrhythmias, nausea, hyperkalemia (see digoxin toxicity in Chapter 1)	(hypertrophic cardiomyopathy) May also be used to control rate in those with atrial fibrillation who have CHF
Digoxin Fab	See Chapter 1	See Chapter 1			
Diltiazem	Adolescents: use adult dose Not indicated in pediatrics	Angina: 30 mg PO QID and advance as needed IV 0.25 mg/kg first dose; second dose 0.35 mg/kg; administer over 5 minutes			CD is once a day SR is BID; can convert from QID directly to CD or SR
Diphenhydramine	5 mg/kg/24h divided Q6h not to exceed 300 mg IV or PO	Adult: 25-50 mg PO Q6h IV or PO	300 mg	Sedation, anticholinergic	

Continued

TABLE 20-1
Commonly prescribed medications—cont'd

Drug	Pediatric dose	Adult dose	Maximum dose	Important side effects	Indications and notes
Dipyridamole	Not indicated in neonates Use 5 mg/kg divided QID as antiplatelet drug	PO: 75-100 mg QID IV for use with thallium scanning: 0.142 mg/min for 4 minutes (0.57 mg/kg total)			
Divalproex	See valproic acid	See valproic acid			
Doxycycline	>8 years: 4.4 mg/kg on day one followed by 2.2 mg/day Maximum is adult dose Not indicated for younger children	200 mg on day 1 followed by 100 mg QD (see Chapter 11 for doses for STD)	200 mg/day	Photosensitivity, decreased renal function	
Droperidol	Not recommended in neonates Anesthesia: 0.088-0.165 mg/kg IM or IV For nausea: 0.025-0.04 mg/kg dose Q6h	For acute control of agitation or combative behavior: 5-10 mg IV or IM For nausea: 1.25-2.5 mg IV or IM Q6h	Generally 10 mg, but larger doses may be needed to treat agitation		Potent sedative Well absorbed IM Little respiratory depression occurs Use with caution in those with renal or hepatic dysfunction

Enalapril	Not indicated in children	2.5-40 mg PO divided QD-BID 0.625-1.25 mg IV Q6h Administer over 5 minutes	40 mg/day PO	Same as captopril	Same as captopril
Enoxaparin	See specific indication in text	See specific indication in text			
Epinephrine	For stridor and bronchiolitis: 5 ml of 1:1000 nebulized; repeat PRN SQ: 1:1000 0.01 ml/kg/dose SQ for asthma every 15-20 minutes × 3 (maximum 0.5 ml)	Asthma: 1:1000 0.3-0.5 ml SQ Q15-20 min	0.5 ml	Tachycardia, arrhythmia, tremor Rebound does not occur but will return to baseline state	Inhaled epinephine works as well as or better than racemic epinephrine and is easier to make dose
Epinephrine in sesame oil (Sus-Phrine)	Asthma or urticaria: SQ only: 0.005 ml/kg/dose (maximum 0.3 ml, 0.15 ml in those <30 kg)	Asthma or urticaria: SQ only: 0.005 cc/kg/dose for 1 dose only Usual adult dose is 0.1-0.3 ml		Not rapid acting Use only for maintenance	

Continued

TABLE 20-1
Commonly prescribed medications—cont'd

Drug	Pediatric dose	Adult dose	Maximum dose	Important side effects	Indications and notes
Erythromycin These dosages are for the base. See last column to calculate erythromycin ethylsuccinate (EES) dose.	PO: 0-7 days 20 mg/kg/12h >1 month: 30-50mg/kg/day divided dose IV: Neonatal: 10 mg/kg/24h given divided Q12h >1 month: 10 mg/kg/24h divided Q8-12h	PO: 250 mg QID or 500 mg BID IV: 500 mg QID	1 g/day PO		To convert to EES, 400 mg of EES = 250 mg of base Multiply base by dose by factor of 1.6 to equal EES dose EES available 200 mg and 400 mg/5 ml
Estrogen, conjugated	Vaginal cream for adhesions: apply BID sparingly	For hormone replacement see Chapter 7 For dysfunctional uterine bleeding: 25 mg IV or IM; may repeat in 6 to 12 hours		Observe for uterine hyperplasia if uterus intact	

Ethacrynic acid	Not indicated in infants Children: PO: 25 mg/dose Q24h and increase by 25 mg/day until desired effect IV: 0.5-1.0 mg/kg/dose	PO: 50-200 mg/day in 1 dose or divided BID IV: 25-100 mg		In adults start low (50-100 mg) and increase by 25 mg/day	
Ethosuximide	Not indicated in neonates: PO: 10-20 mg/kg/dose Q12h Start 250 mg/day in 3-6 years of age 500 mg/day>6 years and adjust up as needed	500 mg PO Q12h	1.5 g/day		Increase dose by 125-250 mg Q4-7 days Therapeutic level 40-100 μg/ml Suspension preferable (250 mg/5 ml)
Famciclovir	Not indicated	Herpes zoster: 500 mg TID × 7 days started within 48 hours of appearance of rash			
Famotidine	Not indicated	Duodenal ulcer: 40 mg PO QD as single dose or divided BID Gastric ulcer: 40 mg PO QHS IV dose: 20 mg IV Q12h	Up to 160 mg Q6h has been used for Zollinger-Ellison syndrome		Available as suspension of 40 mg/5 ml

Continued

TABLE 20-1
Commonly prescribed medications—cont'd

Drug	Pediatric dose	Adult dose	Maximum dose	Important side effects	Indications and notes
Felbamate	Not indicated <2 years of age 2-14 years: initiate at 15 mg/kg/day divided TID-QID Increase by 15 mg/kg every 2 weeks until 45 mg/kg maximum	>14 years: start 1200 mg divided TID-QID; increase by 600 mg/week to 3600 mg/day maximum	3600 mg/day		Reduce doses of other anti-epileptics 20% to 33% to reduce side effects Felbamate increases levels of phenytoin, carbamazepine, and valproic acid Available in 600 mg/5 ml suspension
Fluconazole	Not established but doses of 3-6 mg/kg QD in 3 to 13 year olds has been given without complications	Oral and esophageal candidiasis: 200 mg on day 1 and then 100 mg QD (up to 400 mg has been used) Cryptococcal meningitis:			

		400 mg IV on day 1 followed by 200 mg/day for life Vaginal candidiasis: 150 mg PO once			
Flumazenil	To reverse sedation: 0.2 mg (2 ml) IV over 15 seconds; may give additional dose to 1 mg	For sedation: same as pediatric For overdose: 0.2-5 mg IV *See precautions in Chapter 1 under coma*		*May induce seizures if patient has mixed overdose with tricyclics!*	May need additional doses because is short acting Maintain monitor until fully awake and no possibility of recurrent sedation
Fluoxetine	Not indicated in children	10-80 mg PO QD or divided BID	80 mg	May cause tremor, psychomotor activation	Available as 20 mg/5 ml
Folic acid	PO: 1 mg/day Maintenance: Infants: 0.1 mg/day Up to 0.3 mg/day for children up to 4 years Adult doses >4 years	PO: 1 mg/day 0.4 mg/day maintenance but 1 mg/day for pregnancy			

Continued

TABLE 20-1
Commonly prescribed medications—cont'd

Drug	Pediatric dose	Adult dose	Maximum dose	Important side effects	Indications and notes
Furosemide	1-2 mg/kg as single dose with increase by 1-2 mg/kg Q6h until get diuresis Doses >6 mg/kg not recommended	PO: 20-80 mg QD or more IV: 20 mg or more (give at least patients total daily dose if want acute diuresis)		May cause deafness at high IV dose as well as hypokalemia	Start in adults with 20 mg and titrate up as needed
Gabapentin	See Chapter 14	See Chapter 14			
Gentamicin	Premature (>1200 g): 5 mg/kg/day divided Q12h Neonates/infants: 7.5 mg/kg/day Children: 6.0-7.5 mg/kg/day	Adults: 2 mg/kg loading and then 1.0-1.7 mg/kg Q8h Can give single dose of 5.1 mg/kg/day (but not in endocarditis) See adjustment for renal failure Consider pharmacy consultation to determine dose		Adjust dose for renal failure: roughly multiply 8 by serum creatinine and use this for for dosing interval; don't change loading dose.	Administration with 24-hour dosing interval may reduce side effects, cost, with no change in efficacy Follow creatinine and levels Peak levels 4-8 μg/ml with trough <2 μg/ml

Glipizide	Not indicated	Glucotrol XL: 5-20 mg once daily Non–extended release: 5-40 mg/day divided QD-TID before meals		Not indicated in pregnancy	May dose non–extended release QD or BID depending on dose and response Can change to Glucotrol XL from non-sustained mg for mg
Glucagon	Children: 0.025 mg/kg/dose	For hypoglycemia not secondary to alcohol (with depleted liver glucagon) 1 mg IM or IV			See text for other indications
Glyburide	Not indicated	Micronase/DiaBeta: 2.5-5 mg start and titrate to maximum 20 mg Glynase: 1.3-3 mg start and titrate to maximum 12 mg/day; dose all QD or BID			Not indicated in pregnancy

Continued

TABLE 20-1
Commonly prescribed medications—cont'd

Drug	Pediatric dose	Adult dose	Maximum dose	Important side effects	Indications and notes
Griseofulvin	Micronized only: 10-15 mg/kg/day	Micronized only: 500 mg to 1 g/day		Periodic CBC; liver enzymes should be checked	Tinea capitis: 4-6 weeks Tinea corporis: 2-4 weeks Tinea pedis: 4-8 weeks
Haloperidol	Not indicated in infants. PO: 3-12 years: 0.05 mg/kg/day divided BID-TID increased by 0.5 mg every week until desired effect IV/IM for psychosis: 0.05-0.15 mg/kg/24h divided with single dose of 1-10 mg depending on severity and patient history of exposure to antipsychotics	PO: 0.5-2.0 mg BID or TID increasing up to 20 mg/day IV/IM: 1-10 mg aliquots until behavior controlled	Doses of up to 200 mg/day have been used	Watch for extrapyramidal side effects, neuroleptic malignant syndrome	Monitor vital signs in those who are rapidly sedated

Heparin	50 U/kg with drip at 25 U/kg/hour	"Traditional": 5000-unit bolus with drip at 1000 U/hour Weight-based dosing: bolus 80 U/kg Drip at 18 U/kg/hour SQ prophylaxis: 5000 U SQ Q12h			Weight-based dosing reaches therapeutic levels faster than standard dosing and is preferable
Hydrochlorothiazide	Neonates: 2 mg/kg Q24h PO Older: 2 mg/kg/24h PO	6.25-50 mg PO QD		Watch for hypokalemia	Unlikely to get much more response beyond 25 mg/day
Hydrocortisone	2-10 mg/kg/day depending on illness (PO, IV)	100-500 mg PO or IV depending on disease state			
Hydroxyzine	0.25-0.5 mg/kg/dose Q4-6h	PO: 25-100 mg Q6h IM: 25-100 mg			Must be given deep IM May cause tissue necrosis if given SQ

Continued

TABLE 20-1
Commonly prescribed medications—cont'd

Drug	Pediatric dose	Adult dose	Maximum dose	Important side effects	Indications and notes
Ibuprofen	Not indicated in neonates 10-40 mg/kg divided TID-QID For fever generally 10 mg/kg/dose Q6h JRA: 20-40 mg/kg/day divided TID-QID	200-800 mg Q6h	3200 mg/day		May cause GI ulceration, other GI symptoms Inhibits platelets
Imipramine	6-12 years: 25-50 mg PO QHS >12 years 50-75 mg PO QHS Don't exceed 2.5 mg/kg/day	50-150 mg PO QHS		Sedation, anticholinergic side effects, prolonged QT interval	Be careful in the elderly; may cause falls, mental status changes, constipation
Indomethacin	Neonates to close patent ductus: IV: 0.1-0.3 mg/kg/dose Q12-24h up to total of 3 doses >14 years: 25-50 mg PO Q6-8h	25-50 mg PO Q6h SR tablets: 75 mg PO BID			May have GI side effects similar to those of other NSAIDs.

Isosorbide dinitrate	Not indicated	SL: 2.5-5.0 mg for acute angina PO: 5-40 mg Q6h for angina, CHF			See nitroglycerin for warnings
Ketorolac	Not indicated	15-30 mg IV or 60 mg IM PO: 10 mg Q6h			Oral only indicated for follow-up study of parenteral drug Oral use limited to 5 days!
Labetalol	Not recommended in children Adolescents: start oral at 100 mg BID Otherwise as adult	IV: 20 mg IV with 20-80 mg IV Q10 min. Titrate to blood pressure Alternative method: 20 mg IV and then 2 mg/min to effect PO: 200-400 mg BID	Maximum oral: 2400 mg/24h Maximum IV: 300 mg/24h		
Lactulose	Not indicated in neonates Infants <2 years: 2.5-10 ml/day divided >2 years: 40-90 ml/day divided	30-45 ml (20-30 g of lactulose) TID-QID titrated to effect			May give rectally

Continued

TABLE 20-1
Commonly prescribed medications—cont'd

Drug	Pediatric dose	Adult dose	Maximum dose	Important side effects	Indications and notes
Levothyroxine	Oral: neonates: 8-10 µg/kg 6-12 months: 6-8 µg/kg 1-5 years: 5-6 µg/kg 6-12 years: 4-5 µg/kg IV: 75% of oral dose	PO: 0.0125-0.2 mg/day titrated to normalize TSH IV: 0.05-0.1 mg for hypothyroidism Myxedema coma: 0.2-0.5 mg IV and then 0.1-0.3 mg IV on day 2			Check TSH Q2-3 months and adjust dose; see text for details
Lidocaine	See Pediatric life support in Chapter 1 Neonates: 1 mg/kg/dose over 2-4 minutes; repeat: maximum of 5 mg/kg Children: 0.5-1.0 mg/kg IV to total of 3 mg/kg Drip at 20-50 µg/kg/min	See Chapter 1 as well IV for arrhythmia: 2 mg/kg IV followed by 1 mg/kg IV slowly Follow by 2-4 mg/min drip			
Lorazepam	IV for seizures: 0.1 mg/kg up to 2 mg/dose; repeat as needed	Oral for anxiety: 2-6 mg/day divided BID-TID with higher dose given at bedtime IV for seizures: 1-2 mg; repeat as needed IM for sedation: 2 mg			May cause apnea when given IV Have intubation equipment available

					Reversible with flumazenil
Lovastatin	Not indicated	20 mg PO QHS with evening meal to maximum of 80 mg			
Magnesium oxide		Mag-Ox 400: for magnesium supplementation 1 PO BID-QID	5-10 tablets per day	May cause diarrhea	Avoid in renal failure
Magnesium sulfate		For arrhythmias and asthma: 2 g IV over 5-10 minutes For obstetrics indications see Chapter 8		Occasional flushing, transient mild hypotension	
Mebendazole	Pinworm: 100 mg once Whipworm, roundworm, hookworm: 100 mg PO BID for 3 days; repeat in 3 weeks if not cured	Same as pediatric dose			Chewable tablet available
Meclizine		12.5-25 mg PO Q6h			
Medroxyprogesterone	See specific indication in text	For anovulation: 10 mg/day for 5 days; uterine bleeding should follow			
Mefenamic acid	Not indicated under 14 years of age See adult dose for >14 years	500 mg initially and then 250 mg PO Q6h		NSAID side effects including gastritis, decreased renal blood flow, etc.	Especially helpful for dysmenorrhea

Continued

TABLE 20-1
Commonly prescribed medications—cont'd

Drug	Pediatric dose	Adult dose	Maximum dose	Important side effects	Indications and notes
Meperidine	Neonates: 0.5-1.0 mg/kg IM or IV Q6h Older children: 1-2 mg/kg IV/IM Q3-4h PRN	25-100 mg IV or IM Q2-3h (1-2 mg/kg)		Sedation, respiratory depression	Reverse with naloxone
Methicillin	<2 weeks 50 mg/kg/24h divided Q12h 2-4 weeks: 100 mg/kg/24 divided Q6h Older: 100-400 mg/kg/24h divided Q4-6h	1-4 g IV Q4-6h	12 g/day		Most indications 1-2 g IV Q6h
Methylergonovine	Not indicated	0.2 mg IM or IV after delivery 0.2 mg PO TID-QID for 1 week			
Methylphenidate	Start with 5 mg before breakfast and lunch Increase by 5-10 mg/week until achieve desired effect	10-60 mg PO $1/2$ h AC; may use SR tablets Q8h			Watch for weight loss Try drug-free periods yearly; generally can discontinue after puberty

Methylprednisolone	IV:1-2 mg/kg for asthma Dose differs for different indications; see text for particular indication	For asthma: 40 mg IV Q6h Some give 125 mg IV for loading dose	High doses for spinal cord injury; see text		
Metoclopramide	Neonate for reflux: 0.1-0.2 mg/kg dose ½ h AC <6 years: of age: 0.1 mg/kg/dose >6 years: 2.5-10 mg/dose For chemotherapeutically induced nausea: 1-2 mg/kg dose given before chemotherapy up to Q2h	For GE reflux and gastric paresis: 5-15 mg PO ½ h AC For nausea: 10 mg IV or PO Q6h For chemotherapeutically induced nausea: 10 mg IV but up to 1-2 mg/kg IV if needed up to Q2h			May cause dystonic reaction Some recommend giving with diphenhydramine in chemotherapeutic doses prevent dystonia
Metolazone (Diulo and Zaroxolyn only)	0.2-0.4 mg/kg/day divided Q12h	2.5-20 mg PO once daily	20 mg/day		May cause profound hypokalemia if given with another agent such as furosemide
Metoprolol	Not indicated in infants or young children >2 years: 1-5 mg PO QD divided BID	PO: 25-100 mg QD; may be divided BID IV: 5 mg IV Q5 min as needed	400 mg	Bradycardia, hypotension	Do not use IV in combination with IV verapamil or diltiazem

Continued

TABLE 20-1
Commonly prescribed medications—cont'd

Drug	Pediatric dose	Adult dose	Maximum dose	Important side effects	Indications and notes
Metronidazole	Pseudomembranous colitis: 35 mg/kg/day PO divided Q6h Amebiasis: 35-50 mg/kg divided TID Giardiasis: 15 mg/kg/day divided TID (maximum 750 mg) for 5-10 days IV: Premature: 15 mg/kg load and then 7.5 mg/kg IV Q12h starting 48 hours after first dose Term: 15 mg/kg load and then 7.5 mg/kg Q12h starting 24 hours after load >7 days of age: same as adult	Trichomoniasis: 2 g given at once or divided BID Amebiasis: 750 mg PO TID for 5-10 days Giardiasis: 250 mg PO TID for 5-10 days IV: 15 mg/kg loading and then 7.5 mg/kg Q6h with: maximum of 4 g/day Pseudomembranous colitis: 500 mg PO TID for 7-10 days	4 g	May cause CNS stimulation when given IV If given for long term, may get reversible neuropathy	

Midazolam	0.05-0.2 mg/kg IV IN/PR/PO: 0.3-0.7 mg/kg	0.07-0.08 mg/kg of base IV	Generally need 5 mg maximum for conscious sedation	Respiratory and CNS sedation	Dose for seizures: see Chapter 1 Reverse with flumazenil
Morphine sulfate	IV/IM: 0.1-0.2 mg/kg	IV/IM: 0.1-0.2 mg/kg		Sedation, respiratory depression	Reverse with naloxone See Chapter 9 for PCA pump dosing
Nafcillin	IV: 10-20 mg/kg IV Q4h or 20-40 mg/kg IV Q8h	IV: 500-1500 mg IV Q4h	Adult: 20 g Children: 200 mg/kg/day divided for severe infections		
Naloxone	0.4-2.0 mg repeated Q2 min	0.4-2.0 mg		May precipitate withdrawal	See text for escalating doses and protocols
Naproxen	For rheumatic disease: 10 mg/kg day divided Q12h	Anti-inflammatory: 500 mg Naprosyn BID up to 1500 mg for brief periods Pain: 550 mg Anaprox and then 275 mg PO Q6h			Available as 125 mg/5 ml solution

Continued

TABLE 20-1
Commonly prescribed medications—cont'd

Drug	Pediatric dose	Adult dose	Maximum dose	Important side effects	Indications and notes
Nifedipine	Not indicated	Hypertension: 30-60 mg extended release up to 120 mg/day Angina: 10 mg PO TID up to 120 mg/day divided TID-QID. Sustained release available	Doses up to 180 mg/day have been used Single-dose maximum is 30 mg (short acting)		
Nitroglycerin		SL tablets: 0.2-0.4 mg Spray: up to 3 activations in 15 minutes Oral (that is, Nitro-Bid): 2.5-6.5 mg Q8h to start and increase as needed Paste: 0.5-2 inches Q6h Patch: 0.2-0.8 mg/hour IV: 10-20 μg/min titrated up to effect		Hypotension, reflex tachycardia	Oral sustained-release tablets (that is, Nitro-Bid) at 2.5, 6.5 and 9 mg tablets Provide drug-free period of 10-12 hours/day with all preparations to prevent tachyphylaxis

Norfloxacin	Ophthalmic drops only approved form for children >1 year of age Same as adult dose	400 mg PO BID for UTI Gonorrhea: 800 mg PO single dose Ophthalmic drops: 1-2 gtt QID			
Nortriptyline	6-12 years: 10-20 mg/day or 1-3 mg/kg/day Adolescents: 30-50 mg or 1-3 mg/kg/day; divided or at once Not indicated in younger children	25-150 mg PO QHS or divided TID-QID; start low and increase		Anticholinergic, sedation	Monitor levels if >100 mg/day Levels of 50-150 ng/ml are therapeutic Available as 10 mg/5 ml solution
Nystatin	Thrush premature: 100,000 units QID Thrush infants: 200,000 units QID Thrush older: see adult dose	GI candidiasis: 1-2 tablets QID Oral: 400,000 to 600,000 units QID			Troches: 200,000 units Tablets: 500,000 units Liquid: 200,000 for 2 ml
Ofloxacin	Not indicated	200-400 mg PO BID Gonorrhea: 400 mg PO single dose			

Continued

TABLE 20-1
Commonly prescribed medications—cont'd

Drug	Pediatric dose	Adult dose	Maximum dose	Important side effects	Indications and notes
Omeprazole		20 mg PO QD	40 mg		Occasionally 80 mg/day used for Zollinger-Ellison syndrome
Ondansetron	Not indicated <4 years of age >4 years of age same as adult dose	0.15 mg/kg IV over 15 minutes × 3 doses; start 1/2 hour before chemotherapy			Doses between 4 and 10 mg have been effective in adults for treating emesis in overdose patients
Oxybutynin	>5 years: 5 mg PO BID-TID	5 mg PO BID-TID	20 mg/day	Anticholinergic side effects common at effective dose	Elixir available 5 mg/5 ml

Oxycodone	6-12 years of age: 0.05-0.15 mg/kg dose up to 10 mg/dose	5-10 mg PO Q6h		Sedation, respiratory depression	
Pediazole	Based on erythromycin dose (50 mg/kg/day divided TID-QID)				Not for use under 2 months of age Supplied as 200 mg/5 ml of erythromycin and 600 mg/5 ml of sulfisoxazole
Penicillin G	See indications in text	See indications in text			
Pentamadine	4 mg/kg IV or IM	4 mg/kg IV or IM Nebulized for PCP prophylaxis: 300 mg nebulized Q4 weeks		Hypoglycemia, bronchospasm, fatigue, chills	
Perphenazine	Not established	Acute psychosis: 4-16 mg PO TID-QID IM: 5-10 mg IM Q6h	64 mg PO, 30 mg IM		

Continued

TABLE 20-1
Commonly prescribed medications—cont'd

Drug	Pediatric dose	Adult dose	Maximum dose	Important side effects	Indications and notes
Phenobarbital	Seizures: PO: 3-6 mg/kg/day divided QD-BID Status epilepticus: 15-20 mg/kg IV over 10 minutes (will achieve therapeutic blood level)	Seizures: 60-200 mg/day PO QD divided QD-BID Status epilepticus: 200-320 mg IV over 10 minutes or IM		Respiratory depression, sedation	Therapeutic blood level is 10-40 μg/ml
Phenytoin	PO: 5 mg/kg/day not to exceed 300 mg IV loading dose: 15-20 mg/kg at 1-3 mg/kg/min	PO: 300 mg/day IV loading dose: 10-15 mg/kg at maximum of 50 mg/min			Therapeutic level: 10-20 μg/ml Suspension: 125 mg/5 ml
Piperacillin	Over 12 years: see adult dose	3-4 g IV Q4-6h	24 g/day		
Prednisolone	0.5-2.0 mg/kg divided BID-TID	5-60 mg/day depending on disease For multiple sclerosis exacerbation: 200 mg/day once a week and then 80 mg PO QOD for 1 month		Weight gain, adrenal suppression, immunosuppression	Once disease is under control, alternate-day therapy is preferable, since it is associated with less

					pression, and immunosuppression
Prednisone	0.5-2.0 mg/kg/day depending on indication	5-60 mg PO QD depending on indication			
Procainamide		PO: about 50 mg/kg divided Q6h (sustained release) IV: 50 mg/kg at maximum rate of 50 mg/min; drip at 2-4 mg/min	1.25 g	Reduce maintenance by 25% for age 50, 50% for for age 75	Check procainamide and *N*-acetylprocainamide levels and adjust dose accordingly
Prochlorperazine	Not indicated <9 kg Children 9-13 kg of body weight: PO 2.5 mg QD-BID, not to exceed 7.5 mg/day Children 14-17 kg of body weight: PO 2.5 mg BID-TID, not to exceed 10 mg/day Children 18-39 kg of body weight: PO 2.5 mg TID or 5 mg BID, not to exceed 15 mg/day	IM/IV: 5-10 mg Q3-4h PO: 5-10 mg Q6h PR: 25 mg Q8h	40 mg maximum in adults for nausea 150 mg/day adults for psychosis	Dystonic reactions	Occasional sedation or hypotension

Continued

TABLE 20-1
Commonly prescribed medications—cont'd

Drug	Pediatric dose	Adult dose	Maximum dose	Important side effects	Indications and notes
Promethazine	Neonates: not indicated Children: 0.25-1 mg/kg/dose Q6-8h IM, IV, or PR	25-100 mg IV or IM or PR or PO		May cause sedation, dystonia	Do not give more than 100 mg/dose; give slowly IV (25 mg/min) No SQ or intra-arterial injection! Syrup: 6.25 mg/5 ml
Propranolol	PO: 0.05-4 mg/kg/24h divided Q6-12h IV: 0.01-0.025 mg/kg/dose over 10 minutes	PO: 40-320 mg divided BID-QID IV: 0.5-1.0 mg/min Up to 3 mg: repeat once 5 minutes later		Bradycardia, hypotension, bronchospasm	Avoid in COPD, heart block among others Long-acting preparations available
Pseudoephedrine	Neonates: not indicated Children: 4-5 mg/kg/24h not to exceed adult dose; divide Q6h	30-60 mg PO Q6h or twice this Q12h (sustained release)		Tachycardia, anxiety, hypertension	

Pyrantel pamoate	Neonate: not indicated, see text 11 mg/kg PO as single dose for all indications	11 mg/kg for all indications	1 g		Elixir: 250 mg/5 ml May repeat in 1 week if needed
Ranitidine	2-4 mg/kg divided BID up to 300 mg/day IV: 2-4 mg/kg BID up to 300 mg	150 mg BID or 300 mg PO QHS IV: 50 mg Q8h or as constant infusion (150 mg over 24 hours)	300 mg	Few significant drug interactions	
Rifampin	PO: <1 month: *Haemophilius influenzae* prophylaxis: 10 mg/kg/24h as single dose for 4 days *Neisseria meningitidis:* 5 mg/kg Q12h for 2 days >1 month: *H. influenzae* prophylaxis: 20 mg/kg/day in 1 dose for 4 days *N. meningitidis* prophylaxis: 3 months to 1 year: 10 mg/kg/day Q12h for 2 days	*H. influenzae* prophylaxis: 600 mg PO QD for 4 days *N. meningitidis* prophylaxis: 600 mg PO BID for 2 days	Maximum dose 600 mg per dose	Adjust dose for liver disease	May turn tears yellow/orange/brown Avoid wearing contact lenses, since these may become stained

Continued

TABLE 20-1
Commonly prescribed medications—cont'd

Drug	Pediatric dose	Adult dose	Maximum dose	Important side effects	Indications and notes
Rimantadine	<10 years old: 5 mg/kg PO once a day not to exceed 150 mg >10 years: use adult dose	PO: 100 mg BID Elderly and nursing home: 100 mg/day		Change dose for renal failure, hepatic failure	Syrup is available 50 mg/5 ml
Salsalate	Pediatric dose not established	3 g/day divided BID-TID			500 and 750 mg tablets available
Sertraline	Dose not yet established	50-200 mg/day; start at 50 mg and increase weekly			Do not use with MAOIs
Simvastatin		5-40 mg PO QHS based on response of LDL			Avoid use with gemfibrozil
Spironolactone	Neonates: 3 mg/kg/24h divided Q12h >3 months: 3 mg/kg/24h divided Q8h	25-200 mg/day depending on response; can give Q6h			May cause hyperkalemia
Succinylcholine	IV: 1-2 mg/kg/dose for rapid paralysis	1 mg/kg IV for rapid paralysis			

Sucralfate	>12 years: 1 g PO 1/2 h AC and QHS	1 g PO 1/2 h AC and HS			Suspension: 500 mg/5 ml
Sumatriptan	Dose not yet established	6 mg SQ with second dose in 1 hour if responded to first dose and now have breakthrough PO: 25 mg at start of headache with second dose at 2 hours if responded to first dose and now have breakthrough	SQ: 12 mg PO: 200 mg though no evidence that more than 25 mg Q2h is any more effective	Vasospasm, tachycardia, flushing, chest pain	Use with caution in those with CAD, peripheral artery disease Do not combine with other vasoconstrictors such as ergot preparations
Terazosin	Not indicated	1-5 mg PO QD but up to 20 mg has been used in divided doses	40 mg		Begin at 1 mg QHS May have orthostatic syncope with first dose.
Terbutaline	<12 years: SQ: 0.005-0.01 mg/kg/dose; maximum of 0.4 mg/dose 12 years >SQ: 0.25 mg; can give dose every 15 minutes × 3	SQ: 0.25 mg/dose Q15 min × 3		Tachycardia	

Continued

TABLE 20-1
Commonly prescribed medications—cont'd

Drug	Pediatric dose	Adult dose	Maximum dose	Important side effects	Indications and notes
Tetracycline	Use for children only >8 years of age 6.25-12.5 mg PO Q6h or double this Q12h	250-500 mg PO Q6h			May stain teeth in children <8 years of age
Thiabendazole	Not indicated in neonates 25-50 mg/kg/day divided Q12h	25-50 mg/kg/day divided Q12h	Limit 3 g/day		Available as 500 mg/5 ml
Thiamine	25 mg IV or IM	100 mg IV or IM			
Thioridazine	>2 years: 1-5 mg/kg/24h Q6-8h	25-100 mg PO TID	800 mg		
Ticarcillin (Timentin based on ticarcillin dose)	<2 kg: 75 mg/kg IV Q12h for 1 week and then Q8h Neonates >2 kg: 100 mg/kg loading and then 75 mg/kg Q8h until 1 week old and then 75 mg/kg IV Q6h Sepsis up to 40 kg: 50-75	Adults and >40 kg: Simple UTI: 1 g IV Q4-6h Sepsis: 3 g IV Q3-6h			

	mg/kg IV Q6h Simple UTI: 12.5-25 mg/kg IV Q6h				
Ticlopidine	Not indicated	250 mg PO BID		May cause thrombocytopenia, granulocytopenia	Check CBC Q2 weeks for first 3 months
Tobramycin	<1 week: 2 mg/kg IV Q12h >1 week: 2.0-2.5 mg/kg Q8-16h based on levels	Load with 2 mg/kg 1-1.7 mg/kg IV Q8h Can give 5.1 mg/kg IV Q24h as single dose (but not in endocarditis) Consider pharmacy consultation	8 mg/kg/day in life-threatening infection Must monitor blood levels!		Reduce dose in renal failure; follow serum levels Peak: 6-12 μg/ml Trough: 1.5-2.0 μg/ml 24-hour dosing interval has been used
Trazodone	Not indicated	Start 75-150 mg QHS; increase by 50 mg every 3-4 days until desired effect; can divide BID-TID	400 mg outpatient, 600 mg inpatient		Sedating; may cause priapism
Triazolam	Not indicated	0.125-0.25 mg PO QHS	0.5 mg PO QHS but rarely need this dose		Causes sedation

Continued

TABLE 20-1
Commonly prescribed medications—cont'd

Drug	Pediatric dose	Adult dose	Maximum dose	Important side effects	Indications and notes
Trimethoprim/ sulfamethoxazole	Not recommended if <2 months of age Oral suspension: 5 ml BID for 10 kg 10 ml BID for 20 kg 15 ml BID for 30 kg 10 ml = 1 single dose tablet	1 DS tablet BID			May cause Stevens-Johnson syndrome May cause hemolysis in those with G6PD deficiency.
Valproic acid	Children: 15 mg/kg 24h divided BID-TID; increase to achieve therapeutic levels (maximum 60 mg/kg/day)	Adult same as pediatric dose			Follow liver enzymes, CBC, Therapeutic levels 50-100 µg/ml
Vecuronium	0.08-0.1 mg/kg IV infusion at 1 µg/kg/min	0.1 mg/kg IV infusion at 1 µg/kg/min		Causes respiratory arrest Must be able to to manage airway!	Do not start infusion until some evidence of recovery from bolus

Venlafaxine	Not indicated	75 mg divided TID-BID and increased up to 225 mg/day			Reduce by 50% in liver and renal failure
Verapamil	Generally not indicated in <1 year of age because of possibility of hemodynamic compromise; however cose is 0.1-0.2 mg/kg IV not to exceed 5 mg >1 year: 0.1-0.3 mg/kg IV not to exceed 5 mg	PO: 40-120 mg TID Extended-release: 120-480 mg PO QAM IV: 5 mg followed by 10 mg IV in 10 minutes; see Chapter 1 for details		May cause bradycardia, heart block, hypotension	Do not use with IV beta-blockers
Warfarin	0.05-0.34 mg QHS adjusted to INR	2-10 mg QHS adjusted to INR		May cause bleeding	INR 2 to 3 for DVT prophylaxis INR 2.5 to 3.5 for artificial heart valves
Zidovudine	<3 months: 2 mg/kg Q8h 3 months to 13 years: 1800 mg/m^2 Q6h >13 years: same as adult	Occupational prophylaxis: see Chapter 16 For HIV/AIDS: 200 mg PO or IV Q8h			

INDEX

D

E

F

M

N

O

U

V

W

X

Z